Review of Sleep Medicine

Review of Sleep Medicine

SECOND EDITION

Edited by

Teri J. Barkoukis, MD, FCCP

Associate Professor of Medicine
Diplomate of the American Board of Sleep Medicine
Fellow of the American Academy of Sleep Medicine
Director, Sleep Medicine Fellowship
Co-Director, Nebraska Medical Center Sleep Center
Pulmonary–Critical Care Sleep Medicine and Allergy Section
University of Nebraska Medical Center, Omaha, Nebraska

Alon Y. Avidan, MD, MPH

Associate Professor of Neurology
Diplomate of the American Board of Sleep Medicine
Diplomate, American Board of Psychiatry and Neurology
Associate Director, Sleep Disorders Center
Medical Director, Neurology Clinic
University of California, Los Angeles, California

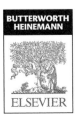

BUTTERWORTH
HEINEMANN

ELSEVIER

BUTTERWORTH
HEINEMANN
ELSEVIER

1600 John F. Kennedy Blvd.
Ste 1800
Philadelphia, PA 19103–2899

REVIEW OF SLEEP MEDICINE   ISBN13: 978-0-7506-7563-5
Second Edition

Notice

Knowledge and best practice in this field are constantly changing. As new research and experience broaden our knowledge, changes in practice, treatment and drug therapy may become necessary or appropriate. Readers are advised to check the most current information provided (i) on procedures featured or (ii) by the manufacturer of each product to be administered, to verify the recommended dose or formula, the method and duration of administration, and contraindications. It is the responsibility of the practitioners, relying on their own experience and knowledge of the patient, to make diagnoses, to determine dosages and the best treatment for each individual patient, and to take all appropriate safety precautions. To the fullest extent of the law, neither the Publisher nor the Editors assume any liability for any injury and/or damage to persons or property arising out of or related to any use of the material contained in this book.

The Publisher

Library of Congress Cataloging-in-Publication Data

Review of sleep medicine / [edited by] Teri J. Barkoukis, Alon Y. Avidan. – 2nd ed.
   p. ; cm.
   Includes bibliographical references and index.
   ISBN-13: 978-0-7506-7563-5   ISBN-10: 0-7506-7563-2
   1. Sleep disorders–Examinations, questions, etc.   2. Sleep–Physiological aspects–Examinations, questions, etc.   I. Barkoukis, Teri J.   II. Avidan, Alon Y.
   [DNLM: 1. Sleep–physiology–Examination Questions.   2. Sleep Disorders–Examination Questions.   WL 18.2 R454 2007]
   RC547.R484 2007
   616.8′4980076–dc22

                                            2006031805

Acquisitions Editor: Susan F. Pioli
Developmental Editor: Joan Ryan
Project Manager: Bryan Hayward
Cover Design Direction: Steven Stave

Printed in the United States of America

Last digit is the print number: 9   8   7   6   5   4   3   2

Contents

SECTION I
HIGHLIGHTS OF SLEEP MEDICINE 1

SECTION II
PRACTICE EXAMS FOR THE ADVENTUROUS . . 209

SECTION **III**

Contributing Authors

AMERICAN SOCIETY OF ELECTRONEURODIAGNOSTIC TECHNOLOGISTS, INC.
Kansas City, Missouri

JON W. ATKINSON, BS, RPSGT
Consultant, Ohio Sleep Consulting and Recording Services, Lancaster, Ohio

ALON Y. AVIDAN, MD, MPH
Associate Professor of Neurology, Diplomate of the American Board of Sleep Medicine, Diplomate, American Board of Psychiatry and Neurology; Associate Director, Sleep Disorders Center, Medical Director, Neurology Clinic, University of California, Los Angeles, California

CHARLES BAE, MD
Associate Staff, Department of Neurology, Cleveland Clinic, Cleveland, Ohio

TERI J. BARKOUKIS, MD, FCCP
Associate Professor of Medicine, Diplomate of the American Board of Sleep Medicine, Fellow of the American Academy of Sleep Medicine; Director, Sleep Medicine Fellowship, Co-Director, Nebraska Medical Center Sleep Center, Pulmonary–Critical Care Sleep Medicine and Allergy Section, University of Nebraska Medical Center, Omaha, Nebraska

CLAUDIO L. BASSETTI, MD
Professor and Vice-Chairman, Department of Neurology, University Hospital of Zürich, Zürich, Switzerland

CARL W. BAZIL, MD, PHD
Associate Professor of Clinical Neurology, Columbia University; Attending Physician, Department of Neurology, New York-Presbyterian Hospital, New York, New York

SRINIVAS BHADRIRAJU, MD, FCCP, D-ABSM
Assistant Professor of Medicine and Associate Division Director, Pulmonary and Critical Care Medicine, Emory University School of Medicine; Chief of Pulmonary and Director, Sleep Clinic, Emory Crawford Long Hospital, Atlanta, Georgia

WYNNE CHEN, MD
Post-Doctoral Fellow, Stanford University Center for Narcolepsy, Stanford Sleep Disorders Center, Palo Alto, California

DEREK J. CHONG, MD, MSC, FRCP(C)
Instructor in Neurology, Neurological Institute, Columbia University; Assistant Attending Neurologist, New York Presbyterian Hospital, New York, New York

DANIEL A. COHEN, MD, MMSC
Clinical Fellow, Harvard Medical School; Staff Neurologist, Beth Israel Deaconess Medical Center; Research Fellow, Division of Sleep Medicine, Brigham and Women's Hospital, Boston, Massachusetts

CAROLYN M. D'AMBROSIO, MD
Assistant Professor of Medicine, Tufts University School of Medicine; Director, The Center for Sleep Medicine, Tufts-New England Medical Center, Boston, Massachusetts

VLAD DIMITRIU, MD
Pulmonary-Critical Care Fellow, Department of Pulmonary, Critical Care, and Sleep Medicine, University of Nebraska Medical Center, Omaha, Nebraska

IOANA DUMITRU, MD
Assistant Professor of Internal Medicine (Cardiology) and Medical Director, Heart Failure and Cardiac Transplant Program, University of Nebraska Medical Center, Omaha, Nebraska

BARUCH EL-AD, MD
Sleep Medicine Center, Technion Institute of Technology, Tel-Aviv, Israel

NANCY FOLDVARY-SCHAEFER, DO
Associate Professor of Medicine, Cleveland Clinic Lerner College of Medicine; Director, Sleep Disorders Center, Cleveland Clinic, Cleveland, Ohio

BRIAN H. FORESMAN, DO, MS
Associate Professor of Clinical Medicine, Indiana University School of Medicine; Medical Director,

Indiana University Center for Sleep Disorders and Director, Indiana University Sleep Medicine and Circadian Biology Program, University Hospital, Indianapolis, Indiana

TERI L. GABEL, PHARMD, BCPP
Assistant Professor of Psychiatry, University of Nebraska Medical Center; Clinical Pharmacy Specialist – Psychiatry, Pharmacy Service, VA Nebraska Western Iowa Healthcare System; Consultant Pharmacist and Co-Founder, Drug Therapy Consultants, PC, Omaha, Nebraska

PIERRE GIGLIO, MD
Assistant Professor of Neurological Sciences, University of Nebraska Medical Center, Omaha, Nebraska

R. CHRIS HAMMOND, MD
Sleep Medicine Fellow, Department of Neurology, Northwestern University Feinberg School of Medicine, Chicago, Illinois

VIKTOR HANAK, MD
Fellow, Pulmonary and Critical Care Medicine, Mayo Clinic Foundation, Rochester, Minnesota

STUART G. HOLTBY, MD, FRCPC, D-ABSM
Director, Northern Nights Sleep Disorder Centre, Thunder Bay, Ontario, Canada

ELIOT S. KATZ, MD
Instructor in Pediatrics, Harvard Medical School; Director, Pediatric Sleep Services, Massachusetts General Hospital, Boston, Massachusetts

SHARON A. KEENAN, PHD, REEGT, RPSGT, D-ABSM
Director, The School of Sleep Medicine, Inc., Palo Alto, California

SURESH KOTAGAL, MD
Professor of Neurology and Pediatrics, Mayo Clinic College of Medicine; Consultant, Sleep Disorders Center, Mayo Clinic, Rochester, Minnesota

LOIS E. KRAHN, MD
Professor and Chair of Psychiatry and Pulmonary, Mayo Clinic, Arizona

JAMES T. LANE, MD
Associate Professor of Internal Medicine – Diabetes, Endocrinology and Metabolism, University of Nebraska Medical Center, Omaha, Nebraska

TEOFILO L. LEE-CHIONG, MD
Associate Professor of Medicine, National Jewish Medical and Research Center, Denver, Colorado

MIKHAEL LOOTS, MPAS, PA-C
Clinical Physicians Assistant, Pulmonary, Critical Care, Sleep Medicine, and Allergy Section, University of Nebraska Medical Center, Omaha, Nebraska

JEAN K. MATHESON, MD, ABSM
Assistant Professor of Neurology, Harvard Medical School; Medical Director, Sleep Disorders Center, Department of Neurology, Beth Israel Deaconess Medical Center, Boston, Massachusetts

EMMANUEL MIGNOT, MD, PHD
Professor of Psychiatry and Behavioral Sciences, Center for Narcolepsy and Principle Investigator, Howard Hughes Medical Institute, Stanford University School of Medicine, Palo Alto, California

VAHID MOHSENIN, MD
Professor of Medicine, Yale University School of Medicine; Attending Physician, Yale-New Haven Hospital, New Haven, Connecticut

CHARLES A. POLNITSKY, MD, FCCP
Associate Clinical Professor of Medicine, Yale University School of Medicine, New Haven; Medical Director, Regional Sleep Lab, Waterbury Hospital Health Center, Waterbury; Adjunct Professor, Graduate School of Nursing, Quinnipiac University, Hamden, Connecticut

GREGORY L. SAHLEM, RPSGT
Medical Student, School of Medicine and Biomedical Sciences, University at Buffalo; Comprehensive Epilepsy Center, New York Presbyterian Hospital; Comprehensive Sleep Disorders Center, Columbia University, New York, New York

PAULA K. SCHWEITZER, PHD
Associate Director, Sleep Medicine and Research Center, St. John's Mercy Medical Center and St. Luke's Hospital, St. Louis, Missouri

MASSIMILIANO M. SICCOLI, MD
Neurologist, Faculty of Medicine, University of Zürich; Neurologist, University Hospital of Zürich, Zürich, Switzerland

CHRISTOPHER M. SINTON, PHD
Assistant Professor of Internal Medicine, University of Texas Southwestern Medical Center, Dallas, Texas; Lecturer, Department of Psychiatry, Harvard Medical School/Brockton VA Medical Center, Brockton, Massachusetts

ROY SMITH, RPSGT
Director of Advanced Technologies, The School of Sleep Medicine, Inc., Palo Alto, California

VIREND K. SOMERS, MD, DPHIL
Professor of Medicine, Division of Cardiovascular
Diseases, Mayo Clinic, Rochester, Minnesota

JUDITH WIEBELHAUS, RPSGT, REEGT
Sleep Disorders Laboratories, University of Michigan,
Ann Arbor, Michigan

SARAH NATH ZALLEK, MD
Clinical Assistant Professor of Neurology, University
of Illinois College of Medicine at Peoria; Vice Chair
and Director, Department of Neurology, OSF Saint
Francis Medical Center, Peoria, Illinois

PHYLLIS C. ZEE, MD, PHD
Professor of Neurology, Northwestern University;
Director, Sleep Disorders Center, Northwestern
Memorial Hospital, Chicago, Illinois

Preface to the Second Edition

Sleep medicine has continued to grow at an astounding rate compared to other medical fields. The transformation of the field has been noted in multiple facets including sharpening clinical practice guidelines with consensus task force committees of the American Academy of Sleep Medicine leading the way, an explosion of research, and significant expansion in the number of sleep trainees and approved fellowship training programs. The major change in sleep medicine fellowship training is a national agreement for accreditation with the Accreditation Council for Graduate Medical Education (ACGME). One major change for sleep board examinations that has already taken place is a shift from a two-day exam (part 1 in the fall and part 2 in the spring) to a one-day exam. Starting in 2007, plans are for a single one-day examination format to continue in a joint agreement with the American Board of Internal Medicine, the American Board of Psychiatry and Neurology, the American Board of Pediatrics, and the American Board of Otolaryngology.

The heart of this second edition of *Review of Sleep Medicine* remains with the purpose of assisting the physician to study for the sleep medicine board examinations. As in the first edition, Section I provides a brief overview of the field of sleep medicine with a continued attempt to emphasize pertinent points. This review, of course, cannot replace keeping abreast of current developments in the field or close attention to the important sleep textbooks that must be mastered to successfully pass the board exams. Critique and suggestions from our trainees and colleagues in the field regarding the first edition has lead to additional chapters that are new to this second edition including *sleep breathing disorders, cardiovascular pathophysiology of sleep apnea, greater expansion of central hypersomnias, introduction of electroencephalography,* and *pediatric sleep-wake disorders.*

Section II remains the major focus of the book with practice exam questions followed by comprehensive answers. As in the first edition, all questions are in multiple choice format with references at the end of each section in alphabetical order rather than referencing each point so as not to distract from using this as a true "mock exam." Many requested more practice questions and as a result this section is greatly expanded with new chapters called *cardiopulmonary disorders, neurological sleep disorders,* and *sleep-wake disorders* that collectively replace the previous chapter, *sleep disorders.* Other new chapters include *electroencephalography, practice parameters,* and a recent *literature review.*

It is our hope that this book review and practice exam will continue to be utilized as an important educational tool among physicians preparing for sleep medicine board examinations. Furthermore this book also serves a critical role in challenging the minds of the sleep trainee by providing questions drawn from actual clinical practice and engaging the reader in active thinking. We therefore hope that this critical educational resource will improve, enhance and stimulate the minds of our colleagues leading to overall better care toward their patients.

Teri J. Barkoukis
and
Alon Y. Avidan

Preface to the First Edition

Sleep medicine is a rapidly growing specialty with a multidisciplinary approach to patient care. Great clinicians and researchers have paved the way for newcomers to this field. There is now an explosion of knowledge in this field that is now more structured with sleep medicine fellowships and national board exams. Knowledge must be mastered in the fields of neurology, pulmonology, pediatrics, psychiatry, psychology, otolaryngology, and others. The task can be formidable with multiple textbooks to read and journals to instruct. For the clinician planning to take sleep medicine board exams, it is hopeful that this book can serve as a guide. The intent is to help guide the student studying for sleep medicine board exams. This is not intended to be a comprehensive textbook of the subject. All students are encouraged to read the excellent textbooks available in the field of sleep medicine as well as spend the many hours of clinical practice to master the "hands-on" experience necessary in this field.

In light of the above goal to emphasize highlights of sleep medicine, the first section recaps major points with multiple tables, figures and lists to guide the sleep medicine student. Even though Section I is emphasizing pertinent points in sleep medicine, the style is still in the form of review chapters with traditional referencing for the student who wants to look up more information on the topic. This is indeed a *Review of Sleep Medicine* with the main intention of serving as a study guide.

Section II is the main portion of this textbook to serve as a mock exam for practice. Certainly, an entire polysomnogram or MSLT cannot be included in any textbook. This becomes somewhat of a limiting factor, for which the student is encouraged to spend those many hours in the sleep laboratory setting mastering the art and science of understanding sleep studies. As much as possible, multiple epochs and polysomnogram segments are present with questions to challenge you. All questions are in multiple choice format with references at the end of each section in alphabetical order rather than referencing each point so as not to distract from using this as a true "mock exam."

This book review and mock exam was my dream when I was studying for sleep medicine boards. My intention was to help people preparing for boards in the same way that I would like to have been helped. Since this was modeled after my own desire to help others in this fashion, I welcome any comments and suggestions for the future.

Teri J. Barkoukis
(formerly Teri Bowman)

Acknowledgments

Thank you to all the contributing authors who supported this project and graciously tolerated my many telephone calls and e-mails. This could not have come together without all of you. I am very grateful to Susan Pioli, Publishing Director, for her friendly demeanor, great encouragement, and wise counsel. She is truly an outstanding publisher who has a great vision for possibilities without losing the keen knowledge for completing each task in this publishing journey. The pulmonary division of the University of Nebraska Medical Center has been supportive throughout this entire process and I couldn't ask for a better and more understanding chief than Dr. Joseph Sisson. I wish to also extend many thanks to the Nebraska Medical Center Sleep Center for their support and encouragement. I am very grateful to Dolores Cunningham, who is not only my main assistant for fielding telephone calls, schedules, and typing, but has become a good friend. She has gone above and beyond the call of duty in working with these many manuscripts in partnership with me. Thanks are also extended to Maralee Gifford and Jeanette Danielsen for assisting with typing, telephone calls, and scheduling. Mikhael Loots is not only an excellent clinical PA, but was wonderful at jumping in to help and compiling all the data for *Section III: Valuable Resources* as well.

Finally, thank you to my parents, Gregory and Louise Barkoukis, who made me believe that nothing was impossible to the one who tries hard enough to succeed. They continue to be supportive in all my achievements.

I again want to personally dedicate this book to God who gives me strength, wisdom, and peace in all of life regardless of the challenges along the way. Psalms 127:2 even gives wisdom on good sleep habits by saying, "It is vain for you to rise up early, to sit up late, to eat the bread of sorrows; for so He gives His beloved sleep." This is my own personal dedication and has nothing to do with the book's content, other authors, or co-editor.

Teri J. Barkoukis

Acknowledgments

I would like to express my gratitude to all of the authors for their outstanding contributions and dedication to this publication. I have already had the pleasure of working with some of them, both as colleagues and as good friends, in the ever-evolving and exciting field of sleep medicine. Special thanks go to Dr. Ronald Chervin, Director of the Michael S. Aldrich Sleep Disorders Center, for his outstanding mentorship during my first years as a member of the faculty at The University of Michigan; to my previous Neurology Chairs at Michigan: Drs. Sid Gilman and David Fink; and to my current Chair at UCLA, Dr. John Mazziotta, for their encouragement and their support of sleep education and publications, such as this, to furthering sleep education and awareness. I deeply appreciate the warm welcome that I have received from the following colleagues at UCLA: Dr. Frisca Yan-Go, Director of the UCLA Sleep Disorders Program, Dr. Ronald M. Harper, Professor in the Department of Neurobiology, and Dr. Michael Irwin, Norman Cousins Professor in the Department of Psychiatry and Biobehavioral Sciences. My thanks also to Ms. Karen Gowen, my administrative assistant at the University of Michigan; Ms. Brenda Livingston, coordinator of the Michael S. Aldrich Sleep Disorders Laboratory, and to my current assistant at UCLA, Ms. Beverly Hill, for their invaluable help.

Finally, I wish to dedicate this book to the late Dr. Michael S. Aldrich: a brilliant, humble, and magnificent teacher who founded the University of Michigan Sleep Disorders Laboratory.

Alon Y. Avidan

Abbreviations

A = auricle
AASM = American Academy of Sleep Medicine
ABG = arterial blood gas
ABIM = American Board of Internal Medicine
ABPN = American Board of Psychiatry and
    Neurology
ABSM = American Board of Sleep Medicine
Ach = acetylcholine
ACT = acid clearance time
ACGME = Accreditation Council for Graduate
    Medical Education
ACTH = adrenocorticotropic hormone
ADHD = attention-deficit hyperactivity disorder
AHI = apnea-hypopnea index
ALTE = apparent life-threatening episode
ANP = atrial natriuretic peptide
ANS = autonomic nervous system
APAP = autotitrating positive airway pressure
APOE = apolipoprotein E
ARAS = ascending reticular activating system
ASD = autistic spectrum disorders
ASPS = advanced sleep phase syndrome
ASPT = advanced sleep phase type
BETS = benign elipeptiform transients of sleep
BF = basal forebrain
BiPAP = bilevel positive airway pressure
BMI = body mass index
BP = blood pressure
BRS = baroreceptor sensitivity
BZ = benzodiazepine
BZRA = benzodiazepine receptor agonist
CAHS = central alveolar hypoventilation syndrome
CAD = coronary artery disease
CBF = cerebral blood flow
CBT = cognitive behavioral therapy
CCHS = congenital central hypoventilation syndrome
CHF = congestive heart failure
CNS = central nervous system
CO = cardiac output
COPD = chronic obstructive pulmonary disease
COX = cyclooxygenase
CPAP = continuous positive airway pressure
CPBS = central periodic breathing in sleep
cps = cycles per second (or Hertz or Hz)
CRH = corticotropin-releasing hormone
CRP = C-reactive protein
CRSD = circadian rhythm sleep disorder
CRY = cryptochrome

CSA = central sleep apnea
CSF = cerebral spinal fluid
CSR = Cheyne-Stokes respiration
CWP = cm H_2O
CYP = cytrochrome P-450
D = decrease
DA = dopamine
DLB = dementia with Lewy bodies
DLMO = dim light melatonin onset
DRG = dorsal respiratory group
DRN = dorsal raphe nucleus
DSIP = delta sleep-inducing peptide
DSPD = delayed sleep phase disorder
DSPS = delayed sleep phase syndrome
DSPT = delayed sleep phase type
dsRNA = Double stranded RNA
Dx = diagnosis
ECG = electrocardiogram
EDS = excessive daytime sleepiness
EEG = electroencephalogram
EKG = electrokardiogram (or electrocardiogram
    or ECG)
EMG = electromyogram
EOG = electrooculogram
ePAP = expiratory positive airway pressure
EPSP = excitatory postsynaptic potentials
ESS = Epworth Sleepiness Score
F = frontal
FDA = federal drug administration
FFI = fatal familial insomnia
FGF = fibroblast growth factor
FIRDA = frontal intermittent rhythmic delta
    activity
5-HT = 5-hydroxytryptamine
Fpz = nasion on EEG mapping
FRC = functional residual capacity
FSH = follicle-stimulating hormone
FSS = Fatigue Severity Scale
GABA = gamma aminobutyric acid
GBS = Guillain-Barré syndrome
GER = gastroesophageal reflux
GH = growth hormone
GHB = gamma hydroxybutyrate
GHRH = growth hormone-releasing hormone
GHT = geniculohypothalamic tract
GLU = glutamate
GND = ground
GnRH = gonadotropin-releasing hormone

GTC = generalized tonic-clonic (seizures)
H = histamine
Hcrtr2 = hypocretin receptor 2 gene
HFF = high-frequency filters
HLA = human leukocyte antigen
HR = heart rate
HRV = heart rate variability
HT = hydroxytryptamine (serotonin)
5-HT = 5-hydroxytryptamine
5-HTP = 5-hydroxytryptophan
Hz = Hertz (or cycles per second or cps)
I = increase
ICSD = *International Classification of Sleep Disorders*
IFN = interferon
IGF-1 = insulin-like growth factor-1
IGL = intergeniculate leaflet
IH = idiopathic hypersomnia
IL = interleukin
IMT = intima-media thickness
iPAP = inspiratory positive airway pressure
IPSP = inhibitory postsynaptic potentials
LC = locus ceruleus
LDT = laterodorsal tegmental nucleus
LFF = low-frequency filters
LGN = lateral geniculate nucleus
LH = luteinizing hormone
L-NAME = N-nitro-L-arginine methyl ester
LOC = outer canthus of the left eye
m = meters
MAD = mandibular advancement devices
MAO-I = monoamine oxidase inhibitor
m-CPP = meta-chlorophenylpiperazine
Mflo = mask flow channel
mm Hg = millimeters of mercury
MRA = mandibular repositioning appliance
MRI = magnetic resonance imaging
MSH = melanocyte-stimulating hormone
MSLT = Multiple Sleep Latency Test
MSL = mean sleep onset latency
MWT = maintenance of wakefulness test
NA = noradrenaline
NBM = nucleus basalis of Meynert
NE = norepinephrine
NFκB = nuclear factor kappa B
NIMV = noninvasive mechanical ventilation
NIPPV = noninvasive positive pressure ventilation
NMDA = *N*-methyl-d-aspartate
NO = nitric oxide
N/O = nasal-oral
NPD = nocturnal paroxysmal dystonia
NPSG = nocturnal polysomnography
NPT = nocturnal penile tumescence
NPY = neuropeptide Y
NREM = non-rapid eye movement sleep
NSAID = nonsteroidal antiinflammatory drugs
NSF = National Sleep Foundation

NTS = nucleus tractus solitarius
O = occipital
OA = obstructive apnea
ODI = oxygen-desaturation index
OH = obstructive hypopnea
OHS = obesity-hypoventilation syndrome
OSA = obstructive sleep apnea
OSAH = obstructive sleep apnea-hypopnea
OSAHS = obstructive sleep apnea-hypopnea
        syndrome
OSAS = obstructive sleep apnea syndrome
Oz = inion on EEG mapping
P = parietal
PAC = premature atrial contraction
PACAP = pituitary adenyl cyclase-activating peptide
PB = periodic breathing
PCO_2 or $PaCO_2$ = arterial partial pressure of
        carbon dioxide
PDR = posterior dominant rhythm
PER = period
PFA = paroxysmal fast activity
PGE = prostaglandin
PGO = ponto-geniculo-occipital
PH = pulmonary hypertension
PLEDS = periodic lateralized epileptiform discharges
PLMD = periodic limb movement disorder
PLMI = periodic limb movement index
PLMS = periodic limb movements during sleep
PO_2 or PaO_2 = arterial partial pressure of oxygen
POA = preoptic area
PPT = pedunculopontine tegmental nucleus
PRC = phase response curve
PRF = pontine reticular formation
PSG = polysomnogram/polysomnography
PT = pars tuberalis
PTSD = post-traumatic stress disorder
PVC = premature ventricular complex
PWS = Prader Willi syndrome
RBD = REM behavior disorder
rCBF = regional cerebral blood flow
RDI = respiratory disturbance index
REM = rapid eye movements
RERA = respiratory effort-related arousals
RGC = retinal ganglion cells
RHT = retinohypothalamic tract
RLS = restless legs syndrome
RMD = rhythmic movement disorder
RME = rapid maxillary expansion
RNT = reticular nucleus of the thalamus
ROC = outer canthus of the right eye
RPO = reticularis pontis oralis
SA = sleep apnea
SaO_2 = arterial oxyhemoglobin saturation
SCN = suprachiasmatic nucleus
SDB = sleep-disordered breathing
SIDS = sudden infant death syndrome

SL = sleep latency
SO = sleep onset
SOAD = sleep-onset association disorder
SOREMP = sleep onset REM periods
SpO_2 = pulse oximetry saturation
SRBD = sleep-related breathing disturbances
SREs = sleep-related erections
SRED = sleep-related eating disorder
SSRI = selective serotonin reuptake inhibitor
SSI = Stanford Center for Narcolepsy Sleep Inventory
SSS = Stanford Sleepiness Scale
SubC = subcoeruleus
SPZ = subparaventricular zone
SVR = systemic vascular resistance
SWS = slow wave sleep
T = temporal
TCA = tricyclic antidepressant
TCS = Treacher Collins syndrome

Th1 = T-helper 1
TIB = time in bed
TMS = transcranial magnetic stimulation
TNF = tumor necrosis factor
TRH = thyrotropin-releasing hormone
TSH = thyroid-stimulating hormone
TST = total sleep time
TMN = tuberomammillary nucleus
TRH = thyrotropin-releasing hormone
TWT = total wake time
UARS = upper airway resistance syndrome
UPPP = uvulopalatopharyngoplasty
VLPO = ventrolateral preoptic nucleus
VRG = ventral respiratory group
VT = ventricular tachycardia
VTA = ventral tegmental area (of the midbrain)
WASO = wake after sleep onset
WSN = warm-sensitive neurons

Highlights of Sleep Medicine

Sleep Medicine and the Boards

TERI J. BARKOUKIS

Board examinations are challenging in any field of medicine, and sleep medicine is no exception. Some have erroneously thought that these board exams had a clinical emphasis similar to board exams in certain disciplines and discovered the first failure of their career. Sleep medicine board exams are extremely challenging. They encompass the extensive multidisciplinary spectrum of this field of medicine in neurology, pulmonary, psychiatry, psychology, otolaryngology, pediatrics, internal medicine, oral surgery, dental, and research scientists. Sleep medicine boards have truly taken an academic approach in the past that covers not only the clinical aspects of this exciting field but also the technical, research, and scientific wealth of information. This rich history paves the road to the mastery of multiple disciplines and provides a unique opportunity that can lead to a satisfying career.

We now have a rich resource of knowledge to draw on that was laid out for us by great leaders in the field to help us improve the sleep-wake cycles of those that come to us for help. Normal sleep and its investigation must first be understood before causes of abnormal sleep-wake patterns are discovered. This chapter focuses on the highlights of normal sleep in light of its history, epidemiology, normal sleep patterns, sleep deprivation, and shift work regulations. For the reader preparing for sleep medicine boards, this chapter may provide some helpful hints.

SLEEP MEDICINE BOARD EXAMS

The American Board of Sleep Medicine (ABSM) was incorporated in 1991 as an independent organization that oversees all examination activity. Originally this was started in 1978 by the Examination Committee of the Association of Sleep Disorders Centers, now the American Academy of Sleep Medicine (AASM). The brochure on guidelines for applicants is available online in .pdf file format that can be downloaded and read through the Acrobat Reader from the ABSM website.[1] Previously, this was given in two parts. Part I,

administered in the fall in a multiple choice format, covered basic sleep science, clinical sleep disorders, and sleep study fragments such as polysomnogram (PSG) epochs. Part II was given in the spring and was slanted toward clinical cases in which the test taker was asked to integrate his or her skills of patient analysis and management. The format of the board exam was changed beginning in fall 2005 to a 1-day examination similar to the style of American Board of Internal Medicine (ABIM) exams but still administered by the ABSM. The guidelines are well described by the ABSM and can be obtained by writing, calling, or simply visiting its website,[1] although changes are likely to be made by the time this book is published.

Starting in fall 2007, there will be a new 1-day board examination under the direction of four boards in the umbrella organization of the American Board of Medical Specialties (ABMS) for the field of sleep medicine. The ABIM, American Board of Psychiatry and Neurology (ABPN), American Board of Pediatrics, and American Board of Otolaryngology are working together in a cooperative venture that allows qualified candidates from each of these areas to sit for the new sleep medicine board examinations according to one of three methods. First, a candidate is eligible simply by already being an ABSM diplomate. Therefore, previous ABSM certification qualifies a clinician to take the new board exam for the first three board exams beginning in 2007. Second, a candidate is eligible by finishing in good standing a 12-month sleep medicine fellowship. This can either be a nonaccredited or accredited program by the Accreditation Council for Graduate Medical Education (ACGME). Beginning July 1, 2009, however, sleep fellowship training must be completed within an ACGME-accredited fellowship. And finally, a candidate who is a graduate of an ACGME training program from internal medicine, neurology, psychiatry, otolaryngology, or pediatrics may qualify if there is a collective practice of sleep medicine that is equivalent to 12 full-time months within the 5-year period before applying for the examination in 2007, 2009, or 2011. All the details are not quite finalized, and the reader is cautioned to log on to the following board web sites for more information that should be available by the fall of 2006:

American Board of Internal Medicine
Web address: http://www.abim.org
American Board of Psychiatry and Neurology, Inc.
Web address: http://www.abpn.com
American Board of Pediatrics
Web address: http://www.abped.org
American Board of Otolaryngology
Web address: http://www.aboto.org

These boards are difficult but easily passed if all aspects of sleep medicine are learned. The major mistake applicants have made is to focus on the most common cause of sleep disorders. Although the most common sleep center case is an analysis for obstructive sleep apnea syndrome, this is *not* the most common emphasis on sleep boards. The recommendation to be familiar with certain books and other sleep medicine resources should be taken very seriously; many resources are listed in the references.[2–22] In addition, it is important to be familiar with the AASM practice parameter guidelines, as well as essential journal articles in the field of sleep medicine.

Many learning styles do not necessarily predict who will do well on an examination. Some candidates have highlighted or underlined text in a book. If this technique is used, it is important to highlight only important points; otherwise the candidate will need to review a large amount of material just before the examination. Many candidates have bought a small, thick notebook and jotted down important points. This strategy forces the writer to streamline learning material. A small notebook can be carried around easily and referred to during any down periods. This method can also be used to organize material in a way that enhances memorization. An example (Table 1-1) is to glean material from the texts on what affects rapid eye movement (REM) sleep and slow wave sleep (SWS), also known as *delta sleep*, and organize it into a quick review table. It is also important to master the many sleep studies that are available in the sleep center.

Postgraduate fellows and other physicians are consistently asking what is important to study for sleep boards. The answer, of course, is that *all* the topics listed here are important. One needs to know *all* the major textbooks in the field of sleep medicine, as well as the major sleep journals and the AASM practice parameters. Neither the editors of this review book nor the authors can tell you exactly what is on the board exams. The following list is only a guide of topics to master. Strictly from a personal point of view, the following topics should not be missed:

1. Neurotransmitter systems, especially as they relate to sleep stage effects and substances that cause change in this system
   a. Acetylcholine (Ach)
   b. Physostigmine interactions
   c. Scopolamine
   d. Norepinephrine (NE)
   e. Monoamine oxidase inhibitors
   f. Reserpine that displaces monoamines
   g. Tricyclics such as desipramine, an NE inhibitor

TABLE 1-1 ■ An Example of Organizing Study Notes: REM and SWS Effects[23–25]			
Decreased REM	**Increased REM**	**Decreased SWS**	**Increased SWS**
Tricyclics	Reserpine	Most benzodiazepines	Ritanserin[d]
Monoamine inhibitors	Cholinergic agonists	Caffeine: 1st 1/2 night	Interleukin-1
Aging	Physostigmine	PGE2	Apomorphine[e]
Acute alcohol	Carbochal	Adenosine antagonists	Adenosine agonists
Stimulants	Acetylcholine	Children with SA	Endogenous hypnogens[f]
Lithium	REM-on neurons[c]	Beta blockers[b]	L-tryptophan[g]
Scopolamine	Methyldopa	Chronic hypercortisolism	
5-HT			
Norepinephrine			
Clonidine[a]			
Phentolamine			
Beta blockers[b]			

HT = hydroxytryptamine (serotonin); SA = sleep apnea; PGE2 = Prostaglandin E2; H = histamine.
[a] Cental anticholinergic activity.
[b] Nonspecific and high affinity for 5-HT receptors such as propranolol.
[c] Located in the cholinergic mesopontine nuclei LDT (laterodorsal tegmental nucleus) and PPT (pedunculopontine tegmental nucleus).
[d] A 5-HT$_2$ receptor antagonist.
[e] A dopamine-2 agonist.
[f] DSIP (delta sleep-inducing peptide) and PGD2 (prostaglandin D2).
[g] 5-HT precursor.

h. Clonidine, a potent alpha-2 agonist

i. Neuroleptics such as chlorpromazine

j. Beta-antagonists such as propranolol

k. Beta-agonists such as isoprenaline

l. 5-Hydroxytryptamine (5-HT) and its precursor, tryptophan, as well as inhibitors such as fluoxetine

m. Amphetamine effects and its derivatives such as methylphenidate and pemoline

n. Histamine

o. Adenosine

p. REM neurophysiology such as neurotransmitters in REM atonia and others

2. Pharmacological effects or disease changes to sleep architecture

a. Antidepressants

b. Neuroleptics

c. Stimulants

d. Anticonvulsants

e. Sedative-hypnotics

f. Antihistamines

g. Antiemetics

h. Cardiovascular medications

i. Alcohol, nicotine, and drugs of abuse

j. Drug withdrawal effects on sleep architecture

k. Caffeine effects and mechanisms

3. Brain lesion studies such as lesion location that produces wake, sleep, or REM

4. Pediatrics

a. Polysomnographic differences in infants

(1) Normal versus abnormal breathing patterns

(2) Active versus quiet sleep

(3) Staging normals

(4) Electroencephalogram (EEG) patterns such as the age of appearance of sleep spindles, K-complexes, or slow eye movements

b. Apnea definitions and etiologies

c. Sudden infant death syndrome (SIDS)

d. Causes of excessive daytime sleepiness (EDS) and sleep fragmentation

e. Parasomnias—REM versus nonrapid eye movement sleep (NREM)

f. Nocturnal enuresis incidence, evaluation, and therapy

5. Polysomnography techniques, scoring, and artifacts

a. Know staging criteria well

b. Stage changes in young adults versus elderly

c. Artifact recognition and technical intervention to resolve

d. Technical set up of filters, time constants, impedence, and calibration

e. Nocturnal penile tumescence techniques and evaluation

f. Understanding the full 10–20 montage and using it to locate a disorder versus artifact

g. Recognizing and understanding EEG patterns such as hypnagogic hypersynchrony or midline theta rhythm (MU rhythm) and others

h. Electrocardiogram rhythm recognition

i. Multiple sleep latency test (MSLT) procedure

j. Maintenance of wakefulness test (MWT) procedure

6. Clinical diagnostics

a. Questionnaires

b. Sleep logs and patterns of recognition of underlying sleep disorders

c. Actigraphy and its analysis for supporting the diagnosis

7. Seizure recognition on EEG and polysomnogram/polysomnography (PSG) monitoring

8. Sleep deprivation

a. Animal research results of total sleep deprivation

b. Human complete and partial sleep loss

9. Endocrinological patterns in the sleep-wake cycle and the circadian rhythm

10. Circadian physiology and genetics

11. Tonic versus phasic REM components in physiology and PSG

12. Cardiopulmonary physiology in sleep versus wake and with arousals

13. Sleep disorders

a. Sleep breathing disorders evaluation, epidemiology, pathogenesis, comorbid conditions, evaluation, and therapies including surgical evaluation and intervention, dental, and positive airway pressure equipment and troubleshooting

b. Narcolepsy presentation, pathophysiology, genetics, diagnostics, and treatment

c. Circadian rhythm disorders and their pathology, genetics, epidemiology, diagnosis, and treatment

d. REM behavior disorder

e. Psychiatric disorders such as schizophrenia or depression and sleep patterns versus drug effects

f. Nocturnal limb movements such as periodic limb movements during sleep (PLMS) and their causes, genetics, epidemiology, and interventions

g. Neurological disorders such as Parkinson's or Alzheimer's disease with sleep changes and subsequent disorders

h. Insomnia diagnostic categories, epidemiology, evaluation, and therapies
i. Disorders associated with alpha intrusion
14. AASM practice guidelines

Make sure you have practiced ahead of time on multiple PSGs and MSLTs quickly and accurately to identify the sleep latency, REM latency, sleep stages, arousals from sleep, PLMS, and apnea types. As in all exams, remember to relax enough to carefully listen to all instructions and check the announcement board, if one is present, to make sure no changes have been made.

BRIEF HISTORICAL OVERVIEW

Sleep is necessary, but its function, physiology, and pathophysiology have been unfolding only in this century. Sleep research has opened the doors to the field of sleep medicine, as we know it today. This section focuses on brief highlights in Table 1-2 of sleep research that has had a major impact on the current

field. Many more bright and talented researchers may not be included but are certainly appreciated.

PREVALENCE OF SLEEP DISORDERS

The National Sleep Foundation (NSF) poll in 2005 discovered that "60% of America's adults who drive or have a license report that, within the past year, they have driven a car or motor vehicle when feeling drowsy... About one-third of the respondents who drive or have a license (37%) report that they have ever nodded off or fallen asleep while driving a vehicle, even just for a brief moment. Among these respondents, 13% say they have done so at least once a month."[26] Drowsiness, fatigue, and insomnia are prevalent in our culture, although there seems to be an increase in public awareness. The overall prevalence of sleepiness is somewhat variable depending on how the survey is completed and the size of the population, but it is estimated to be from 0.5% to 36% overall.[27] In a Swedish study of 10,216 participants, EDS was approximately five times more prevalent in the elderly

		TABLE 1-2 ■ Sleep Medicine History at a Glance	
Year	Investigator	Discovery	Reference
1729	Jean Jacques d'Ortous de Mairan	Chronobiology of heliotrope plant	35
1875	R. Caton	EEG waves in dogs	34
1880	Jean Baptiste Edouard Gelineau	Narcolepsy named and described	35
1928–30	Hans Berger	Human brain surface: alpha waves EEG to differentiate wake versus sleep	34,35
1935	Frederick Bremer	2 cat preps: cerveau isole and encephale isole	35
1937	Loomis, Harvey, Hobart	Stages of sleep reflected in the EEG	34
1949	G. Moruzzi and H. Magoun	Brainstem reticular formation to describe EEG wake versus sleep	35
1951–55	N. Kleitman and E. Aserinsky	REM sleep discovery	34,35
1957	N. Kleitman and W. Dement	Described sleep stages	35
1959–62	Michel Jouvet	REM EMG suppression; pontine brainstem source of REM	35
1960	O. Pompeiano	Cat REM atonia mechanisms	35
1960	G. Vogel	Sleep onset REM periods	35
1960–64	R. Hodes and W. Dement	Depressed "H" reflexes in REM sleep	35
1964	W. Dement and S. Mitchell	First narcolepsy clinic	35
1965	R. Jung and W. Kuhlo Gastaut, Tassinari, and Duron	First clear recognition and description of obstructive sleep apnea	34,35
1965	Oswald and Priest	First sleep tests to evaluate sedatives	35
1966–71	A. Kales and colleagues	Sleep lab to study hypnotics; other illness	35
1968	A. Rechtschaffen and A. Kales	Standard method for scoring sleep stages	18
1970	R. Yoss, N. Moyer, R. Hollenhorst	Pupillometry	38
1970–78	E. Lugaresi and colleagues	Signs, symptoms, and pathophysiology of SA	35
1972	J. Holland and Stanford colleagues	Polysomnography	35
1973	E. Hoddes and colleagues	Stanford Sleepiness Scale	39
1977	C. Guilleminault, W. Dement	Dx/Classification of EDS	36
1976–78	M. Carskadon and colleagues	Studies of sleep latency; MSLT developed	35
1975	Assoc. of Sleep Disorders Centers	Now American Academy of Sleep Med.	35
1981	C. Sullivan and colleagues	CPAP for treatment of SA	37

EEG = electroencephalogram; REM = rapid eye movements; EMG = electromyogram; SA = sleep apnea; Dx = diagnosis; EDS = excessive daytime sleepiness; MSLT = multiple sleep latency test; CPAP = continuous positive airway pressure.

with poor health than in those with good health.[28] That same year (1996) a Finnish study of 11,354 adults ages 33 to 60 years old was published that showed 11% of women and 6.7% of men had EDS nearly every day.[29] More recently, a Japanese study published in 2005 reported EDS in 2.5% of 28,714 participants.[30]

The youth have had an excess of problems with sleepiness as well. The NSF reported (www.sleepfoundation.org) on March 28, 2006 that 45% of adolescents, ages 11 to 17, sleep less than 8 hours on school nights; at least 14% oversleep and 28% fall asleep in school at least once per week. A total of 51% of adolescent drivers have also admitted to driving drowsy within the year preceding this poll.

Sleep problems were also reported in 10.8% of school children ages 4 to 12 years old. In this study, 58.7% of the sleep problems were found to be due to five problems: parasomnias, fatigue, enuresis/gags, insomnia, and noisy sleep.[31]

Insomnia has traditionally been discussed separately from EDS in terms of diagnosis, surveys, and epidemiology and has been thought to be more of a "hyper-aroused" state rather than true EDS. Insomnia prevalence has varied depending on the patient population and type of insomnia evaluated. Prevalence appears to range from 1–2% for chronic insomnia in the general population to 15–20% for acute insomnia.[5] Usually women report more insomnia than men. More traditional disease links with EDS symptoms may actually have insomnia complaints. Sleep-disordered breathing patients are characteristically described as having somnolence rather than insomnia, but in a study of 231 objectively diagnosed patients, half were discovered to have a primary complaint of insomnia.[32] To further complicate how we understand insomnia complaints versus EDS, 22% of insomnia subjects showed evidence of EDS. These authors pointed out that there is indeed a wide spectrum of sleepiness to alertness in patients complaining of insomnia.[33]

For sleep medicine examination purposes, at least some idea of overall prevalence rates may help. The 2005 *International Classification of Sleep Disorders* (ICSD) published by the AASM listed the sleep disorders in the field of sleep medicine.[5] For each sleep disorder, prevalence rates, if known, are listed. Table 1-3 is a compilation of these prevalence rates as known at that time.

NORMAL SLEEP

Human Sleep Patterns

Overall normal sleep patterns for various age groups are discussed in this section. Polysomnography and highlights of sleep scoring fundamentals are addressed in later chapters of this book.

In children over 3 months old and adults, sleep is normally entered through NREM sleep that cycles with REM sleep at an approximate 90-minute interval, with a range of 90 to 110 minutes. There are four to five REM periods throughout the night in young adults. It is *abnormal* for an adult to enter sleep through REM, but within *normal* limits for an infant to have sleep-onset REM periods until around 3 months old. Although sleep spindles begin to appear at approximately 6 to 8 weeks of age,[41,42] NREM does not become clearly demarcated into specific stages until approximately 3 to 6 months.[40,41] Until then, NREM is developed from *quiet* sleep (that can be seen as the trace alternate EEG pattern) and REM from *active* sleep in infants. *Indeterminate or transitional* sleep is an EEG waveform that is not clearly *quiet* or *active* sleep in infants and that disappears with maturation. REM and NREM sleep are fairly equal in concentration for infants compared with a rate of 20–25% of REM for young adults. The 75–80% of sleep that consists of NREM in adults is divided into four stages, stages 1 through 4, with progressively deepening sleep and higher arousal thresholds. Slow wave sleep, also known as *delta sleep*, consists of a combination of stages 3 and 4 sleep that peaks in preadolescence. Slow wave sleep has its largest decline during the second decade of life at the same time that stage 2 sleep increases in concentration to its adult level of around 45–55% of sleep.[43,44] NREM predominates in the first half of sleep and is linked to a prior level of wakefulness that can cause various degrees of "sleep pressure." REM predominates in the last half of sleep and is circadian linked. Table 1-4 summarizes the highlights of sleep patterns in humans.

Mammalian Sleep Patterns

Sleep is present in mammals with NREM (slow-wave sleep, inactive or "quiet sleep") and REM (paradoxical, active, or desynchronized sleep) periods present. The percentages of these stages vary among species. Sleep EEG spindling density also has quite a bit of variability from high-density spindles such as in the 12 to 16 Hz range in primates[47] to no detectable spindles in parakeets.[48,49]

In 1935–1936, Dr. Frederick Bremer reported his research findings of the electrical rhythms in the cat brain.[50,51] The encephale isole, a section in the lower part of the medulla, was used in the study of cortical electrical rhythms responsive to various sensory impulses. The EEG of the encephale isole demonstrated an alternating pattern between the waking and sleeping state. The cerveau isole served to isolate the study of the olfactory and visual impulses. The EEG of this section demonstrated a sleeping state that led to

TABLE 1-3 ■ Prevalence Rates (Estimates) for Sleep Disorders[5]

Sleep Disorder	Prevalence[a,b]
Adjustment insomnia	15–20% approximate
Advanced sleep phase disorder	About 1% of middle-age adults or older
Behavioral insomnia of childhood	10–30% of children
Cheyne-Stokes breathing pattern	25–40% of heart failure; 10% of stroke
Circadian: delayed sleep phase disorder	7–16% of adolescents/young adults
Circadian: free-running type	Likely in over half of blind subjects
Circadian: shift work sleep disorder	2–5% or more
Confusional arousals	17.3% of age 3–13; 2.9–4.2% of age 15
Congenital central alveolar hypoventilation	Rare, with 160 to 180 living children reported
Hypersomnolence–no substance/condition	5–7% of hypersomniacs
Idiopathic insomnia	0.7% of adolescents; <10% of sleep patients
Inadequate sleep hygiene	5–10% of sleep clinic insomniacs
Infant sleep apnea	<31 wks 50–80%; >32 wks 12–15%
Insomnia due to mental disorder	3% of general population
Long sleeper	2% of men; 1.5% of women sleep 10 hours/night
Narcolepsy with cataplexy	0.02–0.18% of US/Western Europe
Narcolepsy without cataplexy	Unknown overall; 10–50% of narcoleptics
Obstructive sleep apnea, adult	4–24% of men; 2–9% of women–depends on study
Obstructive sleep apnea, pediatric	2% of children, usually preschool age
Paradoxical insomnia	<5% of insomniacs
Periodic limb movement disorder	Up to 34% >age 60; 1–15% of insomniacs
Primary sleep apnea of infancy	25% of babies <2.5 kg; <0.5% full-term
Psychophysiological insomnia	1–2% of population; 12–15% of sleep patients
Recurrent hypersomnia	Rare, with 200 reported subjects; male predominance
Recurrent isolated sleep paralysis	5–6% of adults; 15–40% <age 30 of ≥1 episode
REM sleep behavior disorder	About 0.5% of elderly; 0.38% of general population
Restless legs syndrome	10% of N. European adults
Short sleeper	3.6% of men; 4.3% of women sleep 5 hours/night
Sleep enuresis	30% of age 4; 10% of age 6; 5% of age 10
Sleep-related bruxism	14–15% of children; 8% young to middle-age adults
Sleep-related eating disorder	3/4 female; 4.6% of college students in a study
Sleep-related leg cramps	7% of children; nearly all adults >age 50
Sleep-related rhythmic movement disorder	59% of babies; 5% by age 5
Sleep starts	60–70%
Sleep talking	1/2 of young children; 5% of adults
Sleep terrors	1–6.5% of children; 2.2% of adults
Sleep walking	Up to 17% of children; up to 4% of adults
Sleep-related epilepsy	10–45% of epileptics
Snoring (habitual)	10–12% of children; 24% of adult women; 40% of men

[a] Prevalence may not be known for unlisted diagnoses.

[b] Unless otherwise specified, the prevalence rates are of the general population.

the realization that this brain section effectively suppressed nerve impulses necessary for the waking state of the telencephalon. In this brain section the eyeballs turned downward with a progressive miosis along with EEG evidence of a sleeping pattern. This led to the conclusion that sleep is a reversible deafferentation of the cerebral cortex.[50,51] The chronic cerveau isole preparation eventually demonstrated the interactions of paradoxical sleep that were located in the lower brainstem modulated by forebrain structures.[52] This paved the way for further cat and other mammalian experiments that ultimately isolated the REM center to the pontine sections of the brain chiefly at the cholinergic neurons of the laterodorsal and pedunculopontine tegmental nuclei.[53] Characteristics of REM sleep were found to be associated with ponto-geniculo-occipital (PGO) spikes and phasic events such as rapid eye movements, muscle twitches, and middle ear muscle activity. EEG is consistent with a desynchronized, low-amplitude EEG with rapid eye movements and muscle atonia. Animals with implanted electrodes have also demonstrated rhythmic theta waves at 4 to 8 cycles per second (cps). All species have greater REM sleep in early life that tends to decrease with age.[47,53]

TABLE 1-4 ■ Normal Sleep Patterns in Humans[40,44–46]			
	Infants	**Young Adults**	**Elderly**
Wake after sleep onset	<5%	<5%	10–25%
Sleep efficiency	>90%	>90%	75–85%
Stage 1	Quiet sleep[a]	2–5%	5–8%
Stage 2	Quiet sleep	45–55%	57–67%
Stages 3 and 4	Quiet sleep	13–23%	6–17%
Stage REM	50%	20–25%	17–20%
Stage REM:NREM Ratio	50:50	20:80	20:80
Time of REM:NREM cycle	45–60 minutes	90–110 minutes	90–110 minutes
Total sleep time	14–16 hours	7–8 hours	7 hours

[a] Quiet sleep collectively is about 50% of sleep alternating with about 50% active (later developing into stage REM) sleep.

These important neuroscience interactions and discoveries are discussed further in Chapter 2.

Unihemispheric sleep is an interesting sleep pattern unique to dolphins of the order Cetacea, eared seals, manatees, and birds. There is EEG evidence that one hemisphere shows slow wave sleep activity at the same time the opposite hemisphere shows a waking pattern. Unihemispheric sleep serves as a protective feature to allow the mammal or bird to monitor the environment, and in the case of the aquatic mammal, it also permits surfacing to breathe.[54,55]

SLEEP DEPRIVATION

Animal Sleep Deprivation

The classic experiments in total sleep deprivation often quoted are those of the rats on the "moving-platform-over-water" method of study.[56] All rats died or were severely compromised at the time of sacrifice. Interestingly enough, their metabolic rate was extremely high, their body temperature dropped, and weight loss accelerated despite eating as much as they wanted. Their appearance was also debilitated, with severe tail and paw ulcerative and hyperkeratotic lesions. Upon sacrifice, no anatomical or pathological abnormality was found.[57,58]

Selecting a sleep stage for deprivation experiments ended with similar results. Rechtschaffen and colleagues selectively deprived rats of paradoxical sleep that again developed a very high-energy expenditure with weight loss despite increased food intake, as well as skin lesions. The only difference was that these changes occurred more slowly than the totally sleep-deprived rats.[59] Further rat experiments with both complete and selective sleep deprivation that were allowed to have recovery sleep and survived had high paradoxical sleep rebounds that were far above baseline values.[60]

Overall, animal experiments are useful but cannot in all cases be directly extrapolated to the human experience.

Human Sleep Deprivation

Humans who have undergone more than 200 hours of complete sleep deprivation have experienced several physiological changes. Neurological changes were ptosis, hand tremors, mild nystagmus, sluggish corneal reflexes, and yet brisk gag and hyperactive deep tendon reflexes.[61,62] Total sleep deprivation in humans can blunt the secretion of the sleep-linked hormones, growth hormone, and prolactin with a rebound secretion on sleep recovery.[63,64] Although initially there is no significant cortisol change with sleep deprivation, cortisol decreases on the postdeprivation recovery night as a result of rebound slow wave sleep.[65]

Sleep deprivation leads to EEG changes with less ability to sustain alpha activity even with eye closure, an increase in delta and theta waves during wake, and no beta activity change.[63,66] Transient microsleep periods have also been documented with associated performance deficits.

During a study of restorative sleep after 40 hours of sleep deprivation, the slow wave enhancement was most pronounced in the frontal rather than the more parietal derivations.[67] Slow wave sleep predominates on the *first* recovery night after total sleep deprivation in young adults with a subsequent reduction of stages 1, 2, and REM sleep. A REM rebound tends to occur on the *second* recovery night as slow wave sleep nears normal.[63]

Selective sleep deprivation refers to researchers depriving a subject of a particular stage of sleep. In general, the particular stage that is deprived will be the stage that will preferentially rebound on the sleep recovery night. If REM sleep is selectively deprived, then a large REM rebound will occur on the recovery night.[68]

The investigations on the effect of insufficient sleep commonly experienced by the population (about 5 hours of sleep) have shown impairment in psychomotor performance. There are also decreases in the mean sleep latency as recorded on the multiple sleep latency test (MSLT) during this period and shortly beyond the sleep restriction.[69]

ESTABLISHING WORK-HOUR RULES

Overview

There are multiple stories of sleep deprivation resulting in tragedy and loss of life. Sleep deprivation on the job can lead to critical judgment errors and jeopardize the health of not only the worker but others as well. Multiple tragic events have preceded current guidelines to optimize health and safety by developing work-hour rules. For a good summary, please see Chapter 53 by Walsh, Dement, and Dinges in the 2005 edition of *Principles and Practice of Sleep Medicine*.[70]

Total and chronic partial sleep deprivation increases risk for motor vehicle accidents, which have been shown to peak during early morning hours (12 midnight–7 A.M.) and mid-afternoon (around 3 P.M.).[71] Sleep deprivation has a similar impact on daytime sleepiness in commercial truck drivers similar to drivers with severe (apnea-hypopnea index [AHI] = 30) sleep apnea, although driving impairment appears to be more affected by sleep duration of 5 hours sleep per night than by drivers with severe sleep apnea.[72]

In a 2002 "National Survey of Distracted and Drowsy Driving Attitudes and Behaviors" posted on the National Highway Traffic Safety Administration website,[73] 37% of drivers in the general population have fallen asleep while driving at least once in their driving experience, with a greater prevalence (13%) among those 21 to 29 years old. Of these drivers, 48% had drifted off to sleep between 9 P.M. and 6 A.M.

Sleep deprivation in medical training became national news after the well-publicized case of Libby Zion, who died in a New York hospital in 1984. After her death, a court ruled that physician negligence in her care was part of the events that led to her death. A component of this was related to sleep deprivation and lack of attending supervision.[74] This landmark case triggered work-hour changes throughout the country that were initially recommended by the Association of American Medical Colleges to limit the work week to 80 hours, with at least one 24-hour period of nonworking time per week (summarized later). Findings from other studies completed on residency fatigue and subsequent impaired performance were similar to findings from sleep deprivation studies. Baldwin and Daugherty studied 3604 resident surveys and reported that residents averaging 5 hours of sleep per night had more problems with accidents/injuries, professional staff conflict, alcohol, stimulant medications, and significant medical errors. Yet the authors concluded that "capping residents' work hours is unlikely to fully address the sleep deficits and resulting impairments reported by residents." They pointed out that there is a balance between work hours, sleep needs, and personal time outside of work.[75]

Mistakes in an intensive care unit were shown to be linked to intern fatigue on a traditional extended work-hour schedule. There was significant error reduction on a more limited work-hour schedule with shorter shifts.[76] Resident sleep deprivation increases driving risk the same as any other sleep-deprived driver, as pointed out by Barger et al. in a prospective analysis that showed a statistically significant increase in vehicle crashes of interns after extended work hours.[77]

The following sections provide a brief summary of national regulations affecting the trucking industry and the medical profession. These guidelines were developed by task force committees to protect both the worker and the people affected by worker impairment resulting from fatigue.

Trucking Industry

Years of research led to the development of driver-regulated work and sleep schedule rules in 2003. These rules were modified for the commercial truck driver, with new posted regulations[78] effective October 1, 2005:

- The driver may drive a maximum of 11 hours after 10 consecutive hours off duty.
- The driver may drive beyond the 14th hour after coming on duty, after 10 consecutive hours off duty.
- The driver may not drive after 60 hours on duty in 7 consecutive days (70 hours in 8 days) but may restart a 7 consecutive day period after 34 consecutive hours off duty.
- The driver using a sleeper berth must take 8 consecutive hours in the sleeper berth in addition to 2 consecutive hours either in the sleeper berth, off duty, or any combination of the two.

Medical Profession

The ACGME Subcommittee on Duty Hours for residency training recommended changes to the ACGME Board of Directors that were implemented September 2004 with the following summary[79]:

- The resident cannot work more than 80 hours per week that is averaged over 4 weeks.

- There needs to be an adequate rest period of 10 hours between duty periods.
- There is a 24-hour limit on continuous duty with 6 additional hours for continuity of care and didactics.
- It is recommended that 1 out of 7 days, averaged over 4 weeks, be free from patient care or educational responsibilities.
- In-house call should be limited to once every 3 nights, averaged over 4 weeks.

REFERENCES

1. The American Board of Sleep Medicine (ABSM) website is at: www.absm.org. Address: One Westbrook Corporate Center, Suite 920, Westchester, IL 60154. Telephone: 708-492-1290 as of the printing of this book.

2. American Academy of Pediatrics: Section on Pediatric Pulmonology, Subcommittee on Obstructive Sleep Apnea. Clinical practice guideline: Diagnosis and management of childhood obstructive sleep apnea syndrome. Pediatrics 109(4):704–712, 2002.

3. Anders T, Parmalee AH, Emde RN: *A Manual of Standardized Terminology, Technology and Criteria for Scoring of States of Sleep and Wakefulness in New-born Infants.* Los Angeles, CA, UCLA BIS/BRI Publications, 1971.

4. Aldrich MS: *Sleep Medicine.* Contemporary Neurology Series 52, Oxford University Press, 1999.

5. American Academy of Sleep Medicine: *The International Classification of Sleep Disorders: Diagnostic and Coding Manual,* 2nd ed. Westchester, IL, American Academy of Sleep Medicine, 2005.

6. American Thoracic Society: Standards and indications for cardiopulmonary sleep studies in children. Am J Resp Crit Care Med 153(2):866–878, 1996.

7. Butkov N: *Atlas of Clinical Polysomnography,* Vol I & II. Ashland, OR, Synapse Media, 1996.

8. Carskadon MA, Dement WC, Mitler MM, et al: Guidelines for the Multiple Sleep Latency Test (MSLT): a standard measure of sleepiness. Sleep 9(4):519–524, 1986.

9. Chokroverty S (ed): *Sleep Disorders Medicine: Basic Science, Technical Considerations, and Clinical Aspects,* 2nd ed. Boston, Butterworth-Heinemann, 1999.

10. Chokroverty S, Thomas RJ, Bhatt M: *Atlas of Sleep Medicine.* Philadelphia, Elsevier Butterworth-Heinemann, 2005.

11. Culebras A: *Clinical Handbook of Sleep Disorders,* 1st ed. Boston, Butterworth-Heinemann, 1996.

12. Fisch BJ: *Fisch and Spehlmann's EEG Primer: Basic Principles of Digital and Analog EEG,* 3rd ed. New York, Elsevier, 1999.

13. Geyer JD, Payne T, Carney PR, Aldrich M: *Atlas of Digital Polysomnography.* Philadelphia, Lippincott, Williams & Wilkins, 2000.

14. Hauri P (ed): *Case Studies in Insomnia.* New York, Plenum Press, 1991.

15. Kryger MH, Roth T, Dement WC (eds): *Principles and Practice of Sleep Medicine,* 4th ed. Philadelphia, Elsevier Saunders, 2005.

16. Lee-Chiong TL, Sateia MJ, Carskadon MA: *Sleep Medicine.* Philadelphia, Hanley & Belfus, Inc., 2002.

17. Morin CM: *Insomnia. Psychological Assessment and Management,* reissue ed. New York, The Guilford Press, 1996.

18. Rechtschaffen A, Kales A: *A Manual of Standardized Terminology, Techniques, and Scoring System for Sleep Stages of Human Subjects.* Los Angeles, UCLA Brain Information Service/BRI Publications, 1968.

19. Sheldon SH, Ferber R, Kryger MH: *Principles and Practice of Pediatric Sleep Medicine,* 4th ed. Philadelphia, Elsevier Saunders, 2005.

20. Sheldon SH, Riter S, Detrojan M: *Atlas of Sleep Medicine in Infants and Children.* Armonk, NY, Futura Publishing Co., Inc., 1999.

21. Shepard JW (ed): *Atlas of Sleep Medicine.* Mount Kisco, NY, Futura Publishing Co., 1991.

22. Tyner F, Knott JR, Mayer WB: *Fundamentals of EEG Technology, Vol. 1: Basic Concepts and Methods.* New York, Raven Press, 1983.

23. Wooten VD, Buysse DJ: Sleep in psychiatric disorders. (See Table 28-1.) In Chokroverty S (ed): *Sleep Disorders Medicine: Basic Science, Technical Considerations, and Clinical Aspects,* 2nd ed. Boston, Butterworth-Heinemann, 1999, pp 573–586.

24. Schweitzer PK: Drugs that disturb sleep and wakefulness. In Kryger MH, Roth T, Dement WC (eds): *Principles and Practice of Sleep Medicine,* 4th ed. Philadelphia, Elsevier Saunders, 2005, pp 499–518.

25. Zoltoski RK, Cabeza RJ, Gillin JC: Biochemical pharmacology of sleep. In Chokroverty S (ed): *Sleep Disorders Medicine: Basic Science, Technical Considerations, and Clinical Aspects,* 2nd ed. Boston, Butterworth-Heinemann, 1999, pp 63–94.

26. National Sleep Foundation (NSF): Facts about drowsy driving. On the NSF website at http://www.sleepfoundation.org, 1999.

27. Roehrs T, Carskadon MA, Dement WC, Roth T: Daytime sleepiness and alertness. In Kryger MH, Roth T, Dement WC (eds): *Principles and Practice of Sleep Medicine,* 4th ed. Philadelphia, Elsevier Saunders, 2005, pp 39–50.

28. Asplund R: Daytime sleepiness and napping amongst the elderly in relation to somatic health and medical treatment. J Intern Med 239(3):261–267, 1996.

29. Hublin C, Kaprio J, Partinen M, et al: Daytime sleepiness in the adult, Finnish population. J Intern Med 239(5):417–423, 1996.

30. Kaneita Y, Ohida T, Uchiyama M, et al: Excessive daytime sleepiness among the Japanese general population. J Epidemiol 15(1):1–8, 2005.

31. Stein MA, Mendelsohn J, Obermeyer WH, et al: Sleep and behavior problems in school-aged children. Pediatrics 107(4):1–9, 2001.

32. Krakow B, Melendrez D, Ferreira E, et al: Prevalence of insomnia symptoms in patients with sleep-disordered breathing. Chest 120(6):1923–1929, 2001.

33. Day R, Guido P, Helmus T, et al: Self-reported levels of sleepiness among subjects with insomnia. Sleep Med 2(2):153–157, 2001.

34. Chokroverty S: An overview of sleep. In Chokroverty S (ed): *Sleep Disorders Medicine: Basic Science, Technical*

Considerations, and Clinical Aspects, 2nd ed Boston, Butterworth-Heinemann, 1999, pp 7–20.

35. Dement WC: History of sleep physiology and medicine. In Kryger MH, Roth T, Dement WC (eds): *Principles and Practice of Sleep Medicine*, 4th ed. Philadelphia, Elsevier Saunders, 2005, pp 1–12.

36. Guilleminault C, Dement W: 235 cases of excessive daytime sleepiness. Diagnosis and tentative classification. J Neurol Sci 31:13–27, 1977.

37. Sullivan CE, Issa FG, Berthon-Jones M, et al: Reversal of obstructive sleep apnea by continuous positive airway pressure applied through the nares. Lancet 1:862–865, 1981.

38. Yoss RE, Moyer NJ, Hollenhorst RW: Pupil size and spontaneous pupillary waves associated with alertness, drowsiness, and sleep. Neurology 20(6):545–554, 1970.

39. Hoddes E, Zarcone V, Smythe H, et al: Quantification of sleepiness: a new approach. Psychophysiology 10(4):431–436, 1973.

40. Sheldon SH: Polysomnography in infants and children. In Sheldon SH, Ferber R, Kryger MH (eds): *Principles and Practice of Pediatric Sleep Medicine*, 4th ed. Philadelphia, Elsevier Saunders, 2005, pp 49–71.

41. Lenard HG: The development of sleep spindles in the EEG during the first two years of life. Neuropadiatrie 1(3):264–276, 1970.

42. Hughes JR: Development of sleep spindles in the first year of life. Clin Electroencephalogr 27(3):107–115, 1996.

43. Carskadon MA: The second decade. In Guilleminault C (ed): *Sleeping and Waking Disorders: Indications and Techniques*. Boston, Butterworth, 1982, pp 99–125.

44. Carskadon MA, Dement WC: Normal human sleep: an overview. In Kryger MH, Roth T, Dement WC (eds): *Principles and Practice of Sleep Medicine*, 3rd ed. Philadelphia, Saunders, 2000, pp 15–25.

45. Chokroverty S: An overview of sleep. In Chokroverty S (ed): *Sleep Disorders Medicine: Basic Science, Technical Considerations, and Clinical Aspects*, 2nd ed. Boston, Butterworth-Heinemann, 1999, pp 7–20.

46. Bliwise DL: Normal aging. In Kryger MH, Roth T, Dement WC (eds): *Principles and Practice of Sleep Medicine*, 4th ed. Philadelphia Elsevier Saunders, 2005, pp 24–38.

47. Zepelin H, Siegel JM, Tobler I: Mammalian sleep. In Kryger MH, Roth T, Dement WC (eds): *Principles and Practice of Sleep Medicine*, 4th ed. Philadelphia, Elsevier Saunders, 2005, pp 91–100.

48. Ayala-Guerrero F: Sleep patterns in the parakeet *Melopsittacus undulatus*. Physiol Behav 46(5):787–791, 1989.

49. Ayala-Guerrero F, Perez MC, Calderon A: Sleep patterns in the bird *Aratinga canicularis*. Physiol Behav 43(5):585–589, 1988.

50. Bremer F: Cerveau. Nouvelles recherches sur le macanisme du sommeil. C R Soc Biol 122:460–464, 1936.

51. Bremer F: Cerveau "isole" et physiologie du sommeil. C R Soc Biol 118:1235–1241, 1935.

52. Gottesmann C: What the cerveau isole preparation tells us nowadays about sleep mechanisms? Neurosci Biobehav Rev 12(1):39–48, 1988.

53. McCarley RW: Sleep neurophysiology: basic mechanisms underlying control of wakefulness and sleep. In Chokroverty S (ed): *Sleep Disorders Medicine: Basic Science, Technical Considerations, and Clinical Aspects*, 2nd ed. Boston, Butterworth-Heinemann, 1999, pp 21–50.

54. Rattenborg NC, Amlaner CJ, Lima SIBehavioral, neurophysiological and evolutionary perspectives on unihemispheric sleep. Neurosci Biobehav Rev 24(8):817–842, 2000.

55. Rattenborg NC, Lima SL, Amlaner CJ: Facultative control of avian unihemispheric sleep under the risk of predation. Behav Brain Res 105(2):163–172, 1999.

56. Bergmann BM, Kushida CA, Everson CA, et al: Sleep deprivation in the rat: II. Methodology. Sleep 12(1):5–12, 1989.

57. Gilliland MA, Bergmann BM, Rechtschaffen A: Sleep deprivation in the rat: VIII. High EEG amplitude sleep deprivation. Sleep 12(1):53–59, 1989, 1989.

58. Kushida CA, Everson CA, Suthipinittharm P, et al: Sleep deprivation in the rat: VI. Skin changes. Sleep 12(1):42–46, 1989.

59. Kushida CA, Bergmann BM, Rechtschaffen A: Sleep deprivation in the rat: IV. Paradoxical sleep deprivation. Sleep 12(1):22–30, 1989.

60. Everson CA, Gilliland MA, Kushida CA, et al: Sleep deprivation in the rat: IX. Recovery. Sleep 12(1):60–67, 1989.

61. Kollar EJ, Namerow N, Pasnau RO, Naitoh P: Neurological findings during prolonged sleep deprivation. Neurology 18(9):836–840, 1968.

62. Ross JJ: Neurological findings after prolonged sleep deprivation. Arch Neurol 12:399–403, 1965.

63. Bonnet MH: Acute sleep deprivation. In Kryger MH, Roth T, Dement WC (eds): *Principles and Practice of Sleep Medicine*, 4th ed. Philadelphia Elsevier Saunders, 2005, pp 51–66.

64. Von Treuer K, Norman TR, Armstrong SM: Overnight human plasma melatonin, cortisol, prolactin, TSH, under conditions of normal sleep, sleep deprivation, and sleep recovery. J Pineal Res 20(1):7–14, 1996.

65. Vgontzas AN, Mastorakos G, Bixler EO: Sleep deprivation effects on the activity of the hypothalamic-pituitary-adrenal and growth axes: potential clinical implications. Clin Endocrinol 51(2):205–215, 1999.

66. Naitoh P, Pasnau RO, Kollar EJ: Psychophysiological changes after prolonged deprivation of sleep. Biol Psychiatry 3(4):309–320, 1971.

67. Cajochen C, Foy R, Kijk DJ: Frontal predominance of a relative increase in sleep delta and theta EEG activity after sleep loss in humans. Sleep Res Online 2(3):65–69, 1999.

68. Endo T, Roth C, Landolt HP, et al: Selective REM sleep deprivation in humans: effects on sleep and sleep EEG. Am J Physiol 274(4Pt2):R1186–R1194, 1998.

69. Dinges DF, Pack F, Williams K, et al: Cumulative sleepiness, mood disturbance, and psychomotor vigilance performance decrements during a week of sleep restricted to 4–5 hours per night. Sleep 20(4):267–277, 1997.

70. Walsh JK, Dement WC, Dinges DF: Sleep medicine, public policy, and public health. In Kryger MH, Roth T, Dement WC (eds): *Principles and Practice of Sleep Medicine*, 4th ed. Philadelphia, Elsevier Saunders, 2005, pp 648–656.

71. Pack AI, Pack AM, Rodgman E, et al: Characteristics of crashes attributed to the driver having fallen asleep. Accid Anal Prev 27(6):769–775, 1995.

72. Pack AI, Maislin G, Staley B, et al: Impaired performance in commercial drivers: role of sleep apnea and short sleep duration. Am J Respir Crit Care Med 174(4):446–454, 2006.

73. National Highway Traffic Safety Administration (NHTSA): National Survey of Distracted and Drowsy Driving Attitudes and Behaviors: 2002. Posted 2003 on website http://www.nhtsa.dot.gov/people/injury/drowsy_driving1/survey-distractive03/summary.htm.

74. Block AJ: Revisiting the Libby Zion case (editorial). Chest 105(4):977–978, 1994.

75. Baldwin DC Jr, Daugherty SR: Sleep deprivation and fatigue in residency training: results of a national survey of first- and second-year residents. Sleep 27(2):217–223, 2004.

76. Lockley SW, Cronin JW, Evans EE, et al: Effect of reducing interns' weekly work hours on sleep and attentional failures. N Engl J Med 351(18):1829–1837, 2004.

77. Barger LK, Cade BE, Ayas NT, et al: Extended work shifts and the risk of motor vehicle crashes among interns. N Engl J Med 352(2):125–134, 2005.

78. U.S. Department of Transportation's Federal Motor Carrier Safety Administration (FMCSA) Department of Transportation: New rules regulating work and sleep schedules for commercial truck drivers. From websites: (a) http://www.dot.gov/affairs/fmcsa0405.htm (b) http://www.fmcsa.dot.gov/rules-regulations/topics/hos/hos-2005.htm.

79. Subcommittee on Duty Hours. Third Report of the Subcommittee on Duty Hours: Advising ACGME on the Implementation and Monitoring of the Duty Hour Standards. 2004. Website: http://www.acgme.org/acWebsite/dutyHours/dh_index.asp.

Highlights of Sleep Neuroscience

PHYLLIS C. ZEE ■ R. CHRIS HAMMOND

Cycles of rest and activity are ubiquitous among living organisms. Defined from a behavioral standpoint, *sleep* is a reversible state, characterized by decreased responsiveness to the environment and motor activity, and, when deprived, there is a tremendous need for recovery. Sleep is not a static brain state, but rather dynamic states that cycle through stages of biological distinction, divided broadly into rapid eye movement (REM) and non-REM (NREM) sleep. Conventional polysomnographic (PSG) measures distinguish four NREM stages and one REM stage.[1] NREM is subdivided into progressive stages of corresponding deeper states of sleep, stages 1 through 4, with stages 3 and 4 referred to as *slow wave sleep* (SWS). Measurable changes in electrophysiology, neurochemistry, and functional neuroanatomy of the brain accompany these two major sleep states. This chapter summarizes our current understanding of the complex neurobiology of sleep and wake regulation and its implication for the development and treatment of sleep disorders.

REGULATION OF SLEEP-WAKE STATES

Our current understanding of the regulation of the human sleep-wake cycle indicates that sleep and wake behaviors are generated by a complex interaction of endogenous circadian and sleep homeostatic processes, as well as environmental factors.[2,3] The building of sleep pressure, demonstrated as a compensatory response to sleep loss characterized by sleepiness, increased propensity to fall asleep, and increased sleep time once sleep occurs, is referred to as *sleep homeostasis*, or *process S*. The accumulation of process S is proportional to the duration of prior wakefulness.

Physiological sleepiness not only varies with prior waking duration, but also exhibits circadian variation. A circadian regulatory process, or *process C*, is implicated in the temporal organization of sleep-wake cycles, promoting a biphasic tendency for sleep and alertness at specific times of the 24-hour day. Additional regulators of sleep-wake regulation have been described, such as the ultradian process, which promotes the cyclic alternation of NREM and REM sleep, and infradian regulators, which occur beyond the 24-hour cycle.[4] Disruption of the intricate interactions between homeostatic and circadian processes results in serious consequences for sleep, performance, health, and safety (Figure 2-1).

Homeostasis Process S

Homeostatic models propose that a sleep-wake dependent process underlies the rise in sleep pressure during waking and its decay during sleep.[5] Sleep drive is augmented by increasing time spent awake, which results in compensatory changes in sleep duration and intensity during subsequent sleep that is manifested as an elevated arousal threshold and increased delta activity.[6,7] Thus, delta power (calculated EEG activity in the 1–4 Hz range) is thought to reflect SWS need and its underlying homeostatically regulated recovery process.[8] The accumulation of sleep pressure with extended wakefulness is significantly attenuated by intermittent naps measured by delta power and other EEG markers of sleep and wake homeostasis.[9,10]

At present, the exact mechanisms responsible for compensatory sleep after extended waking are not well understood, although recent findings indicate

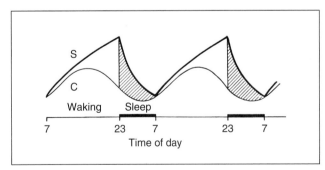

FIGURE 2-1 ■ Schematic representation of the interaction of the sleep homeostatic process (S) and circadian process (C) in the regulation of the sleep-wake cycle. Note that as process S or homeostatic drive for sleep accumulates during the day, the circadian output also increases to promote wakefulness.

that the neuromodulator adenosine contributes to sleep homeostasis. Adenosine accumulates during prolonged wakefulness in the basal forebrain (BF) and in the cerebral cortex, and it returns to baseline levels after sleep recovery.[11,12] Adenosine directly inhibits mesopontine and basal forebrain cholinergic neurons involved in mechanisms of arousal.[13] Furthermore, recent findings demonstrated that adenosine, via activation of adenosine A1 receptors, inhibit inhibitory synaptic inputs to the ventral lateral preoptic nucleus (VLPO)[14] and also via A2 receptors of nearby cell groups activate the VLPO,[15] which in turn promotes sleep. Thus it is not surprising that caffeine, an adenosine receptor antagonist, promotes wakefulness and alters EEG markers of sleep homeostasis, including reducing SWS.[16] Functional polymorphism of the adenosine deaminase gene, which is associated with the reduced metabolism of adenosine, demonstrated both increased duration and intensity of SWS in human subjects.[17] In a study of inbred mouse strains, the delta power was dependent on the duration of prior wakefulness and genotype.[18] In summary, process S increases as a function of prior wakefulness and decreases during sleep. Homeostatic signals include adenosine and other sleep-inducing substances (discussed later) that together influence the state of sleep- and wake-generating centers.

Circadian Process C

Circadian (near 24 hours) rhythms are ubiquitous among living organisms. The most notable circadian rhythm in humans is the recurring cycle of sleep and wakefulness. In addition to governing the 24-hour cycles of sleep and wakefulness, the suprachiasmatic nucleus (SCN) of the hypothalamus also maintains the circadian rhythm of other physiological variables such as temperature, cortisol, and melatonin.[19] Circadian rhythms are endogenous and thus persist under constant conditions with a free-running period (tau) that is close to, but usually not exactly, 24 hours.[20]

Circadian Clock

The SCN, a paired structure composed of approximately 20,000 neurons located in the anterior hypothalamus, contains a master circadian clock.[21–24]

The basic molecular mechanism by which SCN neurons generate and maintain a self-sustaining rhythm is via an autoregulatory feedback loop in which oscillating circadian gene products regulate their own expression through a complex system of transcription, translation, and post-translational processes.[25–27] In mammals, the feedback loop consists of four main proteins: period (PER), cryptochrome (CRY), and the transcriptional factors CLOCK and BMAL1. These two transcription factors combine and form a heterodimer complex that activates the transcription of *Cry* and *Per* genes to increase the production of CRY (CRY1 and CRY2) and PER (PER1, PER2, PER3), which dimerize and inhibit the activity of the CLOCK and BMAL1 heterodimer, which in turn shuts off their own transcription.[28] When CRY and PER levels drop off through degradation by phosphorylation,[29] the cycle is restarted by activation of the CLOCK/ BMAL1 heterodimer. The three PERs are phosphorylated by casein kinase I (CKI) e. There is evidence, however, that CKI e is not the only kinase involved in phosphorylation of clock proteins.[30,31]

Entrainment of Circadian Rhythms

In humans, because the intrinsic circadian period is slightly longer than 24 hours,[20] adaptation to a 24-hour physical environment requires daily synchronization between the endogenously generated circadian rhythm with that of the light/dark or social/physical activity cycle (entrainment). Light, physical activity, and melatonin are the main synchronizing agents or *zeitgebers* (German for "time-giver") for the human circadian clock.[31] Because of their ability to influence the timing of circadian rhythms and sleep, bright light and melatonin are used in clinical practice to treat certain circadian rhythm sleep disorders.

Light is the most important and powerful entraining agent for the circadian clock.[32] Photic information from the retina reaches the SCN via the monosynaptic retinohypothalamic tract (glutamate and pituitary adenylate cyclase-activating polypeptide as neurotransmitters) and also indirectly from the geniculohypothalamic tract derived from the intergeniculate leaflet of the lateral geniculate of the thalamus (neuropeptide Y and GABA as neurotransmitters).[33,34] Recent data indicate that although the rods and cones may contribute to circadian photoreception, neither of these are necessary.[35] The melanopsin-containing retinal ganglion cells, which are most responsive to short wavelength (blue-green) light, are the major photoceptors for the circadian clock.[36–38] Nonphotic information, such as activity via serotoninergic fibers from the dorsal raphe nucleus, are also received by the SCN.[39–41]

Melatonin, produced by the pineal gland, is also an important synchronizing agent for the circadian system. The circadian rhythm of melatonin synthesis and secretion is regulated by the SCN via an indirect pathway from the superior cervical ganglion to the pineal gland.[42,43] Axons of the SCN project to the subventricular zone of the hypothalamus, and from there, via the medial forebrain bundle, these fibers enter the intermediolateral gray column of the spinal cord. Leaving the central nervous system, these projections ascend with the peripheral sympathetic trunk and will synapse at the superior cervical ganglion.[44] Postganglionic fibers from the superior cervical ganglion end in the pineal gland. Melatonin levels begin to rise approximately 2 hours before habitual sleep time, and exposure to bright light will suppress melatonin.[45] Once secreted, melatonin can also influence the timing of the circadian clock by its action on melatonin receptors (MT1 and MT2) located in the SCN.[46]

Role of SCN in Sleep and Wake Regulation

In humans, daily variation in physiological sleep tendency reveals a biphasic circadian rhythm of wake and sleep propensity.[2,10] It has been postulated that in addition to providing temporal organization, another primary role of the circadian pacemaker is to promote wakefulness during the day and thus facilitate the consolidation of sleep during the night.[10,47–49]

Although the mechanisms and neural pathways by which the circadian clock regulates sleep and wake propensity have not been fully established, the SCN likely modulates sleep and wake via its projections to the basal forebrain, thalamus, and the dorsomedial and subparaventricular zones of the hypothalamus, which then project to sleep- and wake-promoting centers such as the VLPO and locus coeruleus.[50,51,84] In addition, direct projections from the SCN to the wake-promoting hypocretin/orexin neurons[42] may be another mechanism for the alerting role of the SCN.

It has also been postulated that the evening rise in melatonin may also play a role in sleep promotion. Intracellular recordings have shown that SCN neurons have a high firing rate in the daytime and low firing rate during the night.[52,53] It has been shown that when applied to SCN neurons, melatonin decreases their firing rate.[54] This effect is primarily mediated by agonism of the subtype MT1 receptors of the SCN.[55] This reduction in SCN neuronal activity has been postulated to be one of the mechanisms by which melatonin promotes sleep.[56]

In summary, evidence for a circadian regulatory process regulating sleep initiation and duration was first obtained in the temporal isolation studies conducted by Aschoff and colleagues.[57] The circadian timing system regulates the timing of the sleep-wake cycle and propensity for sleep and alertness (Figure 2-2). As proposed by Edgar,[21,22] the function of the circadian clock, the SCN, is to promote alertness,[58] thus counteracting the homeostatic drive for sleep during the day and facilitating consolidation of sleep during the night.[10]

Ultradian Process

A third regulator proposed, although less understood, influences oscillation of NREM and REM stages of sleep.[59] Located in the mesopontine area, this oscillator incorporates reciprocal interaction between cholinergic REM-on and aminergic REM-off cell groups (see later). Influence on each of these groups is mediated by interposed excitatory, inhibitory, and autoregulatory circuits that involve multiple neurotransmitters.[60] Timing of REM onset during sleep increases from infancy (60 minutes) to adulthood (90–120 minutes), which may reflect neuronal maturation of ultradian cell groups. Not discussed here are the many infradian (hormonal, seasonal, and other) influences on sleep-wake cycles.

FUNCTIONAL NEUROANATOMICAL BASIS OF AROUSAL AND WAKEFULNESS

The arousal systems of the brain are complex and consist of multiple neuronal circuits, many with significant redundancy. In 1949, Moruzzi and Magoun described the ascending reticular activating system (ARAS).[61] The ARAS originates in the brainstem and exists as a multineuronal, polysynaptic system that is essential for the maintenance of wakefulness and arousal. Early investigators often emphasized the role of the reticular formation in arousal.[43] More recently recognized, however, are multiple pathways that contribute to arousal; these pathways originate among clearly defined cell groups with their respective neurotransmitters located in the brainstem, hypothalamus, thalamus, and basal forebrain. The ARAS contains two major axes: a direct, extrathalamic pathway or ventral tegmental pathway and an indirect, reticulothalamocortical pathway or dorsal tegmental pathway. Activation of the thalamus is necessary for thalamocortical projections that result in low-amplitude, high-frequency EEG patterns characteristic of wakefulness. Activation of the ventral pathway, involving the hypothalamus, may be required for the expression of waking behavior.[62] Several distinct systems involving neurotransmitters such as acetylcholine, histamine, noradrenaline, dopamine, serotonin, glutamate, and the hypocretin/orexin system play fundamental roles in arousal.

The cholinergic pathway is a major element of the ARAS and higher centers of arousal. Acetylcholine

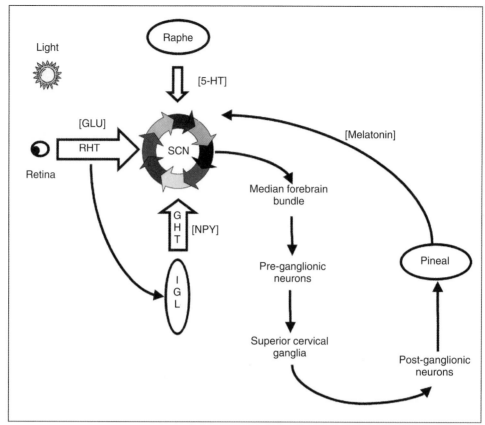

FIGURE 2-2 ■ Schematic diagram of the circadian timing system. The suprachiasmatic nucleus (SCN) operates as the "pacemaker" center. Photic information reaches the SCN through fibers of the retinohypothalamic tract (RHT), which uses glutamate (GLU) as neurotransmitter. A multisynaptic indirect pathway also carries photic information to the SCN. This indirect route arises from the RHT, projects through the intergeniculate leaflet (IGL) of the lateral geniculate nucleus and, finally, the geniculohypothalamic tract (GHT). Neuropeptide Y (NPY) is the neurotransmitter of the GHT. Serotoninergic (5-HT) input to the SCN arrives from the dorsal raphe nuclei. The pathway leading to production of melatonin in the pineal gland is also illustrated in the figure. Melatonin exerts its effect on circadian timing, by directly feeding back onto the SCN.

originates from two major areas: the BF and dorsal brainstem, each activating multiple excitatory signals in the brain that serve as an essential mechanism of vigilance and attention. BF cholinergic neurons project directly to the cortex and are most active during wake and REM sleep.[63] Brainstem projections to the thalamus are mostly cholinergic and comprise the reticulothalamocortical or dorsal tegmental pathway. Isolated cell groups of the ARAS include the cholinergic neurons in the pedunculopontine tegmental (PPT) and laterodorsal tegmental (LDT) nuclei found within the oral pontine–caudal mesencephalic reticular formation. Both PPT and LDT send excitatory signals from the upper brainstem to the lateral hypothalamus, basal forebrain, and the thalamus,[64] including the intralaminar nuclei. The net effect is enhanced excitatory transmission from the thalamus to the cerebral cortex, leading to cortical activation and exerting a tonic facilitatory influence associated with fast cortical activity.[63] During wakefulness, PPT-LDT neurons fire

rapidly, and at the onset of NREM sleep, the rate drops and more so with SWS. During REM sleep, their activity accelerates.[62] Anticholinergic agents decrease vigilance and reduce cortical activation, whereas cholinergic agonists enhance or prolong vigilance and cortical fast activity.

Pontomesencephalic catecholamine (noradrenergic, dopaminergic) neurons project in large numbers up to the forebrain and cerebral cortex and are considered a major component of the ventral tegmental pathway that forms the extrathalamic relay contributing to the regulation of wakefulness.[65] The noradrenaline-producing neurons of the locus ceruleus (LC) of the rostral pontine reticular formation gives robust direct projections to the cerebral cortex and to subcortical structures such as the thalamus and hypothalamus.[66] Similar to the cholinergic PPT-LDT neurons, the noradrenergic neurons also have a state-specific firing rate, with the exception of REM-stage sleep. During REM-stage sleep, the LC firing rate is significantly reduced. Dopamine has long been understood to play a significant role in promoting wakefulness. The ability of stimulants such as amphetamines to promote the state of arousal is mediated by their action on dopaminergic transmission. The ventral tegmental area of the midbrain, with its known dopaminergic projections directly to limbic cortex, prefrontal cortex, and the striatum, is thought to be involved in regulation of wakefulness. Recently recognized is the existence of sleep-state–dependent dopaminergic neurons in the nearby ventral periaqueductal gray.[67]

The monoamine histamine produced by the tuberomammillary nucleus (TMN) of the posterior hypothalamus also plays an important role in the regulation of wakefulness projecting broadly, including the cerebral cortex, striatum, hippocampus, anterior hypothalamus, and the brainstem cholinergic nuclei.[68] *In vivo* recordings from the caudal hypothalamus in freely moving cats have demonstrated the presence of neurons that regularly discharge during wakefulness.[69] These histaminergic neurons, via projection to the anterior hypothalamus, promote wakefulness by their inhibitory effect on the sleep-promoting preoptic region.[70] But similar to norepinephrine, histamine generally moderates excitatory input to thalamic and cortical neurons that are associated with wake and fast cortical activity. Histamine decreases activity during NREM sleep and more so during REM sleep. Antihistaminergic (H1- and H2-receptor antagonists) drugs are well recognized to promote sedation, whereas histamine injected in the cerebral ventricles has an arousing effect in animals.[71] H3-receptor agonists, however, produce sleep, likely through mechanisms of autoinhibition.[72]

The indoleamine serotonin or 5-hydroxytryptamine (5-HT), produced by the dorsal and median raphe nuclei in the midline region of the brainstem reticular formation, provide diffuse innervations to the brain and spinal cord. Serotonin effects on sleep and wake behavior are controversial, with conflicting reports that serotonin promotes sleep and induces wakefulness. In a study, agonists of 5-HT1 type receptors increased wakefulness and the latencies of slow wave and REM sleep, also reducing or abolishing both SWS and REM sleep.[73] In another study, serotonin produced a dose-dependent decrease in high-frequency EEG activity, with no significant change in amounts of wake or slow wave sleep.[74] 5-HT3 receptors are found to promote GABAergic activity,[75] and 5-HT1A postsynaptic inhibitory receptors inhibit cholinergic forebrain neurons.[76] It may be that serotonin acts through concerted activation of multiple different receptors on different cell types influencing sleep-wake cycles.

Glutamate is a major excitatory neurotransmitter found in nearly all areas of the central nervous system. Concentrated in the brainstem reticular formation, it likely serves as the primary neurotransmitter of the ARAS. Cortical activation or evoked stimulation of the midbrain structures releases large amounts of glutamate.[77]

The neuropeptide hypocretin (also called *orexin*) secreted from neurons of the perifornical region of the lateral and posterior hypothalamus plays a significant role in regulating arousal and wakefulness.[78] Widespread projections of hypocretin have been traced to the cerebral cortex, basal forebrain, tuberomammillary nucleus, and brainstem arousal systems.[79,80] The brain region receiving the densest innervation from hypocretin/orexinergic neurons is the locus coeruleus.[81] Two types of excitatory hypocretin peptides are secreted (hypocretin 1 and hypocretin 2), which interact with two receptors (HCRTR1 and HCRTR2). In the model of canine narcolepsy, a mutation of the HCRTR2 gene is responsible for the symptoms of daytime sleepiness, cataplexy, and rapid transitions from wakefulness into REM sleep in these animals.[82,83] Orexin knockout mice have demonstrated behavioral characteristics similar to narcolepsy in humans.[80] In summary, the tonic and coordinated activity of brainstem-activating neurons, intralaminar thalamic nuclei, the posterior hypothalamus, and the basal forebrain is essential for the maintenance of wakefulness and cortical activation (Figure 2-3).

FUNCTIONAL NEUROANATOMICAL BASIS OF SLEEP

Current understanding of the anatomical and physiological basis of sleep indicates that the anterior hypothalamus plays a central role. In the 1930s, von Economo described patients with "encephalitis lethargica" with prominent findings within the anterior hypothalamus who had prominent signs of insomnia, and more recent cases have been reported.[85]

Inhibitory GABAergic mechanisms are pivotal in sleep. GABA is an amino acid, the major inhibitory neurotransmitter in the brain; many sedatives and hypnotics act by binding to GABA receptors. Widespread GABAergic transmission in the brain makes it difficult to isolate individual sleep circuits, but the importance of GABAergic input to thalamocortical circuits has been emphasized.[43,86] Thalamic reticular inhibitory cells release GABA, and their interconnected networks are responsible for the generation of spindle oscillations during sleep.[87] GABAergic neurons inhibit excitatory ARAS neurons. In addition, GABAergic

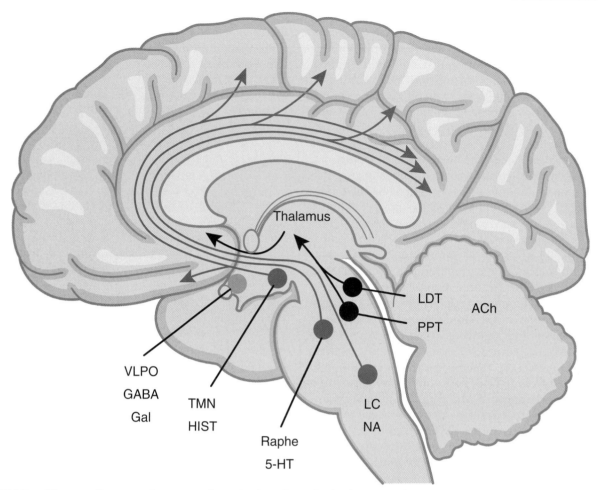

FIGURE 2-3 ■ The *ascending arousal system* sends projections from the brainstem and posterior hypothalamus throughout the forebrain. Neurons of the laterodorsal tegmental nuclei and pedunculopontine tegmental nuclei (LDT and PPT) send cholinergic fibers (Ach) to many forebrain targets, including the thalamus, which then regulate cortical activity. Aminergic nuclei diffusely project throughout much of the forebrain, directly regulating the activity of cortical and hypothalamic targets. Neurons of the tuberomammillary nucleus (TMN) contain histamine (HIST), neurons of the raphe nuclei contain 5-HT, and neurons of the locus coeruleus (LC) contain noradrenaline (NA). Sleep-promoting neurons of the ventrolateral preoptic nucleus (VLPO) contain GABA and galanin (Gal). (From Saper CB, Chou TC, Scammell TE: The sleep switch: hypothalamic control of sleep and wakefulness. Trends Neurosci 24:726–731, 2001; with permission.)

neurons project to sleep-promoting regions of the basal forebrain and hypothalamus,[88,89] thereby depressing cortical fast activity.

A more recently described cluster of GABAergic neurons also containing the inhibitory neuropeptide galanin is the VLPO, located anterior to the hypothalamus. The initiation of NREM sleep is largely influenced by the VLPO, but it also moderates REM sleep. The VLPO contains two main sections, a dense cell cluster that projects to the tuberomammillary nucleus, and extended nuclei that project to the LC and dorsal and median raphe nuclei. In animal studies, lesions of the dense VLPO cluster mainly reduced NREM sleep, seemingly in proportion to the size of the lesion, and lesions of the extended VLPO reduced REM sleep by

half.[90] Recordings of VLPO neurons across wake-sleep states demonstrated a firing rate about twice as fast during sleep as during wakefulness.[91] Input to the VLPO includes circadian influence of the SCN and homeostatic information from endogenous signals such as adenosine and was found to be largely inhibited by noradrenergic and serotoninergic afferents of the brainstem.[92] The tuberomammillary nucleus also projects an inhibitory transmission to the VLPO.[93] The output of the VLPO is broad and thought to initiate sleep onset through reciprocal inhibition of cholinergic, serotoninergic, and noradrenergic arousal systems in the brainstem, as well as histaminergic arousal systems of the posterior hypothalamus and cholinergic systems of the basal forebrain (Figure 2-4).

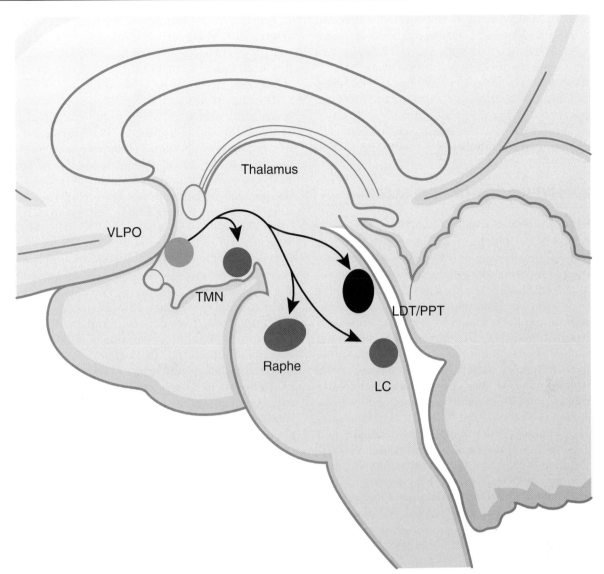

FIGURE 2-4 ■ The projections from the ventrolateral preoptic nucleus (VLPO) to the main components of the ascending arousal system. Axons from the VLPO directly innervate the cell bodies and proximal dendrites of neurons in the major monoamine arousal groups. Within the major cholinergic groups, axons from the VLPO mainly innervate interneurons, rather than the principal cholinergic cells. Abbreviations: LC, locus coeruleus; LDT, laterodorsal tegmental nuclei; PPT, pedunculopontine tegmental nuclei; TMN, tuberomammillary nucleus; VLPO, ventrolateral preoptic nucleus. (From Saper CB, Chou TC, Scammell TE: The sleep switch: hypothalamic control of sleep and wakefulness. Trends Neurosci 24:726–731, 2001; with permission.)

NEUROPHYSIOLOGY OF NREM SLEEP

During sleep onset, responsiveness to external stimuli gradually decreases. This is associated with altered neurotransmission at the level of the thalamus. Long-lasting hyperpolarization resulting from inhibitory postsynaptic potentials (IPSP) can be seen in thalamo-cortical neurons as sleep spindles appear,[94] especially as brainstem nuclei, particularly the cholinergic neurons, diminish their firing rates. Representing the intrinsic activity of reticular nucleus of the thalamus (RNT), sleep spindles present on EEG, occurring more often in stage 2 of sleep, and have a frequency range of 12–14 Hz with progressively increasing and then decreasing amplitude lasting 0.5 to 2 seconds.[95] The rhythmic, inhibitory oscillatory activity generated by the RNT reaches thalamocortical projection neurons, inhibiting their excitatory impulses. The second hallmark of stage 2 sleep is the appearance of K-complexes, which are characterized by a sharp negative wave followed by a slower positive wave with a minimum duration of 0.5 seconds. K-complexes may represent the depolarization of cortical slow wave oscillations.[96] Delta activity (1–4 Hz) is believed to be generated in thalamocortical cells and the cerebral cortex, whereas slow (< 1 Hz) oscillations originate from neocortical neurons with shared synchronous reciprocal input modulating thalamocortical output.[97] As thalamic nuclei become more hyperpolarized, sleep spindles diminish and slower delta waves increase. The appearance of the very-low-frequency slow waves signifies the remarkable depression cholinergic activity originating in the brainstem.[98]

NEUROPHYSIOLOGY OF REM SLEEP

Sleep neurophysiologists refer to REM sleep as *active sleep* because of the high levels of brain activity, such as increased cerebral cortical activity, cerebral blood flow, oxygen consumption, and glucose utilization, as compared with NREM sleep. During REM sleep, autonomic variations occur in respiration, cardiac conduction, and temperature. Early studies by Aserinsky and Kleitman demonstrated EEG findings in REM sleep that were characterized by the appearance of low-amplitude and mixed-frequency activity.[99] The key brain structure for generating REM sleep is the brainstem; early transection studies suggest that the mesencephalopontine junction is a crucial area.[100] REM sleep is accompanied by atonia of the somatic musculature and intermittently emerging rapid eye movements. Typically, the periods of lack of muscle tone and eye movements ("tonic REM") alternate with episodes of fine, intermittent muscle twitches and rapid eye movements ("phasic REM"). Each of these clinical manifestations of REM sleep is under the control of discrete cell groups within the pontine and midbrain reticular formations, often referred to as "REM-on" cells: nucleus reticularis pontis oralis (RPO) and nucleus subcoeruleus (SubC) in addition to the PPT-LDT.[101] Acetylcholine stimulation at this level results in REM sleep,[102] and conversely, neurotoxic lesions result in the disruption of REM sleep.[103,104] These cell groups are generally silent during NREM sleep and begin to depolarize 30 seconds or more before the first sign of REM sleep occurs on EEG.[105,106] The RPO is important for the maintenance of overall arousal state and also for REM. The SubC also is involved in wakefulness but seemingly performs a more significant role in generating REM sleep based on recent lesion studies.[107] Activation of the extended VLPO is most closely associated with REM sleep, and lesions of the extended VLPO cause animals to lose much of their REM sleep, whereas lesions of the VLPO cluster mainly reduce NREM sleep.[106]

SubC excitatory neurons also project to and synapse on cell bodies of the magnocellular nucleus of the medullary reticular formation located in the ventrolateral medulla. Efferents of the lateral portion of this reticular formation form the reticulospinal tract, which synapses on GABAergic and glycinergic neurons to produce hyperpolarization leading to inhibition of alpha motor neurons in the spinal cord and the muscle atonia on REM sleep.[108]

Ponto-geniculo-occipital (PGO) waves are another main feature of REM sleep found in animal studies described in the literature.[109] PGO waves are bursts of large electrical potentials that have been more easily recorded in the lateral geniculate nucleus, originating in the pons, and found with a delayed response in the occipital lobe. They appear a few seconds before REM sleep onset and during phasic activity, usually correlated with rapid eye movements.[110] Triggering neurons for the generation of PGO waves in rats have been localized in the SubC.[111] Important output structures of those PGO-generating cells include not only the occipital cortex but also the entorhinal cortex, piriform cortex, amygdala, hippocampus, and many other thalamic, hypothalamic, and brainstem nuclei that participate in the generation of REM sleep, hypothetically implicating PGO-generating cells in the modulation of cognitive functions.[111] Several groups of neurons in the midbrain reticular formation, including output of the PPT-LDT, are important in mediating REM sleep.

SLEEP DISORDERS AND NEUROSCIENCE

Understanding of the neural basis of sleep disorders continues to evolve. Many sleep disorders involve abnormalities in the regulation of the sleep-wake cycle; others are less clear but are understood to involve complex neurophysiological pathways. Key findings regarding the neuroscience of narcolepsy, circadian disorders, REM behavior disorder, restless legs syndrome, and periodic limb movement disorder are reviewed.

Narcolepsy

Narcolepsy is characterized by symptoms of excessive daytime sleepiness, cataplexy, sleep paralysis, and hypnagogic or hypnopompic hallucinations. Narcolepsy usually develops in the second or third decade of life, although less often it can manifest during early childhood or later in adult life. Narcolepsy is highly associated with HLA genotypes, especially HLA DQB1*0602, but clear autoimmunity is not evident.[83] A breakthrough in understanding the basis of narcolepsy came from the discovery of the hypocretin/orexin neurotransmitter system in the perifornical area of the hypothalamus. Mutation of a hypocretin receptor, HCRTt2, was found in dogs with narcolepsy,[82] and a narcolepsy-like condition was described in hypocretin knockout mice.[80] In addition, the loss of hypocretin neurons in the hypothalamus was reported in brains of deceased narcoleptic patients.[112,113] Hypocretin deficiency in the cerebrospinal fluid was subsequently found in 90% of patients with sporadic narcolepsy with cataplexy, and less commonly in familial narcolepsy.[83] Neuronal loss in the hypothalamus of some narcoleptic patients has been demonstrated by proton magnetic resonance imaging (MRI) spectroscopy.[114] Hypocretin neurons provide excitatory input to the cholinergic, histaminergic, and monoaminergic wake-promoting areas of the brain. Therefore decreased levels of hypocretin or abnormalities of its receptor could lead to a decreased level of alertness.

Beyond daytime sleepiness, a second feature of narcolepsy is the phenomenon of cataplexy, in which there is a sudden loss of muscle tone while awake, provoked by excitement, surprise, or an emotional reaction such as laughing or crying. Typically, the muscles of the jaw, neck, and extremities become suddenly weak in the episode, which can last from a few seconds to minutes with preserved consciousness. Another feature of narcolepsy is sleep paralysis, which occurs during transition from wakefulness to sleep. It is usually a brief episode, between a few seconds to minutes, with the sensation of either partial or entire body paralysis. During wakefulness, brainstem serotoninergic and noradrenergic input inhibits neurons of REM-related activity of the rostral pons and caudal mesencephalon.[115–118] Because monoaminergic neurons normally receive vast excitatory input from the hypocretin/orexin area, decreased hypocretin/orexin input to monoaminergic neurons could facilitate the manifestation of these REM sleep-associated features into wake.

Circadian Rhythm Sleep Disorders

Circadian rhythm sleep disorders (CRSDs) should be considered in the differential diagnosis of patients who present with symptoms of insomnia or hypersomnia. The general criteria for CRSDs include a persistent or recurrent pattern of a sleep disturbance that is thought to be primarily due to either the circadian timing system or a misalignment between endogenous circadian rhythms and external factors that affect the timing of sleep. Also, the sleep disturbance leads to insomnia or hypersomnia and is associated with impairment of function. The International Classification of Sleep Disorders recognizes nine types of CRSDs.[119] The more common types of CRSDs include delayed sleep phase type (DSPT), characterized by delay sleep onset and late morning awakening, and advanced sleep phase type (ASPT), characterized by early morning awakening and early sleep onset. The precise pathophysiology is unknown for these disorders but is likely multifactorial; however, a molecular basis is evident in some familial cases. For example, some specific forms of familial DSPT and polymorphisms in circadian genes such as per3, arylalkylamine N-acetyltransferase, HLA, and CLOCK have been reported in "evening types" and DSPT.[120] Familial studies of ASPT indicate an autosomal dominant mode of inheritance.[121] The most direct evidence for a genetic basis comes from serine to glycine mutation in the human period2 gene on chromosome 2q (per2 gene) in a family with ASPT.[122,123]

REM Sleep Behavior Disorder

REM sleep behavior disorder (RBD) is a parasomnia that occurs in REM sleep. It is seen more often in older individuals and more frequently in males. Rather than the normally expected atonia during REM sleep, muscle tone is increased in patients with RBD, and patients experience dream enactment (hitting, kicking, suddenly leaping out of bed, talking, or yelling) often recalling vivid dream content.[124] Typical findings on PSG include high REM density, intermittent increases in muscle tone during REM, and frequent periodic limb movements in NREM sleep that continues into REM sleep. The pathogenesis of RBD involves the interference with multisynaptic pathways that produce muscle atonia during normal REM sleep.[125]

Acute RBD may be seen in drug withdrawal and medications such as tricyclic antidepressants, monoamine oxidase inhibitors, serotonin-specific reuptake inhibitors, selegiline, and acetylcholinesterases.[126] RBD has been associated with stroke, multiple sclerosis, brain tumors, and other sleep disorders such as narcolepsy. Chronic RBD may be seen in patients as idiopathic or associated with certain neurodegenerative disorders, such as Parkinson's disease,[127] multiple system atrophy,[128,129] dementia with Lewy body disease,[130,131] and progressive supranuclear palsy.[132] Degenerative changes of the dorsal pons or a lesion of the fibers that project to the mesopontine centers may be involved in the development of RBD in these degenerative disorders.

Restless Legs Syndrome and Periodic Leg Movement Disorder

Restless legs syndrome (RLS) is a clinical diagnosis that can disturb sleep onset and sleep maintenance. Approximately 80% of patients with RLS also have periodic leg movements of sleep. Periodic leg movement disorder (PLMD) can be diagnosed by PSG and is also associated with disrupted sleep maintenance and daytime sleepiness. Only about 30% of patients who meet the diagnostic criteria for PLMD have symptoms of RLS.[133]

The clinical picture of RLS typically includes uncomfortable sensations in the extremities associated with a strong urge to move. Movement of the limb usually provides temporary relief of the discomfort. PLMD occurs during sleep and characteristically involves periodic dorsiflexion of the great toe, the foot, and sometimes flexion of the knee. Although the mechanisms that underlie idiopathic RLS or PLMD are not fully understood, there is substantial evidence that dopaminergic dysfunction is likely involved.[134] Neuroimaging studies using positron emission tomography also suggest dopaminergic hypofunction. Decreased dopamine D_2 receptor binding and 6-[^{18}F]fluoro-l-dopa (FDOPA) uptake was shown in the putamen and caudate nuclei in patients with RLS.[135,136] Symptoms of RLS and PLMD are responsive to treatment with dopaminergic agents. With high-resolution functional MRI, symptoms of sensory leg discomfort were associated with bilateral cerebellar and contralateral thalamic activation in patients with RLS.[137] In this study, patients with RLS who also had PLMD had additional activation in the red nucleus and areas close to the reticular structures of the brainstem. These findings imply that activation in the cerebellum and thalamus is associated with sensory discomfort in the extremities and that the red nucleus and certain areas of the brainstem are responsible for generation of periodic limb movements in patients with RLS.

RLS can be idiopathic or familial. One study showed 63% of 133 patients with RLS reported the presence of similar symptoms in at least one first-degree relative.[138] Compared with patients without a family history, individuals with familial RLS have a younger age of onset.[139] In one large French-Canadian family with RLS, a major susceptibility locus was identified on chromosome 12q.[140] Secondary RLS or PLMD has been seen in association with iron deficiency, folate deficiency, chronic renal failure, peripheral vascular disease, myelopathy, peripheral neuropathy, and rheumatoid arthritis. During pregnancy, the prevalence of RLS may be as high as 23%. In these affected women, RLS was associated with low serum folate and/or ferritin levels.[141] The association of RLS with iron deficiency is intriguing. It is known that iron is necessary for tyrosine hydroxylation, which is the rate-limiting step in the biosynthesis of dopamine. Furthermore, decreased iron content was shown with MRI techniques in the nigrostriatal areas in RLS patients. The degree of nigrostriatal iron depletion was correlated with the severity of the disease.[142] RLS can present itself or may worsen in susceptible individuals if serum ferritin level is <50 µg/liter.[143] Reduced ferritin level has also been reported in the cerebrospinal fluid of RLS patients.[144]

REFERENCES

1. Rechtschaffen A, Kales A: *A Manual of Standardized Terminology, Techniques, and Scoring System for Sleep Stages of Human Subjects.* US Department of Health, Education, and Welfare Public Health Service, NIH/NIND, 1968.
2. Borbely AA: Sleep: circadian rhythm vs. recovery process. In KMLDaA J (ed): *Functional States of the Brain: Their Determinants.* Amsterdam, Elsevier/North-Holland, 1980, pp 151–161.
3. Achermann P, Borbely AA: Mathematical models of sleep regulation. Front Biosci 8:s683–s693, 2003.
4. Schibler U, Naef F: Cellular oscillators: rhythmic gene expression and metabolism. Curr Opin Cell Biol 17(2):223–229, 2005.
5. Daan S, Beersma DGM, Borbély AA: Timing of human sleep: recovery process gated by a circadian pacemaker. Am J Physiol 246:R161–R178, 1984.
6. Dijk DJ, Beersma DG, van den Hoofdakker RH: All night spectral analysis of EEG sleep in young adult and middle-aged male subjects. Neurobiol Aging 10:677–682, 1989.
7. Jenni OG, Achermann P, Carskadon MA: Homeostatic sleep regulation in adolescents. Sleep 28(11):1446–1454, 2005.
8. Puente-Munoz AI, Perez-Martinez DA, Villalibre-Valderrey I: The role of slow wave sleep in the homeostatic regulation of sleep. Rev Neurol 34(3):211–215, 2002.
9. Knoblauch V, Kräuchi K, Renz C, et al: Homeostatic control of slow-wave and spindle frequency activity during human sleep: effect of differential sleep pressure and brain topography. Cerebral Cortex 12(10):1092–1100, 2002.
10. Dijk DJ, Czeisler CA: Paradoxical timing of the circadian rhythm of sleep propensity serves to consolidate sleep and wakefulness in humans. Neurosci Lett 166:63–68, 1994.
11. Porkka-Heiskanen T, Strecker RE, Thakkar M, et al: Adenosine: a mediator of the sleep-inducing effects of prolonged wakefulness. Science 276:1265–1268, 1997.
12. Basheer R, Porkka-Heiskanen T, Strecker RE, et al: Adenosine as a biological signal mediating sleepiness following prolonged wakefulness. Biol Signals Recept 9(6):319–327, 2000.
13. Rainnie DG, Grunze HC, McCarley RW, Greene RW: Adenosine inhibition of mesopontine cholinergic neurons: implications for EEG arousal. Science 263:689–692, 1994.
14. Chamberlin NL, Arrigoni E, Chou TC, et al: Effects of adenosine on GABAergic synaptic inputs to identified ventrolateral preoptic neurons. Neuroscience 119:913–918, 2003.
15. Scammell TE, Gerashchenko DY, Mochizuki T, et al: An adenosine A2a agonist increases sleep and induces

Fos in ventrolateral preoptic neurons. Neuroscience 107(4):653–663, 2001.

16. Landolt H, Rétey J, Tönz K, et al: Caffeine attenuates waking and sleep electroencephalographic markers of sleep homeostasis in humans. Neuropsychopharmacology 29:1933–1939, 2004.

17. Rétey J, Adam M, Honegger E, et al: A functional genetic variation of adenosine deaminase affects the duration and intensity of deep sleep in humans. PNAS 102(43):15676–15681, 2005.

18. Franken P, Chollet D, Tafti M: The homeostatic regulation of sleep need is under genetic control. J Neurosci 21(8):2610–2621, 2001.

19. Moore RY: A clock for the ages. Science 284:2102–2103, 1999.

20. Czeisler CA, Duffy JF, Shanahan TL, et al: Stability, precision, and near-24-hour period of the human circadian pacemaker. Science 284:2177–2181, 1999.

21. Edgar D: Circadian control of sleep/wakefulness: implications in shiftwork and therapeutic strategies. In Shiraki K (ed): *Physiological Basis of Occupational Health: Stressful Environments.* Amsterdam, Academic Publishing, 1996, pp 253–265.

22. Edgar D: Functional role of the suprachiasmatic nuclei in the regulation of sleep and wakefulness. In Guilleminault C, Montagna P, Gambetti P (eds): *Fatal Familial Insomnia: Inherited Prion Diseases, Sleep and the Thalamus.* New York, Raven Press, 1994, pp 203–213.

23. Meijer JH, Rietveld WJ: Neurophysiology of the suprachiasmatic circadian pacemaker in rodents. Physiol Rev 69:671–707, 1989.

24. Mistberger RaR B: Mechanisms and models of the circadian timekeeping system. In Herzog ED, Takahashi JS, Block GD (eds): Clock controls circadian period in isolated suprachiasmatic nucleus neurons. Nat Neurosci 1:708–713, 1989.

25. Dunlap JC: Molecular bases for circadian clocks. Cell 96:271–290, 1999.

26. Liu C, Weaver DR, Strogatz SH, Reppert SM: Cellular construction of a circadian clock: period determination in the suprachiasmatic nuclei. Cell 91:855–860, 1997.

27. Herzog ED, Takahashi JS, Block GD: Clock controls circadian period in isolated suprachiasmatic nucleus neurons. Nat Neurosci 1:708–713, 1998.

28. Field MD, Maywood ES, O'Brien JA, et al: Analysis of clock proteins in mouse SCN demonstrates phylogenetic divergence of the circadian clockwork and resetting mechanisms. Neuron 25(2):437–447, 2000.

29. Miyazaki K, Nagase T, Mesaki M, et al: Phosphorylation of clock protein PER1 regulates its circadian degradation in normal human fibroblasts. Biochem J 380:95–103, 2004.

30. Constance CM, Fan JY, Preuss F, et al: The circadian clock-containing photoreceptor cells in *Xenopus laevis* express several isoforms of casein kinase I. Mol Brain Res 20(136[1–2]):199–211, 2005.

31. Kavanau JL, Peters CR: Activity of nocturnal primates: influences of twilight *zeitgebers* and weather. Science 191(4222):83–86, 1976.

32. Richardson G, Tate B: Hormonal and pharmacological manipulation of the circadian clock: recent developments and future strategies. Sleep Suppl 3:S77–S85, 2000.

33. Card JP, Moore RY: Organization of lateral geniculate-hypothalamic connections in the rat. J Comp Neurol 284:135–147, 1989.

34. Harrington ME: The ventral lateral geniculate nucleus and the intergeniculate leaflet: interrelated structures in the visual and circadian systems. Neurosci Biobehav Rev 21:705–727, 1997.

35. Beaule C, Robinson B, Lamont EW, Amir S: Melanopsin in the circadian timing system. J Mol Neurosci. 21(1): 73–89, 2003.

36. Lockley SW, Brainard GC, Czeisler CA: High sensitivity of the human circadian melatonin rhythm to resetting by short wavelength light. Neurosci Lett 342:37–40, 2003.

37. Bellingham J, Foster RG: Opsins and mammalian photoentrainment. Cell Tissue Res 309(1):57–71, 2002.

38. Moore RY: Retinohypothalamic projection in mammals: a comparative study. Brain Res 49:403–409, 1973.

39. Kiss J, Leranth C, Halasz B: Serotoninergic endings on VIP-neurons in the suprachiasmatic nucleus and on ACTH-neurons in the arcuate nucleus of the rat hypothalamus. A combination of high resolution autoradiography and electron microscopic immunocytochemistry. Neurosci Lett 44:119–124, 1984.

40. Medanic M, Gillette MU: Serotonin regulates the phase of the rat suprachiasmatic circadian pacemaker in vitro only during the subjective day. J Physiol 450:629–642, 1992.

41. Dudley TE, Dinardo LA, Glass JD: In vivo assessment of the midbrain raphe nuclear regulation of serotonin release in the hamster suprachiasmatic nucleus. J Neurophysiol 81:1469–1477, 1999.

42. Abrahamson EE, Leak RK, Moore RY: The suprachiasmatic nucleus projects to posterior hypothalamic arousal systems. Neuroreport 12:435–440, 2001.

43. Carpenter M: *Core Text of Neuroanatomy.* Baltimore, Williams & Wilkins, 1999.

44. Isobe Y, Fujioi J, Nishino H: Circadian rhythm of melatonin release in pineal gland culture: arg-vasopressin inhibits melatonin release. *Brain Res* 918(1–2):67–73, 2001.

45. Mistberger RE: Circadian rhythms in mammals, formal properties, and environmental influences. In Kryger M, Roth T, Dement WC (eds): *Principles and Practice of Sleep Medicine,* 4th ed. Philadelphia, Saunders, 2005, pp 321–334.

46. Turek FW, Gillette MU: Melatonin, sleep, and circadian rhythms: rationale for development of specific melatonin agonists. Sleep Med 5(6):523–532, 2004.

47. Czeisler CA, Weitzman E, Moore-Ede MC, et al: Human sleep: its duration and organization depend on its circadian phase. Science 210:1264–1267, 1980.

48. Wever RA: Influence of physical workload on free-running circadian rhythms of man. Pflugers Arch 381:119–126, 1979.

49. Zulley J, Wever R, Aschoff J: The dependence of onset and duration of sleep on the circadian rhythm of rectal temperature. Pflugers Arch 391:314–318, 1981.

50. Chou TC, Bjorkum AA, Gaus SE, et al: Afferents to the ventrolateral preoptic nucleus. J Neurosci 22(3):977–990, 2002.

51. Deurveilher S, Semba K: Indirect projections from the suprachiasmatic nucleus to major arousal-promoting cell groups in rat: implications for the circadian control of behavioural state. Neuroscience 130(1):165–183, 2005.

52. Green DJ, Gillette R: Circadian rhythm of firing rate recorded from single cells in the rat suprachiasmatic brain slice. Brain Res 245:198–200, 1982.

53. Bos NP, Mirmiran M: Circadian rhythms in spontaneous neuronal discharges of the cultured suprachiasmatic nucleus. Brain Res 511:158–162, 1990.

54. van den Top M, Buijs RM, Ruijter JM, et al: Melatonin generates an outward potassium current in rat suprachiasmatic nucleus neurones in vitro independent of their circadian rhythm. Neuroscience 107(1):99–108, 2001.

55. Reppert SM, Weaver DR, Ebisawa T: Cloning and characterization of a mammalian melatonin receptor that mediates reproductive and circadian responses. Neuron 13:1177–1185, 1994.

56. Rajaratnam SM, Middleton B, Stone BM, et al: Melatonin advances the circadian timing of EEG sleep and directly facilitates sleep without altering its duration in extended sleep opportunities in humans. J Physiol 561:339–351, 2004.

57. Aschoff J: Circadian rhythms in man. Science 148:1427–1432, 1965.

58. Edgar DM, Dement WC, Fuller CA: Effect of SCN lesions on sleep in squirrel monkeys: evidence for opponent processes in sleep-wake regulation. J Neurosci 13:1065–1079, 1993.

59. Terzano MG, Parrino L, Smerieri A, et al: CAP and arousals are involved in the homeostatic and ultradian sleep processes. J Sleep Res 4:359–368, 2005.

60. Pace-Schott EF, Hobson JA: The neurobiology of sleep: genetics, cellular physiology and subcortical networks. Nat Rev Neurosci 8:591–605, 2002.

61. Moruzzi G, Magoun HW: Brain stem reticular formation and activation of the EEG. Electroencephalogr Clin Neurol 1:455 (abstract), 1949.

62. España R, Scammell TE: Sleep neurobiology for the clinician. Sleep 27:811–820, 2004.

63. Mesulam M-M: Attentional networks, confusional states, and neglect syndromes. In Mesulam M-M (ed): *Principles of Behavioral and Cognitive Neurology,* 2nd ed. New York, Oxford University Press, 2000, pp 174–238.

64. Hallanger AE, Levey AI, Rye DB, Wainer BH: The origins of cholinergic and other subcortical afferents to the thalamus in the rat. J Comp Neurol 262:105–124, 1987.

65. Jones BE, Cuello AC: Afferents to the basal forebrain cholinergic cell area from pontomesencephalic—catecholamine, serotonin, and acetylcholine—neurons. Neuroscience 31(1):37–61, 1989.

66. Jones BE, Yang TZ: The efferent projections from the reticular formation and the locus coeruleus studied by anterograde and retrograde axonal transport in the rat. J Comp Neurol 242:56–92, 1985.

67. Lu J, Jhou TC, Saper CB: Identification of wake-active dopaminergic neurons in the ventral periaqueductal gray matter. J Neurosci 26(1):193–202, 2006.

68. Lin JS, Hou Y, Sakai K, Jouvet M: Histaminergic descending inputs to the mesopontine tegmentum and their role in the control of cortical activation and wakefulness in the cat. J Neurosci 16:1523–1537, 1996.

69. Vanni-Mercier G, Sakai K, Jouvet M: Specific neurons for wakefulness in the posterior hypothalamus in the cat. C R Acad Sci III 298:195–200, 1984.

70. Lin JS, Sakai K, Jouvet M: Hypothalamo-preoptic histaminergic projections in sleep-wake control in the cat. Eur J Neurosci 6:618–625, 1994.

71. Monnier M, Sauer R, Hatt AM: The activating effect of histamine on the central nervous system. Int Rev Neurobiol 12:265–305, 1970.

72. Monti JM, Jantos H, Ponzoni A, Monti D: Sleep and waking during acute histamine H3 agonist BP 2.94 or H3 antagonist carboperamide (MR 16155) administration in rats. Neuropsychopharmacology 15(1):31–35, 1996.

73. Dzoljic MR, Ukponmwan OE, Saxena PR: 5-HT1-like receptor agonists enhance wakefulness. Neuropharmacology 31:623–633, 1992.

74. Cape EG, Jones BE: Differential modulation of high-frequency gamma-electroencephalogram activity and sleep-wake state by noradrenaline and serotonin microinjections into the region of cholinergic basalis neurons. J Neurosci 18(7):2653–2666, 1998.

75. Morales M, Bloom FE: The 5-HT3 receptor is present in different subpopulations of GABAergic neurons in the rat telencephalon. J Neurosci 17(9):3157–3167, 1997.

76. Khateb A, Fort P, Alonso A, et al: Pharmacological and immunohistochemical evidence for serotonergic modulation of cholinergic nucleus basalis neurons. Eur J Neurosci 5(5):541–547, 1993.

77. Jones BE: Basic mechanisms of sleep-wake states. In Kryger MH, Roth T, Dement WC (eds): *Principles and Practice of Sleep Medicine,* 4th ed. Philadelphia, Saunders, 2005, pp 136–153.

78. Sakurai T, Amemiya A, Ishii M: Orexins and orexin receptors: a family of hypothalamic neuropeptides and G protein-coupled receptors that regulate feeding behaviour. Cell 92:573–585, 1998.

79. Peyron C, Tighe DK, van den Pol AN, et al: Neurons containing hypocretin (orexin) project to multiple neuronal systems. J Neurosci 18:9996–10015, 1998.

80. Chemelli RM, Willie JT, Sinton CM, et al: Narcolepsy in orexin knockout mice: molecular genetics of sleep regulation. Cell 98:437–451, 1999.

81. Hagan JJ, Leslie RA, Patel S, et al: Orexin A activates locus coeruleus cell firing and increases arousal in the rat. Proc Natl Acad Sci 14; 96(19):10911–10916, 1999.

82. Lin L, Faraco J, Li R, et al: The sleep disorder canine narcolepsy is caused by a mutation in the hypocretin (orexin) receptor 2 gene. Cell 98:365–376, 1999.

83. Baumann CR: Hypocretins (orexins) and sleep-wake disorders. Lancet Neurol 4(10):673–682, 2005.

84. Abrahamson EE, Leak RK, Moore RY: The suprachiasmatic nucleus projects to posterior hypothalamic arousal systems. Neuroreport 12:435–440, 2001.

85. Dale RC, Church AJ, Surtees RA, et al: Encephalitis lethargica syndrome: 20 new cases and evidence of basal ganglia autoimmunity. Brain 127:21–33, 2004.

86. Molnar GF, Sailer A, Gunraj CA, et al: Changes in motor cortex excitability with stimulation of anterior thalamus in epilepsy. Neurology 66(4):566–571, 2006.

87. Steriade M: Sleep, epilepsy and thalamic reticular inhibitory neurons. Trends Neurosci 28(6):317–324, 2005.

88. Vincent SR, Hokfelt T, Skirboll LR, Wu JY: Hypothalamic gamma-aminobutyric acid neurons project to the neocortex. Science 220:1309–1311, 1983.

89. Gritti I, Mainville L, Mancia M, Jones BE: GABAergic and other noncholinergic basal forebrain neurons, together with cholinergic neurons, project to the mesocortex and isocortex in the rat. J Comp Neurol 383:163–177, 1997.

90. Lu J, Bjorkum AA, Xu M, et al: Selective activation of the extended ventrolateral preoptic nucleus during rapid eye movement sleep. J Neurosci 22(11):4568–4576, 2002.

91. Szymusiak R, Alam N, Steininger TL, McGinty D: Sleep-waking discharge patterns of ventrolateral preoptic/anterior hypothalamic neurons in rats. Brain Res 803:178–188, 1998.

92. Chou TC, Bjorkum AA, Gaus SE, et al: Afferents to the ventrolateral preoptic nucleus. J Neurosci 22:977–990, 2002.

93. Ericson H, Kohler C, Blomqvist A: GABA-like immunoreactivity in the tuberomammillary nucleus: an electron microscopic study in the rat. J Comp Neurol 305:462–469, 1991.

94. Steriade M: Basic mechanisms of sleep generation. Neurology 42:9–17, 1992.

95. Steriade M, Deschenes M, Domich L, Mulle C: Abolition of spindle oscillations in thalamic neurons disconnected from nucleus reticularis thalami. J Neurophysiol 54:1473–1497, 1985.

96. Amzica F, Steriade M: The K-complex: its slow (<1-Hz) rhythmicity and relation to delta waves. Neurology 49(4):952–959, 1997.

97. Steriade M, Nunez A, Amzica F: A novel slow (<1 Hz) oscillation of neocortical neurons in vivo: depolarizing and hyperpolarizing components. J Neurosci 13:3252–65, 1993.

98. Siegel JM: Brain electrical activity and sensory processing during waking and sleep states. In Kryger MH, Roth T, Dement WC (eds): *Principles and Practice of Sleep Medicine*, 4th ed. Philadelphia, Saunders, 2005, pp 101–119.

99. Aserinsky E, Kleitman N: Regularly occurring periods of eye motility and concomitant phenomena during sleep. Science 118:273–274, 1953.

100. Jouvet M, Delorme F: Locus coeruleus et sommeil paradoxal. C R Soc Biol 159:895 (abstract), 1965.

101. Boissard R, Gervasoni D, Schmidt MH: The rat pontomedullary network responsible for paradoxical sleep onset and maintenance: a combined microinjection and functional neuroanatomy study. Eur J Neurosci 16:1959–1973, 2002.

102. Mazzuchelli-O'Flaherty AL, O'Flaherty JJ, Hernandez-Peon R: Sleep and other behavioural responses induced by acetylcholinic stimulation of frontal and mesial cortex. Brain Res 4:268–283, 1967.

103. Jones BE, Webster HH: Neurotoxic lesions of the dorsolateral pontomesencephalic tegmentum-cholinergic cell area in the cat.I. Effects upon the cholinergic innervation of the brain. Brain Res 451:13–32, 1988.

104. Webster HH, Jones BE: Neurotoxic lesions of the dorsolateral pontomesencephalic tegmentum-cholinergic cell area in the cat.II. Effects upon sleep-waking states. Brain Res 458:285–302, 1988.

105. Sinton CM, McCarley RW: Neurophysiological mechanisms of sleep and wakefulness: a question of balance. Semin Neurol 24:211–223, 2004.

106. Swick T: The neurology of sleep. Neurol Clin 23(4):967–989, 2005.

107. Sanford LD, Yang L, Tang X, et al: Tetrodotoxin inactivation of pontine regions: influence on sleep-wake states. Brain Res 1044(1):42–50, 2005.

108. Holmes CJ, Jones BE: Importance of cholinergic, GABAergic, serotonergic and other neurons in the medial medullary reticular formation for sleep-wake states studied by cytotoxic lesions in the cat. Neuroscience 62:1179–1200, 1994.

109. Morrison AR, Bowker RM: The biological significance of PGO spikes in the sleeping cat. Acta Neurobiol Exp 35(5–6):821 (abstract), 1975.

110. Hunt WK, Sanford LD, Ross RJ, et al: Elicited pontogeniculooccipital waves and phasic suppression of diaphragm activity in sleep and wakefulness. J Appl Physiol 84(6):2106–2114, 1998.

111. Datta S, Siwek DF, Patterson EH, Cipolloni PB: Localization of pontine PGO wave generation sites and their anatomical projections in the rat. Synapse 30(4):409–423, 1998.

112. Thannickal TC, Moore RY, Nienhuis R, et al: Reduced number of hypocretin neurons in human narcolepsy. Neuron 27:469–474, 2000.

113. Nishino S, Ripley B, Overeem S, et al: Hypocretin (orexin) deficiency in human narcolepsy. Lancet 355:39–40, 2000.

114. Lodi R, Tonon C, Vignatelli L: In vivo evidence of neuronal loss in the hypothalamus of narcoleptic patients. Neurology 63:1513–1515, 2004.

115. Jones BE: Paradoxical sleep and its chemical/structural substrates in the brain. Neuroscience 40:637–656, 1991.

116. Honda T, Semba K: Serotonergic synaptic input to cholinergic neurons in the rat mesopontine tegmentum. Brain Res 647:299–306, 1994.

117. Williams JA, Reiner PB: Noradrenaline hyperpolarizes identified rat mesopontine cholinergic neurons in vitro. J Neurosci 13:3878–3883, 1993.

118. Luebke JI, Greene RW, Semba K, et al: Serotonin hyperpolarizes cholinergic low-threshold burst neurons in the rat laterodorsal tegmental nucleus in vitro. Proc Natl Acad Sci 89:743–747, 1992.

119. International Classification of Sleep Disorders: *Diagnostic & Coding Manual*. American Academy of Sleep Medicine, 2nd ed, 2005.

120. Iwase T, Kajimura N, Uchiyama M: Mutation screening of the human Clock gene in circadian rhythm sleep disorders. Psychiatry Res 109(2):121–128, 2002.

121. Reid KJ, Chang AM, Dubocovich ML: Familial advanced sleep phase syndrome. Arch Neurol 58(7):1089–1094, 2001.

122. Ando K, Kripke DF, Ancoli-Israel S: Estimated prevalence of delayed and advanced sleep phase syndromes. Sleep Res 24:509, 1995.

123. Toh KL, Jones CR, He Y: An hPer2 phosphorylation site mutation in familial advanced sleep phase syndrome. Science 291:1040–1043, 2001.

124. Schenck CH, Bundlie SR, Patterson AL, Mahowald MW: Rapid eye movement sleep behavior disorder. A treatable parasomnia affecting older adults. JAMA 257:1786–1789, 1987.

125. Olson EJ, Boeve BF, Silber MH: Rapid eye movement sleep behaviour disorder: demographic, clinical and laboratory findings in 93 cases. Brain 123:331–339, 2000.

126. Schenck CH, Mahowald MW: Rapid eye movement sleep parasomnias. Neurol Clin 23(4):1107–1126, 2005.

127. Comella CL, Nardine TM, Diederich NJ, Stebbins GT: Sleep-related violence, injury, and REM sleep behavior disorder in Parkinson's disease. Neurology 51:526–529, 1998.

128. Septien L, Didi-Roy R, Marin A, Giroud M: REM-sleep behavior disorder and olivo-ponto-cerebellar atrophy: a case report. Neurophysiol Clin 22:459–464, 1992.

129. Plazzi G, Corsini R, Provini F, et al: REM sleep behavior disorders in multiple system atrophy. Neurology 48:1094–1097, 1997.

130. Schenck CH, Mahowald MW, Anderson ML, et al: Lewy body variant of Alzheimer's disease (AD) identified by postmortem ubiquitin staining in a previously reported case of AD associated with REM sleep behavior disorder. Biol Psychiatry 42:527–528, 1997.

131. Boeve BF, Silber MH, Ferman TJ, et al: REM sleep behavior disorder and degenerative dementia: an association likely reflecting Lewy body disease. Neurology 51:363–370, 1998.

132. Arnulf I, Andreu M, Bloch F: REM sleep behavior disorder and REM sleep without atonia in patients with progressive supranuclear palsy. Sleep 28(3):349–354, 2005.

133. Phillips B: Movement disorders: a sleep specialist's perspective. Neurology 62(5 Suppl 2):S9–S16, 2004.

134. Comella CL: Restless legs syndrome: treatment with dopaminergic agents. Neurology 58:S87–S92, 2002.

135. Turjanski N, Lees AJ, Brooks DJ: Striatal dopaminergic function in restless legs syndrome: 18F-dopa and 11C-raclopride PET studies. Neurology 52:932–927, 1999.

136. Ruottinen HM, Partinen M, Hublin C, et al: An FDOPA PET study in patients with periodic limb movement disorder and restless legs syndrome. Neurology 54:502–504, 2000.

137. Bucher SF, Seelos KC, Oertel WH, et al: Cerebral generators involved in the pathogenesis of the restless legs syndrome. Ann Neurol 41:639–645, 1997.

138. Montplaisir J, Boucher S, Poirier G, et al: Clinical, polysomnographic, and genetic characteristics of restless legs syndrome: a study of 133 patients diagnosed with new standard criteria. Mov Disord 12:61–65, 1997.

139. Winkelmann J, Wetter TC, Collado-Seidel V, et al: Clinical characteristics and frequency of the hereditary restless legs syndrome in a population of 300 patients. Sleep 23:597–602, 2000.

140. Desautels A, Turecki G, Montplaisir J, et al: Identification of a major susceptibility locus for restless legs syndrome on chromosome 12q. Am J Hum Genet 69:1266–1270, 2001.

141. Lee KA, Zaffke ME, Baratte-Beebe K: Restless legs syndrome and sleep disturbance during pregnancy: the role of folate and iron. J Womens Health Gend Based Med 10:335–341, 2001.

142. Allen RP, Barker PB, Wehrl F, et al: MRI measurement of brain iron in patients with restless legs syndrome. Neurology 56:263–265, 2001.

143. Sun ER, Chen CA, Ho G, et al: Iron and the restless legs syndrome. Sleep 21:371–377, 1998.

144. Earley CJ, Connor JR, Beard JL, et al: Abnormalities in CSF concentrations of ferritin and transferrin in restless legs syndrome. Neurology 54:1698–1700, 2000.

Sleep Physiology

PIERRE GIGLIO ■ JAMES T. LANE ■ TERI J. BARKOUKIS ■ IOANA DUMITRU

Sleep physiology is discussed here in a succinct style for sleep medicine board review for normal cardiovascular physiology, thermoregulation, immunology, endocrine physiology, and pulmonary physiology. Central nervous system regulation of sleep and subsequent neurology mechanisms are presented in Chapter 2.

THERMOREGULATION

There are three important facets of the sleep-temperature interaction that one must consider. The first is the regulation of body temperature during sleep, which is what is strictly meant by sleep thermoregulation. A second aspect is the effect of ambient temperature on sleep architecture. The third aspect is important reciprocal influences between the circadian rhythms affecting sleep and thermoregulation.

As is true in the waking mammal, thermoregulation during sleep is orchestrated by hypothalamic centers, especially the preoptic area. Heat loss mechanisms (sweating, panting in the animal, and skin vasodilation) and heat production or conservation (thermogenesis, vasoconstriction) are under autonomic nervous system control. During non-rapid eye movement sleep (NREM), sleep thermoregulatory mechanisms are operative, although less so than during wakefulness. In rapid eye movement (REM) sleep, they are blunted or absent.[1]

Cerebral metabolism, on the other hand, shows a significant increase during REM sleep in humans when compared with NREM sleep. The most vivid demonstrations of this are probably the positron emission tomography (PET) studies performed on human volunteers.[2] When normal volunteers were studied with PET during the awake, relaxed state, as well as REM and NREM sleep, metabolic rates were higher in REM than in NREM sleep, and metabolic rates in the awake state were intermediate between those of REM and NREM sleep.[2] The differences in metabolic rates were most prominent in the cingulate cortex, frontal cortex, thalamus, and visual association areas.[2]

Ambient temperature can influence the total sleep time and sleep architecture. Both REM and NREM sleep times are decreased in situations of temperature stress.[3] Conversely, exposures to warm environments before sleep increases slow wave sleep.[3] Table 3-1 summarizes the sleep-temperature relationships discussed previously.

There is a circadian variability in body temperature of the order of 1° C with a parallel variation in brain temperature.[4] Higher body temperatures are associated with improved neurobehavioral performance in humans when one controls for circadian phase and number of hours awake.[4] In experimental conditions of desynchrony, with subjects isolated from time cues and free to sleep or wake up ad lib, sleep occurs close to the body temperature nadir, and the subject tends to wake up with a rise in body temperature. This would suggest that thermoregulation may act as a sleep signaling system, with temperature changes affecting somnogenic brain areas to initiate or discontinue sleep.[5]

This functional interaction is mirrored by anatomical proximity of the centers involved in circadian control of sleep and temperature. The subparaventricular zone (SPZ) in the hypothalamus receives input from the suprachiasmatic nucleus, well recognized as the clock for circadian rhythms.[6] The dorsal portion of the SPZ organizes circadian rhythms of body temperature, and the ventral portion is necessary for sleep circadian rhythms.[6,7] Lesion experiments in rats have demonstrated that ventral SPZ lesions cause reduction in the measures of circadian index of sleep, whereas dorsal SPZ lesions cause more reduction of circadian index of body temperature.[7]

IMMUNOLOGY AND SLEEP

Sleep is believed to be essential for normal immune function. In turn, immunity serves the vital roles of host protection against pathogens and cancer cells. Sleep deprivation affects the immune responses to the hepatitis A[8] and influenza vaccines.[9] In both cases substantial decreases in antibody responses were noted in sleep-deprived subjects.

TABLE 3-1 ■ Thermoregulation, Cerebral Metabolism, and Ambient Temperature Changes During Sleep and Awake State

	Awake	NREM	REM	Comments
Thermoregulation	Thermoregulation fully operative with hypothalamic (preoptic) control over autonomic nervous system operating at effectors (sweat glands, blood vessels, etc.)	Thermoregulation operative at a lower level than when awake; same mechanisms as in the awake state	Thermoregulation blunted or absent	
Cerebral metabolism and sleep	Cerebral metabolism is intermediate to that of REM and NREM sleep	Cerebral metabolism is decreased compared with the awake state	Cerebral metabolism is higher in REM than NREM	A PET study suggests a higher metabolic rate in REM sleep than the awake state[2]
Ambient temperature effect on sleep		Temperature stress (high or low) decreases NREM sleep	Temperature stress (high or low) decreases REM sleep	Warm environment before sleep enhances SWS

NREM, non-rapid eye movement; REM, rapid eye movement; PET, positron emission tomography; SWS, slow wave sleep.

Sleep influences cellular (T-cell) immunity, with significant shifts in T-helper 1 (Th1) versus T-helper 2 (Th2) cells noted in healthy human volunteers during different sleep phases.[10] Dimitrov et al looked at shifts in these T-cell populations across the night by empirically splitting total sleep time (TST) equally into early sleep (first half) and late sleep (second half of TST). In early sleep a moderate relative Th1 cell population is noted, and this is replaced by Th2 dominance in late sleep.[10] It is likely that sleep mediates these effects through changes in the human endocrine profile, consisting mainly of increased prolactin and growth hormone concentrations, as well as decreased cortisol levels during early nocturnal sleep.[11]

Sleep and the immune system are also linked through proinflammatory cytokines, intercellular signaling proteins that regulate immune and inflammatory responses. Sleep deprivation increases interleukin-1 (IL-1), tumor necrosis factor-α (TNF-α) and interferon levels.[12] Interleukin 6 (IL-6) elevations are noted during stages 1, 2, and REM sleep.[13] Cytokines play key roles in inflammatory responses and host defense, and IL-6 also has a potent stimulatory effect on the hypothalamic-pituitary axis.[14]

IL-1, interleukin-2 (IL-2), IL-6, interleukin-8 (IL-8), inteleukin-18 (IL-18), and tumor necrosis factor-α (TNF-α) promote NREM sleep while interleukin-4 (IL-4), interleukin-10 (IL-10), interleukin-13 (IL-13), and TGF-β inhibit NREM sleep.[15] At least some cytokines appear to influence sleep by acting directly at cerebral somnogenic areas. There is experimental evidence in animals to suggest that IL-1β plays a role in sleep regulation by modulating activity of neurons in the preoptic area (POA) and basal forebrain (BF).[16] Direct injection of IL-1β in these rat

TABLE 3-2 ■ Cytokines and NREM Sleep

NREM Sleep Promotion	NREM Sleep Inhibition
Interleukin (IL)-1	IL-4
IL-2	IL-10
IL-6	IL-13
IL-8	TGF-β
IL-18	
TNF-α	

TNF, tumor necrosis factor; TGF, tumor growth factor.

brain areas decreases the discharge rate of POA and BF neurons with differential effects on wake-related versus sleep-related neurons. It is hypothesized that the cytokine suppresses wake-related neurons and activates sleep-related ones, thus promoting sleep.[16] Similarly, direct IL-1β administration into the dorsal raphe nucleus (DRN) of rats increases NREM sleep, possibly by inhibition of serotonergic neurons.[17] Table 3-2 summarizes the effects of the different cytokines on NREM sleep.

Cytokines also mediate effects on sleep though nitric oxide (NO) and hormones of the hypothalamic-pituitary axis such as growth hormone-releasing hormone (GHRH) and corticotrophin-releasing hormone (CRH).[15] Cytokines induce nitric oxide synthase resulting in increased NO production: NO and GHRH, a hypothalamic hormone, have NREM sleep-promoting properties; CRH promotes arousal.[15]

From the foregoing discussion, it would be expected that infections and the inflammatory response they evoke have important consequences on sleep patterns. Endotoxin administration to healthy human volunteers increased NREM sleep while increasing levels of TNF-α, IL-6, soluble TNF receptors, and IL-1 receptor antagonist in a dose-dependent fashion.[18]

Sleep and the immune system therefore appear to be closely linked through endocrine and cytokine mechanisms. Sleep may be modulating the humoral and cell-mediated immune responses through such mediators; conversely, immune responses have an effect on sleep stages, as discussed previously.

ENDOCRINE FUNCTION AND SLEEP

Organization of Endocrine Rhythms Affected by Sleep

The interface for control of endocrine function affected by sleep is at the level of the hypothalamus. This is where the center for circadian rhythms in the suprachiasmatic nucleus interface input from sleep-wake centers and where global control of the autonomic nervous system rests.[19, 20] Sleep-wake input has variable effects on endocrine rhythms depending on the amount, quality, and timing of sleep. Some endocrine axes are more strongly affected by sleep-wake patterns than others. Sleep-wake centers and circadian rhythms have input on centers within the hypothalamus that secrete releasing and inhibitory hormones in a pulsatile fashion and affect the release of glycoprotein hormones from the anterior pituitary gland that have intrinsic effects on target tissues or serve as modulators of other endocrine hormone production at distant sites. Figure 3-1 highlights selected 24-hour hormone profiles from normal men. Notice the solid black bar on the x-axis representing time of sleep.

In general, this section refers to adult human physiology, as differences between human and animal sleep and endocrine patterns exist across species. Human sleep occurs in larger blocks of time compared with multiple interrupted courses of sleep in animals. In addition, differences within humans exist between children and adults, as well as between males and females.

FIGURE 3-1 ■ Plasma levels of ACTH, cortisol, TSH, testosterone, growth hormone, and prolactin (mean + SEM) from 8 to 12 normal men studied at 15-minute intervals over 24 hours. Figure compiled from multiple references.[21–24] (Reproduced with permission from Van Cauter E: Diurnal and ultradian rhythms in human endocrine function: a minireview. Horm Res 34:45–53, 1990.)

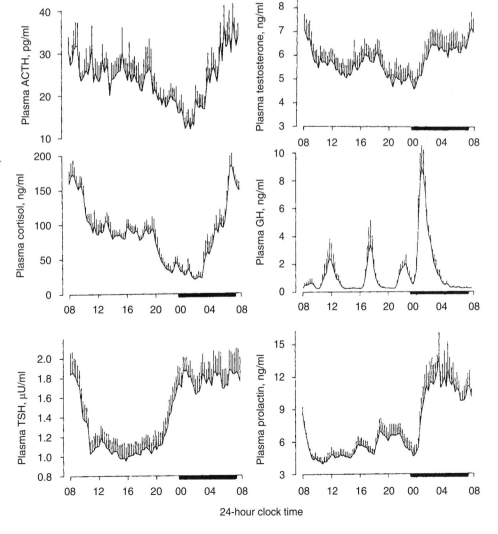

24-hour clock time

The Somatotropic Axis

Growth hormone is positively stimulated by growth hormone–releasing hormone and inhibited by somatostatin. These hypothalamic-releasing factors are not usually measurable in the serum but act locally within the pituitary to provide pulses of growth hormone secretion throughout the day. Growth hormone's biologic effects are mediated through insulin-like growth factor-1 (IGF-1) produced in the liver and growth hormone itself. Growth hormone levels are labile, whereas IGF-1 levels represent an integrated growth hormone effect.

In men, onset of sleep, in concert with the first phase of slow-wave sleep, results in the largest growth hormone pulse of the day.[25] Although other growth hormone pulses may occur, the first pulse is usually the greatest in magnitude. Young premenopausal women demonstrate a slightly different pattern, with larger pulses during the day and a less prominent pulse with onset of slow-wave sleep.[26] During the luteal phase, growth hormone pulses increase during the day and are positively associated with the rise in progesterone seen during this portion of the menstrual cycle. Aging is associated with decreased levels of growth hormone and parallels decreases in slow-wave sleep, decreased responsiveness to GHRH, and increased somatostatin tone.[27] IGF-1 levels also fall with age. Although there appears to be a circadian pattern of growth hormone secretion, the major determinant of growth hormone secretion appears to be the sleep-related increase in GHRH.

Ghrelin has been found to be an endogenous growth hormone secretagogue.[28] It is produced in the stomach, induces appetite, and has positive effects on energy balance. Ghrelin administration has also been shown to increase slow-wave sleep and growth hormone secretion in humans.[29]

Growth hormone secretion is abnormal in a variety of illnesses. In acromegaly, a disease associated with elevated growth hormone and IGF-1 levels, there is loss of the usual pattern of an initial growth hormone spike at sleep onset. In addition, there are unpredictable spikes of growth hormone secretion throughout the day, with generally higher basal levels of secretion compared with normal.[30] Obesity is associated with suppressed growth hormone release.[31] Diabetes is associated with elevated growth hormone secretion during both sleep and daylight hours that can be normalized with improved glycemic control.[32] With depression, the major growth hormone pulse may occur before sleep, rather than after the onset of sleep.[33]

The Lactotropic Axis

Prolactin levels are primarily controlled by tonic inhibition from dopamine arising from the hypothalamus. Dopaminergic drugs may increase prolactin, but the opposite occurs with drugs that have antidopaminergic properties. Prolactin levels rise after sleep onset.[34] Maximum levels occur before rising in the morning. The lowest levels are around noon. The nocturnal rise in prolactin is associated with higher pulse amplitudes and frequency of prolactin during these times compared with daytime. Similar to growth hormone secretion, prolactin secretion is more strongly related to sleep onset, although some circadian input occurs.[35] Prolactin levels are associated with slow-wave sleep, and interrupted sleep results in blunting of the nighttime rise.[36] Similarly, shift workers who superimpose usual sleep and wake times have a rise in prolactin after sleep, but the amplitude of the rise is blunted. Prolactin levels are also higher in premenopausal women, compared with postmenopausal women, and are related to estrogen levels.[37] With aging, there is a dampening of the nocturnal prolactin rise. During pregnancy, prolactin levels rise while the nocturnal rise in prolactin persists. Patients with hyperprolactinemia associated with pituitary adenomas also have a persistent nocturnal rise in prolactin.

The Corticotropic Axis

Plasma adrenocorticotropic hormone (ACTH) and cortisol levels demonstrate a strong circadian pattern, with highest levels during the early morning and lowest levels around midnight. ACTH, in turn, responds to changes in corticotropin-releasing hormone (CRH) at the level of the hypothalamus. Unlike the somatotropic and lactotropic axis that are primarily controlled by the onset of sleep, this axis is primarily controlled by circadian input; however, a short-term fall in cortisol with sleep onset occurs. Later, during the second half of the sleep period, there is an increase in cortisol secretion coincident with the transition from sleep to wake. Sleep deprivation is associated with a rebound elevation of cortisol secretion on the first night of recovery sleep.[38] Aging is associated with a rise in cortisol over time.[27]

Disease can alter circadian cortisol secretion. Cushing's syndrome, associated with elevated levels of cortisol, may be produced by ACTH-producing pituitary tumors, ectopic production of ACTH, or autonomous adrenal adenomas. With adrenal adenomas and ectopic production, there is loss of diurnal variation. Patients with ACTH-producing pituitary tumors, however, may still demonstrate diurnal variation in cortisol secretion.[39] Depression is associated with increased pulsatility and elevated cortisol levels.[40] The circadian rhythm remains with depression, however, with a later onset and earlier peak cortisol with sleep. The amplitude of the cortisol rise with sleep may be blunted with liver disease and hypothyroidism because of decreased clearance.[41,42]

The Thyrotropic Axis

The hypothalamic releasing hormone, thyrotropin-releasing hormone (TRH), stimulates thyrotropin (also known as *thyroid-stimulating hormone*, TSH) release from the anterior pituitary. In humans with usual sleeping patterns at night, TSH levels are low during the day, rise during the afternoon and early evening, and are maximal before onset of sleep.[43] TSH levels decline slowly throughout the night. With recovery sleep, there is a sharper decline in TSH secretion. The rise in TSH during the evening appears to be circadian-linked. Aging is associated with a decrease in TSH secretion.[27] Nonthyroidal illness results in a decreased nocturnal rise in TSH.[44]

The Gonadotropic Axis

Luteinizing hormone (LH) and follicle-stimulating hormone (FSH) do not show a consistent diurnal variation in young men.[45] This is so despite the observation that testosterone exhibits a diurnal rhythm with levels lowest in the late evening and highest in the early morning.[46] With aging, testosterone levels fall, with asynchrony of gonadotropin secretion.[47] In premenopausal women, there is a variability in LH pulse amplitude and frequency, depending on the time of the menstrual cycle.[48] Early follicular phase demonstrates large, infrequent pulses. By the mid-follicular phase, pulse amplitude is decreased and pulse frequency is increased. In the early luteal phase, pulse amplitude is high and pulse frequency increases. By the late luteal phase, pulse amplitude and frequency are markedly decreased. In premenopausal women, the most pronounced sleep-linked effect on gonadotropins is during the early follicular phase. During this time, sleep is associated with decreased frequency of pulses. Lesser inhibition in pulse frequency occurs during the luteal phase. LH and FSH pulse frequency increase with age.[49] With menopause, gonadotropin levels are high but have no circadian pattern.[50]

Glucose and Insulin Levels

Glucose tolerance varies throughout the day. Glucose levels are higher during the evening compared with morning.[51] These differences appear to be modulated by cortisol and growth hormone.[52] As noted previously, these hormones are elevated during sleep, and both have anti-insulin effects. Growth hormone levels are high at onset of sleep, and cortisol rises during the second half of sleep. Insulin resistance is induced through mechanisms mediated through hormones interacting with their respective receptors at the level of the target cells. Therefore glucose tolerance has both a sleep-linked and a circadian-linked component through interactions with other hormone secretory patterns. Insulin levels follow changes in glucose and would be expected to parallel glucose levels throughout the day. NREM sleep is associated with less glucose tolerance than REM sleep, with the latter being more common in the second half of sleep.[53] To some degree, this may be mediated by sleep-associated changes in insulin secretion, independent of glucose. Obesity abolishes the nocturnal variation in glucose and insulin levels.[54]

For a summary of endocrine function and sleep, please see Table 3-3.

Pulmonary Physiology in Sleep

Physiology research into the control of breathing and respiratory mechanisms has advanced over many years from scientists using animal models. The following section represents only a brief summary of the vast amount of publications available. The interested reader can also find more expanded summaries in several review resources,[55–59] to name only a few.

Central Nervous System (CNS) Control of Breathing

Ventilation is controlled by two central mechanisms of automatic control and voluntary control. Automatic control of ventilation is centered in the pons and medulla, which controls breathing regardless of whether the subject is awake or asleep. Animal studies have shown that the pons pneumotaxic center is at the rostral pons in the area of the nucleus parabrachialis and Kölliker-Fuse nuclei.[60,61] The dorsolateral area of the lower pons has been referred to as the *apneustic center*, which may be the location of the inspiratory "off-switch" to medullary inspiratory neurons.[60] The medulla control is centered in two basic areas: (1) the dorsal respiratory group (DRG) and (2) the ventral respiratory group (VRG). The medullary responses for inhalation are principally controlled by the DRG in the nucleus tractus solitarius (NTS). Both inhalation and exhalation are controlled in the medulla ventral respiratory center in the nucleus ambiguus and retro-ambigualis.[60–63] The VRG is believed to be the center of intrinsic respiratory rhythm generation at the pre-Bötzinger complex. The neurotransmitter crucial in respiratory rhythm generation interacting principally at the non-*N*-methyl-D-aspartate (NMDA) receptors is *glutamate*, which also connects the transmission of this

TABLE 3-3 ■ Summary of Endocrine Function

Axis-Hormone	Sleep- or Circadian-Linked	Hypothalamic Input	Peripheral Effector(s)	Normal Pattern
Somatotropic-growth hormone	Sleep-linked	GHRH (+) Somatostatin (−) Ghrelin (+)	IGF-1	Largest pulse with onset of sleep and slow wave sleep
Lactotropic-prolactin	Sleep-linked	Dopamine (−) TRH (+)	Prolactin	Low during the day. Followed by rise after sleep onset and slow wave sleep
Corticotropic–ACTH	Circadian-linked	CRH (+) Vasopressin (+)	Cortisol	Diurnal pattern with lowest levels at midnight, highest in AM
Thyrotropic–TSH	Circadian-linked	TRH (+)	L-T4	Low during day and maximal before sleep onset
Gonadotropic–LH/FSH	Women: related to menstrual cycle with some phases sleep-linked	GnRH (+)	Women: estrogen, progesterone	Women: dependent on menstrual cycle
	Men: circadian-linked		Men: testosterone	Men: diurnal pattern with lowest levels at night and highest in the early AM
Peripheral–Insulin/glucose	Both sleep- and circadian-linked			Glucose levels rise slightly during the evening and return to normal by AM

GHRH, growth hormone-releasing hormone; IGF, insulin-like growth factor; TRH, thyrotropin-releasing hormone; ACTH, adrenocorticotropic hormone; CRH, corticotropin-releasing hormone; TSH, thyroid-stimulating hormone; LH, luteinizing hormone; FSH, follicle-stimulating hormone; GnRH, gonadotropin-releasing hormone.

rhythm to the phrenic motoneurons.[63] Orexin, expressed by pre-Bötzinger neurons and phrenic nuclei, may also be involved in respiratory regulation.[64]

Behavioral control of breathing involves aspects of the respiratory system, such as reflexive control of breathing manifested as coughing or sneezing, and voluntary control of breathing as in singing or speech during the awake period. The voluntary control center is in the cerebral cortex that sends descending neurons with the corticospinal tract, eventually joining the fibers from the medullary respiratory neurons of the automatic respiratory system.[60–62]

Other sites have also been found in the fastigial nucleus, caudal raphe, locus coeruleus, and nucleus ambiguous within the brainstem.[59]

If hypoxia occurs, this is sensed through the carotid body chemoreceptors as the PO$_2$ drops below 60, with a response of increased ventilation. Afferents connect the carotid body through the ninth cranial nerve to the medulla. The carotid body chemoreceptor to medullary control can be blunted in extreme hypoxia conditions if the PO$_2$ drops below 40.[66] Overall, hypoxic triggers to ventilation decrease in NREM sleep compared with wakefulness, with a further reduction in REM sleep.[67]

Metabolic Respiratory Mechanisms

The carotid body chemoreceptors mediate hypoxic ventilatory responses, whereas the hypercapnic ventilatory trigger is primarily through the medullary chemoreceptors, with some carotid body chemoreceptor responses as well. The chemoreceptors operate to keep the carbon dioxide and oxygen levels in homeostasis. If the PCO$_2$ drops below the PCO$_2$ threshold, this relative hypocapnea is sensed chiefly at the medullary chemoreceptor level, with subsequent hypoventilation or an apneic response until the PCO$_2$ rises again to trigger resumption of minute ventilation. This trigger to ventilation as PCO$_2$ rises will decrease in NREM sleep, with a further reduction in stage REM.[65] Animal studies have shown CO$_2$ chemosensitive sites to be important in respiratory homeostatic control, primarily in the ventral medulla and NTS.

Peripheral Respiratory Mechanisms

Chest wall receptors connect via afferents to the medulla. Pulmonary stretch receptors trigger vagal afferents that lead to termination of inhalation. The medullary respiratory centers send efferent signals out to the intercostal muscles and diaphragm for modulation of the respiratory pattern during both wake and sleep.[68] These inflation-deflation reflexes have been referred to as the *Hering-Breuer reflex*. There is a reduction in airway dilator muscle tone, intercostal muscle tone, and diaphragm function during NREM sleep. The motorneuron hyperpolarization of REM sleep causes muscle tone suppression and leads to a significant drop in intercostal muscle activity. In contrast, the diaphragm continues functioning with a tendency to increase activity in phasic REM, although the overall efficiency is reduced.[57] Whether awake or in NREM sleep, the rib cage contributes 44% to the tidal volume in the supine position, with a 19% drop in stage REM owing to loss of tidal volume contribution of intercostal muscle function.[69]

NREM Respiratory Responses

Central control of ventilation tends to decrease during transition into NREM sleep compared with wakefulness, with medullary neurons firing more weakly and with greater variability.[70] Minute ventilation falls by about 0.5 to 1.5 L/min primarily as a consequence of a reduction in tidal volume, with only a slight decrease in respiratory rate.[56] This effective sleep hypoventilation subsequently causes a slight increase in PCO_2 by about 2–3 mm Hg (2–3 additional mm Hg, in stage REM), a reduction in PO_2 by 3–10 mm Hg and oxygen saturation decreases by 0–2%.[56,59,71] During light sleep in stage 1 and early stage 2, variation in breathing can become evident, with brief segments of periodic breathing[72] and possible central apneas as well. A total of 40–80% of normal subjects have periodic breathing at sleep onset, with predominance in men who have a greater hypercapnic ventilatory response.[57] The latter part of stage 2 sleep, as well as stages 3 and 4 sleep, are characterized by the most regular breathing patterns when compared with stage 1, the transitional (early) part of stage 2 sleep and REM sleep.

In the advent of hypoxia, ventilatory responses are slowed during NREM sleep and further reduced or unchanged during REM sleep. In fact, with normal alveolar CO_2, hypoxia has been shown to be a poor arousal trigger in human subjects.[73] Likewise, there is also a reduction in the hypercapnic ventilatory response during NREM sleep, with a further REM reduction to about 33% of that during the awake state.[65]

REM Respiratory Responses

Irregular breathing is characteristic of REM, caused in part by erratic firing patterns of medullary neurons to phrenic motor neurons. Activation of the behavioral control of breathing is thought to combine with chemical regulation during periods of dreaming. Intercostal muscle atonia, in combination with a sharp reduction in upper airway muscle tone, causes an increase in airway resistance, but diaphragm function continues intact. Tidal volume is decreased over wakefulness and the respiratory rate becomes irregular, leading to an overall reduction in minute ventilation. This erratic breathing pattern of REM sleep, particularly in phasic REM, can lead to transient apneas or hypopneas. Gould et al[74] observed an increase in breathing frequency and reduction in tidal volume in phasic REM. Oxygen saturation decreases during stage REM sleep

because of this effective hypoventilation compared with wakefulness.

Airway Responses During Sleep

Cat studies previously showed an increase in upper airway resistance during sleep compared with wakefulness, with a further increase in REM over NREM sleep.[75] More extensive cat research demonstrated waking reticular activation of laryngeal abduction, via the posterior cricoarytenoid muscles, responsible for helping maintain airway patency, that is reduced during sleep with a maximal reduction in stage REM.[76] Diaphragm stimulation is stronger than the activation of laryngeal abduction during sleep. This combination of events is thought to result in higher airway resistance compared with the waking state.

Likewise, in human subjects, there is a relative increase in upper airway resistance during sleep owing to a combination of dynamic changes in the respiratory muscle function during sleep affected by a reduction in tone of the airway dilator muscles. There are at least 20 upper airway muscles. Of these, the genioglossus moves the tongue forward, the geniohyoid elevates the hyoid bone, the tensor veli palatini moves the soft palate away from the posterior pharyngeal wall, and the posterior cricoarytenoid muscle triggers laryngeal abduction. During sleep, there is a reduction in the muscle tone of the genioglossus, geniohyoid, tensor veli palatini, and posterior cricoarytenoid muscles (airway dilator muscles),[77,78] as well as the diaphragm and intercostal muscles (respiratory pump muscles).[79] Subsequently, airway resistance rises and minute ventilation decreases relative to the level of this increased airway resistance.[80] Hypotonia of the airway dilator group of muscles, as well as the intercostal muscles of breathing, occurs during NREM sleep. In REM sleep, the intercostal muscles become atonic, with continued diaphragmatic contraction with respiration, especially in phasic stage REM. With arousals from sleep, airway dilator muscle tone abruptly increases, with a reduction in upper airway resistance.

Upper airway resistance has been shown to be higher in men than in women,[81–83] middle-age to older men than in young men,[84,85] and in users of alcohol[86,87] or sedative-hypnotics[88,89] than in nonusers.

Other Respiratory Responses During Sleep

Animal studies have shown that the cough reflex is depressed during NREM sleep, with a further reduction in REM sleep, and that coughing secondary to an airway irritant does not occur apart from an arousal from sleep.[90,91] This can become an important factor in gastroesophageal reflux clearance.

TABLE 3-4 ■ Physiologic Variations in the Respiratory System During Sleep

Parameter	Waking	Slow Wave Sleep	REM Sleep
Minute ventilation	Varies with activity	Mildly decreased	Variable
Respiratory rate	Varies with activity	Mildly decreased	Variable
$PaCO_2$	Stable	Mildly increased	Increased
PaO_2	Stable	Mildly decreased	Decreased
Hypercapnic ventilatory response	Sensitive to elevation in carbon dioxide	Mildly decreased response	Decreased to a greater extent when compared with wake and SWS
Hypoxic ventilatory response	Sensitive to decreases in oxygen tension	Mildly decreased response	Decreased to a greater extent when compared with wake and SWS

REM, rapid eye movement; $PaCO_2$, arterial carbon dioxide tension; PaO_2, arterial oxygen tension; SWS, slow-wave sleep. (Reprinted with permission from Sheldon SH: Physiologic variations during sleep in children. In Sheldon SH, Ferber R, Kryger MH (eds): *Principles and Practice of Pediatric Sleep Medicine*. Philadelphia, Elsevier Saunders, p 78, 2005.)

Finally, sighs naturally occur during the waking period that serve to avoid atelectasis by increasing functional residual capacity. Sighs continue during sleep, although at a decreased rate in NREM and REM sleep. During sleep, many but not all are associated with an electroencephalogram (EEG) arousal. A dog study showed a larger volume sigh during the awake than the sleep period, with a postsigh breathing pattern that was reduced but returned to control levels within three breaths and remained intact in NREM and REM sleep.[92] Postsigh respiratory activity in humans demonstrate central apneas, hypopneas, or a slowed respiratory rate.[93]

Summary

For a nice summary of respiratory changes in sleep, please see Table 3-4.

CARDIOVASCULAR PHYSIOLOGY IN SLEEP

NREM sleep is characterized by homeostasis of somatic and visceral activity resulting from *closed-loop* neural mechanisms. This is a result of balanced excitatory and inhibitory influences between the brainstem and forebrain at the hypothalamic level causing close autonomic regulation of cardiac and vascular systems during sleep. This leads to a decrease in the tissue metabolic rate facilitating energy regeneration.[94]

REM sleep is characterized by poikilostasis (great variability) of somatic and visceral activity resulting from *open-loop* neural mechanisms. This is the result of a lack in hypothalamic integration between the CNS, autonomic nervous system, and the local tissue influences and leads to sudden changes in somatic and visceral activity.[94]

Heart and Coronary Circulation During Sleep

Autonomic regulation of the cardiovascular system is characterized by relative stability during NREM sleep as a result of the predominance of parasympathetic tone. In contrast, there is marked sympathetic activation during REM sleep with profound changes in heart rate (HR) and circulation.[94–96]

Vagal tone increases during NREM sleep, leading to physiologic bradycardia and a decrease in blood pressure (BP).[95,98] As a result, cardiac output and systemic vascular resistance decrease, facilitating metabolic regeneration of the heart. Coronary blood flow also decreases.[94,96]

HR varies cyclically during NREM sleep (accelerates during inspiration and decelerates during expiration).[94–96] The increase in vagal activity during NREM sleep stimulates local (thoracic) baroreceptors and leads to stimulation of both the respiratory center and the cardiac center in the brainstem. This is called *respiratory sinus arrhythmia*, also known as *heart rate variability* (HRV), and it is a function of normal cardiac activity.[95,96,99–101] Loss of HRV is associated with cardiac pathology and aging.[102] In children, loss of respiratory sinus arrhythmia may be associated with sudden infant death syndrome (SIDS) and congenital central hypoventilation syndrome.[103,104]

Baroreceptor sensitivity (BRS) is increased in the initial stages of NREM sleep when compared with the awake state.[95,96,106] This leads to an increase in arterial as well as venodilation, a decrease in cardiac contractility, and bradycardia. It is thought that increased vagal tone at the beginning of NREM stage decreases cortical reticular influences and also increases local carotid and aortic baroreceptor reflexes.

During REM sleep the baroreceptors attenuate the increase in the sympathetic stimuli at the level of the sinus node. Therefore there is a significant increase in

BRS to hypertensive stimuli when compared with the NREM and awake state.[107,112]

Bradycardia and heart pauses can occur either during transition from NREM to REM sleep or during stage REM.[95,96,105,108]

Transitions from NREM to REM sleep may be accompanied by severe bradycardia, transient heart block, and possible asystole as observed in canines. During this transition, sympathetic activation increases HR and BP, leading to indirect aortic and carotid baroreceptor stimulation and vagal surges in an attempt to balance the sympathetic discharges. This results in heart pauses from 1–8 seconds and an increase in coronary blood flow[111] and vasodilation independent of the cardiac metabolic needs, suggesting neurogenic influences. Similar activity was documented in humans.[105,113]

During tonic REM sleep, bradycardia in humans may be explained by centrally mediated autonomic activity of the heart, which may result in a decrease in sympathetic drive, increase in vagal drive, or both. This is the result of CNS activation during stage REM with alterations in ponto-geniculo-occipital and hippocampal activity.[94,96]

Coronary blood flow and coronary vascular resistance vary with the sleep state. In canines, NREM vagal drive leads to a decrease in HR and therefore a decrease in coronary blood flow and an increase in coronary vascular resistance.[110,111] During the transition between NREM and REM, the rhythm pauses induced by vagal surges (see previous discussion) lead to an increase in coronary blood flow and a decrease in coronary vascular resistance. During stage REM, an increase in HR resulting from sympathetic predominance leads to an increase in coronary blood flow and coronary vasodilation with this elevated cardiac metabolism. Coronary blood flow during stage REM is regulated via the apneustic center in the dorsolateral pons and is independent of BP.[95,96,108]

On the surface electrocardiogram, RR variability and QTc vary during NREM and REM sleep and also with age and gender. In men, RR variability increases and QTc remains stable throughout sleep, whereas in women the reverse is true.

Cardiac ventricular arrhythmia during sleep is mediated by sympathetic activation and requires an intact vagal system.[95,96,108,109,113]

In REM sleep, an increase in sympathetic tonus creates the substrate for ventricular tachyarrhythmias in normal or ischemic myocardium via several pathways:

- Stimulates central and peripheral adrenergic structures and facilitates the release of cathecolamines, which act directly at the level of the myocardial adrenergic receptors, triggering ventricular arrhythmias

- Produces tissue hypoxia via the increase in cardiac metabolic demands and vasoconstriction, altering the supply-demand ratio in a vessel with altered endothelium
- Stimulates cardiac beta-adrenergic receptors, increasing the intracellular influx of Ca^{++} and therefore altering repolarization and decreasing the threshold for ventricular fibrillation

In addition to the increased sympathetic tonus, the parasympathetic surges during REM sleep can result in sinus pauses, which facilitate ventricular arrhythmias via triggered activity as a ventricular escape mechanism.

Peripheral Circulation During Sleep

Cerebral Blood Flow (CBF)

Cerebral blood flow decreases during NREM sleep and increases during REM sleep, overall decreasing throughout the night. CBF fluctuations are the result of changes in vascular resistance and are independent of systemic hemodynamic changes.

The regulation of cerebral circulation involves three mechanisms[97,114]:

- *Flow-metabolism coupling*: O_2 is the link between cerebral perfusion and cerebral activity during sleep; it is the main mechanism of CBF regulation and ensures the restorative function of sleep. Spectroscopy studies showed no change in oxyhemoglobin from the awake state to NREM sleep and an increase in oxyhemoglobin from NREM to REM sleep as a result in increase CBF.
- *Chemical regulation* involves local CBF regulation by changes in PCO_2.
- *Autonomic regulation* ensures an adequate CBF during sleep, independent of the systemic hemodynamic changes.

CBF changes meet the metabolic needs of brain activity and protect the brain from sudden systemic fluctuations.

Cutaneous Circulation

Skin vasodilation occurs at the onset of NREM sleep as a result of a drop in the thermostatic set point. The sympathetic skin activity does not change during NREM sleep.[97]

Skin blood flow during REM sleep depends on the environment temperature and is mediated through neuronal vasomotor activity as the result of an increase in the sympathetic skin activity (skin blood flow increases during a cold environment and decreases during a warm environment with the exception of acute blood loss when there is skin vasoconstriction).[115,116] Overall there is an increase in the skin blood flow during sleep when compared with the awake state.

Renal Circulation

Renal circulation is unchanged during sleep. When there is a generalized thermoregulatory vasomotor reaction, however, renal vasoconstriction ensues.[97]

Splanchnic Circulation

Splanchnic circulation is unchanged during sleep. This may be due to local regulatory mechanisms.[97,117]

Muscle Circulation

Muscle blood flow changes very little between wakefulness and NREM sleep.

Sympathetic tone decreases during NREM sleep, facilitating vasodilation and a reduction in BP. It increases during REM sleep, resulting in changes in the local vasculature as well as changes in the muscle activity. Muscle blood flow during REM sleep is regulated by local metabolic factors, as well as by neuronal influences.

During tonic REM, sympathetic stimulation produces muscle twitches and leads to local muscle vasodilation as a result of the release of local metabolic factors. During phasic REM, sympathetic stimulation produces muscle atonia and local vasoconstriction via direct cathecolamine release, as well as local metabolic factors.[97]

The hypothalamus integrates the autonomic control of sleep stages and environmental influences. Because REM sleep is a closed-loop mechanism, changes in the surroundings during sleep affect the duration of NREM sleep and transition to REM sleep. This is a result of autonomic and central system regulation in an attempt to maintain homeostasis. During REM sleep these complex vasomotor adaptive mechanisms are impaired.[97]

REFERENCES

1. Parmeggiani PL: Thermoregulation and sleep. Front Biosci 8:557–567, 2003.
2. Buchsbaum MS, Hazlett EA, Wu J, et al: Positron emission tomography with deoxyglucose-F18 imaging of sleep. Neuropsychopharmacology 25(5 Suppl):S50–S56, 2001.
3. Bach V, Telliez F, Libert JP: The interaction between sleep and thermoregulation in adults and neonates. Sleep Med Rev 6(6):481–492, 2002.
4. Wright KP, Hull JT, Czeisler CA: Relationship between alertness, performance, and body temperature in humans. Am J Physiol Regul Integr Comp Physiol 283:1370–1377, 2002.
5. Gilbert SS, van den Heuvel CJ, Ferguson SA, et al: Thermoregulation as a sleep signaling system. Sleep Med Rev 8(2):81–93, 2004.
6. Saper CB, Lu J, Chou TC, et al: The hypothalamic integrator for circadian rhythms. Trends Neurosci 28(3):152–157, 2005.
7. Lu J, Zhang YH, Chou TC, et al: Contrasting effects of ibotenate lesions of the paraventricular nucleus and subparaventricular zone on sleep-wake cycle and temperature regulation. J Neurosci 21(13):4864–4874, 2001.
8. Lange T, Perras B, Fehm HL, et al: Sleep enhances the human antibody response to hepatitis A vaccination. Psychosom Med 65:831–835, 2003.
9. Spiegel K, Sheridan JF, Van Cauter E: Effect of sleep deprivation on response to immunization. JAMA 288(12):1471–1472, 2002.
10. Dimitrov S, Lange T, Tieken S, et al: Sleep associated regulation of T helper1/T helper 2 cytokine balance in humans. Brain Behav Immun 18(4):341–348, 2004.
11. Dimitrov S, Lange T, Fehm HL, et al: A regulatory role of prolactin, growth hormone, and corticosteroids for human T–cell production of cytokines. Brain Behav Immun 18(4):368–374, 2004.
12. Majde JA, Krueger JM: Host defense. In Kryger MH, Roth T, Dement WC (eds): *Principles and Practice of Sleep Medicine*, 4th ed. Philadelphia, Saunders, 2005, pp 256–265.
13. Redwine L, Hauger RL, Gillin JC, et al: Effects of sleep and sleep deprivation on interleukin-6, growth hormone, cortisol, and melatonin levels in humans. J Clin Endocrinol Metab 85:3597–3603, 2000.
14. Papanicolaou DA, Wilder RL, Manolagas SC, et al: The pathophysiologic roles of interleukin-6 in human disease. Ann Intern Med 128(2):127–137, 1998.
15. Kapsimalis F, Richardson G, Opp MR, et al: Cytokines and normal sleep. Curr Opin Pulmon Med 11:481–484, 2005.
16. Alam MN, McGinty D, Bashir T, et al: Interleukin-1β modulates state-dependent discharge activity of preoptic area and basal forebrain neurons: role in sleep regulation. Eur J Neurosci 20(1):207–216, 2004.
17. Manfridi A, Brambilla D, Bianchi S, et al: Inteleukin-1β enhances non-rapid eye movement sleep when microinjected into the dorsal raphe nucleus and inhibits serotonergic neurons *in vitro*. Eur J Neurosci 18(5):1041–1049, 2003.
18. Mullington J, Korth C, Hermann DM, et al: Dose-dependent effects of endotoxin on human sleep. Am J Physiol Reg Integrat Comp Physiol 278:R947–R955, 2000.
19. Van Cauter E, Copinschi G, Turek F: Endocrine and other biologic rhythms. In DeGroot L, Jameson J (eds): *Endocrinology*. Philadelphia, Saunders, 2001, pp 235–256.
20. Turek F: Circadian rhythms. Horm Res 49:103–113, 1998.
21. Golstein J, Cauter EV, Desir D, et al: Effects of "jet lag" on hormonal patterns. IV. Time shifts increase growth

hormone release. J Clin Endocrinol Metab 56:433–440, 1983.

22. Van Coevorden A, Laurent E, Decoster C, et al: Decreased basal and stimulated thyrotropin secretion in healthy elderly men. J Clin Endocrinol Metab 69:177–185, 1989.

23. Lejeune-Lenain C, Van Cauter E, Desir D, et al: Control of circadian and episodic variations of adrenal androgens secretion in man. J Endocrinol Invest 10:267–276, 1987.

24. Van Cauter E, L'Hermite M, Copinschi G, et al: Quantitative analysis of spontaneous variations of plasma prolactin in normal man. Am J Physiol 241:E355–E363, 1981.

25. Van Cauter E, Plat L, Copinschi G: Interrelations between sleep and the somatotropic axis. Sleep 21:553–566, 1998.

26. Ho K, Evans W, Blizzard R, et al: Effects of sex and age on the 24-hour profile of growth hormone secretion in man: importance of endogenous estradiol concentrations. J Clin Endocrinol Metab 64:51–58, 1987.

27. Van Coevorden A, Mockel J, Laurent E, et al: Neuroendocrine rhythms and sleep in aging men. Am J Physiol 260:E651–E661, 1991.

28. Ghigo E, Broglio F, Arvat E, et al: Ghrelin: more than a natural GH secretagogue and/or an orexigenic factor. Clin Endocrinol 62:1–17, 2005.

29. Weikel J, Wichniak A, Ising M, et al: Ghrelin promotes slow-wave sleep in humans. Am J Physiol 284:E407–E415, 2003.

30. Hartman M, Veldhuis J, Vance M, et al: Somatotropin pulse frequency and basal concentrations are increased in acromegaly and are reduced by successful therapy. J Clin Endocrinol Metab 70:1375–1384, 1990.

31. Veldhuis J, Iranmanesh A, Ho K, et al: Dual defects in pulsatile growth hormone secretion and clearance subserve the hyposomatotropism of obesity in man. J Clin Endocrinol Metab 72:51–59, 1991.

32. Edge J, Dunger D, Matthews D, et al: Increased overnight growth hormone concentrations in diabetic compared with normal adolescents. J Clin Endocrinol Metab 71:1356–1362, 1990.

33. Mendlewicz J, Linkowski P, Kerkhofs M, et al: Diurnal hypersecretion of growth hormone in depression. J Clin Endocrinol Metab 60:505–512, 1986.

34. Sassin J, Frantz A, Kapen S, Weitzman E: Human prolactin: 24-hour pattern with increased release during sleep. Science 177:1205, 1972.

35. Sassin J, Frantz A, Kapen S, Weitzman E: The nocturnal rise of human prolactin is dependent on sleep. J Clin Endocrinol Metab 37:436–440, 1973.

36. Spiegel K, Luthringer R, Follenius M, et al: Temporal relationship between prolactin secretion and slow-wave electroencephalographic activity during sleep. Sleep 18:543–548, 1995.

37. Katznelson L, Riskind P, Saxe V, Klibanski A: Prolactin pulsatile characteristics in postmenopausal women. J Clin Endocrinol Metab 83:761–764, 1998.

38. Spiegel K, Leproult R, Van Cauter E: Impact of sleep debt on metabolic endocrine function. Lancet 354:1435–1439, 1999.

39. Van Cauter E, Refetoff S: Evidence for two subtypes of Cushing's disease based on the analysis of episodic cortisol secretion. N Engl J Med 312:1343–1344, 1985.

40. Linkowski P, Mendlewicz J, Leclercq R, et al: The 24-hour profile of adrenocorticotropin and coritsol in major depressive illness. J Clin Endocrinol Metab 61:429–438, 1985.

41. Rosman P, Farag A, Benn R, et al: Modulation of pituitary-adrenal function: decreased secretory episodes and blunted circadian rhythmicity in patients with alcoholic liver disease. J Clin Endocrinol Metab 55:709–717, 1981.

42. Iranmanesh A, Lizarralde G, Johnson M, Veldhuis J: Dynamics of 24-hour endogenous cortisol secretion and clearance in primary hypothyroidism assessed before and after partial thyroid hormone replacement. J Clin Endocrinol Metab 70:155–161, 1990.

43. Behrends J, Prank K, Dogu E, Brabant G: Central nervous system control of thyrotropin secretion during sleep and wakefulness. Horm Res 49:173–177, 1998.

44. Romjin J, Wiersinga W: Decreased nocturnal surge of thyrotropin in nonthyroidal illness. J Clin Endocrinol Metab 70:35–42, 1990.

45. Spratt D, O'Dea L, Schoenfeld D, et al: Neuroendocrine-gonadal axis in men: frequent sampling of LH, FSH, and testosterone. Am J Physiol 254:E658–E666, 1988.

46. Bremner W, Vitiello M, Prinz P: Loss of circadian rhythmicity in blood testosterone levels with aging in normal men. J Clin Endocrinol Metab 56:1278–1280, 1983.

47. Pincus S, Mulligan T, Iranmanesh A, et al: Older males secrete luteinizing hormone and testosterone more irregularly, and jointly more asynchronously, than younger males. Proc Natl Acad Sci USA 93:14100–14105, 1996.

48. Filicori M, Santoro N, Merriam G, Crowley W: Characterization of the physiological pattern of episodic gonadotropin secretion throughout the menstrual cycle. J Clin Endocrinol Metab 62:1136–1144, 1986.

49. Reame N, Kelch R, Beitins I, et al: Age effects of follicle-stimulating hormone and pulsatile luteinizing hormone secretion across the menstrual cycle of premenopausal women. J Clin Endocrinol Metab 81:1512–1518, 1996.

50. Turek F, Van Cauter E: Rhythms in reproduction. In Knobil E, Neill J (eds): *The Physiology of Reproduction.* New York, Raven Press, 1993, pp 1789–1830.

51. Van Cauter E: Diurnal and ultradian rhythms in human endocrine function: a minireview. Horm Res 34:45–53, 1990.

52. Plat L, Byrne M, Sturis J, et al: Effects of morning cortisol elevation on insulin secretion and glucose regulation in humans. Am J Physiol 270:E36–E42, 1996.

53. Scheen A, Byrne M, Plat L, Van Cauter E: Relationships between sleep quality and glucose regulation in normal humans. Am J Physiol 271:E261–E270, 1996.

54. Van Cauter E, Polonsky K, Blackman J, et al: Abnormal temporal patterns of glucose tolerance in obesity: relationship to sleep-related growth hormone and circadian cortisol rhythmicity. J Clin Endocrinol Metab 79:1797–1805, 1994.

55. Bolton CF, Chen R, Wijdicks EFM, Zifko UA: *Neurology of Breathing*. Philadelphia, Butterworth Heinemann Elsevier, 2004.

56. Chokroverty S: Physiologic changes in sleep. In Chokroverty S (ed): *Sleep Disorders Medicine: Basic Science, Technical Considerations, and Clinical Aspects*, 2nd ed. Boston, Butterworth-Heinemann, 1999, pp 95–126.

57. Krieger J: Respiratory physiology: breathing in normal subjects. In Kryger MH, Roth T, Dement WC (eds): *Principles and Practice of Sleep Medicine*, 4th ed. Philadelphia, Elsevier Saunders, 2005, pp 232–244.

58. Sheldon SH: Physiologic variations during sleep in children. In Sheldon SH, Ferber R, Kryger MH (eds): *Principles and Practice of Pediatric Sleep Medicine*. Philadelphia: Elsevier Saunders 2005, pp 73–84.

59. Krimsky WR, Leiter JC: Physiology of breathing and respiratory control during sleep. Semin Respir Crit Care Med 26(1):5–12, 2005.

60. Berger AJ, Mitchell RA, Severinghaus JW: Regulation of respiration. N Engl J Med 297(3):138–143, 1977.

61. Mitchell RA: Neural regulation of respiration. Clin Chest Med 1:3–12, 1980.

62. Mitchell RA, Berger AJ: Neural regulation of respiration. Am Rev Respir Dis 111(2):206–224, 1975.

63. Bolton CF, Chen R, Wijdicks EFM, Zifko UA: Anatomy and physiology of the nervous system control of respiration. In Bolton CF, Chen R, Wijdicks EFM, Zifko UA (eds): *Neurology of Breathing*. Philadelphia, Butterworth Heinemann Elsevier, 2004, pp 19–36.

64. Young JK, Wu M, Manaye KF, et al: Orexin stimulates breathing via medullary and spinal pathways. J Appl Physiol 98(4):1387–1395, 2005.

65. Douglas NJ, White DP, Weil JV, et al: Hypercapnic ventilatory response in sleeping adults. Am Rev Respir Dis 126(5):758–762, 1982.

66. Douglas NJ: Respiratory physiology: control of ventilation. In Kryger MH, Roth T, Dement WC (eds): *Principles and Practice of Sleep Medicine*, 4th ed. Philadelphia, Elsevier Saunders, 2005, pp 224–231.

67. Douglas NJ, White DP, Weil JV, et al: Hypoxic ventilatory response decreases during sleep in normal man. Am Rev Respir Dis 125:286–289, 1982.

68. Hudgel DW, Martin RJ, Johnson B, et al: Mechanics of the respiratory system and breathing during sleep in normal humans. J Appl Physiol 56(1):133–137, 1984.

69. Tusiewicz K, Moldofsky H, Bryan AC, Bryan MH: Mechanics of the rib cage and diaphragm during sleep. J Appl Physiol 43(4):600–602, 1977.

70. Orem J, Montplaisir J, Dement WC: Changes in the activity of respiratory neurons during sleep. Brain Res 82(2):309–315, 1974.

71. Rist KE, Daubenspeck JA, McGovern JF: Effects of non-REM sleep upon respiratory drive and the respiratory pump in humans. Respir Physiol 63(2):241–256, 1986.

72. Webb P: Periodic breathing during sleep. J Appl Physiol 37(6):899–903, 1974.

73. Berthon-Jones M, Sullivan CE: Ventilatory and arousal responses to hypoxia in sleeping humans. Am Rev Respir Dis 125(6):632–639, 1982.

74. Gould GA, Gugger M, Molloy J, et al: Breathing pattern and eye movement density during REM sleep in humans. Am Rev Respir Dis 138(4):874–877, 1988.

75. Orem J, Netick A, Dement WC: Increased upper airway resistance to breathing during sleep in the cat. Electroencephalogr Clin Neurophysiol 43(1):14–22, 1977.

76. Orem J, Lydic R: Upper airway function during sleep and wakefulness: experimental studies on normal and anesthetized cats. Sleep 1(1):49–68, 1978. Reprinted in Sleep 25(5):49–68, 2002.

77. Ayappa I, Rapoport DM: The upper airway in sleep: physiology of the pharynx. Sleep Med Rev 7(1):9–33, 2003.

78. Series F: Upper airway muscles awake and asleep. Sleep Med Rev 6(3):229–242, 2002.

79. Worsnop C, Kay A, Pierce R, et al: Activity of respiratory pump and upper airway muscles during sleep onset. J Appl Physiol 85(3):908–920, 1998.

80. Wiegand L, Zwillich CW, White DP: Collapsibility of the human upper airway during normal sleep. J Appl Physiol 66(4):1800–1808, 1989.

81. Block AJ, Boysen PG, Wynne JW, Hunt LA: Sleep apnea, hypopnea and oxygen desaturation in normal subjects. A strong male predominance. N Engl J Med. 300(10):513–517, 1979.

82. Pillar G, Malhotra A, Fogel R, et al: Airway mechanics and ventilation in response to resistive loading during sleep: influence of gender. Am J Respir Crit Care Med 162(5):1606–1607, 2000.

83. Trinder J, Kay A, Kleiman J, Dunai J: Gender differences in airway resistance during sleep. J Appl Physiol 83(6):1986–1997, 1997.

84. Worsnop C, Kay A, Kim Y, et al: Effect of age on sleep onset-related changes in respiratory pump and upper airway muscle function. J Appl Physiol 88(5):1831–1839, 2000.

85. Hudgel DW, Hamilton HB: Respiratory muscle activity during sleep-induced periodic breathing in the elderly. Appl Physiol 77(5):2285–2290, 1994.

86. Robinson RW, White DP, Zwillich CW: Moderate alcohol ingestion increases upper airway resistance in normal subjects. Am Rev Respir Dis 132(6):1238–1241, 1985.

87. Dawson A, Bigby BG, Poceta JS, Mitler MM: Effect of bedtime alcohol on inspiratory resistance and respiratory drive in snoring and nonsnoring men. Alcohol Clin Exp Res 21(2):183–190, 1997.

88. Nozaki-Taguchi N, Isono S, Nishino T, et al: Upper airway obstruction during midazolam sedation: modification by nasal CPAP. Can J Anaesth 42(8):685–690, 1995.

89. Schneider H, Grote L, Peter JH, et al: The effect of triazolam and flunitrazepam—two benzodiazepines with different half-lives—on breathing during sleep. Chest 109(4):909–915, 1996.

90. Sullivan CE, Murphy E, Kozar LF, Phillipson EA: Waking and ventilatory responses to laryngeal stimulation in sleep dogs. J Appl Physiol 45(5):681–689, 1978.

91. Sullivan CE, Kozar LF, Murphy E, Phillipson EA: Arousal, ventilatory, and airway responses to bronchopulmonary stimulation in sleeping dogs. J Appl Physiol 47(1):17–25, 1979.

92. Issa FG, Porostocky S: Effect of sleep on changes in breathing pattern accompanying sign breaths. Respir Physiol 93(2):175–187, 1993.

93. Perez-Padilla R, West P, Kryger MH: Sighs during sleep in adult humans. Sleep 6(3):234–243, 1983.

94. Parmeggiani PL: Physiologic regulation in sleep. In Kryger MH, Roth T, Dement WC (eds): *Principles and Practice of Sleep Medicine*, 4th ed. Philadephia, Elsevier Saunders, 2005, pp 185–191.

95. Verrier RL: Cardiac physiology during sleep. In Lee-Chiong TL, Sateia MJ, Carskadon MA (eds): *Sleep Medicine*. Philadelphia, Hanley & Belfus, Inc., 2002, pp 53–57.

96. Verrier RL, Harper RM, Hobson JA: Cardiovascular physiology: central and autonomic regulation. In Kryger MH, Roth T, Dement WC (eds): *Principles and Practice of Sleep Medicine*, 4th ed. Philadephia, Elsevier Saunders, 2005, pp 192–202.

97. Franzini C: Cardiovascular physiology: the peripheral circulation. In Kryger MH, Roth T, Dement WC (eds): *Principles and Practice of Sleep Medicine*, 4th ed. Philadephia, Elsevier Saunders, 2005, pp 203–212.

98. Murali NS, Svatikova A, Somers VK: Cardiovascular physiology and sleep. Frontiers Biosci 8:s636–s652, 2000.

99. George CF, Kryger MH: Sleep and control of heart rate. Clin Chest Med 6(4):595–601, 1985.

100. Baust W, Bohnert B: The regulation of heart rate during sleep. Exp Brain Res 7:169–180, 1969.

101. Zemaityte D, Varoneckas G, Sokolov E: Heart rhythm control during sleep. Psychophysiology 21(3):279–290, 1984.

102. Guilleminault CP, Pool P, Motta J, et al: Sinus arrest during REM sleep in young adults. N Engl J Med 311:1006–1010, 1984.

103. Massin MM, Maeyns K, Withofs N, et al: Circadian rhythm of heart rate and heart rate variability. Arch Dis Child 83:179–182, 2000.

104. Task Force of the European and North American Society of Pacing and Electrophysiology: Heart rate variability: standards of measurement, physiological interpretation, and clinical use. Circulation 93(5):1043–1065, 1996.

105. Vanoli E, Adamson PB, Ba-Lin, et al: Heart rate variability during specific sleep stages—a comparison of healthy subjects with patients after myocardial infarction. Circulation 91(7):1918–1922, 1995.

106. Legramante JM, Marciani MG, Placidi F, et al: Sleep-related changes in baroreflex sensitivity and cardiovascular autonomic modulation. J Hypertens 21(8):1555–1561, 2003.

107. Lombardi F, Parati G: An update: cardiovascular and respiratory changes during sleep in normal and hypertensive subjects. Cardiovasc Res 45:200–211, 2000.

108. Verrier RL, Muller JE, Hobson JA: Sleep, dreams, and sudden death: the case for sleep as an autonomic stress test for the heart. Cardiovasc Res 31:181–211, 1996.

109. Lown B, Verrier RL: Neural activity and ventricular fibrillation. N Engl J Med 294(21):1165–1170, 1976.

110. Kirby DA, Verrier RL: Differential effects of sleep stages on coronary hemodynamic function. Am J Physiol 256:H1378–H1383, 1989.

111. Dickerson LW, Huang AH, Nearing BD, Verrier RL: Primary coronary vasodilatation associated with pauses in heart rhythm during sleep. Am J Physiol 264:186–196, 1993.

112. Smith HS, Sleight P, Pickering GW: Reflex regulation of arterial pressure during sleep in man. Circ Res 24:109–121, 1969.

113. Somers VK, Phil D, Dyken ME, et al: Sympathetic-nerve activity during sleep in normal subjects. N Engl J Med 328(5):303–307, 1993.

114. Grant DA, Franzini C, Wild J, Walker AM: Cerebral circulation in sleep: vasodilatory response to cerebral hypotension. J Cerebral Blood Flow Metab 18:639–645, 1998.

115. Cianci T, Zoccoli G, Lenzi P, Franzini C: Regional splanchnic blood flow during sleep in the rabbit. Eur J Physiol 415:594–597, 1990.

116. Cianci T, Zoccoli G, Lenzi P, Franzini C: Loss of integrative control of peripheral circulation during desynchronized sleep. Am J Physiol 261:R373–R377, 1991.

117. Noll G, Elam M, Kunimoto M, et al: Skin sympathetic nerve activity and effector function during sleep in humans. Acta Physiol Scand 151:319–329, 1994.

Sleep Breathing Disorders

TEOFILO L. LEE-CHIONG ■ CHARLES A. POLNITSKY

The snoring person has been historically portrayed in literature as one peacefully at rest in deepest sleep, perhaps disturbing his companions, but usually regarded with humor. There was no concern for the health of the individual. The past several decades have produced an entirely new picture, in which sleep-disordered breathing, ranging from snoring and mild increases in upper airway resistance to apnea with profound hypoxemia, actually causes profound physiologic reactions. Furthermore, the conditions are now recognized in both genders and at all ages. The incidence appears to be increasing beyond what would be expected from newfound awareness alone. Obesity, allergic upper airway conditions, and other influences, including survival advantages conferred by better health care, have combined to make sleep-disordered breathing one of the new epidemics of this millennium.

OBSTRUCTIVE SLEEP APNEA

Terminology centered around obstructive sleep apnea continues to evolve. In general, an obstructive apnea (OA) occurs when there is complete, or nearly complete, cessation of airflow, *accompanied by preservation of respiratory drive manifested by persistent respiratory muscle activity* (Figure 4-1). If there is partial reduction in airflow, of >30% of baseline, *with preservation of respiratory effort*, the event is defined as an obstructive hypopnea (OH) (Figure 4-2). Although OA and OH have different specific definitions, their pathophysiology and physiologic consequences are essentially similar, and in clinical polysomnographic reporting they are combined as a single result, the apnea-hypopnea index (AHI). The American Academy of Sleep Medicine standard, in fact, does not call for distinction between OA and OH under routine circumstances.[1] The magnitude of the AHI generally reflects the severity of excessive daytime sleepiness (EDS), cardiovascular risk, and general metabolic consequences of sleep-disordered breathing. It also provides cut points for treatment reimbursement. When respiratory effort-related arousals (RERAs, see later) are included in the total number of events, the convention is to report the sum as the respiratory disturbance index (RDI).

The term *obstructive sleep apnea* (OSA) is properly reserved to describe the *objective* documentation of OA and OH events. When an individual is diagnosed as having psychological or physiologic *manifestations* of OSA(s), that is person is considered to have the obstructive sleep apnea syndrome (OSAS), sometimes also termed the *obstructive sleep apnea/hypopnea syndrome*.[1]

Epidemiology

OSA is thought to affect approximately 5% of the adult US population.[2] Depending on how OSA and OSAS are defined, estimates of prevalence are as high as 20% of adults for OSA.[3] A general population study of randomly chosen, middle-age, State of Wisconsin employees found mild apnea (AHI ≥ 5) in 17% and moderate-severe apnea (AHI ≥ 20) in 7%.[4] Age, gender, and body mass index (BMI) have an important impact on prevalence in various cohorts. Apnea is present in 60% or more of individuals who have had a stroke (CVA)[5] and is increased in context of other chronic conditions such as congestive heart failure, polycystic ovary syndrome, and asthma. Although obesity-related, OSA is also found in context of normal weight, and its prevalence may be markedly underestimated because of failure of caregivers to consider the diagnosis in thin individuals.[6] A similar concern has been raised for the female gender.[7] OSA is not uncommon in children, although specific diagnostic criteria are not as clearly defined as in adults.[8,9]

Definitions

An OA/OH event is scored if there is a >50% reduction in flow, lasting ≥10 seconds. If the reduction is clearly visible but <50%, it must be accompanied by either or both of the following: a drop in oxygen saturation

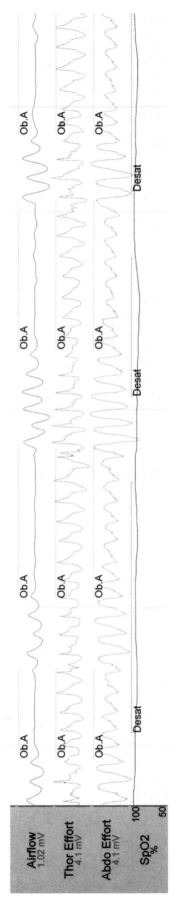

FIGURE 4-1 ■ Obstructive apnea. 2-minute screen. Complete cessation of airflow ≥10 seconds in duration, accompanied by persisting respiratory effort (Thor effort, Abdo effort). The associated desaturation is not essential for the events to be scored as OAs.

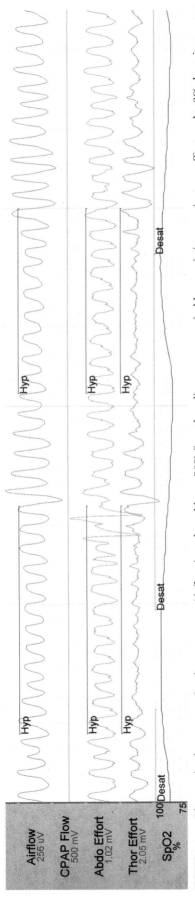

FIGURE 4-2 ■ Obstructive hypopnea. 2-minute screen. Airflow is reduced by ~ 50% from baseline, accompanied by persisting respiratory effort and >3% drop in oxygen saturation.

>3% or an electroencephalogram (EEG) arousal ≥ 3 seconds.[1] (Qualification is made for some instances in which a lesser reduction in airflow occurs.) It should be noted that there is considerable variation in the interpretation of data in both research and clinical laboratories, based on an evolving understanding of sleep-disordered breathing.[10] For Medicare treatment reimbursement, however, scoring of an OH is allowed only when there is a desaturation $\geq 4\%$.

Physiologic Consequences

With each OA or OH, as upper airway resistance increases, tidal volume falls, oxygen saturation drops, and CO_2 rises. Increased sympathetic activity causes vasoconstriction and frequently tachycardia, yielding an increase in blood pressure. As respiratory efforts against a narrowed or occluded airway increase, there may be reflex bradycardia and atrioventricular block. Once the apnea has terminated, there may be recovery tachycardia. Supraventricular and ventricular ectopy can occur in susceptible individuals.

A combination of increased preload, leftward shift of the intraventricular septum, reduction of left ventricular compliance, and increased afterload occurs. As a result, there may be an exacerbation of preexisting congestive heart failure (CHF).[11,12]

The physiologic stress imposed by each event causes a number of pathological responses. These include release of inflammatory mediators,[13–17] elevation of leptin,[18] increases in platelet adhesiveness[19] and fibrinogen levels, and reduced fibrinolytic activity.[20] Insulin resistance is also increased. In females, hyperinsulinemia shifts the androgen-estrogen balance of ovarian hormone synthesis more toward the androgen side.[21] Atrial naturetic peptide secretion is augmented by a false volume-overload signal, causing nocturia.[22] There also is cyclic elevation of microvascular resistance[23] and generalized persistent endothelial dysfunction.[24,25] Sympathetic responses to the stress of apnea can lead to diurnal persistence of hypertension[26–30] and worsening of CHF.[31,32] There appears to be an increased propensity toward development of atrial fibrillation and a 50% reduction in maintenance of normal sinus rhythm if the OSA is not corrected.[33]

Pulmonary artery pressure may become transiently elevated, and in a small percentage of individuals, fixed pulmonary hypertension occurs.[34] During periods of intense apnea and hypoxia, elevated right-sided cardiac pressures can lead to opening of a patent foramen ovale, exacerbating systemic hypoxia and increasing the risk of embolic stroke.[35]

Long-term intermittent hypoxia results in oxidative stress[15,36] and may further worsen pharyngeal muscle dilator function[37] (see Pathophysiology). Repetitive

mechanical trauma to the muscles can lead to inflammation and denervation, yielding a similar effect.[38] The final common physiologic pathway is increased atherogenesis.[39] There is evidence for acceleration of coronary artery disease,[40] the appearance of new clinical cardiovascular morbidity (recurrent atrial fibrillation, fatal and nonfatal myocardial infarction, and pulmonary hypertension), and an association with stroke.[41,42] Furthermore, studies have also shown that the progression of cardiovascular disease is retarded when OSA is corrected.[43–45]

Repetitive EEG arousals result in sleep fragmentation and in some cases suppression of normal sleep staging, especially stage rapid eye movement (REM). The failure to achieve restorative sleep and effects of oxidative stress are thought to be responsible for excessive daytime somnolence and affective complaints such as increased irritability, depression, and cognitive dysfunction, including deterioration of memory and ability to concentrate.

Pathophysiology

OSA can develop in any given individual as a result of the summation of a variety of predisposing anatomical and physiologic aberrations in the maintenance of upper airway patency during sleep. Determinants range from central nervous system drive to pharyngeal size and muscle control. Maintenance of upper airway patency reflects the balance of those forces that foster collapse (extraluminal tissue pressure and negative intraluminal pressure generated by inspiratory airflow) or maintenance of patency (action of pharyngeal dilator muscles, primarily the genioglossus, and traction from inspiratory lengthening).[46]

Although central apnea (CA) (see later) is categorized as a distinct and separate condition, there is evidence for abnormal central respiratory drive that is present in OSA as well.[47,48] Inspiration is marked by phasic increases in pharyngeal muscle tone, as well as in the diaphragm and accessory muscles of respiration. When there is instability in ventilatory control (*high loop gain*, a term that describes increased sensitivity and response to change in physiologic state in systems governed by feedback control), the ability of the controller to offset the mechanical forces leading to airway collapse may be overcome, resulting in OA.[46,49] Conversely, pharyngeal instability may contribute to the development of CA.[50]

Phasic increases in pharyngeal dilator tone are necessary to offset the tendency toward collapse. There is evidence of sleep stage-dependent compromised maintenance of pharyngeal tone during stage 2 and REM in children with OSA, pointing to an underlying alteration in mechanoreceptor/chemoreceptor control.[47] To overcome airway floppiness, pharyngeal dilator tone is increased even during wakefulness in children and adults[51,52] to counteract the diurnal increase in collapsibility.[53]

Sex hormone levels also play a role. There is an overall male predominance of OSA, but the association goes beyond simple gender influence. Testosterone replacement therapy in men has been reported to induce or worsen OSA.[54] Variation in OSA severity in women has been demonstrated through the menstrual cycle and during pregnancy.[55] It is also seen in women with polycystic ovary syndrome in excess of the prevalence that would be expected if caused by obesity alone.[21] Furthermore, the prevalence of OSA in females is approximately tripled after menopause,[56,57] thought to result from a drop in female hormone levels and a relative increase in androgen. This observation holds even with correction for age and BMI.[57]

Reduction of luminal diameter by hyperplastic tonsils and other tissues also increases collapsability. Also, increased pharyngeal length[58] and diameter appear to be factors in the development of OSA.[59] Obesity is a major factor, and historically, the phenotypic obesity-hypoventilator (pickwickian) was thought to represent most cases of OSA. There are various mechanisms by which an increased BMI predisposes to OSA. The simple reduction in upper airway diameter by retropharyngeal fat deposition has been seen in imaging studies.[60] Inspiratory resistive loading associated with increased thoracic and abdominal mass plays a role in effort-related airway collapse. There is evidence that autonomic dysfunction such as seen in diabetes may have an etiological role.[61] Whatever the mechanism, weight reduction can eliminate or reduce OSA severity in some individuals.[62,63]

In children, hyperplasia of tonsils and adenoids is responsible for most cases of OSA, although craniofacial abnormalities of various types may be etiological. Tonsillectomy is frequently curative, although exceptions commonly occur.[64] Furthermore, it is interesting to note that in a small but significant number of children successfully treated by surgery, OSA returns in puberty or adulthood, once again calling attention to the multifactorial etiology.[65]

Nasal obstruction in young children with allergy or congenital nasopharyngeal abnormalities can play a role.[66] Mouth breathing predisposes to snoring and increases the risk of apnea. In the long run, it also results in mandibular developmental insufficiency. Whether acquired, hereditary, or congenital, micrognathia and retrognathia cause pharyngeal narrowing. The same is true for macroglossia. With increasing age and BMI, even relatively subtle upper airway structural abnormalities predispose to OSA development. Table 4-1 contains a more comprehensive list of predisposing conditions.

TABLE 4-1 ■ Factors Associated with Development of OSA

Ear, nose, and throat	Seasonal allergic rhinitis
	Perennial rhinitis/sinusitis
	Nasal septal deviation
	Hyperplasia of tonsils/adenoids
	Retrognathia
	Micrognathia
	Incisor overjet
	Dental mandibular crowding
	Macroglossia
	High arched hard palate
	Extended soft palate
	Enlarged/elongated uvula
	Vocal cord paralysis
	Anatomically reduced pharyngeal area
	Increased pharyngeal length
	Heredofamilial craniofacial syndromes
	Treacher-Collins
	Pierre Robin
Metabolic/endocrine	Obesity
	Testosterone predominance
	Iatrogenic androgen supplementation
	Male gender
	Female postmenopausal state
	Pregnancy
	Hypothyroidism
Medical/constitutional conditions	Stroke
	Congestive heart failure
	Autonomic dysfunction
	Familial predisposition–multiple
	Charcot-Marie-Tooth syndrome
	Myotonic dystrophy
	Cervical spine injury
	Sedative use
	Alcohol consumption
	Tobacco smoking

Clinical Evaluation

The often cited medical maxim—unless a specific condition is considered as a possibility, its timely identification is unlikely—is especially true for OSA. The obese middle-age male who snores profoundly at night and falls asleep readily during the day does not pose a diagnostic challenge. In this circumstance, excessive daytime sleepiness (EDS) should always raise the possibility of OSA. An Epworth Sleepiness Score (ESS) > 10 is considered abnormal, but the ESS lacks sufficient specificity and sensitivity to be relied on exclusively. An elevated BMI in either gender and at any age increases the likelihood of a positive diagnosis; however, an increasing number of people with BMIs in the normal or minimally elevated range are being diagnosed with OSA now that the possibility is being considered.[6] A wide array of presenting complaints and comorbidities should prompt the clinician to perform an extended sleep-oriented history, physical examination, and laboratory evaluation. In addition to some highlights in the following paragraphs, Table 4-2 summarizes the clinical presentations that may suggest consideration of an OSA diagnosis.

Sleep-wake patterns and complaints may vary. The typical male with OSA will report feeling groggy in the morning (despite the perception of having had a good night's sleep) and may indicate nodding off while sitting quietly or driving; women are more likely to complain of insomnia, generalized daytime fatigue, and a variety of psychological and somatic complaints such as depression and headache.[7,67] Sleep fragmentation is sometimes accompanied by paroxysmal nocturnal dyspnea, palpitations, anxiety attacks, or dreams of physical exertion. Children may respond to sleep fragmentation from sleep-disordered breathing with hyperactivity, a report of behavioral difficulties, or diagnosis of attention deficit–hyperactivity disorder that should prompt a consideration of OSA.[68]

Hypertension, especially when relatively refractory to conventional treatment,[69] has been linked to OSA via cyclic episodes of apnea-associated hypoxia and augmented sympathetic discharge. Unexpected nocturia in both genders occurs when apnea results in alterations in circulatory dynamics causing inappropriate nocturnal secretion of atrial naturetic peptide. Gastroesophageal reflux symptoms, especially with nocturnal regurgitation, may be caused or exacerbated by OSA. The recurrent microaspiration of nasopharyngeal secretions and/or gastric contents associated with the inspiratory gasps following airway closure can lead to persistent hoarseness, tickle in the throat, and chronic cough. Male erectile dysfunction can be caused by OSA as well as by the many comorbidities that apnea sufferers may also have, such as hypertension and diabetes.

The presence of several specific endocrine abnormalities should raise a suspicion of OSA. There is an association with hypothyroidism,[70] probably multifactorial and based on reduction in metabolic rate; macroglossia; mucosal abnormalities; obesity; and other influences. Women with polycystic ovary syndrome have an increased prevalence of OSA in excess of that expected in context of obesity alone.[21] There is also an increased incidence of OSA in pregnancy. Unexpected difficulty with glycemic control may be an OSA marker. Most individuals with the metabolic syndrome should at least be queried about symptoms and signs that might raise suspicion for OSA, especially because of the cardiovascular risks.

Physical examination can also provide clues. A neck circumference greater than 17 inches has been identified as an OSA predictor. The examiner should also look for the craniofacial features discussed previously

TABLE 4-2 ■ Presenting Complaints and Physical Findings Suggesting OSA Diagnosis	
Sleep-related	Excessive sleep need
	Snoring
	Restless sleep
	Insomnia
	Bruxism
	Nonrestorative sleep
	Gasping arousals
	Nocturnal gastroesophageal reflux disease
	Nocturnal panic attacks
	Nocturia
	Parasomnias
	Dreams of exertion or suffocation
	Daytime complaints
	Morning somnolence
	Morning headache
	Morning dry mouth
	Excessive daytime somnolence
	Reduced quality of life
	Impaired job performance
	Generalized fatigue
	Drowsy driving
	Cognitive impairment
	Mood disorders
	Intense menopausal complaints
	Reduced libido/erectile dysfunction
	Somatic syndrome symptoms
	Fibromyalgia
	Chronic fatigue syndrome
	Irritable bowel syndrome
	Headache
	Refractory asthma
Miscellaneous conditions	Attention deficit disorder
	Dysglycemia
	Metabolic syndrome
	Polycystic ovary syndrome
	Refractory systemic hypertension
	Angiotensin converting enzyme
	Polymorphism
	Chronic renal failure
	Stroke
	Recurrent or unexpected atrial fibrillation
	Unexplained pulmonary hypertension
	Congestive heart failure
	Acromegaly
	Myotonic dystrophy
	Parkinson's disease
	Multiple system atrophy
	Down syndrome
	Postpolio syndrome
	Difficult intubation or anesthesia recovery

as well as the presence of significant nasal obstruction, a high arched palate, tonsillar hyperplasia, engorgement of pharyngeal tissues, and uvular prominence. Approximately 70% of individuals with Down syndrome will have OSA either by history or on polysomnography. There is also a significantly increased incidence in persons with neuromuscular diseases and parkinsonism.

A history of difficult endotracheal intubation, slow postoperative recovery from anesthesia, unexplained postoperative hypoxemia, or need for reintubation after anesthesia should raise the suspicion of underlying OSA.[71]

Reports from family members or bed partner should also be elicited. Witnesses often report persistent nodding off, especially under inappropriate social circumstances. Bed partners may have taken to sleeping in another room or have banished the patient from the bedroom because of disruptive snoring.

Diagnosis

Attended in-laboratory polysomnography remains the reference standard for diagnosis.[10] OA and OH are detected by various sensors of oronasal airflow and thoracic and abdominal excursion. Integrated airflow signals are supplementing or replacing thermistor-generated data because their sensitivity and response times are better.[1] In addition, they provide information about more subtle events such as RERAs (see later).[72]

Transcutaneous oximetry provides data on depth and duration of apnea-associated hypoxia and response to treatment. An oximeter with appropriate sensitivity and response time is necessary to avoid overdiagnosis or underdiagnosis of desaturations.[73] Pediatric sleep laboratories also frequently monitor transcutaneous CO_2 because the identification of OSA is significantly more challenging and less well defined in children than in adults.[9]

Three or four EEG channels are commonly used to identify sleep stage and document arousals. Extraocular motion and peripheral leg electromyogram channels assist in the definition of stage REM.

An AHI < 5 is considered normal, although there is strong evidence that persistent snoring and the upper airway resistance syndrome (UARS) confer similar adverse health consequences, modifying a negative polysomnogram (PSG) interpretation in this context (see UARS, later). An AHI of 5–14 is arbitrarily ranked as mild, 15–30 as moderate, and ≥30 as severe disease, but the designations vary among laboratories. A case can be made for designating an AHI > 15–20 as having increased physiologic significance because it is at this approximate level that some of the adverse consequences (such as increased blood coagulability and platelet adhesion) appear.

Current Medicare guidelines for treatment are generally accepted by most commercial insurance providers. These are an AHI ≥ 5, determined over a minimum of 2 hours of actual sleep time, in context of at least one of the following: hypertension, cardiac disease, history of stroke, insomnia, excessive daytime somnolence, depression, or cognitive dysfunction. Medicare also calls for treatment of individuals with an AHI ≥ 15 even in the absence of the additional modifiers. As emphasized previously, the guidelines specifically require that an OH be defined by an oxygen desaturation ≥ 4% and exclude the diagnosis based on an arousal without desaturation.[74]

The definition of pediatric OSA is not as precise.[9,68] The current accepted PSG criterion is an AHI ≥ 1 for children and adolescents up to the age of 16.[8]

Numerous lower-level diagnostic approaches are available. They range from snoring recorders[75] and recording oximetry to multichannel home PSG systems. As a screening technique, overnight oximetry has adequate sensitivity but may lack specificity and is not recommended.[10,76] Various multichannel data collectors, used in both attended and unattended settings, have been used in an attempt to substitute for formal PSG, but data are difficult to compare, and the accuracy of the testing continues to be evaluated.[77] American Academy of Sleep Medicine (AASM) guidelines continue to call for attended, in-lab PSG under most circumstances.[78,79] Simple problems such as loss of electrode contact can be easily repaired. Sleep staging is provided. Diagnosis of other significant conditions such as limb movement disorders, parasomnias, seizure activity, and cardiac dysrhythmias is facilitated. In-lab PSG also affords an opportunity for continuous positive airway pressure (CPAP) titration in the second half of the night. Studies have demonstrated the equivalence of the split-night study to a full-night PSG followed by a second night devoted to CPAP titration.[80]

Therapy

CPAP remains the definitive treatment for essentially all individuals.[81,82] Current AASM practice standards call for the initial titration to be performed in-laboratory to facilitate mask fitting, patient training, and desensitization where needed, as well as to document the achievement of well-consolidated sleep under positive airway pressure circumstances. Ideally, a CPAP pressure is determined that achieves essentially total elimination of apneas, with the patient in supine stage REM sleep (Figure 4-3).

The mechanism by which CPAP reverses airway collapse is generally considered to be via the generation of a "pneumatic splint" to the upper airway.[83] Since inspiration generates a pressure drop that causes the airway to collapse, and persons with OSA have an abnormally elevated critical closing pressure, pressurization of the airway is thought to counteract

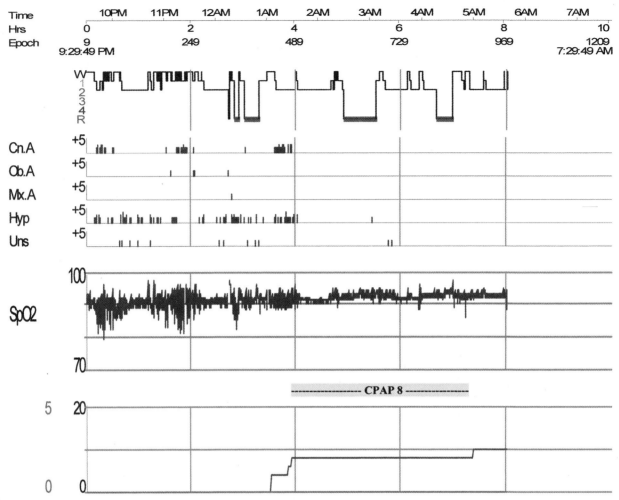

FIGURE 4-3 ■ Split-night polysomnography. This individual has a combination of respiratory effort–related arousals (Uns), obstructive hypopneas (Hyp), a mixed apnea (Mx.A), obstructive apneas (ObA.), and central apneas (Cn.A), with associated desaturation. Nearly all events are eliminated by CPAP titration done in the second half of the night.

inspiratory collapse. An alternative recent suggestion invokes the increased lung volume effect of CPAP as a reason for CPAP effectiveness.[84] The usual therapeutic range for CPAP is 4–20 cm H_2O. Use of CPAP appears to reduce the development of cardiovascular disease possibly in proportion to nightly duration of use.[43,44]

When a patient experiences high CPAP pressure intolerance, alternative modes such as bilevel positive airway pressure (BiPAP) may be used.[85] In this instance, the inspiratory pressure (iPAP) is usually maintained at ~3–5 CWP above the expiratory (ePAP) setting and pressures are sequentially elevated to provide control of apnea at the lowest possible setting. Although there are proponents of BiPAP as an important technique to improve overall CPAP compliance, studies have failed to demonstrate consistent benefit.[81,86] BiPAP, however, may be of use in massively obese individuals with marked reduction in chest wall compliance who require a degree of noninvasive mechanical respiratory assist that the modality provides.[81]

Similarly, there is scant evidence that autotitrating positive airway pressure (APAP) devices[87] provide major benefit to most CPAP-intolerant persons.[88] In controlled studies, the mean APAP pressure needed to control apnea has not been shown to be consistently much lower than the fixed setting that was determined during lab titration, and nightly duration of use has only slightly increased in most studies.[89] In general, there is no indication for APAP devices to be prescribed as first-line therapy.[90] APAP devices differ in the sensor array and algorithms for apnea detection, and units from different manufacturers are not necessarily comparable.[91] They are not indicated for use in persons with CHF, chronic obstructive pulmonary disease, or hypoxemic respiratory failure or in nonsnorers. APAP devices may be used during attended in-lab titration but should not be used for initial titration at home.[82,91] A small number of persons, however, show a strong preference for APAP as their standard mode of airway pressurization and can be thus maintained. CPAP generators that feature expiratory pressure relief are also being offered as alternatives to standard CPAP. They have not been subjected to sufficient objective study to demonstrate their therapeutic equivalence or superiority to the conventional CPAP.[92,93]

At the other end of the therapeutic spectrum, tracheostomy is also universally effective. Because of the surgical risk and potential for long-term complications, tracheostomy is usually reserved for certain specific cases: (1) when death from hypoxia or cor pulmonale is considered imminent and CPAP is not effective; (2) morbid obesity with hypoventilation that requires nocturnal mechanical ventilation; and (3) in cases of fixed upper airway obstruction where CPAP is ineffective. Individuals who do not require a cuffed tube to permit mechanical ventilation can be fitted with a low-profile flanged device that can be plugged during the daytime to allow normal respiration and speech.

For individuals with genuine CPAP intolerance whose apnea is based on pharyngeal narrowing at the level of the base of the tongue, mandibular advancement devices (MAD; also referred to as *anterior mandibular positioners*) provide an alternative, but often less effective, option.[94] When given the opportunity to try both CPAP and MAD, more people have preferred the MAD and have used it more consistently, but the therapeutic response has not been equivalent.[95] Whereas CPAP is nearly always close to 100% effective, mandibular advancement has a wide range of response. Some individuals experience little or no reduction in AHI. An adjustable device, rather than one made from a fixed mold, should be used, and the degree of advancement may need to be titrated over time. PSG confirmation of effectiveness is essential to avoid a situation in which snoring has been silenced but apnea remains.[96] Adaptation to MAD use is difficult for some people who experience excessive salivation or temporomandibular joint discomfort. In contrast to CPAP, which has been extensively studied since its inception in 1981, MAD experience is limited both in case size and length of follow-up. Application continues to be evaluated.[97]

There is a wide range of variously invasive surgical procedures for the control of OSA,[98] but their indications and effectiveness continue to be debated.[99,100] The current consensus is as follows. Minor procedures such as laser-assisted uvuloplasty (LAUP) have no role in the treatment of OSA, although they may silence simple snoring at least temporarily.[101] Procedures with increasing complexity such as uvulopalatopharyngoplasty (UPPP), genioglossus advancement/hyoid fixation, and mandibulo-maxillary advancement yield increasingly better results but have unpredictable effectiveness on an individual basis, involve some amount of risk and discomfort, and may have permanent untoward sequelae. The most consistent positive results are found in cases of pharyngeal narrowing with an anatomical etiology that can be specifically corrected. More detailed description is beyond the scope of this chapter but may be found in recent summary statements and reviews.[98,102]

Weight loss can lessen OSA. The most quoted projection is that a 10% reduction in weight results in a 26% drop in the AHI, based on a cohort of mildly overweight individuals.[103] A somewhat less favorable result was recently reported.[104] Results in morbid obesity may be more dramatic.[105] Except in context of bariatric surgery, however, maintenance of the loss is difficult.[106] Open and laparoscopic gastric bypass, gastric banding, and intragastric balloon techniques are the most common procedures.[107,108] Because OSA is multifactorial in etiology, several series of patients have shown that OSA can recur in some individuals, even if the weight loss has been maintained.[105,108]

There is no evidence that noninvasive treatments and devices have a therapeutic role.[109] Nasopharyngeal lubricants and sprays, nasal dilators, oral dietary supplements, and magnetic therapy have failed to show a beneficial effect on OSA. Plastic soft palate stents, radiofrequency tongue volume reduction, and soft palate chemical and radiofrequency ablation have also been used, but datasets are small and results not encouraging. Research is underway on medications that modify neurotransmitter activity[110,111] and on hypoglossal nerve stimulation.[112]

Some individuals who have had OSA eliminated by effective treatment fail to experience the expected relief from excessive daytime somnolence. For them, the judicious use of modafinil as a maintenance of wakefulness agent has been approved by the Food and Drug Administration.[113] It should be stressed that recourse to stimulants is only indicated and justified if OSA control has been verified. Because most persons are being treated with CPAP, there must be documentation via surveillance download data from the CPAP generator that compliance is consistent and the CPAP setting is appropriate. Pharmacological treatment of daytime somnolence in lieu of prescribed CPAP use is not medically defensible.[114]

CENTRAL SLEEP APNEA

CA results from an instability of central nervous system controller mechanisms. In contrast to OSA, central apneas occur when there is a temporary cessation of signaling to inspiratory muscles. Airway collapse may also occur,[115] but it is not the pivotal event or necessary for diagnosis. Rather, gradual or abrupt cessation of airflow results from a lapse in controller signaling. Thus no inspiratory efforts accompany central apneas (Figure 4-4). CA frequently causes oxygen desaturation but is usually terminated by the increased PCO_2 that results from the apnea. As with OSA, sleep fragmentation is common. Because CA may occur under a diverse set of pathological conditions, a unifying underlying mechanism is unlikely to be found.

Pathophysiology

CA occurs in a number of distinct patterns. Random events meeting the preceding criteria can be seen in many individuals undergoing PSG. Because an instability of ventilatory control is thought to underlie *all* forms of apnea, it has been proposed that there is an overlap in the mechanisms by which central and obstructive apneas occur.[116] In the awake state, control of ventilation is a function of responses to changes in $PaCO_2$ and PO_2, as well as input from behavioral and wakefulness activity.[46] In sleep, most of the modulating influence originates from changes in $PaCO_2$ and PaO_2. Hypoxic and hypercapnic responses in general are blunted in sleep, especially in stage REM, although some gender-specific variation has been described.[117] Changes in PaO_2 within the normal physiologic range do not cause a large respiratory variation. Relatively small changes in $PaCO_2$, however, result in brisk, inversely proportionate responses in minute ventilation. $PaCO_2$ variation is considered to be the dominant respiratory controller in sleep.[116] Because CO_2 responsiveness falls during sleep, sleep-onset central apneas are commonly seen.

CAs can also occur as CPAP pressures reach therapeutic levels during titration for OSA. This is thought to result from reflex controller inhibition as partial pharyngeal closure occurs.[50] CA has been described following tracheostomy for OSA, illustrating the overlap between the two forms of apnea. Occasionally, mixed apneas are encountered. There is an apparent initial CA event in which the terminal portion is marked by a return of respiratory efforts in what appears to have become an OA (Figure 4-5). The specific underlying mechanism has not been fully resolved.[118,119] Other, more significantly pathological forms of CA are outlined next.

Cheyne-Stokes Respiration

When an alternating hyperventilation/hypoventilation cycle is evident, the term *periodic breathing* (PB) is applied. The most commonly recognized form of PB is Cheyne-Stokes respiration (CSR), typically seen in the context of CHF. Individuals with CHF-linked CSR generally have a *reduced* baseline $PaCO_2$ secondary to hyperventilation associated with heightened sympathetic activity and pulmonary vagal stimulation[120] in the context of increased controller responsiveness to CO_2, although some disagreement about specifics exists.[46] Any source of a further increase in minute ventilation pushes the $PaCO_2$ below the apneic threshold and a CA occurs. As $PaCO_2$ rises, respirations resume. It appears that the prolonged circulation time in CHF results in an overshoot of the hyperpnea and an extension of the periodic breathing cycle, yielding the characteristic cyclic crescendo-decrescendo pattern of CSR with a periodicity of about 1 minute[121] (Figure 4-6). Thus a rhythmic oscillation between hyperpnea and hypopnea/apnea around the apneic threshold occurs. CSR is usually seen in NREM sleep. A more subtle but similar pattern can be seen during wakefulness in some CHF-afflicted individuals.

CSR has also been described in stroke, but in most cases it is now thought to be a manifestation of coexisting occult or subclinical left ventricular dysfunction.[122] The hyperpneic phase of CSR has also been shown to be the origin of ventricular ectopy that persists even if associated hypoxia is corrected.[123] The presence of CSR in CHF increases mortality risk, and its correction reduces this trend.[124]

High-Altitude Periodic Breathing

Hypoxic drive is augmented by the reduced barometric pressure at high altitude, yielding hyperpnea and consequent hypocapnia. As in CSR, hyperpnea is only retarded when $PaCO_2$ falls sufficiently to trigger alkalosis-induced apnea. Increasing hypoxia and rising $PaCO_2$ will propagate the cycle, which is more pronounced in sleep. Periodic breathing at sea level, having a similar disorder of respiratory control, can also occur[125] (Figure 4-7).

Idiopathic Central Sleep Apnea

Idiopathic central sleep apnea is a relatively uncommon condition afflicting individuals who have an inherent high chemoreceptor responsiveness that drives ventilation and results in hypocapnia even at sea level.[46] As with high-altitude PB, the cycling is exaggerated during sleep; the smooth crescendo-decrescendo pattern of CRS and PB, however, is frequently absent, and apneas may be abruptly terminated. This observation indicates that additional mechanisms may also exist.

Central Apnea Associated with Baseline Hypercapnia

A wide variety of conditions, having different etiologies, comes under this heading. The most common is

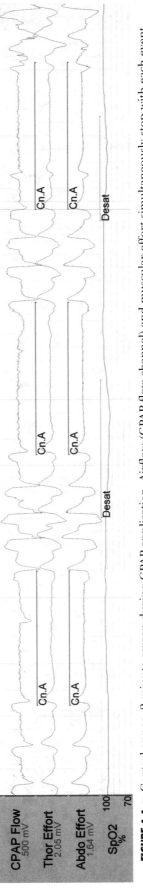

FIGURE 4-4 ■ Central apnea. 2-minute screen during CPAP application. Airflow (CPAP flow channel) and muscular effort simultaneously stop with each event.

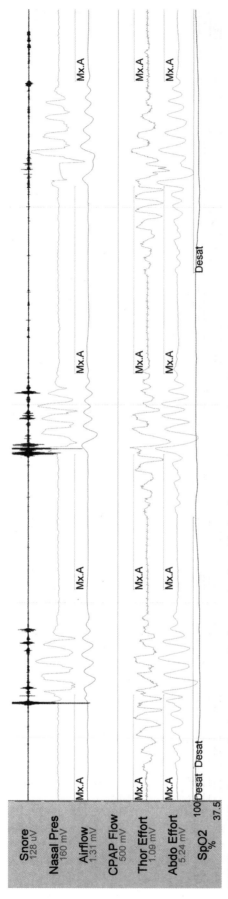

FIGURE 4-5 ■ Mixed apnea. 2-minute screen. Each event begins with simultaneous interruption of both airflow and muscular effort, resembling a CA, but resumption of effort precedes reestablishment of respiration, characteristic of OA.

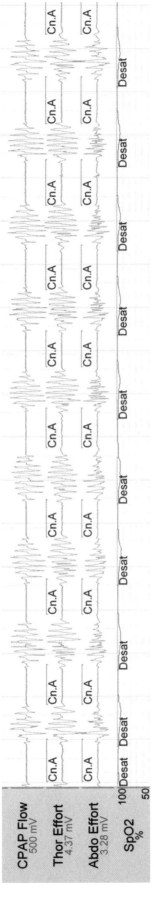

FIGURE 4-6 ■ Central sleep apnea/Cheyne-Stokes respiration. 10-minute screen. Persisting CAs with a waxing and waning pattern and a periodicity of ∼1 minute. Oxygen desaturations accompany each event.

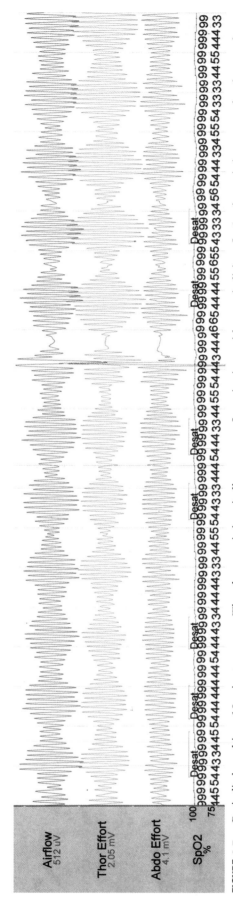

FIGURE 4-7 ■ Periodic breathing. 10-minute screen. The characteristic spindle pattern of respirations with a periodicity of ~1 minute is interrupted only once by an airflow cessation. Desaturations accompany most events (values are read vertically).

TABLE 4-3 ■ Central Apnea Classification	
Nonhypercapnic	Central sleep apnea/Cheyne-Stokes respiration
	Idiopathic central sleep apnea
	High-altitude central apnea
	Periodic breathing at sea level
	Incidental (e.g., at sleep onset)
Hypercapnic	Obesity/hypoventilation syndrome
	Congenital central apnea
	Neuromuscular diseases

the obesity-hypoventilation syndrome, discussed later. Other neuromuscular diseases compromising mechanical gas exchange and leading to chronic hypercapnia can result in CA, but upper airway instability may also result in OSA in these instances. Central alveolar hypoventilation secondary to various acquired neurological abnormalities or lesions, especially in the brainstem, may be accompanied by CA. Table 4-3 summarizes the classification of CA.

MIXED CENTRAL AND OBSTRUCTIVE APNEA

Some individuals show combined OSA and CA. As control of airway stability is established with CPAP, they develop intractable CA, especially during NREM sleep. Once again, this phenomenon reflects common underlying pathophysiology.[126]

Clinical Manifestations

As partially considered previously, the manifestations of CA vary in the context of the specific form and underlying etiology.[116] In general, a considerably smaller database on CA has been collected compared with the extensive literature on OSA. Obesity-hypoventilators are typically plethoric and lethargic, and show signs of congestive heart disease. Those with idiopathic central apnea present with a variety of complaints, including fatigue and other problems found with OSA, but more commonly these patients complain of insomnia or sleep fragmentation. They are often not obese. As CA also results in hypoxic periods, as with OSA, it can result in pulmonary and systemic hypertension.

Diagnosis

PSG is the primary diagnostic tool for CA of any etiology. The current standards vary somewhat but generally call for an AI > 5 in pure CA, or for ~80% of apneas to be central in cases of mixed disease. Central apneas

are scored when airflow and thoracoabdominal movement simultaneously pause for ≥10 seconds.[1] Central hypopneas are scored if there is a 30–80% drop in airflow and muscle effort channels for the same duration. Refinements in diagnosis are based on clinical context and patterns of frequency, such as are seen in CSR.

Treatment

The underlying etiology of the specific form of CA often determines specific treatment.[127] For CSR, the use of CPAP has become established. The mechanism appears to be indirect, via augmentation of cardiac output. CPAP produces this result via a number of effects, including improvement in afterload and shifting of the interventricular septum. CPAP also effects a slight increase in $PaCO_2$ (possibly by reducing hyperventilation caused during apnea recovery or by increased lung water), pushing the value beyond the apneic threshold and triggering the resumption of controller signaling. CPAP improves left ventricular function parameters, but it remains unclear whether mortality is reduced.[128] BiPAP has also been used, but recent evidence indicates that it may in fact worsen CSR by inducing further controller instability.[129] Noninvasive adaptive positive pressure ventilation has also been reported to be effective.[130] Oxygen therapy has also been shown to cause a significant reduction in the AHI[131] but does not appear to improve left ventricle (LV) function[132] or arrhythmia.[133] When neuromuscular disease is the underlying etiology, BiPAP has also been used.[134]

Idiopathic central sleep apnea is not responsive to a specific treatment approach. Oxygen administration, respiratory stimulants, and metabolic agents such as acetazolamide have been used with variable success. In some cases in which OSA and CA are combined, CPAP has been shown to control both forms. For refractory mixed disease unresponsive to conventional approaches, continuously controlled CO_2 added to positive airway pressure has shown promise.[135]

Patients with hypercapnic cental sleep apnea may require nocturnal ventilation. Most are currently managed with the use of noninvasive positive pressure ventilation. Historically, and in selected cases today, there is a role for external ventilatory assist devices or mechanical ventilation via tracheostomy.

SNORING

Vibration of upper airway structures, including the soft palate, uvula, and lateral walls of the pharynx, during sleep causes snoring. The character and timbre of the audible sound produced is influenced by the site(s) of vibration. Although snoring is often noted during inspiration, it can also occur during exhalation. There is a male predominance in snoring prevalence. Women may develop snoring during pregnancy. A positive family history can often be elicited.

The upper airway, from the nares to the larynx, is a flexible collapsible tube that performs various functions in respiration, swallowing, and phonation. In anatomically susceptible upper airways, snoring is produced when the inspiratory luminal negative pressure exceeds the distending activity of the upper airway muscles.[136] Collapsibility increases during sleep as a result of a reduction in upper airway muscle tone. Differences in collapsibility of the upper airway, defined by its critical closing pressure (P_{crit}), determine whether snoring, hypopneas, or apneas result.[137] Sleep disordered breathing can also stem from, or be made worse by, nasal obstruction. Nasal congestion may give rise to oronasal breathing that further compromises the upper airway.[138]

Data from the Wisconsin Sleep Cohort Study revealed that habitual snorers tend to have a higher prevalence of apnea-hypopnea indices of 15 or higher.[139] Nonetheless, snoring by itself lacks specificity for obstructive sleep apnea syndrome.

Snorers may present for evaluation and management when snoring is causing significant disruption of the bed partner's or roommate's sleep or when there is concern that snoring is associated with obstructive sleep apnea syndrome.

The bed partner should be asked about duration, frequency, and intensity of snoring. Risk factors for snoring include a supine sleep position, nasal congestion, and the ingestion of alcohol, muscle relaxants, opioid analgesics, and sedative-hypnotic agents close to bedtime, as well as smoking. In one study, current smokers had a significantly greater risk of snoring compared with never smokers and former smokers.[140] Snoring can also worsen with sleep deprivation.

Snoring should be differentiated from stridor resulting from laryngeal narrowing, incoherent sleep talking, and expiratory groaning during sleep (catathrenia) in which groaning usually occurs during the second part of the night during REM and non-REM (NREM) stage 2 sleep. Otorhinolaryngological and neurological evaluation is normal in patients with catathrenia.[141]

Snorers share many of the upper airway features of patients with OSA. Examination may demonstrate swollen nasal mucosa; enlargement of the tonsils, uvula, and tongue; narrowing of the airway by the lateral pharyngeal walls; a low palate; and retrognathia. Referral to an otorhinolaryngologist for fiberoptic pharyngoscopy may provide additional information that might be useful for patients with incomplete

response to medical therapy or those who are considering surgery for their snoring. However, pharyngoscopic features do not reliably predict responses to surgical interventions for snoring.

PSG is not routinely indicated in the evaluation of snorers, but it might be helpful in patients undergoing upper airway surgery, especially if other symptoms suggestive of obstructive sleep apnea, such as daytime sleepiness, are present. Snoring is identified during PSG either by using microphones or sound/vibration sensors placed either on the neck or near the oronasal opening, or from reports of audible snoring by the sleep technologists.

Patients with problematic snoring should be advised to maintain optimal weight, avoid smoking and alcohol consumption, and restrict the use of muscle relaxants and sedatives. If snoring is present only, or is worse, during a supine sleep position, measures to maintain a nonsupine posture during sleep may be beneficial. The bed partner can be offered noise-reducing therapies, such as the use of earplugs. Needless to say, appropriately titrated CPAP therapy will eliminate snoring, but this therapy is not universally covered by medical insurers.

Causes of nasal congestion, if present, should be identified and addressed appropriately. Medical therapies for nasal congestion might include avoidance of allergens, oral antihistamines, nasal decongestants, nasal anticholinergic agents, or nasal corticosteroids. A report by the Clinical Practice Committee of the AASM indicated that there is limited data available on the beneficial effect of external nasal dilator strips, internal nasal dilator devices, and oral-nasal lubricants for snoring; therefore there is currently insufficient information to provide standards of practice recommendations.[142]

An oral device constructed to advance the mandible or tongue is an effective treatment option for snoring,[94] and clinical guidelines for its use in patients with snoring or obstructive sleep apnea have been published.[143]

Surgical approaches to snoring include radiofrequency surgery of the soft palate,[144] LAUP,[101] UPPP, and palatal implants to reduce palatal flutter.[145] Specific nasal surgery (septoplasty for nasal septal deviation, polypectomy for nasal polyps, and turbinectomy for engorged nasal turbinates) can be considered for patients with considerable nasal narrowing or obstruction.

UPPER AIRWAY RESISTANCE SYNDROME

As its name implies, UARS is characterized by repetitive episodes of increase in resistance to airflow in the upper airways associated with arousals from sleep. Frequent arousals, in turn, result in sleep fragmentation and complaints of hypersomnolence.[146] Other associated features include fatigue and a higher prevalence of systemic hypertension.[147] Snoring may or may not be present. Patients may also present with less-specific somatic complaints including headaches, irritable bowel syndrome, and sleep-onset insomnia.[148]

Accurate identification of UARS is hampered by the lack of standardized diagnostic criteria. Definitions commonly include the presence of EEG arousals after one to three breaths with increased inspiratory effort (more negative peak end-inspiratory esophageal pressure [Pes] swings) and decrement in airflow. Pes is an indicator of respiratory effort. This is then followed by less negative Pes excursions as airflow increases during arousals. The apnea-hypopnea index should be less than five events per hour, and there is no oxygen desaturation. Respiratory events may be accompanied by increases in heart rate and systolic and diastolic pressures and changes in electrocardiographic R-R intervals.[149]

Two types of breathing patterns have been described in patients with UARS. A crescendo pattern, seen commonly during stages 1 and 2 NREM sleep, consists of a more negative peak end-inspiratory Pes. In contrast, regular and continuous high respiratory efforts are seen during stages 3 and 4 NREM sleep.[150]

Nasal cannula/pressure transducers may capture a pattern of airflow limitation with an inspiratory "plateauing" or flattened contour of the tracing corresponding with the increasingly negative pleural pressure excursions, followed by a rounded contour during arousals.[151] Although more accurate than thermistors, nasal cannula/pressure transducers may, nonetheless, fail to detect all abnormal breathing episodes during sleep.[150]

Mild upper airway abnormalities may be appreciated during physical examination. There is no apparent gender difference.

Polysomnography often demonstrates a longer duration of wake after sleep onset and decreased duration of slow wave sleep.[147]

The proper identification of UARS might be particularly important in patients with a presumptive diagnosis of idiopathic hypersomnia.[152]

Therapies proposed for patients with UARS have included nasal CPAP[146] and anterior mandibular positioning devices.[153] A variety of surgical interventions, including tonsillectomy and adenoidectomy for pediatric cases and palatal surgery, have been described. Novel treatment options such as internal jaw distraction osteogenesis are being investigated.[154]

OBESITY HYPOVENTILATION SYNDROME

Obesity hypoventilation syndrome is characterized by the presence of severe obesity (defined as a BMI[3]

> 40 kg/m^2) and hypercapnia (elevated arterial partial pressure of carbon dioxide [PaCO$_2$]) during wakefulness. Hypercapnia develops as a result of increased production of carbon dioxide owing to greater work of breathing and decreased ventilation (e.g., decreased expiratory reserve volume, decreased tidal volume, increased resistive load, and increased dead space). In addition, ventilatory response to hypercapnia and hypoxemia is decreased.

Although weight is a significant factor in the pathogenesis of OHS, even among obese persons, OHS is uncommon. In one study of hospitalized patients with severe obesity, hypoventilation was present in 31% of subjects who did not have other reasons for hypercapnia. These patients required greater intensive care, long-term care at discharge, and mechanical ventilation, and they had higher mortality at 18 months after hospital discharge compared with patients with simple obesity without OHS.[155]

Patients may present with complaints of hypersomnolence, decreased objective attention or concentration, peripheral edema, or cyanosis. Evaluation may disclose the presence of periodic respiration, hypoxemia, pulmonary hypertension, and polycythemia. Severe obesity can be associated with mild-to-moderate degrees of restrictive ventilatory impairment.

Although OSA is present in most cases of OHS, patients may present without OSA. Diurnal arterial blood gas measurements are worse and pulmonary artery hypertension is more frequent in those with OHS compared with patients with OSA.[156]

Other causes of chronic hypoventilation, such as severe chronic obstructive pulmonary disease, neuromuscular disorders, or diaphragmatic paralysis, should be excluded.

Nasal CPAP therapy and nasal noninvasive mechanical ventilation (NIMV) during sleep are effective therapies for patients with OHS.[157] The use of NIMV in patients with OHS has resulted in improvements in hypersomnolence, dyspnea, morning headache, leg edema, and arterial blood gas parameters.[158] Gastric surgery for morbid obesity has also been shown to improve symptoms, increase PaO$_2$, and decrease PaCO$_2$.[159] No pharmacological agent has, thus far, been found to be effective for OHS.

CONGENITAL CENTRAL HYPOVENTILATION SYNDROME

Hypoventilation and failure of the autonomic respiratory control in patients with congenital central hypoventilation syndrome (CCHS) is present from birth. Ventilatory responses to hypoxia and hypercarbia are impaired because of a disorder of central chemoreceptor responsiveness.

Hypoventilation during sleep can be severe with lack of ventilatory or arousal response. In one study, significant abnormalities of arterial blood gas parameters were observed with $PaCO_2$ (mean ± structural equation modeling) of 62 ± 2.5 mm Hg and a hemoglobin saturation of $65\% \pm 3.3\%$.[160] Hypoventilation is characteristically most severe during REM sleep.

Activity and exercise can result in worsening gas exchange with greater hypoxemia and hypercarbia and a lesser increase in heart rate.[161] Affected patients have no subjective sensation of dyspnea.[162] Despite the absence of chemoreceptor function, however, hyperpnea can occur during exercise with increasing respiratory frequency rather than an augmentation of tidal volume responsible for the increase in minute ventilation.[163]

Clinical manifestation, including tachycardia, diaphoresis, and cyanosis, vary depending on disease severity. Onset is typically during the newborn period with episodic apnea, cyanosis, feeding difficulties, or bradycardia. Proper diagnosis might be delayed until infancy when apparent life-threatening events, respiratory arrest, or pulmonary hypertension may develop.

Children with CCHS can develop arrhythmias (e.g., heart block and sick sinus syndrome), seizures, syncope, heat intolerance, esophageal dysmotility, and ophthalmological abnormalities. Hirschsprung disease and tumors of neural-crest derivatives (i.e., ganglioneuromas and neuroblastomas) have been reported.[160] Growth may be impaired with hypotonia or major motor delay.[160] Impaired mental processing may be present. CCHS patients may also have dysfunction of the autonomic nervous system control of the heart with decreased heart rate variability.[164] This potentially life-threatening disorder appears to be rare.

The exact pathophysiological mechanisms remain incompletely defined.[165] Heterozygous de novo mutations in PHOX2B have been described in patients with CCHS and associated autonomic dysfunction. A majority of mutations consist of 5–9 alanine expansions within a 20-residue polyalanine tract (exon 3).[166] There was an association between repeat mutation length and severity of the CCHS phenotype. Diagnosis of CCHS is aided by genetic testing for mutations of the polyalanine expansion sequence of the PHOX2b gene. Less commonly, patients may demonstrate an EDN3 frameshift point mutation.[167]

CCHS should be distinguished from other congenital syndromes that are associated with abnormalities in respiratory control, such as Prader-Willi syndrome and familial dysautonomia. Other causes of chronic hypoventilation, such as cardiopulmonary, neuromuscular, and metabolic disorders, should also be excluded.[168]

Patients require either continuous 24-hour ventilatory support or, if they are able to maintain adequate spontaneous respiration while awake, ventilatory support during sleep.[160] Ventilatory support can be provided at home with positive-pressure ventilation (via a tracheostomy or a nasal/oronasal mask), bi-level positive airway pressure device, negative-pressure ventilation, or diaphragm pacers using phrenic nerve stimulation.[162]

REFERENCES

1. Sleep-related breathing disorders in adults: recommendations for syndrome definition and measurement techniques in clinical research: The report of an American Academy of Sleep Medicine Task Force. Sleep 22(5):667–689, 1999.
2. Caples SM, Gami AS, Somers VK: Obstructive sleep apnea. Ann Intern Med 142(3):187–197, 2005.
3. Young T, Skatrud J, Peppard PE: Risk factors for obstructive sleep apnea in adults. JAMA 291(6):2013–2016, 2004.
4. Young T, Peppard PE, Gottlieb DJ: Epidemiology of obstructive sleep apnea: a population health perspective. Am J Resp Crit Care Med 165(9):1217–1239, 2002.
5. Bassetti C, Aldrich MS: Sleep apnea in acute cerebrovascular diseases: final report on 128 patients. Sleep 22(2):217–223, 1999.
6. Lettieri CJ, Eliasson AE, Andrada T, et al: Obstructive sleep apnea syndrome: are we missing an at-risk population? J Clin Sleep Med 1(4):381–385, 2005.
7. Young T, Peppard PE: Clinical presentation of OSAS: gender does matter. Sleep 28(3):293–295, 2005.
8. Uliel S, Tauman R, Greenfield M, Sivan Y: Normal polysomnographic respiratory values in children and adolescents. Chest 125(3):872–878, 2004.
9. Carroll JL: Obstructive sleep-disordered breathing in children: new controversies, new directions. Clin Chest Med 24(2):261–282, 2003.
10. Kushida CA, Littner MR, Morgenthaler T, et al: Practice parameters for the indications for polysomnography and related procedures: an update for 2005. Sleep 28(4):499–521, 2005.
11. Pinsky MR: Sleeping with the enemy: the heart in obstructive sleep apnea. Chest 121(4):1022–1024, 2002.
12. Bradley TD, Hall MJ, Ando S, Floras JS: Hemodynamic effects of simulated obstructive apneas in humans with and without heart failure. Chest 119(6):1827–1835, 2001.
13. Hatipoglu U, Rubenstein I: Inflammation and obstructive sleep apnea syndrome. Chest 126(1):1–2, 2004.
14. Terramoto S, Yamamoto H, Yamaguchi Y, et al: Obstructive sleep apnea causes systemic inflammation and metabolic syndrome. Chest 127(3):1074, 2005.
15. Minoguchi K, Tazaki T, Yokoe T, et al: Elevated production of tumor necrosis factor-a by monocytes in patients with obstructive sleep apnea syndrome. Chest 126(5):1473–1479, 2004.
16. Parish JM, Somers VK: Obstructive sleep apnea and cardiovascular disease. Mayo Clin Proc 79(8):1036–1046, 2004.
17. Goldbart AD, Goldman JL, Li RC, et al: Differential expression of cysteinyl leukotriene receptors 1 and 2 in

tonsils of children with obstructive sleep apnea syndrome or recurrent infection. Chest 126(1):13–18, 2004.

18. Phillips BG, Kato M, Narkiewicz K, et al: Increases in leptin levels, sympathetic drive, and weight gain in obstructive sleep apnea. Am J Physiol Heart Circ Physiol 279:H234–H237, 2000.

19. Hui DS, Ko FW, Fok JP, et al: The effects of nasal continuous positive airway pressure on platelet activation in obstructive sleep apnea syndrome. Chest 125(5):1768–1775, 2004.

20. von Kanel R, Dimsdale JE: Hemostatic alterations in patients with obstructive sleep apnea and the implications for cardiovascular disease. Chest 124(5):1956–1967, 2003.

21. Ehrmann DA: Polycystic ovary syndrome. N Engl J Med 352(12):1223–1236, 2005.

22. Umlauf MG, Chasens E, Greevy RA, et al: Obstructive sleep apnea, nocturia, and polyuria in older adults. Sleep 27(1):139–144, 2004.

23. Shamsuzzaman ASM, Gersh BJ, Somers VJ: Obstructive sleep apnea. Implications for cardiac and vascular disease. JAMA 290(14):1906–1914, 2003.

24. Ip MS, Tse HF, Lam B, et al: Endothelial function in obstructive sleep apnea and response to treatment. Am J Resp Crit Care Med 169(3):348–353, 2004.

25. Nieto FJ, Herrington DM, Redline S, et al: Sleep apnea and markers of vascular endothelial function in a large community sample of older adults. Am J Resp Crit Care Med 169(3):354–360, 2004.

26. Budhiraja R, Sharief I, Quan S: Sleep disordered breathing and hypertension. J Clin Sleep Med 1(4):401–404, 2005.

27. Phillips C, Hedner J, Berend N, Grunstein R: Diurnal and obstructive sleep apnea influences on arterial stiffness and central blood pressure in men. Sleep 28(5):604–609, 2005.

28. Peppard PE, Young T, Palta M, Skatrud J: Prospective study of the association between sleep-disordered breathing and hypertension. N Engl J Med 342(19):1378–1384, 2000.

29. Nieto FJ, Young TB, Lind BK, et al: Association of sleep-disordered breathing, sleep apnea, and hypertension in a large community-based study. Sleep Heart Health Study. JAMA 283(14):1829–1836, 2000.

30. Hla KM, Skatrud JB, Finn L, et al: The effect of correction of sleep-disordered breathing on BP in untreated hypertension. Chest 122(4):1125–1132, 2002.

31. Kaneko Y, Floras JS, Usui K, et al: Cardiovascular effects of continuous positive airway pressure in patients with heart failure and obstructive sleep apnea. N Engl J Med 348(13):1233–1241, 2003.

32. Laaban J-P, Pascal-Sebaoun S, Block E, et al: Left ventricular systolic dysfunction in patients with obstructive sleep apnea syndrome. Chest 122(4):1133–1138, 2002.

33. Kanagala R, Murali NS, Friedman PA, et al: Obstructive sleep apnea and the recurrence of atrial fibrillation. Circulation 107(20):2589–2594, 2003.

34. Marrone O, Bonsignore MR: Pulmonary haemodynamics in obstructive sleep apnoea. Sleep Med Rev 6(3):175–193, 2002.

35. Beelke M, Angeli S, Del Sette M, et al: Obstructive sleep apnea can be provocative for right-to-left shunting through a patent foramen ovale. Sleep 25(8):856–862, 2002.

36. Lavie L, Vishnevsky A, Lavie P: Evidence for lipid peroxidation in obstructive sleep apnea. Sleep 27(1):123–128, 2003.

37. Veasey SC, Zhan G, Fenik P, Pratico D: Long term intermittent hypoxia. Reduced excitatory hypoglossal nerve output. Am J Resp Crit Care Med 170(6):665–672, 2004.

38. Boyd JH, Petrof BJ, Hamid Q, et al: Upper airway muscle inflammation and denervation changes in obstructive sleep apnea. Am J Resp Crit Care Med 170(5):541–546, 2004.

39. Drager LF, Bottolotto LA, Lorenzi MC, et al: Early signs of atherosclerosis in obstructive sleep apnea. Am Resp Crit Care Med 172(5):613–618, 2005.

40. Leineweber C, Kecklund G, Janszky I, et al: Snoring and progression of coronary artery disease: the Stockholm Female Coronary Angiography Study. Sleep 27(7):1344–1349, 2004.

41. Arzt M, Young T, Finn L, et al: Association of sleep-disordered breathing and the occurrence of stroke. Am J Resp Crit Care Med 172(11):1442–1447, 2005.

42. Yaggi HK, Concato J, Kernan WN, et al: Obstructive sleep apnea as a risk factor for stroke and death. N Engl J Med 353(19):2034–2041, 2005.

43. Doherty LS, Kiley JL, Swan V, McNichols WT: Long-term effects of nasal continuous positive airway pressure therapy on cardiovascular outcomes in sleep apnea syndrome. Chest 127(6):2076–2084, 2005.

44. Campos-Rodriguez F, Pena-Grinan N, Reyes-Nunez N, et al: Mortality in obstructive sleep apnea-hypopnea patients treated with positive airway pressure. Chest 128(2):624–633, 2005.

45. Marin JM, Carrizo SJ, Vicente E, Agusti AGN: Long-term cardiovascular outcomes in men with obstructive sleep apnoea-hypopnoea with or without treatment with continuous positive airway pressure: an observational study. Lancet 365(9464):1046–1053, 2005.

46. White DP: Pathogenesis of obstructive and central sleep apnea. Am J Resp Crit Care Med 172(11):1363–1370, 2005.

47. Katz ES, White DP: Genioglossus activity during sleep in normal control subjects and children with obstructive sleep apnea. Am J Resp Crit Care Med 170(5):553–560, 2004.

48. Onal E, Lopata M, O'Connor T: Pathogenesis of apneas in hypersomnia-sleep apnea syndrome. Am Rev Resp Dis 125(2):167–174, 1982.

49. Wellman A, Jordan AS, Malhotra A, et al: Ventilatory control and airway anatomy in obstructive sleep apnea. Am J Resp Crit Care Med 170(11):1225–1232, 2004.

50. Issa FG, Sullivan CE: Reversal of central sleep apnea using nasal CPAP. Chest 90(2):165–171, 1986.

51. Katz ES, White DP: Genioglossus activity in children with obstructive sleep apnea during wakefulness and sleep onset. Am Rev Resp Dis 168(6):664–670, 2003.

52. Fogel RB, Malhotra A, Pillar G, et al: Genioglossal activity in patients with obstructive sleep apnea versus

control subjects. Am Rev Resp Dis 164(11):2025–2030, 2001.

53. Gozal D, Burnside MM: Increased upper airway collapsibility in children with obstructive sleep apnea during wakefulness. Am Rev Resp Dis 169(2):163–167, 2003.

54. Rhoden EL, Morgentaler A: Medical progress: risks of testosterone-replacement therapy and recommendations for monitoring. N Engl J Med 350(5):482–492, 2004.

55. Polnitsky CA: Sleep in women. In Shigley L, Jones-Parker M, Lee-Chiong T (eds): *Textbook of Polysomnography.* Philadelphia, Lippincott, Williams & Wilkins, 2006.

56. Young T, Finn L, Austin D, Peterson A: Menopausal status and sleep-disordered breathing in the Wisconsin sleep cohort study. Am J Resp Crit Care Med 167(9):1181–1185, 2003.

57. Bixler EO, Vgontzas AN, Lin H-O, et al: Prevalence of sleep disordered breathing in women: effects of gender. Am J Resp Crit Care Med 163(3):608–613, 2001.

58. Malhotra A, Huang Y, Fogel RB, et al: The male predisposition to pharyngeal collapse. Importance of airway length. Am J Resp Crit Care Med 166:1388–1395, 2003.

59. Jordan A, Malhotra A: The pharyngeal lumen: both length and size matter. J Clin Sleep Med 1(3):264–265, 2005.

60. Olson EJ, Moore WR, Morgenthalerr TI, et al: Obstructive sleep apnea-hypopnea syndrome. Mayo Clin Proc 78:1545–1552, 2003.

61. Sanders MH, Givelber R: Sleep disordered breathing may not be an independent risk factor for diabetes, but diabetes may contribute to the occurrence of periodic breathing in sleep. Sleep Med 4(4):349–350, 2003.

62. Peppard PE, Young T, Palta M, et al: Longitudinal study of moderate weight change and sleep-disordered breathing. JAMA 284:3015–3021, 2000.

63. Newman AB, Foster G, Givelber R, et al: Progression and regression of sleep-disordered breathing with changes in weight. Arch Intern Med 165(20):2048–13, 2005.

64. Guilleminault C, Biol D, Li K, et al: A prospective study on the surgical outcomes of children with sleep-disordered breathing. Sleep 27(1):95–100, 2004.

65. McNamara F, Sullivan CE: Pediatric origins of adult lung diseases. 3: The genesis of adult sleep apnea in childhood. Thorax 55(11):964–969, 2000.

66. Meltzer EO: Introduction: Stuffy is also related to Sleepy and Grumpy: the link between rhinitis and sleep-disordered breathing. J Allergy Clin Immunol 114:S133–S134, 2004.

67. Shepertycky MR, Banno K, Kryger MH: Differences between men and women in the clinical presentation of patients diagnosed with obstructive sleep apnea syndrome. Sleep 28(3):309–314, 2005.

68. Gottlieb DJ: The future risks of childhood sleep-disordered breathing. Sleep 28(7):796–797, 2005.

69. Logan AG, Perlikowski SM, Mente A, et al: High prevalence of unrecognized sleep apnoea in drug-resistant hypertension. J Hypertension 19(12):2271–2277, 2001.

70. Kapur VH, Koepsell TD, deMaine J, et al: Association of hypothyroidism and obstructive sleep apnea. Am J Resp Crit Care Med 158(5 Pt 1):1379–1383, 1998.

71. den Herder C, Schmeck J, Appelboom DJK, de Vries N: Risks of general anaesthesia in people with obstructive sleep apnoea. BMJ 329(7472):955–959, 2004.

72. Hosselet JJ, Norman RG, Ayappa I, Rapoport DM: Detection of flow limitation with a nasal cannula/pressure transducer system. Am J Resp Crit Care Med 157(5 Pt 1):1461–1467, 1998.

73. Zafar S, Ayappa I, Norman RG, et al: Choice of oximeter affects apnea-hypopnea index. Chest 127(1):80–88, 2005.

74. Department of Health and Human Services Centers for Medicare and Medicaid Services: *Medicare Coverage Issues Manual 12-26-2001:* transmittal 150, section 60-17. Washington, DC, Department of Health and Human Services.

75. Liesching TN, Carlisle C, Marte A, et al: Evaluation of the accuracy of SNAP technology sleep sonography in detecting obstructive sleep apnea in adults compared to standard polysomnography. Chest 125(3):886–891, 2004.

76. Magalang UJ, Dmochowski J, Veeramachaneni S, et al: Prediction of the apnea-hypopnea index from overnight pulse oximetry. Chest 124(5):1694–1701, 2003.

77. Flemons WW, Littner MR, Rowley JA, et al: Home diagnosis of sleep apnea: a systematic review of the literature. Chest 124(4):1543–1579, 2003.

78. Chesson AL Jr, Berry RB, Pack A: Practice parameters for the use of portable monitoring devices in the investigation of suspected obstructive sleep apnea in the adult. Sleep 26(7):907–913, 2003.

79. Iber C: Home portable monitoring and obstructive sleep apnea. J Clin Sleep Med 1(1):11–13, 2005.

80. Sanders MH, Constantino JP, Strollo PJ, et al: The impact of split-night polysomnography for diagnosis and positive pressure therapy titration on treatment acceptance and adherence in sleep apnea/hyopopnea. Sleep 23(1):17–24, 2000.

81. Loube DI, Gay PC, Strohl KP, et al: Indications for positive airway treatment of adult obstructive sleep apnea patients: a consensus statement. Chest 115(3):863–866, 1999.

82. Littner M, Hirshkowitz M, Davila D, et al: Practice parameters for the use of auto-titrating continuous positive airway pressure devices for titrating pressures and treating adult patients with obstructive sleep apnea syndrome. An American Academy of Sleep Medicine Report. Sleep 25(2):143–147, 2002.

83. Abbey N, Cooper K, Kwentus J: Benefit of nasal CPAP in obstructive sleep apnea is due to positive pharyngeal pressure. Sleep 12:420–422, 1989.

84. Heinzer RC, Stanchina ML, Malhotra A, et al: Lung volume and continuous positive airway pressure requirements in obstructive sleep apnea. Am J Resp Crit Care Med 172(1):114–117, 2005.

85. Sanders MH, Kern N: Obstructive sleep apnea treated by independently adjusted inspiratory and expiratory positive airway pressures via nasal mask. Chest 98(2):317–324, 1990.

86. Reeves-Hoche MK, Kudgel DW, Meck R, et al: Continuous versus bilevel positive airway pressure for obstructive sleep apnea. Am J Resp Crit Care Med 151(2 Pt 1):443–449, 1995.

87. Roux FJ, Hilbert J: Continuous positive airway pressure: new generations. In Lee-Chiong TL, Mohsenin V (eds): *Clinics in Chest Medicine,* Philadelphia, Saunders, pp 315–342, 2003.

88. Berry RB, Parish JM, Hartse KM: The use of autotitrating continuous positive airway pressure for treatment of adult sleep apnea: an American Academy of Sleep Medicine review. Sleep 25(2):148–173, 2002.

89. Noseda A, Kempenaers C, Kerkhofs M, et al: Constant vs auto-continuous airway pressure in patients with sleep apnea hypopnea syndrome and a high variability in pressure requirement. Chest 126(1):31–37, 2004.

90. Ayas NT, Patel SR, Malhotra A, et al: Autotitrating versus standard continuous positive airway pressure for the treatment of obstructive sleep apnea: results of a meta-analysis. Sleep 27(2):249–253, 2004.

91. Kessler R, Weitzenbaum E, Chaouat A, et al: Evaluation of unattended automated titration to determine therapeutic continuous positive airway pressure in patients with obstructive sleep apnea. Chest 123(3):704–710, 2003.

92. Gay PC, Herold DL, Olson EJ: A randomized, double-blind clinical trial comparing continuous positive airway pressure with a novel bilevel pressure system for treatment of obstructive sleep apnea syndrome. Sleep 26(7):864–869, 2003.

93. Aloia MS, Stanchinaa M, Arendt JT, et al: Treatment adherence and outcomes in flexible vs standard continuous positive airway pressure therapy. Chest 127(6):2085–2093, 2005.

94. Ferguson KA: The role of oral appliance therapy in the treatment of obstructive sleep apnea. In Lee-Chiong T, Mohsenin V (eds): *Clinics in Chest Medicine.* Philadelphia, Saunders, 2003, pp 355–364.

95. Randerath WJ, Heise M, Hinz R, Ruehle K-H: An individually adjustable oral appliance vs continuous positive airway pressure in mild-to-moderate obstructive sleep apnea syndrome. Chest 122(2):569–575, 2002.

96. Marklund M, Franklin KA, Sahlin C, Lundgren Rune: The effect of a mandibular advancement device on apneas and sleep in patients with obstructive sleep apnea. Chest 113(3):707–713, 1998.

97. Marklund M, Stenlund H, Franklin KA: Mandibular advancement devices in 630 men and women with obstructive sleep apnea and snoring. Chest 125(4):1270–1278, 2004.

98. Li KK: Surgical therapy for adult obstructive sleep apnea. Sleep Med Rev 9:201–209, 2005.

99. Powell N: Upper airway surgery does have a major role in the treatment of obstructive sleep apnea. J Clin Sleep Med 1(3):236–240, 2005.

100. Phillips B: Upper airway surgery does not have a major role in the treatment of sleep apnea. J Clin Sleep Med 1(3):241–245, 2005.

101. Littner M, Kushida CA, Hartse K, et al: Practice parameters for the use of laser-assisted uvuloplasty: an update for 2000. Sleep 24(5):603–619, 2001.

102. Li KK: Surgical therapy for obstructive sleep apnea syndrome. Sem Resp Crit Care Med 26(1):80–88, 2005.

103. Peppard PE, Young T, Palta M, et al: Longitudinal study of moderate weight change and sleep-disordered breathing. JAMA 284(23):3015–3021, 2000.

104. Newman AB, Foster G, Givelber R, et al: Progression and regression of sleep-disordered breathing with changes in weight. Arch Intern Med 165(20):2408–2413, 2005.

105. Busetto L, Enzi G, Inelmen EM, et al: Obstructive sleep apnea syndrome in morbid obesity. Chest 128(2):618–623, 2005.

106. Brolin RE: Bariatric surgery and long-term control of morbid obesity. JAMA 128(22):2793–2796, 2002.

107. Steinbrook R: Surgery for severe obesity. N Engl J Med 350(11):1075–1079, 2004.

108. Verse T: Bariatric surgery for obstructive sleep apnea. Chest 128(2):485–487, 2005.

109. Meoli AL, Rosen CL, Kristo D, et al: Nonprescription treatments of snoring or obstructive sleep apnea: an evaluation of products with limited scientific evidence. Sleep 26(5):619–624, 2003.

110. Fenik VB, Davies RO, Kubin L: REM sleep-like atonia of hypoglossal (XII) motoneurons is caused by loss of noradrenergic and serotonergic inputs. Am J Resp Crit Care Med 172(10):1322–1330, 2005.

111. Berry RB, Koch GL, Hayward LF: Low-dose mirtazapine increases genioglossus activity in the anesthetized rat. Sleep 28(1):78–84, 2005.

112. Bellemare F, Pecchiari M, Bandini M, et al: Reversibility of airflow obstruction by hypoglossus nerve stimulation in anesthetized rabbits. Am J Resp Crit Care Med 172(5):606–612, 2005.

113. Schwartz JRL, Hirshkowitz M, Erman MK, Schmidt-Nowara W: Modafanil as adjunct therapy for daytime sleepiness in obstructive sleep apnea. Chest 124(6):2192–2199, 2003.

114. Vastag B: Poised to challenge need for sleep, "wakefulness enhancer" rouses concerns. JAMA 291:167–168, 2004.

115. Badr MS, Toiber F, Skatrud JB, Dempsey J: Pharyngeal narrowing/occlusion during central sleep apnea. J Appl Physiol 78(5):1806–1815, 1995.

116. White DP: Central sleep apnea. In Kryger MH, Roth T, Dement WC (eds): *Principles and Practice of Sleep Medicine,* 4th ed. Philadelphia, Elsevier Saunders, 2005, pp 969–982.

117. Douglas NJ: Respiratory physiology: control of ventilation. In Kryger MH, Roth T, Dement WC (eds): *Principles and Practice of Sleep Medicine,* 4th ed. Philadelphia, Elsevier Saunders, 2005, pp 224–231.

118. Sanders MH, Rogers RM, Pennock BE: Prolonged expiratory phase in sleep apnea: a unifying hypothesis. Am Rev Resp Dis 131(3):401–408, 1985.

119. Gold AR, Bleeker ER, Smith PL: A shift from central and mixed sleep apnea to obstructive sleep apnea resulting from low–flow oxygen. Am Rev Resp Dis 132(2):220–223, 1985.

120. Mansfield DR, Solin P, Roebuck T, et al: The effect of successful heart transplant treatment of heart failure on central sleep apnea. Chest 124(5):1675–1681, 2003.

121. Bradley TD, Floras JS: Sleep apnea and heart failure. Part II: central sleep apnea. Circulation 107:1822–1826, 2003.

122. Nopmaneejumruslers C, Kaneks Y, Hajek V, et al: Cheyne-Stokes respiration in stroke. Relationship to hypocapnia and occult cardiac dysfunction. Am J Resp Crit Care Med 171(9):1048–1052, 2005.

123. Leung RS, Diep TM, Bowman ME, et al: Provocation of ventricular ectopy by Cheyne-Stokes respiration in patients with heart failure. Sleep 27(7):1337–1343, 2004.

124. Sin DD, Man GCW: Cheyne-Stokes respiration. A consequence of a broken heart? Chest 124(5):1627–1628, 2003.

125. Krieger J: Respiratory physiology: breathing in normal subjects. In Kryger MH, Roth T, Dement WC (eds): *Principles and Practice of Sleep Medicine*, 4th ed. Philadelphia, Elsevier Saunders, 2005, pp 232–243.

126. Dempsey J, Skatrud J, Smith C: Powerful stabilizing effects of CO_2 treatment. Sleep 28(1):12–13, 2005.

127. Brown L: "Dephlogisticated air" revisited: oxygen treatment for central sleep apnea syndrome. Chest 111(2):269–271, 1997.

128. Bradley TD, Logan AG, Kimoff RJ, et al: Continuous positive airway pressure for central sleep apnea and heart failure. N Engl J Med 353(19):2025–2033, 2005.

129. Johnson KG, Johnson DC: Bilevel positive airway pressure worsens central apneas during sleep. Chest 128(4):2141–2150, 2005.

130. Pepperel JCT, Maskell NA, Jones DR, et al: A randomized controlled trial of adaptive ventilation for Cheyne-Stokes breathing in heart failure. Am J Resp Crit Care Med 168:1109–1114, 2003.

131. Franklin KA, Eriksson P, Sahlin C, Lundgren R: Reversal of central sleep apnea with oxygen. Chest 111:163–169, 1997.

132. Krachman SL, Nugent T, Crocetti J, et al: Effects of oxygen therapy on left ventricular function in patients with Cheyne-Stokes respiration and congestive heart failure. J Clin Sleep Med 1(3):271–276, 2005.

133. Javaheri S, Ahmed M, Parker TJ: Effects of nasal O_2 on sleep-related disordered breathing in ambulatory patients with stable heart failure. Sleep 22(8):1101–1106, 1999.

134. Guilleminault C, Philil P, Robinson A: Sleep and neuromuscular disease: bilevel positive airway pressure by nasal mask as a treatment for sleep disordered breathing in patients with neuromuscular disease. J Neurol Neurosurg Psychiatry 65(2):225–232, 1998.

135. Thomas RJ, Daly RW, Weiss JW: Low-concentration carbon dioxide is an effective adjunct to positive airway pressure in the treatment of refractory mixed central and obstructive sleep-disordered breathing. Sleep 28(1):69–77, 2005.

136. Ayappa I, Rapoport DM: The upper airway in sleep: physiology of the pharynx. Sleep Med Rev 7(1):9–33, 2003.

137. Gleadhill IC, Schwartz AR, Schubert N, et al: Upper airway collapsibility in snorers and in patients with obstructive hypopnea and apnea. Am Rev Respir Dis 143(6):1300–1303, 1991.

138. Rappai M, Collop N, Kemp S, deShazo R: The nose and sleep-disordered breathing: what we know and what we do not know. Chest 124(6):2309–2323, 2003.

139. Young T, Palta M, Dempsey J, et al: The occurrence of sleep-disordered breathing among middle-aged adults. N Engl J Med 328(17):1230–1235, 1993.

140. Wetter DW, Young TB, Bidwell TR, et al: Smoking as a risk factor for sleep-disordered breathing. Arch Intern Med 154(19):2219–2224, 1994.

141. Vetrugno R, Provini F, Plazzi G, et al: Catathrenia (nocturnal groaning): a new type of parasomnia. Neurology 56(5):681–683, 2001.

142. Meoli AL, Rosen CL, Kristo D, et al: Nonprescription treatments of snoring or obstructive sleep apnea: an evaluation of products with limited scientific evidence. Sleep 26(5):619–624, 2003.

143. Practice parameters for the treatment of snoring and obstructive sleep apnea with oral appliances: American Sleep Disorders Association. Sleep 18(6):511–513, 1995.

144. Stuck BA, Sauter A, Hormann K, et al: Radiofrequency surgery of the soft palate in the treatment of snoring. A placebo-controlled trial. Sleep 28(7):847–850, 2005.

145. Maurer JT, Hein G, Verse T, et al: Long-term results of palatal implants for primary snoring. Otolaryngol Head Neck Surg 133(4):573–578, 2005.

146. Guilleminault C, Stoohs R, Duncan S: Snoring (I). Daytime sleepiness in regular heavy snorers. Chest 99(1):40–48, 1991.

147. Lofaso F, Coste A, Gilain L, et al: Sleep fragmentation as a risk factor for hypertension in middle-aged non-apneic snorers. Chest 109(4):896–900, 1996.

148. Gold AR, Dipalo F, Gold MS, O'Hearn D: The symptoms and signs of upper airway resistance syndrome: a link to the functional somatic syndromes. Chest 123(1):87–95, 2003.

149. Lofaso F, Goldenberg F, d'Ortho MP, et al: Arterial blood pressure response to transient arousals from NREM sleep in nonapneic snorers with sleep fragmentation. Chest 113(4):985–991, 1998.

150. Guilleminault C, Poyares D, Palombini L, et al: Variability of respiratory effort in relation to sleep stages in normal controls and upper airway resistance syndrome patients. Sleep Med 2(5):397–405, 2001.

151. Ayappa I, Norman RG, Krieger AC, et al: Non-invasive detection of respiratory effort-related arousals (REras) by a nasal cannula/pressure transducer system. Sleep 23(6):763–771, 2000.

152. Guilleminault C, Stoohs R, Clerk A, et al: A cause of excessive daytime sleepiness. The upper airway resistance syndrome. Chest 104(3):781–787, 1993.

153. Yoshida K: Oral device therapy for the upper airway resistance syndrome patient. J Prosthet Dent 87(4):427–430, 2002.

154. Bao G, Guilleminault C: Upper airway resistance syndrome—one decade later. Curr Opin Pulm Med 10(6):461–467, 2004.

155. Nowbar S, Burkart KM, Gonzales R, et al: Obesity-associated hypoventilation in hospitalized patients: prevalence, effects, and outcome. Am J Med 116(1):1–7, 2004.

156. Kessler R, Chaouat A, Schinkewitch P, et al: The obesity-hypoventilation syndrome revisited: a prospective study of 34 consecutive cases. Chest 120(2):369–376, 2001.

157. Sullivan CE, Berthon-Jones M, Issa FG: Remission of severe obesity-hypoventilation syndrome after short-term treatment during sleep with nasal continuous positive airway pressure. Am Rev Respir Dis 128(1):177–181, 1983.

158. Masa JF, Celli BR, Riesco JA, et al: The obesity hypoventilation syndrome can be treated with noninvasive mechanical ventilation. Chest 119(4):1102–1107, 2001.

159. Sugerman HJ, Fairman RP, Sood RK, et al: Long-term effects of gastric surgery for treating respiratory insufficiency of obesity. Am J Clin Nutr 55(2 Suppl):597S–601S, 1992.

160. Weese-Mayer DE, Silvestri JM, Menzies LJ, et al: Congenital central hypoventilation syndrome: diagnosis, management, and long-term outcome in thirty-two children. J Pediatr 120(3):381–387, 1992.

161. Silvestri JM, Weese-Mayer DE, Flanagan EA: Congenital central hypoventilation syndrome: cardiorespiratory responses to moderate exercise, simulating daily activity. Pediatr Pulmonol 20(2):89–93, 1995.

162. Paton JY, Swaminathan S, Sargent CW, Keens TG: Hypoxic and hypercapnic ventilatory responses in awake children with congenital central hypoventilation syndrome. Am Rev Respir Dis 140(2):368–372, 1989.

163. Paton JY, Swaminathan S, Sargent CW, et al: Ventilatory response to exercise in children with congenital central hypoventilation syndrome. Am Rev Respir Dis 147(5):1185–1191, 1993.

164. Woo MS, Woo MA, Gozal D, et al: Heart rate variability in congenital central hypoventilation syndrome. Pediatr Res 31(3):291–296, 1992.

165. Gozal D: Congenital central hypoventilation syndrome: an update. Pediatr Pulmonol 26(4):273–282, 1998.

166. Amiel J, Laudier B, Attie-Bitach T, et al: Polyalanine expansion and frameshift mutations of the paired-like homeobox gene PHOX2B in congenital central hypoventilation syndrome. Nat Genet 33(4):459–461. Epub 2003 Mar 17, 2003.

167. Weese-Mayer DE, Berry-Kravis EM, Zhou L, et al: Idiopathic congenital central hypoventilation syndrome: analysis of genes pertinent to early autonomic nervous system embryologic development and identification of mutations in PHOX2b. Am J Med Assoc 123(3):267–278, 2003.

168. Weese-Meyer DE, Shannon DC, Keens TG, Silvestri JM: American Thoracic Society consensus statement. Idiopathic congenital central hypoventilation syndrome. Diagnosis and management. Am J Respir Crit Care Med 160:368–373, 1999.

Cardiovascular Pathophysiology of Sleep Apnea

VIKTOR HANAK ■ VIREND K. SOMERS

NORMAL CARDIOVASCULAR RESPONSES TO SLEEP

The autonomic nervous system has an important role in regulating blood pressure and heart rate during sleep. In non-rapid eye movement (NREM) sleep there is an approximately 20% reduction in blood pressure and heart rate, which is associated with a decrease in sympathetic nervous activity.[1,2] Heart rate and blood pressure also decrease throughout the NREM sleep stages, with the lowest values in stage 4 NREM sleep. One exception to this trend is the K-complex of stage 2 NREM sleep, when blood pressure and heart rate increase momentarily. In rapid eye movement (REM) sleep there are abrupt increases in blood pressure and heart rate, with activation of the sympathetic system, to levels similar to those during wakefulness.[2] The bursts in sympathetic activity and the surges in blood pressure are more prominent during phasic than tonic REM sleep, corresponding with rapid eye movements and "REM twitches."[2,3]

CARDIOVASCULAR EFFECTS OF OBSTRUCTIVE SLEEP APNEA (OSA)

Blood Pressure Changes

The apneic episodes represent a significant hemodynamic stress.[4,5] During the apnea, cardiac preload is reduced as a result of impaired venous return. At the same time, sympathetic activation in response to hypoxemia and apnea increases afterload by peripheral vasoconstriction. The combination of decreased preload and increased afterload results in low cardiac output during the apnea. Upon resumption of breathing, the cardiac output increases. The biggest surge in blood pressure is seen at apnea termination, when the restored cardiac output enters the still-constricted vascular system. Peripheral vasoconstriction is subsequently attenuated by the baroreceptors, which sense the blood pressure increase and reflexively inhibit sympathetic activity. The relatively lower blood pressure during the apnea with subsequent blood pressure elevation in the immediate postapneic period is the simplified hemodynamic cycle that is repeated with each apneic event (Figure 5-1).

Heart Rate Changes

During the apnea itself, parasympathetic stimulation of the heart, resulting from activation of the diving reflex, leads to bradycardia.[5,6] The heart rate slowing is vagally mediated and is often evident if the apnea is long enough and leads to oxygen desaturation. The bradycardia normally lasts only for the duration of the apnea and is then followed by sinus tachycardia on resumption of ventilation (Figure 5-2). The combination of bradycardia with peripheral vasoconstriction forms the "diving-reflex" response to hypoxemia and apnea (this helps preserve oxygen in sea mammals during the dive).[5,6]

Arousals from Sleep

Arousal is by definition shorter than 15 seconds; otherwise it is labeled as *awakening*. The arousal from sleep is accompanied by a rapid increase in heart rate and blood pressure mediated by activation of the sympathetic nervous system and rapid parasympathetic withdrawal.[7] The average arousal causes a 20 mm Hg increase in systolic and 15 mm Hg increase in diastolic blood pressure, with a heart rate increase of 10 beats per minute.[8] When inducing arousals experimentally by noise, cortical arousal is sometimes not detectable on electroencephalogram (EEG). Instead, the arousal is only "autonomic," with sympathetic activation. The autonomic nervous system appears sensitive to both external and internal arousal stimuli (Figure 5-3). Adverse cardiovascular effects can infrequently be triggered by acute changes in autonomic balance on arousal in subjects with vulnerable substrates, such as the long QT syndrome.[9]

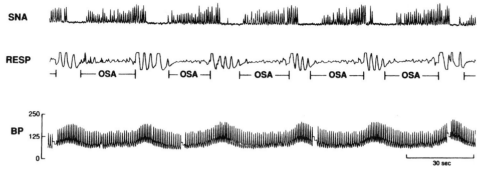

FIGURE 5-1 ■ Blood pressure (BP) oscillation in response to obstructive apnea episodes (OSA). Blood pressure is reduced during the apneic period but increases in the postapneic period. The reduced blood pressure during the apnea is the result of reduced venous return. The increase in blood pressure in the postapneic period corresponds with arousal. Note the cyclic variation in the sympathetic nervous activity (SNA) during apnea. (Adapted from Somers VK, Dyken ME, Clary MP, Abboud FM. Sympathetic neural mechanisms in obstructive sleep apnea. J Clin Invest 96[4]:1897–1904, 1995.)

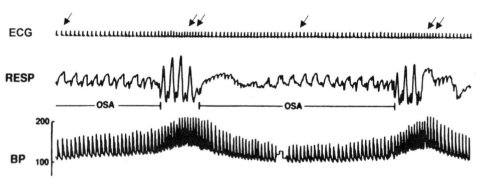

FIGURE 5-2 ■ Heart rate changes during obstructive apnea. During the apneic episode itself, the vagal nerve causes slowing of heart rate, seen as slight prolongation of the R-R intervals on the ECG strip (*arrow*). Bradycardia normally lasts only for the duration of the apnea. Sinus tachycardia brought about by resumption of ventilation upon arousal is seen as slight crowding of the R-R intervals on the ECG strip (*double arrow*). (Adapted from Somers VK, Dyken ME, Clary MP, Abboud FM. Sympathetic neural mechanisms in obstructive sleep apnea. J Clin Invest 96[4]:1897–1904, 1995.)

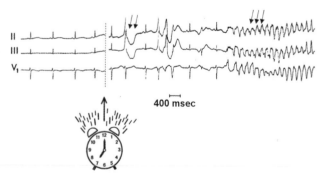

FIGURE 5-3 ■ Anecdotal case of ventricular fibrillation in an otherwise healthy woman after an external auditory stimulus. Alarm clock (*arrow*) elicits arousal with increased sympathetic stimulation leading to ventricular ectopic beats (*double arrows*) and ultimately ventricular fibrillation (*triple arrows*). Despite this case being anecdotal, it illustrates the potential arrhythmogenic effect of arousal mediated sympathetic activation. (Adapted from Wellens HJ, Vermeulen A, Durrer D: Ventricular fibrillation occurring on arousal from sleep by auditory stimuli. Circulation 46[4]:661–665, 1972.)

MECHANISMS LEADING TO CARDIOVASCULAR PATHOLOGY IN OSA

Various neural, humoral, thrombotic, metabolic, hemodynamic, and inflammatory mechanisms contribute to cardiovascular pathology in OSA.[4]

Sympathetic Activation

Desaturations during apnea lead to chemoreflex activation with reflex surges in sympathetic activity and elevated catecholamine levels.[10,11] The increased sympathetic drive persists during the daytime[5] and is accompanied by tachycardia and higher blood pressures. Heart rate variability is decreased as a result of subtle autonomic imbalance.[12] Decreased heart rate variability is an important marker of risk for future hypertension.[13] Continuous positive airway pressure

(CPAP) treatment has been shown to reduce not only nighttime sympathetic activation and blood pressure, but also to lower daytime measurements of muscle sympathetic nerve activity in patients with hypertension.[14] In normotensive subjects, CPAP does not appear to have any significant effects on daytime blood pressure levels.

Vascular Endothelial Dysfunction

The response to vasodilators such as acetylcholine is impaired, suggesting small or resistance vessel endothelial dysfunction.[15,16] Acetylcholine stimulates nitric oxide production by the endothelial cells, and the magnitude of the vasodilator response to acetylcholine is taken as an index of endothelial function. Impaired endothelial function is usually evident in patients with hypertension, hyperlipidemia, or diabetes and in smokers. In the absence of any of these risk factors, otherwise healthy patients with OSA have impaired endothelial function when compared with similarly obese individuals without OSA.[16] In these otherwise healthy OSA subjects, however, brachial artery or conduit vessel endothelial function does not appear to be consistently impaired.[16] In the long term, endothelial dysfunction may be associated with future risk of vascular disease.

Oxidative Stress and Inflammation

The repetitive apneic episodes may cause oxidative stress,[17,18] although the evidence is not consistent.[19] The oxygen radicals may promote inflammation and tissue damage. Chronic sleep deprivation also leads to production of inflammatory cytokines. C-reactive protein,[20] tumor necrosis factor, and other inflammatory mediators are elevated in OSA patients; may correlate with the apnea-hypopnea index; and are reportedly reduced by CPAP treatment.[21]

Metabolic Effects

OSA is linked to glucose intolerance and to increased leptin levels.[22–25] Leptin is an adipokine produced by the fat cells and mediates appetite suppression. Obese patients have high leptin levels but are resistant to the appetite-suppressant effects (analogous to insulin resistance in type 2 diabetics). OSA patients have even higher leptin levels than similarly obese individuals without OSA, suggesting that OSA is accompanied by heightened leptin resistance. Treatment with CPAP reduces the elevated leptin levels, decreases the abdominal fat accumulation, and improves glucose tolerance.[22,26]

Hypercoagulability

Increased platelet aggregation, increased activity of clotting factors, and elevated levels of fibrinogen and hematocrit may contribute to hypercoagulability in OSA.[27] Evidence implicating OSA as a cause of increased risk for intravascular thrombosis, however, is very limited, and much of the existing data are confounded by significant comorbidities in OSA patients.

CLINICAL CARDIOVASCULAR DISEASE AND OSA

Hypertension

The association of OSA with hypertension is well established. In prospective epidemiological studies, an increased apnea-hypopnea index at baseline predicts the risk of hypertension in the years to come in a dose-response manner.[28,29] Daytime hypertension in OSA may be a carryover of the nighttime effects. CPAP lowers blood pressure in these hypertensive patients.[30–34] Patients with OSA do not have the normal nighttime blood pressure reduction ("dipping"); instead their blood pressure may stay elevated at night.[33] The higher nighttime pressures ("nondipping") have been prospectively linked to adverse cardiovascular outcomes. There is also a high incidence of undiagnosed OSA in patients with hypertension refractory to medical treatment (resistant hypertension). OSA needs to be considered in patients resistant to antihypertensive medications and in patients who are "nondippers" on ambulatory monitoring.

Stroke

In patients with stroke, there is a high prevalence of OSA.[34] OSA is a strong risk factor for stroke even after adjustment for important confounders, such as hypertension, smoking, alcohol use, body-mass index, diabetes mellitus, hyperlipidemia, and atrial fibrillation.[35,36] Nevertheless, the relationship between sleep apnea and increased risk of future stroke has not yet been proven to be causal. Snoring is by itself also an independent predictor of stroke.[37] In addition to a higher incidence of strokes, there are also structural abnormalities of the gray and white matter seen by magnetic resonance imaging in apnea patients.[38] The damage to brain parenchyma might be a result of repetitive cerebral ischemia (Figure 5-4).[39,40] Once stroke occurs, it may often make any preexisting OSA worse, especially if it involves the brainstem and cranial nerves affecting the tonus of upper airways.[41–43] Central sleep apnea is usually a result of the stroke rather than a risk factor and typically resolves within a

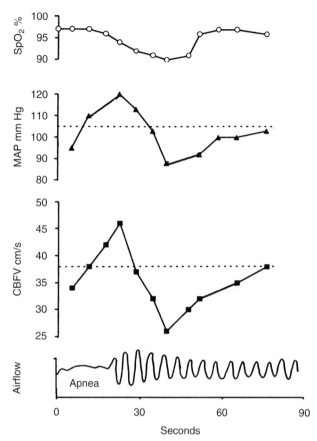

FIGURE 5-4 ■ During the apnea itself, the values of mean arterial (MAP) and cerebral perfusion pressure (CBFV) are lower than normal. In the immediate postapneic period, mean arterial pressure and cerebral blood flow are increased. (Adapted from Balfors EM, Franklin KA: Impairment of cerebral perfusion during obstructive sleep apneas. Am J Respir Crit Care Med 150[6 Pt 1]:1587–1591, 1994.)

few months in stroke survivors.[34] In patients with OSA that is present and severe after stroke, there is decreased functional capability, and some data suggest increased risk of early mortality.[44]

Cardiac Ischemia

OSA has been identified as an independent predictor of coronary artery disease in prospective studies. OSA also indicates a poor prognosis in patients with established coronary artery disease (CAD).[45,46] In long-term observational studies, cardiac events were especially increased in patients with severe OSA who were not treated. In those OSA patients who were treated, the risk for cardiac events was lower. As with studies of other cardiovascular disease conditions and OSA, however, conclusive evidence of any etiological relationship awaits the conduct of randomized, controlled treatment studies. OSA may cause nocturnal angina

with ST depressions, especially during REM sleep where apneas are longer and desaturations greater.[47,48] Cardiac ischemia may be explained by severe hypoxemia, carbon dioxide retention, acidosis, sympathetic activation, and heightened blood pressure. Nocturnal angina can be successfully relieved by CPAP treatment.

Patients with OSA are more likely to die suddenly during the nighttime hours as compared with those without OSA, who are more likely to die in the early morning after waking from sleep.[49] Whether nocturnal sudden cardiac death in OSA patients is linked to cardiac ischemia and myocardial infarction remains to be determined.

Heart Failure

Patients with systolic heart failure have a high likelihood of central sleep apnea (CSA) (between 40% and 50%). About 10% of systolic heart failure patients are thought to have OSA, although the prevalence is likely to be increasing, given the current epidemic of obesity. CSA in heart failure is known to be associated with a poorer prognosis.[50,51] The recent Continuous Positive Airway Pressure for Patients with Central Sleep Apnea and Heart Failure (CANPAP) study, however, showed no evidence of any mortality benefit in heart failure patients with CSA randomized to CPAP therapy as compared with those who are not treated.[52] This may in part be due to incomplete efficacy of CPAP in treating CSA in heart failure.[36]

In patients with heart failure, the presence of OSA and associated sympathetic surges, pressor increases, and so forth would be expected to worsen heart failure. Indeed several small studies have suggested improved functional capacity after treating OSA in these patients. Surrogates of outcome that have demonstrated improvement include lower blood pressures and increased left ventricular ejection fractions. However, no studies have been conducted to examine whether patients with heart failure and OSA randomized to CPAP treatment have improved survival or other outcome measures.

In patients with diastolic heart failure, obstructive sleep apnea may also be present and may indeed potentially contribute to hypertension and cardiac hypertrophy in these patients.[53,54] Heart failure itself may directly exacerbate OSA by edema formation in the soft tissues of the neck and by the fact that periodic breathing may trigger an upper airway closure.

Pulmonary Hypertension

Acute episodes of hypoxemia occurring during sleep apnea may be associated with pulmonary vasoconstriction and increased pulmonary artery pressures;

however, whether OSA is an important cause of established pulmonary hypertension remains unknown.[55,56] OSA may be especially important in those patients with pulmonary hypertension with daytime hypoxemia. There are very few data examining the effects of treatment of OSA in patients with pulmonary hypertension. Available information suggests that treating OSA may have only modest effects in lowering pulmonary artery pressures.[57] Nevertheless, patients with pulmonary hypertension suspected of having concomitant OSA should undergo sleep studies and receive treatment as appropriate.

ARRHYTHMIAS

Cyclic Variation in Heart Rate During OSA

Patients with OSA have typical cyclic variations of heart rate during sleep. Heart rate is reduced during the apnea, with increases in the postapneic period. This cyclic variation is the result of periodic parasympathetic and sympathetic activation and does not represent a true arrhythmia, as heart rate usually stays within normal range.[58]

Bradyarrhythmia

Bradyarrhythmias are common in OSA. The vagally mediated sinus bradycardia is the physiologic response to combined apnea and hypoxemia.[6,59-61]

The combination of sinus bradycardia and peripheral vasoconstriction is sometimes referred to as the "diving reflex" and is more pronounced with increasing apnea severity. Bradycardia occurs in longer apneas, typically toward the end of the apnea when the hypoxemia is most pronounced. Various forms of nodal heart block are common, especially in REM sleep where the apneas are often more severe (Figures 5-5 and 5-6).[61]

Bradycardia in patients with OSA may be discovered incidentally (such as when these patients are monitored in the hospital for unrelated medical problems) and responds to CPAP.[62] Severe bradyarrhythmias, surprisingly not associated with apnea, have been described during phasic REM sleep in some young, otherwise healthy subjects tested for dysautonomia.[63]

Atrial Fibrillation

Atrial fibrillation is another common arrhythmia evident in patients with OSA.[64] About 50% of patients with atrial fibrillation undergoing cardioversion have a high risk of severe sleep apnea.[65] It has not been proven prospectively that OSA causes atrial fibrillation, but the recurrence rate of atrial fibrillation after successful cardioversion is much higher in untreated compared with treated patients with OSA.[65]

Premature Ventricular Complexes

Premature ventricular complexes (PVCs), or extrasystoles, are common in the OSA patient population. There is no clear relationship between sleep PVC

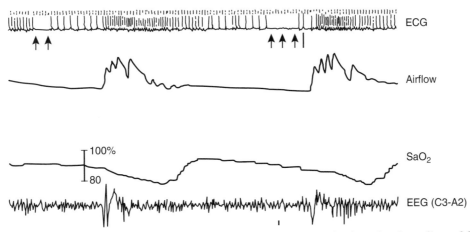

FIGURE 5-5 ■ Vagal activation elicited by the diving reflexes during the apnea leads to bradycardia and bradyarrhythmia. Bradycardia is a physiologic response to apnea, but more severe forms of bradyarrhythmia occur (*arrows*), particularly with apneas of longer duration and pronounced desaturation. Note the characteristic timing of the bradyarrhythmia that occurs at the end of the apnea. The most common forms of bradyarrhythmia are sinoatrial and atrioventricular conduction blocks. (Adapted from Grimm W, Koehler U, Fus E, et al: Outcome of patients with sleep apnea-associated severe bradyarrhythmias after continuous positive airway pressure therapy. Am J Cardiol 86[6]:688–692, A9, 2000.)

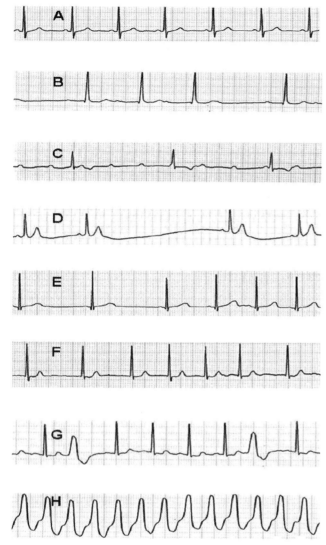

FIGURE 5-6 ■ Examples of various ECG rhythms that might be seen during sleep. **A,** Normal sinus rhythm. **B, C,** Atrioventricular conduction block. P wave is not followed by the QRS complex. **D,** Sinus pause. **E,** Atrial fibrillation. No P waves are visible. **F,** Sinus arrhythmia. **G,** Isolated extrasystoles. **H,** Ventricular tachycardia. Note that the QRS complex is narrow in the supraventricular arrhythmias, differentiating them from ventricular arrhythmias (in the absence of preexisting bundle branch block).

frequency and sleep apnea, except in the most severe apnea cases.[60]

Ventricular Tachycardia

Ventricular tachycardia is an uncommon observation on the polysomnographic rhythm.[66] Whether ventricular tachycardia or other arrhythmia is implicated in the heightened occurrence of sudden cardiac death during the nighttime in patients with OSA remains to be determined.[49]

SUMMARY

1. Heart rate, blood pressure, and sympathetic activity are lowest in stage 4 NREM sleep. These increase during REM sleep, especially in phasic REM.

2. Blood pressure and heart rate are relatively lower during the apneic episode itself, followed by sharp increases on resumption of ventilation. The "diving reflex" refers to simultaneous parasympathetic bradycardia and sympathetic peripheral vasoconstriction during the apnea.

3. A number of cardiovascular disease mechanisms may contribute to established cardiac and vascular disease in patients with OSA. These mechanisms include sympathetic activation, endothelial dysfunction, and systemic inflammation.

4. Patients with OSA have elevated levels of the appetite-suppressant hormone leptin but may be resistant to its action. Patients with OSA appear predisposed to weight gain, and CPAP treatment of OSA lowers leptin and may decrease visceral fat.

5. OSA needs to be considered in patients resistant to antihypertensive therapy (resistant hypertension) and those who do not have nighttime blood pressure reduction on ambulatory monitoring (nondippers). The apnea-hypopnea index may predict the future risk of hypertension development.

6. OSA may be a risk factor for stroke, even after adjustment for other confounders. Once stroke occurs, it generally worsens preexisting OSA. Development of CSA after stoke is not predicted by involvement of any particular brain region and typically resolves in months.

7. OSA may cause nocturnal ischemia in cardiac patients and precipitate paroxysmal nocturnal dyspnea.

8. Bradyarrhythmias are common in OSA. Atrial fibrillation is more prevalent in patients with OSA. Recurrence of atrial fibrillation after cardioversion may occur more frequently in those with untreated OSA, compared with those on CPAP treatment.

REFERENCES

1. Murali NS, Svatikova A, Somers VK: Cardiovascular physiology and sleep. Front Biosci 8:S636–S63652, 2003.
2. Somers VK, Dyken ME, Mark AL, Abboud FM: Sympathetic-nerve activity during sleep in normal subjects. N Engl J Med 328(5):303–307, 1993.
3. Dickerson LW, Huang AH, Thurnher MM, et al: Relationship between coronary hemodynamic changes and

the phasic events of rapid eye movement sleep. Sleep 16(6):550–557, 1993.

4. Shamsuzzaman AS, Gersh BJ, Somers VK: Obstructive sleep apnea: implications for cardiac and vascular disease. JAMA 290(14):1906–1914, 2003.

5. Somers VK, Dyken ME, Clary MP, Abboud FM: Sympathetic neural mechanisms in obstructive sleep apnea. J Clin Invest 96(4):1897–1904, 1995.

6. Leung RS, Bradley TD: Sleep apnea and cardiovascular disease. Am J Respir Crit Care Med 164(12):2147–2165, 2001.

7. Catcheside PG, Chiong SC, Orr RS, et al: Acute cardiovascular responses to arousal from non-REM sleep during normoxia and hypoxia. Sleep 24(8):895–902, 2001.

8. Morgan BJ, Crabtree DC, Puleo DS, et al: Neurocirculatory consequences of abrupt change in sleep state in humans. J Appl Physiol 80(5):1627–1636, 1996.

9. Wellens HJ, Vermeulen A, Durrer D: Ventricular fibrillation occurring on arousal from sleep by auditory stimuli. Circulation 46(4):661–665, 1972.

10. Somers VK, Mark AL, Zavala DC, Abboud FM: Influence of ventilation and hypocapnia on sympathetic nerve responses to hypoxia in normal humans. J Appl Physiol 67(5):2095–2100, 1989.

11. Dimsdale JE, Coy T, Ziegler MG, et al: The effect of sleep apnea on plasma and urinary catecholamines. Sleep 18(5):377–381, 1995.

12. Narkiewicz K, Montano N, Cogliati C, et al: Altered cardiovascular variability in obstructive sleep apnea. Circulation 98(11):1071–1077, 1998.

13. Singh JP, Larson MG, Tsuji H, et al: Reduced heart rate variability and new-onset hypertension: insights into pathogenesis of hypertension: the Framingham Heart Study. Hypertension 32(2):293–297, 1998.

14. Narkiewicz K, Kato M, Phillips BG, et al: Nocturnal continuous positive airway pressure decreases daytime sympathetic traffic in obstructive sleep apnea. Circulation 100(23):2332–2335, 1999.

15. Carlson JT, Rangemark C, Hedner JA: Attenuated endothelium-dependent vascular relaxation in patients with sleep apnoea. J Hypertens 14(5):577–584, 1996.

16. Kato M, Roberts-Thomson P, Phillips BG, et al: Impairment of endothelium-dependent vasodilation of resistance vessels in patients with obstructive sleep apnea. Circulation 102(21):2607–2610, 2000.

17. Schulz R, Mahmoudi S, Hattar K, et al: Enhanced release of superoxide from polymorphonuclear neutrophils in obstructive sleep apnea. Impact of continuous positive airway pressure therapy. Am J Respir Crit Care Med 162(2 Pt 1):566–570, 2000.

18. Dyugovskaya L, Lavie P, Lavie L: Increased adhesion molecules expression and production of reactive oxygen species in leukocytes of sleep apnea patients. Am J Respir Crit Care Med 165(7):934–939, 2002.

19. Svatikova A, Wolk R, Lerman LO, et al: Oxidative stress in obstructive sleep apnoea. Eur Heart J 26(22):2435–2439, 2005.

20. Shamsuzzaman AS, Winnicki M, Lanfranchi P, et al: Elevated C-reactive protein in patients with obstructive sleep apnea. Circulation 105(21):2462–2464, 2002.

21. Chin K, Nakamura T, Shimizu K, et al: Effects of nasal continuous positive airway pressure on soluble cell adhesion molecules in patients with obstructive sleep apnea syndrome. Am J Med 109(7):562–567, 2000.

22. Chin K, Shimizu K, Nakamura T, et al: Changes in intra-abdominal visceral fat and serum leptin levels in patients with obstructive sleep apnea syndrome following nasal continuous positive airway pressure therapy. Circulation 100(7):706–712, 1999.

23. Elmasry A, Lindberg E, Berne C, et al: Sleep-disordered breathing and glucose metabolism in hypertensive men: a population-based study. J Intern Med 249(2):153–161, 2001.

24. Punjabi NM, Sorkin JD, Katzel LI, et al: Sleep-disordered breathing and insulin resistance in middle-aged and overweight men. Am J Respir Crit Care Med 165(5):677–682, 2002.

25. Phillips BG, Kato M, Narkiewicz K, et al: Increases in leptin levels, sympathetic drive, and weight gain in obstructive sleep apnea. Am J Physiol Heart Circ Physiol 279(1):H234–H237, 2000.

26. Ip MS, Lam B, Ng MM, et al: Obstructive sleep apnea is independently associated with insulin resistance. Am J Respir Crit Care Med 165(5):670–676, 2002.

27. Wessendorf TE, Thilmann AF, Wang YM, et al: Fibrinogen levels and obstructive sleep apnea in ischemic stroke. Am J Respir Crit Care Med 162(6):2039–2042, 2000.

28. Peppard PE, Young T, Palta M, Skatrud J: Prospective study of the association between sleep-disordered breathing and hypertension. N Engl J Med 342(19):1378–1384, 2000.

29. Nieto FJ, Young TB, Lind BK, et al: Association of sleep-disordered breathing, sleep apnea, and hypertension in a large community-based study. Sleep Heart Health Study. JAMA 283(14):1829–1836, 2000.

30. Suzuki M, Otsuka K, Guilleminault C: Long-term nasal continuous positive airway pressure administration can normalize hypertension in obstructive sleep apnea patients. Sleep 16(6):545–549, 1993.

31. Dimsdale JE, Loredo JS, Profant J: Effect of continuous positive airway pressure on blood pressure: a placebo trial. Hypertension 35(1 Pt 1):144–147, 2000.

32. Pepperell JC, Ramdassingh-Dow S, Crosthwaite N, et al: Ambulatory blood pressure after therapeutic and sub-therapeutic nasal continuous positive airway pressure for obstructive sleep apnoea: a randomised parallel trial. Lancet 359(9302):204–210, 2002.

33. Portaluppi F, Provini F, Cortelli P, et al: Undiagnosed sleep-disordered breathing among male nondippers with essential hypertension. J Hypertens 15(11):1227–1233, 1997.

34. Culebras A: Cerebrovascular disease and sleep. Curr Neurol Neurosci Rep 4(2):164–169, 2004.

35. Yaggi HK, Concato J, Kernan WN, et al: Obstructive sleep apnea as a risk factor for stroke and death. N Engl J Med 353(19):2034–2041, 2005.

36. Somers VK: Sleep—a new cardiovascular frontier. N Engl J Med 353(19):2070–2073, 2005.

37. Hu FB, Willett WC, Manson JE, et al: Snoring and risk of cardiovascular disease in women. J Am Coll Cardiol 35(2):308–313, 2000.

38. Kamba M, Inoue Y, Higami S, et al: Cerebral metabolic impairment in patients with obstructive sleep apnoea: an independent association of obstructive sleep apnoea with white matter change. J Neurol Neurosurg Psychiatry 71(3):334–339, 2001.

39. Balfors EM, Franklin KA: Impairment of cerebral perfusion during obstructive sleep apneas. Am J Respir Crit Care Med 150(6 Pt 1):1587–1591, 1994.

40. Hayakawa T, Terashima M, Kayukawa Y, et al: Changes in cerebral oxygenation and hemodynamics during obstructive sleep apneas. Chest 109(4):916–921, 1996.

41. Parra O, Arboix A, Bechich S, et al: Time course of sleep-related breathing disorders in first-ever stroke or transient ischemic attack. Am J Respir Crit Care Med 161(2 Pt 1):375–380, 2000.

42. Mohsenin V, Valor R: Sleep apnea in patients with hemispheric stroke. Arch Phys Med Rehabil 76(1):71–76, 1995.

43. Bassetti C, Aldrich MS: Sleep apnea in acute cerebrovascular diseases: final report on 128 patients. Sleep 22(2):217–223, 1999.

44. Good DC, Henkle JQ, Gelber D, et al: Sleep-disordered breathing and poor functional outcome after stroke. Stroke 27(2):252–259, 1996.

45. Marin JM, Carrizo SJ, Vicente E, Agusti AG: Long-term cardiovascular outcomes in men with obstructive sleep apnoea-hypopnoea with or without treatment with continuous positive airway pressure: an observational study. Lancet 365(9464):1046–1053, 2005.

46. Mooe T, Franklin KA, Holmstrom K, et al: Sleep-disordered breathing and coronary artery disease: long-term prognosis. Am J Respir Crit Care Med 164(10 Pt 1):1910–1913, 2001.

47. Schafer H, Koehler U, Ploch T, Peter JH: Sleep-related myocardial ischemia and sleep structure in patients with obstructive sleep apnea and coronary heart disease. Chest 111(2):387–393, 1997.

48. Hanly P, Sasson Z, Zuberi N, Lunn K: ST-segment depression during sleep in obstructive sleep apnea. Am J Cardiol 71(15):1341–1345, 1993.

49. Gami AS, Howard DE, Olson EJ, Somers VK: Day-night pattern of sudden death in obstructive sleep apnea. N Engl J Med 352(12):1206–1214, 2005.

50. Lofaso F, Verschueren P, Rande JL, et al: Prevalence of sleep-disordered breathing in patients on a heart transplant waiting list. Chest 106(6):1689–1694, 1994.

51. Lanfranchi PA, Braghiroli A, Bosimini E, et al: Prognostic value of nocturnal Cheyne-Stokes respiration in chronic heart failure. Circulation 99(11):1435–1440, 1999.

52. Bradley TD, Logan AG, Kimoff RJ, et al: Continuous positive airway pressure for central sleep apnea and heart failure. N Engl J Med 353(19):2025–2033, 2005.

53. Fung JW, Li TS, Choy DK, et al: Severe obstructive sleep apnea is associated with left ventricular diastolic dysfunction. Chest 121(2):422–429, 2002.

54. Niroumand M, Kuperstein R, Sasson Z, Hanly PJ: Impact of obstructive sleep apnea on left ventricular mass and diastolic function. Am J Respir Crit Care Med 163(7):1632–1636, 2001.

55. Bady E, Achkar A, Pascal S, et al: Pulmonary arterial hypertension in patients with sleep apnoea syndrome. Thorax 55(11):934–939, 2000.

56. Sajkov D, Wang T, Saunders NA, et al: Daytime pulmonary hemodynamics in patients with obstructive sleep apnea without lung disease. Am J Respir Crit Care Med 159(5 Pt 1):1518–1526, 1999.

57. Sajkov D, Wang T, Saunders NA, et al: Continuous positive airway pressure treatment improves pulmonary hemodynamics in patients with obstructive sleep apnea. Am J Respir Crit Care Med 165(2):152–158, 2002.

58. Lattimore JD, Celermajer DS, Wilcox I: Obstructive sleep apnea and cardiovascular disease. J Am Coll Cardiol 41(9):1429–1437, 2003.

59. Zwillich C, Devlin T, White D, et al: Bradycardia during sleep apnea. Characteristics and mechanism. J Clin Invest 69(6):1286–1292, 1982.

60. Guilleminault C, Connolly SJ, Winkle RA: Cardiac arrhythmia and conduction disturbances during sleep in 400 patients with sleep apnea syndrome. Am J Cardiol 52(5):490–494, 1983.

61. Koehler U, Becker HF, Grimm W, et al: Relations among hypoxemia, sleep stage, and bradyarrhythmia during obstructive sleep apnea. Am Heart J 139(1 Pt 1):142–148, 2000.

62. Grimm W, Koehler U, Fus E, et al: Outcome of patients with sleep apnea-associated severe bradyarrhythmias after continuous positive airway pressure therapy. Am J Cardiol 86(6):688–692, A9, 2000.

63. Guilleminault C, Pool P, Motta J, Gillis AM: Sinus arrest during REM sleep in young adults. N Engl J Med 311(16):1006–1010, 1984.

64. Mooe T, Gullsby S, Rabben T, Eriksson P: Sleep-disordered breathing: a novel predictor of atrial fibrillation after coronary artery bypass surgery. Coron Artery Dis 7(6):475–478, 1996.

65. Gami AS, Friedman PA, Chung MK, et al: Therapy insight: interactions between atrial fibrillation and obstructive sleep apnea. Nat Clin Pract Cardiovasc Med 2(3):145–149, 2005.

66. Fichter J, Bauer D, Arampatzis S, et al: Sleep-related breathing disorders are associated with ventricular arrhythmias in patients with an implantable cardioverter-defibrillator. Chest 122(2):558–561, 2002.

Narcolepsy and Hypersomnia of Central Origin: Diagnosis, Differential Pearls, and Management

WYNNE CHEN ■ EMMANUEL MIGNOT

The focus of this chapter is the evaluation, differential diagnosis, and management of hypersomnia as defined in the newly updated *International Classification of Sleep Disorders* (ICSD-2), "Hypersomnia of Central Origin Not Due to a Circadian Rhythm Sleep Disorder, Sleep Related Breathing Disorder, or Other Cause of Disturbed Nocturnal Sleep" (Table 6-1).[1] Sleep-disordered breathing (SDB), a major cause of excessive daytime sleepiness, is the principal differential diagnosis and will not be discussed. It is assumed that hypersomnia in the presence of SDB can be confirmed only after SDB has been properly treated. Insufficient sleep and normal variants can also be involved and will similarly only be briefly mentioned.

Historically, the term *hypersomnia* has been used to characterize a rare condition characterized by "increased sleep amounts."[2–4] More recently, however, the term has been used more broadly to include all conditions characterized by a primary, centrally mediated excessive daytime sleepiness.[5,6] In this context, hypersomnia as defined in the ICSD-2 also includes patients with normal sleep amounts but with a documented and unexplained complaint of excessive daytime sleepiness.[1,6] Narcoleptic subjects, for example, do not typically have increased daily sleep amounts yet are included in this broad "hypersomnia" category.

THE CHARACTERISTICS OF SLEEPINESS AND ASSOCIATED SYMPTOMS

Sleepiness, also called *somnolence*, is determined by multiple factors including the quantity and quality of prior sleep, circadian time, drugs, attention, motivation, environmental stimuli, and various medical, neurological, and psychiatric conditions.[7,8] Oftentimes, patients with excessive daytime sleepiness do not use the word *sleepiness* to describe their symptoms. They may use vague words such as *tired, fatigue, decreased daytime vitality or energy*, or other similar terminology. These alternate terms may reflect either genuine sleepiness or fatigue.[9] Fatigue (or "being easily fatigued") is a feeling of tiredness that may be both physical and psychological and typically occurs in psychiatric conditions such as depression and in other conditions such as fibromyalgia and multiple sclerosis.[8,9] Pure fatigue is not associated with sleepiness[8–10]; unfortunately, however, it is used in some contexts as a reflection of sleepiness (for example, in discussing transportation and driving regulations).[11] In patients with pure fatigue, there is no physiologic drive for sleep that occurs when they lie down to rest, as they do not fall asleep. In contrast, those with true sleepiness will be able to fall asleep in situations that are conducive to sleep and, when severe enough, even during situations that are not soporific in nature.[10]

Sleepiness and fatigue have different causes. Indeed, if the sleepiness is the main focus, then attention will be directed toward sleep at night or specific sleep disorders, whereas if the primary problem is fatigue, then the focus might be on a possible underlying medical or psychological problem that is not producing any specific sleep disruption.[10] In addition, some diagnoses may be associated with either or both fatigue and sleepiness; for example, in multiple sclerosis[12,13] and Parkinson's disease.[14,15] Patients with multiple sclerosis are typically fatigued but may also suffer from narcolepsy or a concomitant sleep-disordered breathing that may lead to superimposed sleepiness.[12–16] Similarly, patients with Parkinson's disease may be left with residual fatigue despite treatment of sleepiness.[10,14] Finally, in sleep apnea, unresolved fatigue after continuous positive airway pressure (CPAP) treatment may reveal either a central nervous system–mediated residual hypersomnia or a comorbid depression.[17,18]

Sleepiness manifests in several ways. The first is an ability to fall asleep in any circumstance, sometimes called *sleepability*.[19] The second is a general feeling of *decreased subjective alertness*, often worse after lunchtime.[7] The third is the inability to function normally while awake; errors are made and performance is not optimal.[20,21] Other important manifestations are sleep attacks, sudden occurrence of irresistible sleep, leading to unintentional sleep episodes during wakefulness or frequent naps if circumstances permit.[7,22]

TABLE 6-1 ■ International Classification of Sleep Disorders (ICSD2): Diagnosis Pertaining to Commonly Encountered Hypersomnias

Condition	Symptoms	Diagnostic Criteria		
Narcolepsy with cataplexy	Complaint of EDS, recurrent naps, or lapses into sleep for at least 3 months.	A definite history of cataplexy is present; cataplexy defined as sudden and transient episodes of loss of muscle tone triggered by strong emotions (most reliably laughing or joking; bilateral and brief; <2 minutes; consciousness preserved).	No medical or mental disorder accounts for the symptom.	The diagnosis of narcolepsy should, whenever possible, be confirmed by nocturnal polysomnography (TST >6 hr) followed by an MSLT (MSL ≤8 min; ≥2 SOREMPs). Alternatively, CSF hypocretin-1 may be measured and found to be low (≤110 pg/ml or 1/3 of mean normal control values).
Narcolepsy without cataplexy	Complaint of EDS, recurrent naps, or lapses into sleep for at least 3 months.	Typical cataplexy is not present, although doubtful or atypical cataplexy-like episodes may be reported.	No medical or mental disorder accounts for the symptom.	Supporting evidence is required, typically in the form of a positive MSLT, as described above for narcolepsy with cataplexy.
Idiopathic hypersomnia with long sleep time	Complaint of EDS for at least 3 months.	Prolonged nocturnal sleep time (≥10 hours), documented by interviews, actigraphy, or sleep logs. Waking up in the morning or at the end of naps is almost always laborious.	No medical (most notably head trauma) or mental disorder is present that could account for the symptoms. Symptoms do not meet the diagnostic criteria of other sleep disorders causing excessive sleepiness.	PSG excludes other causes of sleepiness. It demonstrates a short sleep latency and a major sleep period that is prolonged to more than 10 hours. If an MSLT is performed, it should show a mean sleep latency of less than two SOREMPs.
Idiopathic hypersomnia without long sleep time	Complaint of EDS for at least 3 months.	Nocturnal sleep of normal habitual duration (>6 but <10 hours). Need documentation by interviews, actigraphy, or sleep logs.	No medical or mental disorder accounts for the symptom. Symptoms do not meet the diagnostic criteria of other sleep disorders causing excessive sleepiness.	PSG must be performed and demonstrate a major sleep period of normal durations (>6 but <10 hours). Sleep efficiency is usually more than 85%. An MSLT performed following a PSG must show: (1) MSL ≤8 minutes; (2) <2 SOREMPs.
Recurrent hypersomnia (includes Kleine-Levin syndrome and menstrual-related hypersomnia)	The patient experiences episodes of EDS lasting a minimum of 2 days to a maximum of 4 weeks.	Episodes recur at least once or twice per year.	The hypersomnia is not associated with other medical or mental disorders, such as tumors of the central nervous system or bipolar disorder.	The patient has normal alertness, cognitive functioning, and behavior between attacks.

CSF, Lumbar sac cerebrospinal fluid; EDS, excessive daytime sleepiness; MSLT, Multiple Sleep Latency Test; PSG, polysomnography; SOREMP, sleep-onset rapid eye movement period; TST, total sleep time.

When severe, sleepiness may also manifest as *automatic behavior*.[22,23] In automatic behavior, sleep attacks and microsleep episodes occur in the middle of a purposeful activity, leading to dramatically impaired performance and no memory of the event. In a typical event, a sleepy patient on the phone may continue to talk but in an unintelligible way. The special case of *sleep drunkenness* should also be mentioned.[5,7,24] In sleep drunkenness, there is sleepiness in extreme when emerging from sleep, leading to confusion. Sleep drunkenness is an extreme form of sleep inertia. Whether or not somnolence can be alleviated by sleeping is also important (i.e., is sleep "refreshing"?).[22] In some sleep disorders such as narcolepsy, sleepiness is typically reversed temporarily by short naps.[23] In others, for example in many patients with sleep-disordered breathing or idiopathic hypersomnia, it is not.[3] Of note, however, is that there is significant clinical overlap in the clinical presentation of sleepiness between these conditions.[4,5]

The severity, duration, and timing of sleepiness are also important. The subjective severity of the somnolence was taken into account in the diagnostic criteria of the former ICSD-1 1997 classification.[25] In this classification, excessive sleep was considered mild if it occurred during rest or when little attention is required (e.g., reading) and was associated with minor impairment of social and occupational function; moderate if occurring occasionally during physical activities that involved only a mild to moderate degree of attention (e.g., eating or driving) and was associated with a moderate impairment in social or occupational function; and severe if sleepiness occurred daily and during activities that required a moderate degree of attention (e.g., group meeting or conference call) and was associated with marked impairment of social or occupational function. In the revised classification, it was noted that it is difficult to quantify impairment. In the context of an ICSD-2 defined sleep disorder, sleepiness must have occurred almost daily for at least 3 months and be significant enough to "impair daytime functioning."[1] A notable exception are periodic hypersomnia cases, a combination of rare disorders in which hypersomnia is episodic and the patient is normally functioning between episodes. It was also noted that severity of sleepiness is typically higher in cases with narcolepsy-cataplexy, periodic hypersomnia (in episodes), and idiopathic hypersomnia with long sleep time.[1]

CATAPLEXY

Cataplexy is almost pathognomonic for narcolepsy-cataplexy.[22,26,27] Cataplexy is a brief (seconds, rarely more than minutes), bilateral loss of muscle tone elicited by emotions.[27,28] The existence of a typical trigger is crucial to the recognition of genuine cataplexy. It is usually produced by humor or laughter; for example, when the patient is telling a joke or relating a funny story.[27,29] Less commonly, anger, surprise, elation, or playful excitement are involved.[27,29] Other emotions such as stress, sexual activity, and embarrassment may also be involved, but occur in addition to more typical triggers.[27,29] Cataplexy may present more atypically without any emotional trigger at the beginning of narcolepsy, around disease onset, when the disorder is still developing. There is no sensory component or loss of consciousness. Attacks can be mild, such as an inability to retain facial muscle tone, or severe, leading to complete collapse. Reflexes are abolished,[28,30] but the episodes are rarely long enough to evaluate by physical examination.

Cataplexy must be differentiated from physiologic reactions (cataplexy-like events), syncope, sleep attacks, and seizures.[27,29] Syncope, sleep attacks, and generalized seizures all involve a loss of consciousness. The bilateral distribution of weakness and temporal course are inconsistent with most strokes. The short duration and lack of correlation with intense exercise are inconsistent with episodic or fluctuating neuromuscular disorders. The lack of positive phenomena rules out most seizures. Because startle alone is not a typical trigger, hyperekplexia can be excluded. It is also important to differentiate genuine cataplexy from normal physiologic reactions.[31] For example, a person may laugh so hard that his or her face hurts or feels weak. When laughing hard, non-narcoleptic patients might also feel "rubber knees" or roll onto the floor. In true cataplexy, muscle weakness is obvious and must occur more than a few times in a lifetime.[27,29] A large portion of the general population reports cataplexy-like events, but those are rare, mild, and often not triggered by typical emotions.[29,32] Curiously, however, these cataplexy-like events are significantly correlated in population samples with daytime sleepiness and depression.[32–34]

The existence of definite cataplexy alone, together with sleepiness (over 3 months in duration), is sufficient to diagnose narcolepsy-cataplexy in the ICSD-2, although it is suggested to proceed with a multiple sleep latency test (MSLT)[1] (see Table 6-1). Because of this, cataplexy must be definite and typical to diagnose narcolepsy-cataplexy. If cataplexy is atypical (e.g., occurring only during sex or while stressed) or is very rare or mild (cataplexy-like events), it is best to consider cataplexy as absent and to classify the patient as narcolepsy without cataplexy. As discussed later, this may be helpful in case drug response is unsatisfactory.

Other Symptoms

Sleep paralysis is an inability to move that occurs most commonly on awakening and occasionally at sleep onset.[22,27,35] Hypnagogic and hypnopompic hallucinations are dreamlike visual or auditory perceptions that occur at sleep onset and on awakening, respectively.[22,27,36] These symptoms can be severe and bothersome in patients with narcolepsy.[26,27] In these cases the symptom is often frightening and may deserve clinical attention. Importantly, however, is the fact that these symptoms can also be found in normal individuals, idiopathic hypersomnia, or obstructive sleep apnea in some circumstances.[33–36] In the other cases, however, it is often milder, and may occur at times where rapid eye movement (REM) sleep is normally present, in the middle of the night.

The special case of insomnia in the context of hypersomnia and narcolepsy deserves special mention. Disturbed nocturnal sleep is present in approximately 50% of patients with narcolepsy-cataplexy and can be very disabling.[7,22,26,37–39] In narcolepsy, it is usually not characterized by difficulty falling asleep but rather by recurrent nighttime awakenings and a feeling of restlessness during the night.[7,22,26] Nightmares and increased periodic limb movements are often seen.[37,38] The situation becomes more complex when insomnia is associated with a complaint of excessive daytime sleepiness, as sleepiness could be the result of insufficient sleep. In these cases, it is typically recommended to treat the insomnia first. As mentioned previously, it is also generally recommended to treat sleep-disordered breathing first before diagnosing centrally mediated hypersomnias, keeping in mind that these conditions may be associated.

PERIODIC HYPERSOMNIA

In periodic hypersomnia, the somnolence or increased sleep lasts 2 days to 4 weeks, recur at least once a year and is separated by periods with normal alertness and cognitive functioning (see Table 6-1). The major differential diagnoses are medical conditions, bipolar disorder, seasonal affective disorder, or other recurrent psychiatric conditions. Periodic hypersomnia is a rare condition, and diagnosis is primarily clinically based. If the hypersomnia occurs in association with menstruation, a diagnosis of menstrual-related hypersomnia may be made.[40,41] This extremely rare condition is typically reactive to hormonal therapy. More commonly, symptoms suggestive of Kleine-Levin syndrome (KLS) may be present, typically in an adolescent male.[42] KLS is a rare disease characterized by recurrent episodes of hypersomnia and, to various degrees, behavioral or cognitive disturbances, compulsive eating behavior, and hypersexuality. In addition, in KLS, one or more of the associated features may apply: (1) binge eating; (2) hypersexuality; (3) abnormal behavior such as irritability, aggression, or other odd behavior; and/or (4) cognitive abnormalities such as a feeling of unreality, confusion, and hallucinations. KLS is a difficult disorder to treat; only lithium has been suggested to be effective in some cases.[42] This contrasts with the lack of effect of other thymoregulators such as carbamazepine.[42] Median duration for KLS was 8 years in a recent meta-analysis of 186 cases.[42] The best course of action is often education and passive surveillance rather than pharmacological treatment.

CLASSIFICATION OF THE DISORDERS ASSOCIATED WITH HYPERSOMNIA

There are multiple ways in which to classify the disorders associated with daytime sleepiness (and equivalents), as reflected in Tables 6-1 to 6-3. Such classification can also serve as a basis for studying for the sleep medicine board exams and may facilitate differential diagnoses. The most intuitive method may be to categorize them by etiology or mechanism. At the most basic level, these can be separated into those in which sleepiness is presumably the result of a primary centrally mediated abnormality (see Table 6-1), those in which sleepiness is secondary to a known medical or psychiatric conditions (Table 6-2), and those that are typically an extension of a normal physiology, for example, sleep restriction or long sleeper (Table 6-3). Sleepiness may also be due to disturbed nocturnal sleep secondary to sleep apnea (see Table 6-3) or seizures of other conditions disturbing nocturnal sleep. Another diagnosis where sleepiness may be a critical component is circadian rhythm disorders, most commonly in the context of shift work disorder (see Table 6-3). Of note, the observation of isolated periodic leg movements together with sleepiness is not considered a diagnostic entity in the new ICSD-2 (in contrast to the former ICSD-1) owing to lack of evidence of a correlation with sleepiness.[43,44]

Disorders can also be separated by those seen more often in children, adolescents or young adults, and those seen in predominantly in older adults. For example, narcolepsy and KLS (see Table 6-1) tend to occur in adolescents or young adults, whereas advanced sleep phase disorder tends to occur in the elderly. Furthermore, disorders with a significant behavioral component can also be identified, in particular with regard to insomnia and the circadian rhythm disorders.

When specifically examining the diagnoses under the category of hypersomnias of central origin, separating the 11 main diagnoses into those causing persistent symptoms versus those causing intermittent symptoms of hypersomnolence may help to simplify organization of the details and characteristics of each disorder (see Table 6-3). Most commonly, however, the

TABLE 6-2 ■ Secondary Hypersomnia and Narcolepsy Diagnoses

Condition	Diagnostic Criteria	
Narcolepsy resulting from a medical condition (secondary to neurological or medical disorders)	Complaint of EDS for at least 3 months. Possible cataplexy. A significant underlying medical or neurological disorder accounts for the daytime sleepiness.	If cataplexy is not present or is very atypical, polysomnographic monitoring performed over the patient's habitual sleep period followed by an MSLT must demonstrate a mean sleep latency of ≤8 minutes with 2 or more SOREMPs, despite sufficient nocturnal sleep prior to test (minimum 6 hours).
	The hypersomnia is not better explained by another sleep disorder, mental disorder, medication use, or substance use disorder.	Hypocretin-1 levels in the CSF are less than 110 pg/ml (or 30% of normal control values), provided the patient is not comatose.
Hypersomnia due to a medical condition (neurological and medical disorders)	The patient has a complaint of EDS present almost daily for at least 3 months. A significant underlying medical or neurological disorder accounts for the daytime sleepiness. The hypersomnia is not better explained by another sleep disorder, mental disorder, medication use, or substance use disorder.	If an MSLT is performed, the mean sleep latency is <8 minutes with no more than one SOREMP following polysomnographic monitoring performed over the patient's habitual sleep period.
Hypersomnia resulting from drug or substance (drug abuse and adverse effects of a medication)	The patient has a complaint of EDS or excessive sleep. The complaint is believed to be secondary to current use, recent discontinuation, or prior prolonged use of drugs or prescribed medication.	The hypersomnia is not better explained by another sleep disorder, medical or neurological disorder, mental disorder, or medication use or substance use disorder.
Hypersomnia not resulting from substance or a physiological condition (resulting from a psychiatric condition but not substance abuse disorder)	The patient has a complaint of EDS or excessive sleep. The complaint is temporally associated with a psychiatric diagnosis. The hypersomnia is not better explained by another sleep disorder, medical or neurological disorder, medication use, or substance use disorder.	Polysomnographic monitoring demonstrates both: Reduced sleep efficiency and increased frequency and duration of awakenings. Variable, often normal, mean sleep latencies on the MSLT.

CSF, Lumbar sac cerebrospinal fluid; EDS, excessive daytime sleepiness; MSLT, Multiple Sleep Latency Test; SOREMP, sleep-onset REM period.

patient can be evaluated following the chart described in Figure 6-1.

CLINICAL INTERVIEW OF THE SLEEPY PATIENT

The severity and nature of the primary complaint of excessive daytime sleepiness should be evaluated. Questions should include ability to fall asleep in any circumstances, whether the patient dozes easily or feels sleepy in quiet or monotonous situations (such as while driving or eating), how frequently the patient has irresistible sleep attacks, how many naps are taken (during the work week and during weekends), and whether the patient generally feels rested in the morning or after naps (if routinely taken).

The clinician should also explore typical duration of sleep during the night when working and when on vacation (ideal duration of sleep). The use of an alarm clock and how difficult it is to wake up should be noted (sleep inertia). This is primarily important to exclude insufficient sleep but may also suggest idiopathic hypersomnia. Timing (and regularity) of the major sleep episodes should also be evaluated for the possibility of circadian abnormalities. A list of the patient's current medications (prescription and over-the-counter) should be taken, and a note should be made if these have sedation as side effects (for example, antiepileptic medications). Finally, the patient should be evaluated for other possible sleep disorders, such as SDB (snoring, breathing pauses, etc.), parasomnia, or sleep-related movement disorders. As mentioned, patients are often unaware of their true sleepiness, and simply observing their tendency to fall asleep (in the waiting room or examining room) can verify the true extent of their symptoms.

The natural evolution of the symptoms should also be explored. Symptoms are stable for most primary disorders of excessive daytime sleepiness, except for

TABLE 6-3 ■ Normal Variants, Sleep-Related Breathing Disorders, Parasomnia, and Circadian Rhythms Sleep Disorders That May Be Confused with Hypersomnia Diagnoses

Condition	Diagnostic Criteria	
Sleep-related breathing disorders	See chapter on sleep-related breathing disorder.	The major differential diagnosis for hypersomnia.
	Most typically obstructive sleep apnea syndromes.	May contribute only partially to overall daytime sleepiness.
		Must be treated first before a diagnosis of hypersomnia or narcolepsy without cataplexy can be made (except if cataplexy is present).
Behaviorally induced insufficient sleep syndrome	Complaint of excessive daytime sleepiness or, in prepubertal children, of behavioral abnormalities suggesting sleepiness.	When habitual sleep schedule is not maintained (weekends or vacation), patients will sleep considerably longer than usual.
	The abnormal sleep pattern is present for at least 3 months.	May be only one of the components contributing to overall daytime sleepiness.
Long sleeper	The daily total sleep time is ≥10 hours.	The sleep pattern typically has been present since childhood.
		Habitual sleep episode is usually shorter than expected from age-norms except for long sleepers, where it may be within normal limits. This should be established using history, a sleep log, or actigraphy.
	Excessive daytime sleepiness occurs if the patient does not obtain that amount of sleep.	Polysomnography not required; sleep must first be extended. If polysomnography is done, sleep efficiency >90%; multiple sleep latency test (MSLT) may be abnormal.
Circadian rhythm sleep disorders	Persistent or recurrent sleep disturbances caused by either an alteration of the circadian time-keeping system or a misalignment between the endogenous circadian rhythms and exogenous factors affecting sleep timing or duration.	May be only one of the components contributing to daytime sleepiness. With sleepiness, most commonly involve delayed or advanced sleep phase disorder and shift work disorders.
	Must lead to insomnia, sleepiness, or both to be considered a disorder.	The sleep disturbance is not explained by another sleep disorder, medical or neurological disorder, mental disorder, medication use, or substance use disorder. May be technically difficult to differentiate from idiopathic hypersomnia.
	Must be associated with an impairment of social, occupational, or other areas of functioning.	More rarely: irregular sleep–wake rhythm disorder, free running type, jet lag type, and secondary to a medical or psychiatric condition.
Recurrent isolated sleep paralysis	Inability to move at sleep onset or on awakening (a few seconds to a few minutes).	A parasomnia explained by narcolepsy, hypersomnia (with sleepiness and abnormal MSLT), or another medical condition.
		Sleepiness is not the key associated feature, otherwise an hypersomnia diagnosis should be considered. Should be considered as a normal variant if mild or infrequent. May be familial.
Nightmare disorder REM sleep behavior disorders	See chapter on parasomnia.	When not explained by narcolepsy, hypersomnia, or another condition.
		Sleepiness is not the key associated feature, otherwise a hypersomnia diagnosis should be considered.

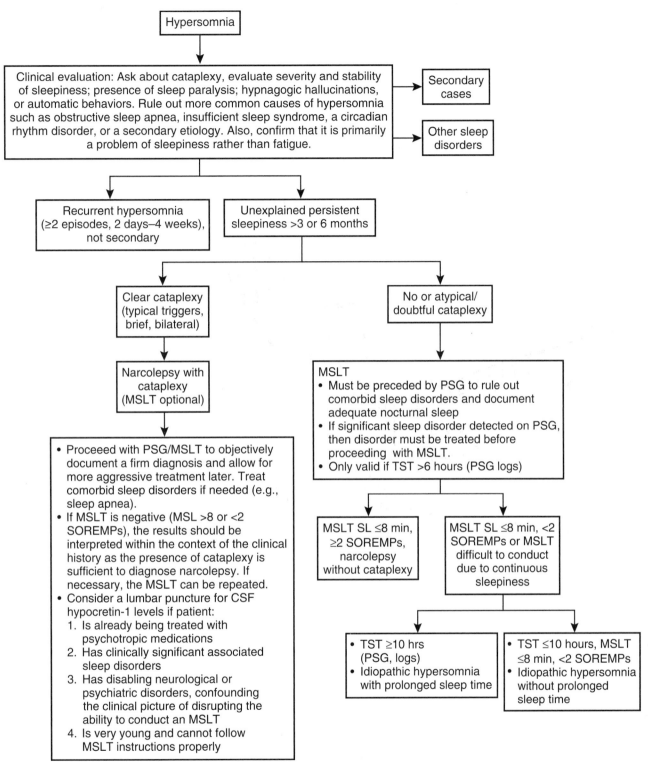

FIGURE 6-1 ■ Diagnostic flow chart for most commonly encountered types of hypersomnia. MSL, Multiple sleep latency; MSLT, multiple sleep latency test; CSF, cerebrospinal fluid; PSG, polysomnography; SOREMP, sleep onset REM period; TST, total sleep time.

periodic hypersomnia and in some cases of psychiatric hypersomnia. It is also important to have the patient describe disease onset (especially when mediations were not confounding the clinical picture). An abrupt onset is more likely to be organically based. If onset is recent, with weight gain, or in a child or an adolescent, it may suggest evolving narcolepsy.[45,46] Timing of sleepiness and the presence of concomitant insomnia may also be helpful. Although most sleepiness occurs throughout the day or on awakening (before medications or caffeine is consumed), advanced sleep phase disorder is associated with sleepiness in the evening and early morning awakening with insomnia. Conversely, those with delayed sleep phase disorder experience evening insomnia and morning sleepiness and "sleep drunkenness."[1]

Because of its importance to the diagnosis, questions regarding cataplexy should be asked carefully to avoid leading the patient. Cataplexy is rarely observed during interviews, although small facial attacks are sometimes observed when severely affected patients recount emotional events. A question such as "Does anything unusual happen when you are laughing?" is more appropriate than "Do you feel weak when you are laughing?" Similarly, the clinician should not be satisfied with a simple affirmative response. Rather, the patient should be asked to recall specific circumstances. In this regard, it is useful to ask for a description of the first or last episode experienced. Patients describing unclear events, or events that have occurred only once, should be considered without cataplexy for the purpose of further evaluation and treatment strategies (Figures 6-1 and 6-2).

Nocturnal sleep disruption or symptoms suggestive of REM behavior disorder,[47,48] periodic limb movements, nightmares, or other parasomnia may be associated with several sleep disorders, including narcolepsy.* There may also be an association with sleep-disordered breathing. A particularly long nocturnal sleep duration (>10 hours) suggests idiopathic hypersomnia with long sleep time[3,4,6] (or simply a long sleeper, based on reversibility with reasonable sleep amounts; see Table 6-3). The presence and severity of sleep paralysis and/or hypnagogic hallucinations should be noted. As noted previously, however, presence of these symptoms is not predictive of diagnosis,[33–36] but if severe, it has some limited diagnostic value and may require therapeutic attention.[22,27]

Driving should be discussed, and, if needed, the patient should be instructed to stop driving.[50,51] Risk of accidents is higher in those who are chronically sleepy[52,53] or have a sleep disorder such as narcolepsy[54,55] or sleep apnea.[56] Patients may be reluctant to discuss their symptoms fully for fear of losing their driver's license or, in the case of typical narcolepsy, because of the strange and often bizarre nature of their symptoms.[57]

A detailed medical history, with emphasis on cardiovascular, endocrinological, and nasopharyngeal problems, as well as neurological and psychiatric problems, should be taken. Significant neurological or psychiatric symptomatology should lead to formal consultations

with appropriate services if needed. Thyroid evaluation and red blood cell counts may be needed. Social history should include information about any alcohol or drug use/abuse, as well as use of caffeine or nicotine and living environment. For example, the institutionalized elderly individual may be predisposed to circadian sleep disorders such as irregular sleep-wake rhythm owing to lack of consistent exposure to *zeitgebers* (external synchronizing agents such as light, activity, and social schedules).[1] Furthermore, the social history may provide clues to the impact of chronic sleepiness, such as heightened risk for accidents at home or at work, poor performance at the workplace or academically, and social and marital problems.[57] Physical examination of major systems, including blood pressure (stimulants and some antidepressants may interact with blood pressure and heart rate) and nose/upper airway examination (mostly for sleep apnea), is needed.

Family history should elicit information about other family members who may have similar symptoms and/or patterns of sleep; disorders with a genetic component, such as circadian rhythm disorders, narcolepsy and SDB, may run in families.[1,10,58,59]

Subjective Quantification of Sleepiness and Other Symptoms

A number of instruments have been developed to assess daytime sleepiness and cataplexy; the most commonly used in clinical practice are discussed next.

Epworth Sleepiness Scale (ESS)

The Epworth Sleepiness Scale (ESS) is an eight-item, self-rating scale. It assesses the patient's likelihood of falling asleep (dozing behavior) during the course of the day during eight, normal everyday situations of varying soporific nature (sitting, watching TV, in a car, talking to someone). The patient is asked to rate the likelihood of falling asleep on a scale from 0–3, where 0 indicates no chance of falling asleep or dozing, and 3 represents a very high chance of falling asleep. The total ESS score ranges from 0 to 24, with higher scores reflecting a greater sleep propensity.[60] A total score of 10 or more suggests pathologic sleepiness, requiring further evaluation and treatment.[18,61] Most patients with a complaint of excessive daytime sleepiness have scores of 12 or higher (for example, more than 90% of narcoleptic subjects have an ESS $\geq$ 12, personal data in over 1000 narcoleptic subjects). Of importance, however, many control subjects, approximately 25% of a general population sample, score high ($\geq$12) on this scale. High scores on the ESS also do not necessarily correlate well with MSLT mean sleep

*7,22,26,37,38,49.

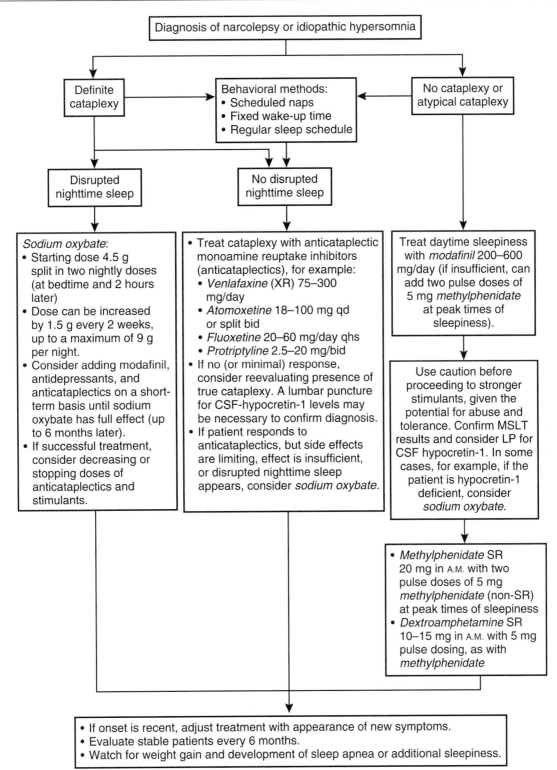

FIGURE 6-2 ■ Suggested treatment strategy for narcolepsy and idiopathic hypersomnia. Note that other strategies for treatment are possible on a case-by-case basis. MSLT, Multiple sleep latency test; CSF, cerebrospinal fluid; SR/XR, slow- or extended-release formula.

latencies.[62–64] A disconnection between the two may suggest fatigue rather than sleepiness,[65] a psychiatric hypersomnia,[66-68] or, in some cases, idiopathic hypersomnia.[5]

Sleep Logs and Actigraphy

Sleep logs document time of sleep onset and waking times, and awakenings during the night, as well as daytime naps, during a period of approximately 2 weeks.[10] It is most useful to document significant sleep restriction or circadian disruption and the frequency and timing of nocturnal events (motor activity or parasomnias).[10] It can be used to document typical amounts of daily sleep over the 24-hour period and should be examined before MSLT testing. Alternatively, actigraphy can be used,[69,70] although it is most accurate in measuring sleep amounts in subjects without disturbed sleep or a sleep disorder.

The Stanford Center for Narcolepsy Sleep Inventory (SSI)

The SSI is a 146-item questionnaire divided into nine sections (http://med.stanford.edu/school/Psychiatry/narcolepsy/). Section I and II report demographic information while the ESS is included in Section III. Section IV includes questions about sleep habits, insomnia, sleep-related breathing disorders, abnormal movements during the night, and napping. Section V contains 51 items on cataplexy; and sections VI, VII, and VIII include questions about hypnagogic hallucinations, sleep paralysis, and automatic behavior, respectively. This questionnaire has been validated in narcoleptic patients.[29] It is most useful to help detect definite cataplexy, as previous validation indicates a high correlation with clinical and biologic findings when the patients reported muscle weakness episodes when "telling and hearing a joke" and, less specifically, with laughing.[27,29]

The Fatigue Severity Scale (FSS)

A self-rated test that assesses the degree of fatigue intensity on various functional and behavioral aspects of life, this questionnaire provides a subjective measurement of daytime fatigue[18] that is largely independent of daytime sleepiness and depression. Each item is rated from 1 (strongly disagree) to 7 (strongly agree). Scoring involves calculating the mean score for all statements, with the range of possible scores being from 1–7 and higher scores reflecting greater fatigue. The FSS provides adequate means of assessing fatigue intensity within a general population, has high internal consistency and strong validation data, and clearly distinguishes between patients and controls. A score of 3 has been used as the cut-off point for normal, above which implied pathological fatigue should be suspected.[18]

There is not always a correlation between subjective and objective measures of sleepiness, but gross disparities should compel the clinician to consider hypersomnia associated with a psychiatric disorder (hypersomnia not due to a substance or known physiologic condition).

Polysomnographic Investigations

A complaint of excessive daytime sleepiness not explained by another medical condition is a clear indication for polysomnography (PSG).[71] Most typically, an overnight sleep study, followed by the MSLT, is required.[72]

Nocturnal Polysomnography (NPSG)

The all-night polysomnogram has its greatest utility in detection of SDB, but it is also useful for determining abnormal events that occur during specific sleep stages, such as parasomnias and nocturnal motor activity. Video monitoring with expanded electroencephalography (EEG) montage can be very helpful in determining the clinical features of an abnormal event that occurs during sleep so that differentiation can be made between a parasomnia and an epileptic disorder.[10] EEG activity is also crucial in making this differentiation.[10] The occurrence of a REM sleep onset (within 20 minutes of sleep onset) during the NPSG occurs in approximately 50% of cases with narcolepsy-cataplexy but is rare in control subjects.[73] A sleep-onset REM period (SOREMP) at night is thus highly predictive of narcolepsy.

Multiple Sleep Latency Testing (MSLT)

Performed during the main period of wakefulness, the MSLT was designed to determine a patient's tendency to fall asleep.[72,74,75] To be valid, an NPSG must have been performed the night before and must show at least 6 hours of total sleep time.[1] Significant sleep-disordered breathing, if present, should have been treated first, using positive pressure therapy or other techniques.[1] For this last criterion, no formal apnea hypopnea index number has been provided in the ICSD-2, and the decision is left to the clinician.

The mean sleep onset latency (MSL) is determined from five naps (ideally, rarely four), and patients who have normal alertness take more than 10 minutes, on average, to fall asleep. Sleepy patients will fall asleep in less than 10 minutes, and those with severe sleepiness in less than 5 minutes. A cut-off of 8 minutes or less is used in the ICSD-2 classification[1] as an indication of documented sleepiness, both in the context of a diagnosis of idiopathic hypersomnia or narcolepsy. It should be noted, however, that up to one third of the general population may have a MSL of 8 minutes or less.[72] The finding of a short MSL alone, without any SOREMP, should be interpreted cautiously together with the clinical picture.[76] Very short sleep latencies are more likely to reflect real central nervous system pathology. The MSLT MSL is known to be sensitive to sleep deprivation.[64,76] The MSLT can also be of some value in detecting sleepiness in patients who might otherwise deny sleepiness.[10]

The finding of multiple REM sleep during the MSLT is more predictive of pathology than a short sleep latency. Current criteria for narcolepsy include MSL of ≤8 minutes and ≥2 SOREMPs. Recent large studies have, however, shown that 4–9% of the general population may have multiple SOREMPs on routine clinical MSLTs,[77–79] with about half (2–4%) reporting daytime sleepiness and meeting MSLT criteria for narcolepsy. This last finding may reflect mild narcolepsy phenotypes in the general population of a higher prevalence of narcolepsy without cataplexy than previously suspected.[79] The occurrence of multiple SOREMPs during the MSLT may be influenced by SDB and sleep deprivation, although data are conflicting in this area.[76–80]

The MSLT is not a validated test in young children (typically less than 8 years old).[1] It may difficult to instruct young children properly and may be more often negative in these subjects[81] (Box 6-1).

Maintenance of Wakefulness Test (MWT)

The MWT is a 40-minute protocol (four trials separated by 2-hour intervals) used to assess an individual's ability to stay awake. It is performed in much the same way as the MSLT (under soporific conditions), but the patient is placed in a semireclining position. As with the MSLT, the latency to onset of sleep is recorded, and healthy alert patients will not fall asleep within a mean of 15 minutes on the four or five nap opportunities.[82,83] One of the advantages of the MWT over the MSLT is the ability to measure and distinguish sleepiness at higher levels of somnolence. Indeed, the MSLT suffers from a significant "floor" effect; a significant number of patients have very short mean sleep latencies, and the very sleepy and extremely sleepy cannot be distinguished from each other. In the MWT, pathological mean sleep latency has a bigger spread of values. For this reason, the MWT is usually performed to assess efficacy of treatment for hypersomnia.[83–85] Unlike the MSLT, the performance of nocturnal polysomnography before the MWT is optional, determined on a case-by-case basis.[10,72,86] The MWT may also be helpful when there is a need to document that the patient is alert and adequately treated; for example in cases of professional or medicolegal inquiry. It does not, however, constitute absolute proof of constant alertness and can be used only as supporting data.[72,76]

Continuous 24-Hour Sleep Recording

Twenty-four-hour ambulatory or in-house PSG/EEG monitoring may be useful in the evaluation of seizure disorders, documentation of cataplexy, or sleep-onset REM period in the evaluation of narcolepsy[87,88] or in documenting a long sleep time for idiopathic hypersomnia cases.[1,2] Although not routinely performed in clinical practice for practical reasons, it is an excellent test. It may also be useful to detect distribution of interictal eplieptiform activity during the sleep-wake cycle.[1]

Standard Daytime 16-Channel to 20-Channel EEG

This test can be performed (with partial or total sleep deprivation the night before) to document seizures if clinically indicated.[1] In some cases, it can be useful to distinguish atonic seizures from cataplexy.

Biologic and Radiological Evaluations

Routine Blood Tests

These have usually been performed by the referring physician before consultation, but the patient should be asked if certain tests have been recently performed.[10] Electrolytes, thyroid-stimulating hormone, and blood cell counts (to exclude anemia and endocrinological abnormalities) are important, especially when the clinical picture suggests a fatigue component.[10] Patients with features suggestive of restless legs syndrome should have ferritin measured. Measuring selected drug of abuse in urine samples is indicated if malingering is suspected.

Human Leukocyte Antigen (HLA) Typing

Narcolepsy is associated with genes of the HLA system, DRB1, DQA1, and HLA-DQB1.[89–91] The HLA complex refers to a collection of more than 20 genes located on chromosome 6. These genes are important for the presentation of antigens to the rest of the immune system and the control of the subsequent immune response. HLA genes are highly polymorphic (i.e., have subtle differences between people), resulting in multiple molecular subtypes.[89] In the past, HLA subtype variants were determined using antibody-based serological techniques (e.g., DR2, DQ1, DQ6). More recently, these subtypes are determined at the deoxyribonucleic acid (DNA) level, using a classification indicated with stars (e.g., DRB1*1501, DQB1*0602). The HLA DRB1, DRA (nonpolymorphic), DQA1, and DQB1 genes encode the alpha and beta chains of the corresponding HLA-DR and DQ protein.

In narcolepsy with cataplexy, 90–95% of the cases are HLA-DRB1*1501, DQA1*0102, and DQB1*0602 positive.[91,92] These three variants are almost always found

BOX 6-1 ■ Multiple Sleep Latency Testing (MSLT) for Narcolepsy

1. The MSLT consists of five nap opportunities performed at 2-hour intervals. The initial nap opportunity begins 1.5–3 hours after termination of the nocturnal recording. The conventional recording montage for the MSLT includes central EEG and occipital derivations, left and right eye electrooculograms (EOGs), mental/submental electromyogram (EMG), and electrocardiogram (ECG).

2. The MLST must be performed immediately after PSG recorded during the patient's major sleep period. The use of MSLT to support a diagnosis of narcolepsy is suspect if total sleep time on the previous night is less than 6 hours or if significant sleep-disordered breathing is noted. The test should not be performed after a split-night sleep.

3. Have the patient maintain a sleep diary for 2 weeks before sleep testing, including the following recommended questions:
   - What time did you go to bed last night?
   - What time did you turn off the light, intending to sleep, last night?
   - How long did it take you to fall asleep?
   - What time did you plan to wake up?
   - What time did you actually wake up?
   - Rate how rested/refreshed you feel now: 1 = very rested; 10 = not at all.
   - Rate the quality of your sleep last night: 1 = excellent; 10 = very poor.
   - How many times did you wake up during the night?
   - Estimate the amount of time you spent awake after you fell asleep (in minutes).
   - How long did you nap yesterday (in minutes)?

4. Obtain a current medication list, including over-the-counter and illicit drugs, particularly stimulants, stimulant-like medications, and REM-suppressing medications. Medications that may suppress REM include carbamazepine, phenytoin, fluoxetine, tricyclic antidepressants, lithium, venlafaxine, chlorpromazine, haloperidol, progesterone, beta blockers, clonidine, diphenhydramine, loratadine, promethazine, barbiturates, and benzodiazepines.

5. Ensure that patients are drug-free for at least 15 days before sleep testing; the ideal length of time off drugs is at least 5 half-lives of the drug or longer-acting metabolite. Urine toxicology screening may be needed to verify the absence of medications and/or illicit drugs on the night of the sleep study or the morning after (morning of the MSLT).

6. Ensure that the patient's use of usual medications, such as antihypertensives, is planned by the sleep clinician before the MSLT so that undesired influences by the stimulating or sedating properties of the medications are minimized.

7. Before each nap opportunity, the patient should be asked if he/she needs to go to the bathroom or needs other adjustments for comfort. Standard instructions for biocalibration before each nap include:
   - Lie quietly with your eyes open for 30 seconds;
   - Close both eyes for 30 seconds;
   - Without moving your head, look to the right, then left, right, and then left;
   - Blink eyes slowly five times;
   - Clench or grit your teeth tightly together.

8. With each nap opportunity, the subject should be given the same instructions: "Please lie quietly, assume a comfortable position, keep your eyes closed, and try to fall asleep." Immediately after these instructions are given, the lights are turned off, signaling the beginning of the test.

9. Between naps, the patient should be out of bed and prevented from sleeping. The patient should also be advised to:
   - Stop smoking at least 30 minutes before each nap opportunity.
   - Avoid vigorous physical activity during the day and stop any stimulating activities at least 15 minutes before each nap opportunity.
   - Abstain from all caffeine and avoid any unusual exposure to bright sunlight.
   - A light breakfast is recommended at least 1 hour before the first trial, and a light lunch is recommended after the termination of the second noon trial.

10. A nap session is terminated after 20 minutes if sleep does not occur. Sleep onset for the clinical MSLT is determined by the time from lights out to the first epoch of any stage of sleep, including stage 1 sleep. Sleep onset is defined as the first epoch of greater than 15 seconds of cumulative sleep in a 30-second epoch. The absence of sleep on a nap opportunity is recorded as a sleep latency of 20 minutes. This latency is included in the calculation of mean sleep latency (MSL). To assess for the occurrence of REM sleep in the clinical MSLT, the test continues for 15 minutes after the first epoch of sleep.

11. The MSLT report should include the start and end times of each nap opportunity, latency from lights out to the first epoch of sleep, MSL, and number of sleep-onset REM periods (defined as >15 seconds of REM sleep in a 30-second epoch).

together in both control subjects and narcolepsy patients. The most specific and likely culprit subtype is DQB1*0602, as association with this variant is strongest across all ethnic groups. This may be most important in African Americans, where DRB1*1501 is not a good marker for narcolepsy.[91] It should be kept in mind, however, that 12–38% of the general population (depending of the specific ethnic group) carry the exact same HLA subtype, DQB1*0602.[91] HLA typing may thus be most helpful to exclude narcolepsy-cataplexy; for example, before cerebrospinal fluid (CSF) hypocretin-1 measurement (see Figure 6-1). Of importance, however, there have been rare reports of DQB1*0602-negative patients with unquestionable narcolepsy; four out of several hundreds tested with low CSF hypocretin-1.[92–95] Other HLA alleles, in particular DQB1*0301, also have a slight effect on narcolepsy predisposition.[91]

In narcolepsy without cataplexy, a slight increase in HLA frequency has been reported. In the United States, for example, approximately 25% of the control population is DQB1*0602 positive, whereas narcolepsy without cataplexy cases are 35–40% DQB1*0602 positive.[92,96] This moderately increased frequency suggests some etiological heterogeneity, with approximately 15% of cases without cataplexy sharing pathophysiological similarities with narcolepsy-cataplexy.[79] This is also in line with the finding suggesting 5–40% hypocretin deficiency reported in such cases (see later).[92] The slight increase in HLA frequency in cases without cataplexy has limited diagnostic value. In this context, HLA typing may only be useful in selected cases; for example, before CSF hypocretin-1 evaluation and/or in the consideration of some aggressive therapeutic strategies (see Figure 6-1).

CSF Hypocretin-1

Decreased hypocretin neurotransmission is known to cause most of the cases of narcolepsy with cataplexy.[93] Animal models with defective hypocretin transmission have a disorder very similar, if not identical, to narcolepsy.[97,98]

Hypocretin (also called *orexin*) neuropeptides (hypocretin-1 and -2) are produced by approximately 70,000 neurons, all located in a subregion of the dorsolateral hypothalamus. Hypocretin neurons project widely throughout the brain, most notably onto monoaminergic and cholinergic neurons also involved in the regulation of sleep.[99,100] These peptides are excitatory in almost all cases. In human narcolepsy brains, most cells producing hypocretin have been destroyed or cannot be detected.[95,101] Although most cases of human narcolepsy are idiopathic, genetic and environmental factors are suspected to play a role in the

development of this disorder.[102] The very tight association with HLA-DQB1*0602 and delayed development suggest that narcolepsy may be caused by an autoimmune-mediated degeneration of hypocretin-producing neurons located in the hypothalamus.[89] This hypothesis remains unproven to date.[103] It is also possible that narcolepsy is caused indirectly and that hypocretin neurons are especially sensitive to excitotoxicity.

Hypocretins cannot yet be reliably measured in the blood,[104] but hypocretin-1 can easily been measured in the CSF.[93] In patients with narcolepsy-cataplexy (typically HLA positive), almost all cases have dramatically decreased CSF hypocretin-1.[37,67,93,105–110] Values below 110 pg/ml or one third of mean normal control values are highly diagnostic for narcolepsy in the absence of a severe brain pathology.[93,111] Unfortunately, however, although this test is highly specific and sensitive for cases with cataplexy, it is only positive in 5–40% of cases without cataplexy (but still highly specific). In more than 300 patients with narcolepsy tested to date by multiple groups, all but 4 cases with low CSF hypocretin-1 have been shown to be DQB1*0602 positive.[92–95] We therefore often advise checking HLA-DQB1*0602 first before testing CSF hypocretin-1, although as often encountered in medicine, rare exceptions can occur[112] (see Figure 6-1).

Considering the difficulty of conducting lumbar punctures, the use of CSF hypocretin-1 in the diagnosis of narcolepsy is typically reserved for complex cases.[111,112] These cases mostly include cases where the MSLT cannot be properly interpreted: young children, patients with both narcolepsy and severe sleep apnea or with very disturbed nocturnal sleep, patients where it is difficult to instruct an MSLT (mental retardation, psychiatric condition), and secondary narcolepsy cases. It may also be useful in patients in whom the presence of cataplexy is atypical, when treatment response has been suboptimal and there is a need to use more forceful treatments (for example, high-dose amphetamine or sodium oxybate). In rare instances, MSLT costs may also be an issue.

Computed Tomography or Magnetic Resonance Imaging of the Brain and Other Secondary Explorations

The tests are indicated if a secondary medical or neurological etiology is suspected or if the clinical picture or therapeutic response is atypical. In narcolepsy with and without cataplexy, examples include all subjects with abnormal neurological findings at clinical examination, HLA-negative subjects with isolated cataplexy, and subjects with a narcolepsy plus other symptoms suggestive of a more complex syndrome.

Secondary narcolepsy cases are more frequent in children than in adults.[113,114] In children, narcolepsy-like features may occur in the context of a complex genetic disorders, often with dysmorphic features, such as Prader-Willi syndrome (with obesity and sleep apnea, mental retardation, and other features), myotonic dystrophy (plus muscle weakness, sleep apnea, cataract, hair loss, mental retardation, or other), Niemann-Pick type-C (with seizures, ataxia, profound mental retardation, hepatosplenomegaly, early death), Coffin-Lowry syndrome (mental retardation, with seizures), Norries disease (ocular atrophy, deafness), and late-onset congenital hypoventilation syndrome (with hypothalamic abnormality).[90,93,111,115] Cataplexy may be difficult to differentiate from atonic seizures in these cases.

In both adults and children, narcolepsy may also be the reflection of a hypothalamic tumor (pontine tumors have also been reported in isolated cataplexy),[116] an inflammatory condition (acute disseminated encephalomyelitis, multiple sclerosis, Guillain-Barré syndrome), or traumatic hypothalamic lesions[117] and other diseases. Finally, it should be mentioned that hypersomnia is a common symptom and is associated with many neurological disorders, including Parkinson's disease and post-traumatic conditions. Investigations have shown low CSF hypocretin-1 in many of these "secondary cases," but it is often difficult to establish if the decreased hypocretin-1 is a cause or consequence.[111] Reversal of decreased CSF hypocretin with treatment of the primary condition has been found in multiple cases.

Psychiatric Evaluation and Psychological Testing

These are helpful when depression, psychosis, malingering, or conversion disorder is suspected.

Management

Treatment strategies are primarily pharmacological (see Figure 6-2). Of importance, however, is that pharmacotherapy should be initiated more carefully in cases where the clinical picture is unclear and the origin of the sleepiness may have multiple causes. For example, it is not uncommon in clinical practice to encounter patients with a picture of idiopathic hypersomnia who also have some sleep apnea, insufficient sleep, and a hieratic sleep-wake schedule. In these complex cases, a step-by-step progressive therapeutic approach is needed. Addressing these issues first is often more fruitful than starting pharmacotherapy. Pharmacotherapy using amphetamine-like stimulant should also proceed cautiously in such patients to avoid the development of addiction. Finally,

as a rule, treatments that are not effective should be withdrawn to avoid accumulating complex drug interactions and side effects.

Behavioral Treatments

Good sleep hygiene, education, and treatment compliance[118] are important to the management of narcolepsy and hypersomnia.[7] Referral to support groups such as the Narcolepsy Network may also be helpful. Fixed wake-up times and regular sleep schedules are recommended. Napping every day at regular time(s), but not excessively, can also be of benefit.[119,120] Timing of meals and avoidance of alcohol and some foods may also be helpful.[121] In some cases of idiopathic hypersomnia, a long period of "sleep" may be reported, but sleep periods are fragmented all through the night and day, largely occurring at the wrong circadian phase. A depressive component may also be present in these cases. Light therapy, sleep restriction, and sleep hygiene can be paradoxically helpful in some of these cases, unlike in genuine narcolepsy.[122] In narcolepsy, obesity may develop, especially in young children when the disease onset is abrupt.[45,46] In these cases, it is useful to restrict diet, encourage exercise, and treat sleepiness aggressively around disease onset.

The risk of driving while sleepy, especially before adequate therapy, must be discussed and, if appropriate, regulatory agencies notified.[50] Patients with narcolepsy or severe hypersomnia must avoid jobs that put others in danger and should consider activities that are less sedentary.[54] Jobs that involve repetitive tasks, or sitting down and looking at a computer all day, can be difficult. Employers or teachers should be asked to accommodate 15- to 30-minute scheduled naps.

Wake-Promoting Therapeutics

Modafinil is now a first-line, standard-of-care treatment for sleepiness associated with hypersomnia or narcolepsy.[123,124] The mode of action of modafinil is not well established but is likely to involve inhibition of dopamine reuptake.[90] Headache can be a problematic side effect but usually resolves and can often be avoided by slowly increasing the dose. Drug-drug interaction, including with oral contraceptives, need to be explored before prescription. The safest starting dose is 100 mg in the morning, which can be gradually increased to a maximum of 400–600 mg. There is a rare patient benefit from higher doses. This may be split into a morning and a noon dose. Modafinil is usually not addictive[125] and can thus be used more easily in cases in which the origin of the somnolence is not well understood or of physiological origin. For example, it is approved for use in the treatment of residual sleepiness in patients with treated sleep apnea[126] and shift work disorder.[127]

Amphetamine-like stimulants, such as methylphenidate, dextroamphetamine, amphetamine racemic mixture, and methylamphetamine, can also be used and are often stronger stimulants but have a number of disadvantages.[90,124] They are potentially addictive and should be reserved for patients with a well-established diagnosis. Also, side effects such as palpitations, hypertension, and nervousness may occur because of their action on the autonomic nervous system.[90,124] The mode of action of amphetamine-like stimulants on wakefulness is thought to involve increased dopaminergic transmission (blocking of reuptake and stimulation of release).[90] Amphetamine (especially methamphetamine) should be used more cautiously than methylphenidate, as animal experiments have shown cytotoxicity on monoaminergic neurons for amphetamine,[128] a compound that depletes dopamine store by interfering with the vesicular monoamine transporter.[129]

The most important concept in using stimulants for treating daytime sleepiness is timing. A typical scenario is to use modafinil or an extended-release methylphenidate or amphetamine formulation in the morning with pulse dosing of short-acting medication at appropriate times throughout the day. For example, a student who still has problems with sleepiness after lunch might take 5–15 mg short-acting methylphenidate at that time in addition to morning modafinil. Although stimulants are used primarily for daytime sleepiness, amphetamines (not modafinil) also have some effect on cataplexy at high doses. Of note, short- and fast-acting stimulants are more likely to be abused, and it may be more difficult to control their administration. In the use of stimulant medications, the specific formulation,[130] isomer,[131] packaging, and brand can make a difference in optimizing efficacy. In rare cases, pemoline (a mild dopaminergic stimulant, but with hepatotoxicity), mazindol (also a dopaminergic reuptake inhibitor stimulant), and selegiline (a monoamine oxidase inhibitor-B inhibitor with metabolism into amphetamine) may also be considered.[131]

Antidepressants

Antidepressants are commonly used to treat cataplexy but can also be useful in some cases to treat other symptoms. For example, they are effective for sleep paralysis and hypnagogic hallucinations, a sometimes disabling symptom.[90,131] Tricyclic agents are very effective but have anticholinergic side effects.[131] Serotonin reuptake specific inhibitors are efficacious, but relatively high doses are generally needed.[131] Newer medications targeting norepinepherine reuptake, such as venlafaxine and atomoxetine, are most effective.[123,129,132]

The dual serotoninergic and noradrenergic reuptake inhibitor venlafaxine (75–300 mg/day) is now a typical first-line treatment.[123,133] The use of an extended-release formulation is critical, or multiple daily doses should used. If this is not helpful, atomoxetine (18–100 mg qd or split bid), fluoxetine (20–60 mg/day), or even tricyclic antidepressants (such as protryptiline 2.5–20 mg/day, clomipramine 25–200 mg/day) can be used. Atomoxetine is unique in being the only medication approved by the Food and Drug Administration (for attention deficit–hyperactivity disorder) that selectively blocks norepinephrine reuptake.[132,134] It is also a mild stimulant and can sometimes be used to treat mild daytime sleepiness, in some cases with idiopathic hypersomnia. Rarely, the use of other compounds, for example monoamine oxidase inhibitors, can be considered.[131] Patients should be forewarned that rebound cataplexy almost always occurs when antidepressant medications are discontinued, changed, or skipped. Compliance is the key to therapeutic efficacy as anticataplectic agents. It is occasionally difficult to wean patients from these medications because of rebound cataplexy.

Sodium Oxybate

Sodium oxybate (gamma hydroxybutyrate or GHB) is unique, as it is efficacious on all symptoms.[85,133,135–137] This naturally occurring compound is a potent but short-acting hypnotic that consolidates slow wave and REM sleep, most likely via gamma aminobutyric acid-receptor B agonist effects.[133,135] It has been available since the 1970s[138] for narcolepsy but was only recently approved for the treatment of cataplexy. It is thought that the consolidation of nocturnal sleep and REM sleep leads to decreased daytime symptoms. The starting dose is 4.5 g per night, divided in two nightly doses (before bedtime and 2–3 hours later, once the first dose has metabolized). The patient should prepare both doses, lie down after taking the drug, and possibly set an alarm for the second dose. The dose can be increased every 2 weeks by 1.5-g increments to a maximum of 9 g per night (rarely 12 g). The most common side effects are dizziness, nausea, and at a higher dose, enuresis. Sodium oxybate should not be taken with alcohol or other central nervous system depressants.

One of its best indications is in cases with narcolepsy-cataplexy and disturbed nocturnal sleep.[135] In this indication, it should be noted that full efficacy is often delayed and occurs over months. Experiments have also shown no acute rebound of cataplexy or other symptoms on withdrawal when properly prescribed in this population,[139] possibly because of the particular nature of the population and the exclusive night use. It should also be noted that the drug can be prescribed in the presence of sleep apnea if treated properly by CPAP (or after surgical treatment). This use can be helpful when a patient with narcolepsy has sleep apnea and insomnia, making it difficult to tolerate CPAP. In this case, however, CPAP compliance should be carefully monitored.

A limitation for the use of sodium oxybate is its abuse potential, toxicity at high dose, and illicit use.[140,141] The drug should probably be used more cautiously in patients without a clear diagnosis. In some of these cases, however, it can be of clear benefit.

Other Sedatives

Some narcolepsy and hypersomnia patients can benefit from GABAergic acting hypnotics, such as zolpidem or a benzodiazepine, to help consolidate nighttime sleep. These may be most helpful when sodium oxybate is not an option.

Treatment of Ancillary and Associated Conditions

In the special case of narcolepsy or hypersomnia caused by other medical or neurological conditions, optimal therapy for the associated condition should be achieved first, with special attention to having adequate control of nocturnal sleep disturbances that could partially or entirely cause the daytime sleepiness. Primary narcolepsy is also frequently associated with other sleep disorders. Obstructive sleep apnea is common and must be treated, especially if sodium oxybate is to be used. Periodic leg movements are also common but rarely need treatment, unless associated with restless legs syndrome.

CONCLUSION AND PERSPECTIVES

The diagnosis and treatment of narcolepsy with cataplexy is well codified. Its pathophysiology is also well understood. Improved therapy for narcolepsy-cataplexy has resulted from the introduction of the novel antidepressants, sodium oxybate and modafinil. In contrast, little is known in the area of narcolepsy without cataplexy, idiopathic hypersomnia, and periodic hypersomnia. Additional research is needed to find the cause of these related disorders. Also, these pathologies are increasingly diagnosed based on the MSLT alone, yet the MSLT is not well validated as a diagnostic tool for these conditions. This is especially true in the context of idiopathic hypersomnia, a condition increasingly diagnosed on the basis of short mean sleep latency alone. With the growth of sleep medicine, patients with hypersomnia symptoms are increasingly identified in the context of other sleep symptoms or disorders, mostly insomnia, depression, circadian abnormalities, sleep deprivation, and obstructive sleep apnea. Clear therapeutic guidelines are absent for these conditions, although it is generally advised to be more cautious with the use of potentially addictive substances such as amphetamine and sodium oxybate. The diagnosis and management of these complex cases remains challenging but may be a next frontier in optimizing diagnosis and clinical care in the field of hypersomnia.

REFERENCES

1. American Academy of Sleep Medicine: *ICSD-2, The International Classification of Sleep Disorders, Diagnostic and Coding Manual*, 2nd ed. Westchester, IL, American Academy of Sleep Medicine, 2005, pp 1–293.
2. Billiard M: Idiopathic hypersomnia. Neurol Clin 14(3):573–582, 1996.
3. Billiard M, Dauvilliers Y: Idiopathic hypersomnia. Sleep Med Rev 5(5):349–358, 2001.
4. Roth B: Narcolepsy and hypersomnia: review and classification of 642 personally observed cases. Schweiz Arch Neurol Neurochir Psychiatr 119(1):31–41, 1976.
5. Bassetti C, Aldrich MS: Idiopathic hypersomnia. A series of 42 patients. Brain 120(Pt 8):1423–1435, 1997.
6. Dauvilliers Y: Differential diagnosis in hypersomnia. Curr Neurol Neurosci Rep 6(2):156–162, 2006.
7. Black JE, Brooks SN, Nishino S: Narcolepsy and syndromes of primary excessive daytime somnolence. Semin Neurol 24(3):271–282, 2004.
8. Guilleminault C, Brooks SN: Excessive daytime sleepiness: a challenge for the practising neurologist. Brain 124(Pt 8):1482–1491, 2001.
9. Pigeon WR, Sateia MJ, Ferguson RJ: Distinguishing between excessive daytime sleepiness and fatigue: toward improved detection and treatment. J Psychosom Res 54(1):61–69, 2003.
10. Thorpy MJ: Approach to the patient with a sleep complaint. Semin Neurol 24(3):225–235, 2004.
11. Dawson D, McCulloch K: Managing fatigue: it's about sleep. Sleep Med Rev 9(5):365–380, 2005.
12. Fleming WE, Pollak CP: Sleep disorders in multiple sclerosis. Semin Neurol 25(1):64–68, 2005.
13. MacAllister WS, Krupp LB: Multiple sclerosis-related fatigue. Phys Med Rehabil Clin North Am 16(2):483–502, 2005.
14. Rye DB, Bliwise DL, Dihenia B, Gurecki P: FAST TRACK, daytime sleepiness in Parkinson's disease. J Sleep Res 9(1):63–69, 2000.
15. Thorpy MJ, Adler CH: Parkinson's disease and sleep. Neurol Clin 23(4):1187–1208, 2005.
16. Tachibana N, Howard RS, Hirsch NP, et al: Sleep problems in multiple sclerosis. Eur Neurol 34(6):320–323, 1994.
17. Black J: Sleepiness and residual sleepiness in adults with obstructive sleep apnea. Respir Physiol Neurobiol 136(2–3):211–220, 2003.
18. Hossain JL, Ahmad P, Reinish LW, et al: Subjective fatigue and subjective sleepiness: two independent consequences of sleep disorders? J Sleep Res 14(3):245–253, 2005.
19. Harrison Y, Horne JA: "High sleepability without sleepiness." The ability to fall asleep rapidly without other signs of sleepiness. Neurophysiol Clin 26(1):15–20, 1996.
20. Durmer JS, Dinges DF: Neurocognitive consequences of sleep deprivation. Semin Neurol 25(1):117–129, 2005.
21. Van Dongen HP, Dinges DF: Sleep, circadian rhythms, and psychomotor vigilance. Clin Sports Med 24(2):237–249, vii–viii, 2005.
22. Overeem S, Mignot E, van Dijk JG, Lammers GJ: Narcolepsy: clinical features, new pathophysiologic insights, and future perspectives. J Clin Neurophysiol 18(2):78–105, 2001.
23. Honda Y: Clinical features of narcolepsy: Japanese experience. In Honda Y, Juji T (eds): *HLA in Narcolepsy*. New York, Springer-Verlag, 1988, pp 24–57.
24. Roth B, Nevsimalova S, Sagova V, et al: Neurological, psychological and polygraphic findings in sleep drunkenness. Schweiz Arch Neurol Neurochir Psychiatr 129(2):209–222, 1981.
25. Disorders AAS: *ICSD-1, The International Classification of Sleep Disorders, Revised: Diagnostic and Coding Manual*. Rochester, MN, American Sleep Disorders Association, 1997.
26. Dauvilliers Y, Billiard M, Montplaisir J: Clinical aspects and pathophysiology of narcolepsy. Clin Neurophysiol 114(11):2000–2017, 2003.
27. Okun ML, Lin L, Pelin Z, et al: Clinical aspects of narcolepsy-cataplexy across ethnic groups. Sleep 25(1):27–35, 2002.
28. Guilleminault C, Wilson RA, Dement WC: A study on cataplexy. Arch Neurol 31(4):255–261, 1974.
29. Anic-Labat S, Guilleminault C, Kraemer HC, et al: Validation of a cataplexy questionnaire in 983 sleep-disorders patients. Sleep 22(1):77–87, 1999.
30. Krahn LE, Boeve BF, Olson EJ, et al: A standardized test for cataplexy. Sleep Med 1(2):125–130, 2000.
31. Overeem S, Lammers GJ, van Dijk JG: Weak with laughter. Lancet 354(9181):838, 1999.
32. Kaprio J, Hublin C, Partinen M, et al: Narcolepsy-like symptoms among adult twins. J Sleep Res 5(1):55–60, 1996.
33. Szklo-Coxe M, Young T, Finn L, Mignot E: Depression: relationship to sleep paralysis and other sleep disturbances in a community sample. Sleep 28 (Abstract supplement):A306, 2005.
34. Szklo-Coxe M, Young T, Finn L, Mignot E: Sleep paralysis, hypnagogic hallucinations, cataplexy: narcolepsy spectrum and aternate etiology. In Bassetti C, Billiard M, Mignot E (eds): *Narcolepsy and Hypersomnia*. New York, Informa Healthcare, 2007, pp 133–148.
35. Ohayon MM, Zulley J, Guilleminault C, Smirne S: Prevalence and pathologic associations of sleep paralysis in the general population. Neurology 52(6):1194–1200, 1999.
36. Ohayon MM, Priest RG, Caulet M, Guilleminault C: Hypnagogic and hypnopompic hallucinations: pathological phenomena? Br J Psychiatry 169(4):459–467, 1996.
37. Hong SC, Leen K, Park SA, et al: HLA and hypocretin studies in Korean patients with narcolepsy. Sleep 25(4):440–444, 2002.
38. Godbout R, Montplaisir J: Nocturnal sleep of narcoleptics: revisited. Sleep 9(1):159–161, 1986.
39. Montplaisir J, Godbout R: Nocturnal sleep of narcoleptic patients: revisited. Sleep 9(1 Pt 2):159–161, 1986.
40. Billiard M, Guilleminault C, Dement WC: A menstruation-linked periodic hypersomnia, Kleine-Levin syndrome or new clinical entity? Neurology 25(5):436–443, 1975.

41. Sachs C, Persson HE, Hagenfeldt K: Menstruation-related periodic hypersomnia: a case study with successful treatment. Neurology 32(12):1376–1379, 1982.

42. Arnulf I, Zeitzer JM, File J, et al: Kleine-Levin syndrome: a systematic review of 186 cases in the literature. Brain 128(Pt 12):2763–2776, 2005.

43. Mendelson WB: Are periodic leg movements associated with clinical sleep disturbance? Sleep 19(3):219–223, 1996.

44. Nicolas A, Lesperance P, Montplaisir J: Is excessive daytime sleepiness with periodic leg movements during sleep a specific diagnostic category? Eur Neurol 40(1):22–26, 1998.

45. Kotagal S, Krahn LE, Slocumb N: A putative link between childhood narcolepsy and obesity. Sleep Med 5(2):147–150, 2004.

46. Daniels L: Narcolepsy. Medicine 13(1):1–122, 1934.

47. Abad VC, Guilleminault C: Review of rapid eye movement behavior sleep disorders. Curr Neurol Neurosci Rep 4(2):157–163, 2004.

48. Schenck CH, Mahowald MW: REM sleep behavior disorder: clinical, developmental, and neuroscience perspectives 16 years after its formal identification in SLEEP. Sleep 25(2):120–138, 2002.

49. Mayer G, Meier-Ewert K: Motor dyscontrol in sleep of narcoleptic patients (a lifelong development?). J Sleep Res 2(3):143–148, 1993.

50. Black JE, Brooks SN, Nishino S: Conditions of primary excessive daytime sleepiness. Neurol Clin 23(4):1025–1044, 2005.

51. Douglas NJ: The psychosocial aspects of narcolepsy. Neurology 50(2 Suppl 1):S27–S30, 1998.

52. Gander PH, Marshall NS, Harris RB, Reid P: Sleep, sleepiness and motor vehicle accidents: a national survey. Aust N Z J Public Health 29(1):16–21, 2005.

53. Philip P: Sleepiness of occupational drivers. Ind Health 43(1):30–33, 2005.

54. Broughton WA, Broughton RJ: Psychosocial impact of narcolepsy. Sleep 17(8 Suppl):S45–S49, 1994.

55. Findley L, Unverzagt M, Guchu R, et al: Vigilance and automobile accidents in patients with sleep apnea or narcolepsy. Chest 108(3):619–624, 1995.

56. Pack AI, Pien GW: How much do crashes related to obstructive sleep apnea cost? Sleep 1 27(3):369–370, 2004.

57. Wise MS: Narcolepsy and other disorders of excessive sleepiness. Med Clin North Am 88(3):597–610, vii–viii, 2004.

58. Taheri S, Mignot E: The genetics of sleep disorders. Lancet Neurol 1(4):242–250, 2002.

59. Tafti M, Maret S, Dauvilliers Y: Genes for normal sleep and sleep disorders. Ann Med 37(8):580–589, 2005.

60. Kim H, Young T: Subjective daytime sleepiness: dimensions and correlates in the general population. Sleep 28(5):625–634, 2005.

61. Doghramji PP: Recognizing sleep disorders in a primary care setting. J Clin Psychiatry 65(Suppl 16):23–26, 2004.

62. Olson LG, Cole MF, Ambrogetti A: Correlations among Epworth Sleepiness Scale scores, multiple sleep latency tests and psychological symptoms. J Sleep Res 7(4):248–253, 1998.

63. Punjabi NM, Bandeen-Roche K, Young T: Predictors of objective sleep tendency in the general population. Sleep 26(6):678–683, 2003.

64. Young TB: Epidemiology of daytime sleepiness: definitions, symptomatology, and prevalence. J Clin Psychiatry 65(Suppl 16):12–16, 2004.

65. Briones B, Adams N, Strauss M, et al: Relationship between sleepiness and general health status. Sleep 19(7):583–588, 1996.

66. Billiard M, Dolenc L, Aldaz C, et al: Hypersomnia associated with mood disorders: a new perspective. J Psychosom Res 38(Suppl 1):41–47, 1994.

67. Bassetti C, Gugger M, Bischof M, et al: The narcoleptic borderland: a multimodal diagnostic approach including cerebrospinal fluid levels of hypocretin-1 (orexin A). Sleep Med 4(1):7–12, 2003.

68. Dolenc L, Besset A, Billiard M: Hypersomnia in association with dysthymia in comparison with idiopathic hypersomnia and normal controls. Pflugers Arch 431(6 Suppl 2):R303–304, 1996.

69. Ancoli-Israel S, Cole R, Alessi C, et al: The role of actigraphy in the study of sleep and circadian rhythms. Sleep 26(3):342–392, 2003.

70. Sadeh A, Acebo C: The role of actigraphy in sleep medicine. Sleep Med Rev 6(2):113–124, 2002.

71. Kushida CA, Littner MR, Morgenthaler T, et al: Practice parameters for the indications for polysomnography and related procedures: an update for 2005. Sleep 28(4):499–521, 2005.

72. Littner MR, Kushida C, Wise M, et al: Practice parameters for clinical use of the multiple sleep latency test and the maintenance of wakefulness test. Sleep 28(1):113–121, 2005.

73. Hong SC, Hayduk R, Lim J, Mignot E: Clinical and polysomnographic features in DQB1*0602 positive and negative narcolepsy patients: results from the modafinil clinical trial. Sleep Med 1(1):33–39, 2000.

74. Mitler MM: The multiple sleep latency test as an evaluation for excessive somnolence. In Guilleminault C (ed): *Sleeping and Waking Disorders: Indications and Techniques*. Menlo Park, CA, Addisson-Wesley, 1982, pp 145–153.

75. Carskadon MA, Dement WC, Mitler MM, et al: Guidelines for the multiple sleep latency test (MSLT): a standard measure of sleepiness. Sleep 9(4):519–524, 1986.

76. Bonnet MH: ACNS Clinical Controversy, MSLT and MWT have limited clinical utility. J Clin Neurophysiol 23(1):50–58, 2006.

77. Singh M, Drake C, Roth T: The prevalence of multiple sleep onset REM periods in a population-based sample. Sleep 29(7):890–895, 2006.

78. Geisler P, Tracik F, Tajana AM, et al: The influence of age and sex on sleep latency in the MSLT-30: a normative study. Sleep 29(5):687–697, 2006.

79. Mignot E, Lin L, Finn L, et al: Correlates of Sleep onset REM periods during the Multiple Sleep Latency Test in community adults. Brain 129(Pt 6):1609–1623, 2006.

80. Chervin RD, Aldrich MS: Sleep onset REM periods during multiple sleep latency tests in patients evaluated for sleep apnea. Am J Respir Crit Care Med 161(2 Pt 1):426–431, 2000.

81. Guilleminault C, Pelayo R: Narcolepsy in children: a practical guide to its diagnosis, treatment and follow-up. Paediatr Drugs 2(1):1–9, 2000.

82. Doghramji K, Mitler MM, Sangal RB, et al: A normative study of the maintenance of wakefulness test (MWT). Electroencephalogr Clin Neurophysiol 103(5):554–562, 1997.

83. Mitler MM, Walsleben J, Sangal RB, Hirshkowitz M: Sleep latency on the maintenance of wakefulness test (MWT) for 530 patients with narcolepsy while free of psychoactive drugs. Electroencephalogr Clin Neurophysiol 107(1):33–38, 1998.

84. Mitler MM, Hajdukovic R: Relative efficacy of drugs for the treatment of sleepiness in narcolepsy. Sleep 14(3):218–220, 1991.

85. Mamelak M, Black J, Montplaisir J, Ristanovic R: A pilot study on the effects of sodium oxybate on sleep architecture and daytime alertness in narcolepsy. Sleep 27(7):1327–1334, 2004.

86. Arand D, Bonnet M, Hurwitz T, et al: The clinical use of the MSLT and MWT. Sleep 28(1):123–144, 2005.

87. Billiard M, Salva MQ, De Koninck J, et al: Daytime sleep characteristics and their relationships with night sleep in the narcoleptic patient. Sleep 9(1 Pt 2):167–174, 1986.

88. Rubboli G, d'Orsi G, Zaniboni A, et al: A video-polygraphic analysis of the cataplectic attack. Clin Neurophysiol 111(Suppl 2):S120–S128, 2000.

89. Lin L, Hungs M, Mignot E: Narcolepsy and the HLA region. J Neuroimmunol 117(1–2):9–20, 2001.

90. Mignot E: Narcolepsy: pharmacology, pathophysiology and genetics. In Kryger M, Roth T, Dement W (eds): *Principles and Practice of Sleep Medicine*, 4th ed. Philadelphia, Elsevier Saunders, 2005, pp 761–779.

91. Mignot E, Lin L, Rogers W, et al: Complex HLA-DR and -DQ interactions confer risk of narcolepsy-cataplexy in three ethnic groups. Am J Hum Genet 68(3):686–699, 2001.

92. Lin L, Mignot E: HLA and narcolepsy: present status and relationship with familial history and hypocretin deficiency. In Bassetti C, Billiard M, Mignot E (eds): *Narcolepsy and Hypersomnia*. New York, Informa Healthcare, 2007, pp 411–424.

93. Mignot E, Lammers GJ, Ripley B, et al: The role of cerebrospinal fluid hypocretin measurement in the diagnosis of narcolepsy and other hypersomnias. Arch Neurol 59(10):1553–1562, 2002.

94. Dalal MA, Schuld A, Pollmacher T: Undetectable CSF level of orexin A (hypocretin-1) in a HLA-DR2 negative patient with narcolepsy-cataplexy. J Sleep Res 11(3):273, 2002.

95. Peyron C, Faraco J, Rogers W, et al: A mutation in a case of early onset narcolepsy and a generalized absence of hypocretin peptides in human narcoleptic brains. Nat Med 6(9):991–997, 2000.

96. Mignot E, Hayduk R, Black J, et al: HLA DQB1*0602 is associated with cataplexy in 509 narcoleptic patients. Sleep 20(11):1012–1020, 1997.

97. Chemelli RM, Willie JT, Sinton CM, et al: Narcolepsy in orexin knockout mice: molecular genetics of sleep regulation. Cell 98(4):437–451, 1999.

98. Lin L, Faraco J, Li R, et al: The sleep disorder canine narcolepsy is caused by a mutation in the hypocretin (orexin) receptor 2 gene. Cell 98(3):365–376, 1999.

99. Peyron C, Tighe DK, van den Pol AN, et al: Neurons containing hypocretin (orexin) project to multiple neuronal systems. J Neurosci 18(23):9996–10015, 1998.

100. Saper CB, Scammell TE, Lu J: Hypothalamic regulation of sleep and circadian rhythms. Nature 437(7063):1257–1263, 2005.

101. Thannickal TC, Moore RY, Nienhuis R, et al: Reduced number of hypocretin neurons in human narcolepsy. Neuron 27(3):469–474, 2000.

102. Mignot E: Genetic and familial aspects of narcolepsy. Neurology 50(2 Suppl 1):S16–S22, 1998.

103. Scammell T: The frustrating and mostly fruitless search for an autoimmune cause of narcolepsy. Sleep, in press.

104. Nishino S, Mignot E: Article reviewed: plasma orexin-A is lower in patients with narcolepsy. Sleep Med 3(4):377–378, 2002.

105. Arii J, Kanbayashi T, Tanabe Y, et al: CSF hypocretin-1 (orexin-A) levels in childhood narcolepsy and neurologic disorders. Neurology 63(12):2440–2442, 2004.

106. Dalal MA, Schuld A, Haack M, et al: Normal plasma levels of orexin A (hypocretin-1) in narcoleptic patients. Neurology 56(12):1749–1751, 2001.

107. Kanbayashi T, Inoue Y, Chiba S, et al: CSF hypocretin-1 (orexin-A) concentrations in narcolepsy with and without cataplexy and idiopathic hypersomnia. J Sleep Res 11(1):91–93, 2002.

108. Krahn LE, Pankratz VS, Oliver L, et al: Hypocretin (orexin) levels in cerebrospinal fluid of patients with narcolepsy: relationship to cataplexy and HLA DQB1*0602 status. Sleep 25(7):733–736, 2002.

109. Tsukamoto H, Ishikawa T, Fujii Y, et al: Undetectable levels of CSF hypocretin-1 (orexin-A) in two prepubertal boys with narcolepsy. Neuropediatrics 33(1):51–52, 2002.

110. Dauvilliers Y, Baumann CR, Carlander B, et al: CSF hypocretin-1 levels in narcolepsy, Kleine-Levin syndrome, and other hypersomnias and neurological conditions. J Neurol Neurosurg Psychiatry 74(12):1667–1673, 2003.

111. Mignot E: CSF hypocretin-1/orexin-A in narcolepsy: technical aspects and clinical experience in the United States. In Bassetti C, Billiard M, Mignot E (eds): *Narcolepsy and Hypersomnia*. New York, Informa Healthcare, 2007, pp 287–297.

112. Mignot E, Chen W, Black J: On the value of measuring CSF hypocretin-1 in diagnosing narcolepsy. Sleep 26(6):646–649, 2003.

113. Challamel MJ, Mazzola ME, Nevsimalova S, et al: Narcolepsy in children. Sleep 17(8 Suppl):S17–S20, 1994.

114. Marcus CL, Trescher WH, Halbower AC, Lutz J: Secondary narcolepsy in children with brain tumors. Sleep 25(4):435–439, 2002.

115. Nishino S, Kanbayashi T: Symptomatic narcolepsy, cataplexy and hypersomnia, and their implications in the hypothalamic hypocretin/orexin system. Sleep Med Rev 9(4):269–310, 2005.

116. Aldrich MS, Naylor MW: Narcolepsy associated with lesions of the diencephalon. Neurology 39(11):1505–1508, 1989.

117. Scammell TE, Nishino S, Mignot E, Saper CB: Narcolepsy and low CSF orexin (hypocretin) concentration after a diencephalic stroke. Neurology 56(12):1751–1753, 2001.

118. Rogers AE, Aldrich MS, Berrios AM, Rosenberg RS: Compliance with stimulant medications in patients with narcolepsy. Sleep 20(1):28–33, 1997.

119. Helmus T, Rosenthal L, Bishop C, et al: The alerting effects of short and long naps in narcoleptic, sleep deprived, and alert individuals. Sleep 20(4):251–257, 1997.

120. Mullington J, Broughton R: Scheduled naps in the management of daytime sleepiness in narcolepsy-cataplexy. Sleep 16(5):444–456, 1993.

121. Pollak CP, Green J: Eating and its relationships with subjective alertness and sleep in narcoleptic subjects living without temporal cues. Sleep 13(6):467–478, 1990.

122. Hajek M, Meier-Ewert K, Wirz-Justice A, et al: Bright white light does not improve narcoleptic symptoms. Eur Arch Psychiatry Neurol Sci 238(4):203–207, 1989.

123. Mignot E: An update on the pharmacotherapy of excessive daytime sleepiness and cataplexy. Sleep Med Rev 8(5):333–338, 2004.

124. Banerjee D, Vitiello MV, Grunstein RR: Pharmacotherapy for excessive daytime sleepiness. Sleep Med Rev 8(5):339–354, 2004.

125. Jasinski DR: An evaluation of the abuse potential of modafinil using methylphenidate as a reference. J Psychopharmacol 14(1):53–60, 2000.

126. Kingshott RN, Vennelle M, Coleman EL, et al: Randomized, double-blind, placebo-controlled crossover trial of modafinil in the treatment of residual excessive daytime sleepiness in the sleep apnea/hypopnea syndrome. Am J Respir Crit Care Med 163(4):918–923, 2001.

127. Czeisler CA, Walsh JK, Roth T, et al: Modafinil for excessive sleepiness associated with shift-work sleep disorder. N Engl J Med 353(5):476–486, 2005.

128. Hanson GR, Rau KS, Fleckenstein AE: The methamphetamine experience: a NIDA partnership. Neuropharmacology 47(Suppl 1):92–100, 2004.

129. Mignot E, Nishino S: Emerging therapies in narcolepsy-cataplexy. Sleep 28(6):754–763, 2005.

130. Wolraich ML, Doffing MA: Pharmacokinetic considerations in the treatment of attention-deficit hyperactivity disorder with methylphenidate. CNS Drugs 18(4):243–250, 2004.

131. Nishino S, Mignot E: Pharmacological aspects of human and canine narcolepsy. Prog Neurobiol 52(1):27–78, 1997.

132. Mignot E, Nishino, S: Perspectives for new treatments: A 2005 update. In Bassetti C, Billiard M, Mignot E (eds): *Narcolepsy and Hypersomnia*. New York, Informa Healthcare, 2007, pp 641–652.

133. Houghton WC, Scammell TE, Thorpy M: Pharmacotherapy for cataplexy. Sleep Med Rev 8(5):355–366, 2004.

134. Niederhofer H: Atomoxetine also effective in patients suffering from narcolepsy? Sleep 28(9):1189, 2005.

135. Arnulf I, Mignot E: Sodium oxybate for excessive daytime sleepiness in narcolepsy-cataplexy. Sleep 27(7):1242–1243, 2004.

136. Xyrem MSG: A randomized, double blind, placebo-controlled multicenter trial comparing the effects of three doses of orally administered sodium oxybate with placebo for the treatment of narcolepsy. Sleep 25(1):42–49, 2002.

137. Xyrem MSG: Sodium oxybate demonstrates long-term efficacy for the treatment of cataplexy in patients with narcolepsy. Sleep Med 5(2):119–123, 2004.

138. Broughton R, Mamelak M: The treatment of narcolepsy-cataplexy with nocturnal gamma-hydroxybutyrate. Can J Neurol Sci 6(1):1–6, 1979.

139. Xyrem MSG: The abrupt cessation of therapeutically administered sodium oxybate (GHB) does not cause withdrawal symptoms. J Toxicol Clin Toxicol 41(2):131–135, 2003.

140. O'Connell T, Kaye L, Plosay JJ 3rd: Gamma-hydroxybutyrate (GHB): a newer drug of abuse. Am Fam Physician 62(11):2478–2483, 2000.

141. Wong CG, Chan KF, Gibson KM, Snead OC: Gamma-hydroxybutyric acid: neurobiology and toxicology of a recreational drug. Toxicol Rev 23(1):3–20, 2004.

Insomnia: Differential Pearls

LOIS E. KRAHN

Insomnia occurs when a patient perceives that he or she has obtained inadequate sleep. Despite trying, sometimes for hours, patients with insomnia get insufficient sleep, in many cases leading to adverse daytime consequences. Affected patients experience significant distress; in part, because of the frustration in lying awake at night when sleep is desired.

BACKGROUND

Classifying insomnia has been challenging because of all the possible causes and subtypes. The definition of insomnia is particularly important for research purposes because observations concerning epidemiology, etiology, natural history, and treatment response may apply primarily to patients with similar characteristics.

Insomnia can be most easily classified in terms of the duration of the condition. This approach has clinical relevance because the treatment options available for insomnia are often studied according to the duration of the symptoms. The treatment options for transient insomnia often differ substantially from the recommendations for chronic insomnia. The classification of transient, short-term, and chronic insomnia was used in a large American epidemiologic study funded by the National Sleep Foundation. In the United States, approximately 30% of adults report transient insomnia once a month and 10% describe chronic insomnia.[1] This study reported adverse consequences of untreated insomnia including impaired concentration, decreased memory, reduced ability to fulfill roles, and decreased enjoyment of interpersonal relationships. Classifying insomnia by the duration of symptoms does present significant challenges because it does not provide any information about the etiology of the sleep disturbance or adequately describe patients with recurrent episodes of insomnia. The International Classification of Sleep Disorders (ICSD)[2] approached insomnia from the perspective of etiology, as is described next.

SIGNS AND SYMPTOMS

Insomnia is defined by a repeated difficulty with sleep initiation, duration, continuity, or quality that occurs despite adequate opportunity for sleep. To be considered a medical disorder, insomnia must result in some degree of daytime impairment. Patients with insomnia typically describe excessive wakefulness during the night in addition to unsatisfactory nighttime sleep. Some patients do not have complaints regarding the quantity of sleep but instead describe nonrestorative or light sleep as their chief complaint.

Patients with insomnia can have a variety of daytime symptoms. For patients with severe insomnia, they may experience difficulty in functioning in occupational or social situations or education. Quality of life overall can be reduced. Patients can experience a variety of medical complaints including headache, gastrointestinal distress, or chronic pain that they attribute to insomnia. Insomnia is a risk factor in certain settings that has been linked to motor vehicle accidents as well as occupational injuries. In milder cases of insomnia, patients may report fatigue, depressed mood, irritability, and cognitive impairment. The ICSD Second Edition includes general criteria for insomnia:

1. A complaint of difficulty initiating sleep, difficulty maintaining sleep, or waking up too early or sleep that is chronically nonrestorative or poor in quality. In children the sleep difficulty is often reported by the caregiver and may consist of observed bedtime resistance or inability to sleep independently.
2. The above sleep difficulty occurs despite adequate opportunity and circumstances for sleep.
3. At least one of the following forms of daytime impairment related to the nighttime sleep difficulties reported by the patient: (a) fatigue or malaise; (b) attention, concentration, or memory impairment; (c) social or vocational dysfunction or poor school performance; (d) mood disturbance or irritability; (e) daytime sleepiness;

(f) motivation, energy, or initiative reduction; (g) proneness for errors or accidents at work or while driving; (h) tension, headaches, or gastrointestinal symptoms in response to sleep loss; (i) concerns or worries about sleep.[2]

CRITERIA FOR THE DIAGNOSIS

A variety of sleep disorders share the common complaint of insomnia. The insomnia can be a primary complaint or can be secondary to primary medical illnesses, psychiatric disorders, or other sleep disorders. Prescription medications and drugs of abuse can lead to unsatisfactory sleep. The next section includes both insomnia that persists as a primary sleep disorder, as well as insomnia secondary to other conditions. Clearly there are differences in the causes, presenting symptoms, and perpetuating factors between the subtypes of insomnia.

Identifying the underlying cause of unsatisfactory nighttime sleep is a challenging task because of the many factors that need to be considered. Although the preference is to select a single diagnosis, sometimes patients have multiple factors that are associated with their poor quality of sleep. In these cases, multiple insomnia diagnoses should be used.

Adjustment Insomnia (Acute Insomnia)

This disorder, which is also known as *short-term* or *transient insomnia*, is the presence of a sleep disturbance in association with an identifiable stressor. The duration should be relatively short, lasting typically a few days to several weeks. The sleep disturbance is expected to resolve once the specific trigger fades or when the patient learns to better cope with the disturbing situation. The stressors that may lead to adjustment insomnia include psychological, social, medical, and environmental factors. Insomnia may be triggered by occupational stress, bereavement, diagnosis of a new medical condition, or relocation. Sometimes modification to the usual sleep environment has been identified as a cause. The changes may represent either positive or negative events in a person's life. Both positive and negative events in a person's life may lead to adjustment insomnia. The patients with this condition most commonly present with poor quality nighttime sleep with fatigue or excessive daytime sleepiness being the primary symptoms and only in rare cases. The clinician should carefully evaluate whether the daytime fatigue appears to be secondary to undesirable changes in the quality of nighttime sleep.

Most patients with adjustment insomnia have additional symptoms such as anxiety, obsessive thinking, or depressed mood. In certain settings patients can have physical complaints that have triggered sleep difficulties, including chronic pain, headaches, gastrointestinal difficulties, or muscle tension.

Adjustment insomnia has been thought to have a 1-year prevalence in adults of 15–20%.[3] This condition can occur across the age spectrum but is felt to be more common in older adults. It has also been thought to be more common in women than men. Patients at risk have a prior history of insomnia and more specifically adjustment insomnia. Vulnerable individuals may have a history of light sleep or poor sleep during times of stress. Individuals with a history of a depressive or anxiety disorder may also be at increased risk. No known familial pattern is known.

The duration of adjustment insomnia should not exceed 3 months. The symptoms may develop abruptly but should be in association with the triggering event. Persons may have recurrent episodes of adjustment insomnia either related to a single stressor or multiple stressors. Complications of adjustment insomnia over time can include excessive use of alcohol, street drugs, or medications in an attempt to self-medicate. In these cases, the use of substances may lead to additional sleep or daytime symptoms.

Sleep studies have been performed on patients who have been deliberately caused to experience short-term insomnia. The findings are fairly nonspecific with a prolonged sleep latency, increased number and duration of awakenings, short total sleep time, and reduced sleep efficiency. This diagnosis is primarily made based on patient report rather than polysomnographic data.

The relationship between this condition and other more persistent types of insomnia is not well understood. The differential diagnosis needs to include psychophysiologic insomnia as well as sleep disorders secondary to medical conditions or substance use. An important part of the differential diagnosis is insomnia secondary to a psychiatric disorder such as an anxiety disorder. In these cases the duration of the sleep difficulties and the presence of an identifiable stressor, as well as the acute onset, help the clinician make an appropriate classification.

Psychophysiologic Insomnia (Conditioned Insomnia)

Psychophysiologic insomnia describes a condition in which patients have heightened arousal. Overall, they develop associations in which they anticipate having poor quality sleep. Affected patients also have decreased functioning during the day. Vulnerable individuals have developed associations that prevent them from falling asleep. Instead of the bedroom being a welcoming place that induces muscle relaxation, affected patients may have a paradoxical arousal response as they prepare to fall asleep at night. The arousal response can include a hypervigilant state in which an individual is thinking about many different issues. Sometimes patients complain of feeling very stimulated as they lie in bed at night trying to sleep. This situation can arise because of a patient's longstanding psychological makeup.

Typically patients are very concerned about their insomnia. An affected patient strives to sleep but becomes more agitated. Accordingly, individuals have even more difficulty falling asleep. Over time, a patient may have negative expectations and no longer assume that they will fall asleep once they get into bed in a familiar environment. Patients with a conditioned response of this type may experience better sleep away from their own bedroom. At times the associations that prevent sleep arise in the course of insomnia that is triggered by another factor such as medication, medical illness, or a disturbed sleep environment. Over time the sleep-preventing associations take hold and even though the precipitating factor is no longer present, the patient is unable to readily fall asleep.

Patients with this condition report decreased quality of life during the day. They often experience decreased mood, decreased attention, suboptimal motivation, decreased vigilance, mild cognitive impairment, and fatigue. However, patients with psychophysiologic insomnia generally are unable to sleep during the day. Excessive daytime sleepiness is not a feature of this disorder.

The prevalence of psychophysiologic insomnia ranges from 1–2% of the general population.[4] For patients who are seen at a sleep disorder center, approximately 12–15% are estimated to have this condition.[5] Women are more likely than men to experience this condition. Patients at increased risk have a pattern of unsatisfactory sleep or episodic poor sleep before they develop the sleep-preventing associations. Unlike adjustment insomnia, this condition may start gradually or acutely. Some patients report insomnia that dates back to their childhood. This psychophysiologic insomnia can be chronic and last for the majority of a patient's lifespan. Over time, patients with this condition are felt to be at higher risk for a major depressive disorder or for overuse of hypnotic agents.

Polysomnographic data reveals increased sleep latency or increased wakefulness after sleep onset. Most patients take at least 30 minutes to fall asleep, although some patients can take considerably longer. Some data indicate an increase in stage 1 sleep and a decrease in slow wave sleep. Multiple sleep latency tests show normal daytime alertness. No pathological sleepiness is found.

The diagnosis of psychophysiologic insomnia is typically based on patient report rather than sleep study data.

The differential diagnosis of psychophysiologic insomnia includes idiopathic insomnia. There can be considerable overlap between psychophysiologic insomnia and inadequate sleep hygiene. At times it is difficult to differentiate between these two conditions. Clinicians should be alert to the possibility that a circadian rhythm disorder with a delayed sleep phase resembles psychophysiologic insomnia. However, if the sleep history indicates that the patient has normal sleep duration as long as he or she is able to have an uninterrupted opportunity to sleep later in the day, then these conditions can be differentiated.

Paradoxical Insomnia (Sleep State Misperception)

A paradoxical insomnia exists when patients have severe insomnia without any objective evidence of sleep disturbance or a daytime impairment that corresponds with the degree of unsatisfactory sleep. In the classic setting, patients describe being fully aware of their sleep environment when trying to fall asleep. Observations of these individuals, however, indicate that they may not be obviously awake but rather lying with their eyes closed with no spontaneous movements. This condition is diagnosed relatively infrequently because of the difficulty in differentiating it from other insomnia states. The key feature is the magnitude of the discrepancy between the patient's report of insomnia and any data obtained from family members, nursing staff, or polysomnography.

The prevalence of this condition in the general population is unknown; however, it is suspected to affect fewer than 5% of patients with insomnia.[6] No data are available concerning the gender ratio, although it is suspected to be more common in women than men. Also, it is thought to be more common in younger rather than older adults. The factors that make predisposed individuals to this disorder are unknown. The duration of the disorder is variable and may last from months to years. Over time, however, the condition can evolve into other sleep disorders. Affected individuals are felt to be at higher risk for depression, anxiety disorders, or hypnotic agent dependency.

Polysomnography is more useful in this condition than other insomnia states. Affected patients will describe poor quality sleep during the sleep study. Yet the sleep studies will yield a total sleep time, initial sleep latency, and awake after sleep onset that are similar to patients without sleep complaints. Patients typically overestimate their sleep latency and wakefulness by

150% of what is measured with polysomnography. They also will underestimate their total sleep time by at least 50%.[7] The multiple sleep latency test yields different findings ranging from normal to mild excessive daytime sleepiness. The etiology of this disorder is poorly understood. The differential diagnosis includes psychophysiologic insomnia as well as idiopathic insomnia. Paradoxical insomnia can be difficult to diagnose because often there are limited objective data against which the patient's subjective report can be compared. Family members and nursing staff have often not been continually observing the patient during the night, making their observations less precise and complicating the recognition of the mismatch between patient report and other data.

Idiopathic Insomnia (Childhood-Onset Insomnia)

This condition is characterized by insomnia that is very longstanding. Affected patients often report poor sleep that started in childhood. Patients describe significant distress or impairment that occurs in the absence of any other condition. Patients with this type of lifelong insomnia have difficulty falling asleep, repeated awakenings, or short overall sleep duration. Typically, the patients have continuous symptoms without periods of remission. In contrast to adjustment insomnia and insomnia secondary to other conditions, this condition occurs in the absence of any triggering or perpetuating factors. Patients with idiopathic hypersomnia can have daytime fatigue or excessive daytime sleepiness, mood symptoms, or cognitive impairment. Associated features include the possibility that patients minimize or deny interpersonal issues. One theory is that they may be expressing emotional distress in terms of a sleep complaint parallel to somatoform disorders in which patients may experience chronic pain that actually represents an unconscious emotional complaint.

The prevalence of idiopathic insomnia is not well understood but is estimated to be 0.7% among adolescents and 1% among young adults. This group is thought to comprise less than 10% of patients with insomnia. No gender data are available. Polysomnographic data reveal prolonged initial sleep latency, increased wakefulness after sleep onset, and reduced total sleep time. The patients may have increased stage 1 and 2 sleep and decreased stage 3 and 4 sleep.[8] The findings are quite similar to those identified in psychophysiologic insomnia.

The differential diagnosis of this condition includes behavioral insomnia of childhood as well as psychophysiologic and paradoxical insomnia. Especially for patients who have medical disorders that can be challenging to differentiate idiopathic insomnia from

insomnia caused by medical condition. The situations where this differentiation is most challenging are for those individuals with medical illnesses that started during childhood, such as cystic fibrosis or asthma. Another important consideration in the differential diagnosis is distinguishing these individuals from those who are short sleepers. Individuals who are short sleepers, however, should not have psychological distress or link daytime consequences to their sleep pattern.

Insomnia Resulting from a Mental Disorder

Insomnia resulting from a mental disorder is triggered by an underlying psychiatric condition. The time course of the psychiatric disorder and the insomnia should be fairly closely linked. Some of the disorders implicated in this condition are major depressive disorder, dysthymic disorder, bipolar disorder, and psychothymia. Many of the anxiety disorders, including generalized anxiety disorder, panic disorder, and obsessive compulsive disorder, can also be responsible. A somatoform disorder such as chronic pain syndrome can also be implicated. This disorder is one of the most frequently encountered by clinicians working in a sleep disorder center. Data estimate that 3% of the population may meet the criteria for insomnia resulting from psychiatric disorder.[9] This condition is less common among older adults and men. There are no specific changes in sleep architecture that have been described using polysomnography. This diagnosis is based on the patient's subjective report of sleep complaints and the coexisting psychiatric disorder.

The differential diagnosis includes the consideration of psychophysiologic insomnia as well as inadequate sleep hygiene. There could be considerable discussion whether the insomnia merits being considered a separate disorder as opposed to being a symptom within the context of a psychiatric disorder. Clinicians have considerable latitude in deciding how they would like to classify patients with these complaints. However, there appears to be increased agreement that treatment plans ought not only target the psychiatric disorder but also try to address the sleep complaint.

Inadequate Sleep Hygiene

Inadequate sleep hygiene is an insomnia that is associated with environmental factors. An affected individual pursues a lifestyle that is inconsistent with good quality nighttime sleep. A patient may experience suboptimal daytime alertness or functioning. This condition is associated with patients who choose a lifestyle that is not as conducive to sleep. The patients pursue activities that increase arousal at a time when sleep is desired or do not make sleep a priority and, therefore, lack adequate opportunity to sleep. Some of the factors that can lead to poor sleep for patients with inadequate sleep hygiene are use of caffeine and nicotine, as well as excessive alcohol use. Patients may have a stressful life situation or may even seek stimulating physical or mental activities close to bedtime. This interferes with the opportunity to relax and unwind. Accordingly, patients then have difficulty falling asleep as desired. Patients often do not make keeping a regular sleep-wake schedule and having an adequate opportunity to sleep sufficient priorities.

This condition has been identified in 1–2% of adolescents and young adults.[10] The prevalence in older age groups are unknown. It is estimated that approximately 5–10% of those who present to sleep disorder centers have this condition.[11] Typically this condition starts early in life and may persist for many years. Some individuals lack a basic understanding of the conditions that are conducive to good quality sleep. Over time, affected individuals are at risk for caffeine dependence, excessive alcohol use, and conditioned insomnia. They may compensate by taking daytime naps that may produce excessive daytime sleepiness and reduce the homeostatic drive for sleep at bedtime.

There is no classic picture based on polysomnographic data for this condition. The diagnosis is based on a careful history of both the patient's sleep pattern and lifestyle.

The differential diagnosis is rather challenging because patients with many types of insomnia can have lifestyles that are not conducive to sleep. The differential diagnosis, at minimum, includes psychophysiologic insomnia, idiopathic insomnia, paradoxical insomnia, and insomnia related to psychiatric or medical conditions. Clinicians should be especially attentive to insomnia secondary to substance use, including caffeine. Lastly, patients who have a primary sleep disorder such as sleep-related breathing disorder, restless legs syndrome, or circadian rhythm disorder may appear to have primary inadequate sleep hygiene. The clinician needs to carefully assess the relative contribution of the primary sleep disorder versus lifestyle factors when clarifying the situation.

Behavioral Insomnia of Childhood (Sleep-Onset Association Disorder)

Individuals with behavioral insomnia of childhood have difficulty falling asleep or staying asleep. This often results because of inadequate limits put on their bedtime routine or inappropriate sleep associations. A child may become dependent on a specific setting to fall asleep. Children may repeatedly refuse to go to bed or come up with delaying tactics that have not been adequately addressed by a caregiver. This condition is separated into two main subtypes of sleep-onset association type versus limit-setting type.

The prevalence of this disorder is estimated to be 10–30% of children, without any known gender predominance.[12] This disorder should not be diagnosed before 6 months of age, as the human brain has not matured satisfactorily to permit continuous sleep until this point at the earliest. A major risk factor for this condition is the behaviors of the child's caregivers. Cultural factors can play a role here as well. The clinician needs to carefully evaluate both the child's sleep pattern and the parenting style. Children who have a demanding temperament or active medical problem such as colic are also at higher risk. Over time, caregivers may try many different techniques to soothe a child who is aroused at bedtime. Not surprisingly, sometimes the child becomes dependent on a particular toy, presence of an adult, or other factors before sleep can happen.

No specific pattern is found on polysomnographic studies. Sleep studies are typically done in a very specific setting, especially when sleep-onset association disorder is suspected. Generally, this disorder resolves with time as the child matures and becomes more independent. However, sometimes the sleep disorder leads to ongoing complications such as decreased attention, hyperactive behavior, irritability, and decreased school performance. Caregivers may experience significant sleep loss that can lead to family tensions.

The differential diagnoses include circadian rhythm sleep disorder, delayed sleep-wake type, and irregular sleep-wake type. Inadequate sleep hygiene can overlap with this disorder. Clinicians should carefully investigate the possibility of a coexisting psychiatric disorder, such as an anxiety disorder, or a medical disorder. Lastly, consideration should be given to the presence of a coexisting primary sleep disorder such as obstructive sleep apnea or restless legs syndrome.

Insomnia Resulting from Drug or Substance Use

This category includes a variety of sleep disorders including alcohol-dependent sleep disorder, stimulant-dependent sleep disorder, substance abuse, rebound insomnia, prescription medication side effect, prescription medication reaction, food allergy insomnia, and toxic-induced sleep disorder. In general, the affected patient has sleep disruption related to the consumption of a prescription medication or other substance. Typically, the substances act as central nervous system (CNS) stimulants; however, CNS depressants can also be implicated. The disorder is more common when individuals use substances with a half-life that is long enough to interfere with sleep. The prevalence of this disorder indicates that insomnia related to substance abuse or dependencies is found in approximately 0.2% of the general population but in 3.5% of sleep disorder samples.[13] This disorder can commonly coexist with other sleep disorders. This disorder can develop at any age. The polysomnographic findings vary depending on the substance involved. The differential diagnosis includes inadequate sleep hygiene and psychophysiologic insomnia.

Insomnia Resulting from a Medical Condition

In this state, affected patients have insomnia that is caused by a coexisting medical disorder or physiologic factor. The most common causes are hot flashes or night sweats, as well as dyspnea, wheezing, coughing, and chest tightness with anxiety as seen in sleep-related asthma. Numerous neurological disorders can cause sleep complaints, including Parkinson's disease, other movement disorders, and seizure disorders.

This disorder can occur at any age. No data exist concerning a male/female distribution. Polysomnographic data findings depend on the underlying medical disorder.

The differential diagnosis, in particular, should address the possibility of insomnia resulting from a drug or substance, as well as psychophysiologic insomnia or inadequate sleep hygiene.

TREATMENT

Sleep Hygiene

Sleep hygiene is a necessary but typically not sufficient approach for a patient with insomnia. Patients should be asked to identify behaviors that they find to be stimulating versus relaxing and deliberately plan ones that help them unwind in the 30 to 60 minutes before going to bed. An emphasis on engaging in relaxing behaviors before bedtime is helpful. The focus should be on reinforcing the importance of a regular sleep-wake schedule, with the patient encouraged to have a structured day with regular exercise and consistent meal times. Optimizing sleep hygiene may be particularly helpful for patients who have sleep-onset insomnia. All subsequent treatments for insomnia will be less effective if sleep hygiene issues go unaddressed.

Behavioral Treatment

Behavioral techniques have proven valuable for the treatment of insomnia (Table 7-1). These can be used in combination, with several different techniques used simultaneously. Several reviews of behavioral techniques for insomnia indicate the efficacy of these techniques.[14] The various behavioral treatments have been critically reviewed in a practice parameter published by the American Academy of Sleep Medicine.[15] This committee concluded that stimulus control was the most well-accepted management strategy. Biofeedback, progressive muscle relaxation, and asking patients to avoid trying to fall asleep (paradoxical intention) were also strategies that had value. More controversial therapies included sleep restriction and cognitive therapy addressing multiple issues. Cognitive behavioral therapy has been viewed to be useful for patients in a more recent study.[16] The advantage of cognitive behavioral therapy is that it can address many behaviors that may be perpetuating insomnia, including lack of confidence in the ability to sleep, daytime naps, irregular sleep scheduling issues, and anxiety. Unfortunately, access to behavioral therapies can be limited for some patients. Communities often lack appropriate therapists, or insurance coverage can be restrictive. For that reason, pharmacological treatment often needs to be used while searching for behavioral treatment or in place of behavioral treatment.

TABLE 7-1 ■ Recommended Behavioral Therapies for Insomnia	
Therapy	**Comment**
Stimulus control	Reassociate the bed with rapid sleep initiation.
Sleep restriction	Reduce time in bed to decrease amount of fragmented sleep.
Paradoxical intention	Coach the patient to not try to fall asleep but rather to engage in other activities.
Progressive muscle relaxation	Reduce muscle tension to decrease mental arousal.
Biofeedback	Use EEG monitoring to reinforce success with relaxing.
Multicomponent behavioral therapy	Understand and modify attitudes not conducive to sleep.

PHARMACOLOGICAL TREATMENT

General Principles

Sedative-hypnotic medications are widely used. Many agents have been used to induce sleep without being carefully researched or receiving approval by the Food and Drug Administration (FDA) as a hypnotic. More recently a variety of agents have received FDA approval based on extensive studies of their hypnotic properties.

The clinician should not prescribe a hypnotic without first performing a comprehensive sleep assessment. Sleep hygiene issues should always be addressed even when it is clear that a medication will be initiated. The goal of hypnotic therapy is to improve subjective sleep quality and quantity, decrease daytime fatigue, improve concentration, and enhance global daytime functioning. Good medical practice calls for using the lowest effective dose for the shortest possible duration. Table 7-2 lists several important features of hypnotics. The onset of action of medications is determined by the rate of absorption and distribution. The onset of action is important for patients with prominent complaints about initial insomnia. Especially for aging patients or those with hepatic disease, prolonged elimination time increases the risk of excessive sedation. This places the patient at increased risk for falls and cognitive impairment.

Hypnotics with longer half-lives also increase the risk of a hangover effect leading to undesired morning sedation. Some patients interpret morning sleepiness as a need for more sleep and elect to increase the dose of the hypnotic, thereby exacerbating the problem. Hypnotics with short half-lives raise a different set of concerns because the sedation can wear off before dawn. Patients therefore may experience early morning awakenings or rebound insomnia. Triazolam, in particular, has been associated with amnesia because of its short half-life, leading to possible abrupt drug withdrawal.

The challenge of tolerance is another important general pharmacological consideration. When a medication used long-term ceases to induce sleep, patients may increase the dose. Newer agents have been developed to minimize the risks of tolerance and dose escalation. The barbiturates and benzodiazepines are known to produce tolerance at a higher rate than the newer medications. These older agents also can cause physical dependence in which patients experience withdrawal symptoms when these agents are abruptly discontinued. The ideal hypnotic could be used long-term without developing tolerance to the sedative qualities or experiencing withdrawal on discontinuation.

Modern Hypnotics

The FDA has approved several benzodiazepines to treat primary insomnia, including flurazepam, triazolam, quazepam, estazolam, and temazepam. Of this group, the medication that is the most useful is temazepam because of its half-life and lack of active metabolite, ranging between 6 and 16 hours, which is useful for inducing sleep.[17] The dosage ranges has been extended to 7.5–30 mg. Temazepam increases total sleep time with decreased initial sleep latency and reduction in wakefulness after sleep onset. If a benzodiazepine is specifically required for sleep, temazepam may be a reasonable choice (Table 7-3).

Nonbenzodiazepine agents are increasingly used as the first-line treatment option for insomnia. Initially, the agents of zaleplon and zolpidem were approved only for the short-term treatment of insomnia. Because many patients with insomnia have chronic symptoms, this was an unfortunate mismatch of short-term treatment with a chronic disorder. Newly available medications such as eszopiclone, zolpidem-CR, and ramelteon have been approved for the treatment of chronic insomnia without any specification of the time period. The FDA guidelines allowing longer-term use of these medications significantly aid the clinician in treating affected patients.

The benzodiazepine receptor agonists interact with the GABA-A alpha subunit that opens chloride channels. These agents are more selective than the benzodiazepines. As a result they cause less rebound insomnia and have a lower risk of being abused or contributing to respiratory depression when given at the recommended therapeutic doses. All have relatively short half-lives that minimize excessive daytime sleepiness. Zolpidem is a selective agonist of the type 1 GABA-A alpha subunit (see Table 7-3). This agent is primarily used to treat sleep-onset insomnia because of its short half-life. The newer form of zolpidem-CR now has a biphasic release, allowing this new compound to address both sleep-onset and sleep maintenance insomnia. This agent does not appear to significantly alter normal sleep architecture.[18] Zaleplon acts on a similar site and has a shorter half-life

---

TABLE 7-2 ■ Relevant Characteristics of Hypnotic Medication[22]

Rate of absorption
Rapidity of distribution to the central nervous system
Action on specific neurotransmitters
Duration of elimination half-life
Site of metabolism
Presence of inactive metabolites
Likelihood of tolerance
Risk of dependence

of approximately 1 hour. Like zolpidem, it is primarily used for sleep initiation. This agent can be used partway through the night to help patients with middle insomnia because of its long half-life. Like zolpidem, zaleplon does not appear to alter normal sleep architecture. The most recent addition to this group with a similar mechanism is eszopiclone. This was the first medication approved for longer-term use based on a study that lasted 6 months. Eszopiclone is not associated with significant tolerance or morning sedation. Sleep is improved with respect to decreased sleep latency, increased sleep efficiency, and increased total sleep time. The medication has been associated with an unpleasant taste.[19]

The most recently approved agent for the treatment of insomnia is ramelteon, which is an agonist on the MT_1 and MT_2 melatonin receptors. This agent has a novel mechanism compared with the other agents available in the United States. It is the only prescription hypnotic that is not classified as a controlled substance. The medication has shown to be beneficial in improving insomnia. What its role may be with respect to circadian rhythm issues remains unclear.

A variety of agents (including antidepressant medications) that are not officially classified as hypnotics have been used for sleep over time (Table 7-4). Clinicians at times view antidepressants as a convenient

TABLE 7-3 ■ Nonbenzodiazepine Hypnotics

Agent	Initiates Sleep	Maintains Sleep	Appropriate for Limited Time in Bed	Required Sleep Time
Zolpidem	X	X		7–8 hr
Zaleplon	X		X	4 hr
Eszopiclone	X	X		8 hr
Zolpidem CR	X	X		7–8 hr
Ramelteon	X			$\cong$ >5 hr[23]

TABLE 7-4 ■ Other Medication Options

Agent	Class	Duration of Action	Dose	Indications	Concerns
Temazepam	Benzodiazepines	8–15 hours	7.5–30 mg	Benzodiazepines-dependent insomnia, insomnia with existing RBD, insomnia with treatment-resistant RLS	Incoordination, falls, cognitive impairment
Clonazepam	Benzodiazepines	8–15 hours	0.5–2 mg	Same	Same
Trazodone	Antidepressant	8 hours	25–100 mg	Need to minimize chemical dependence risk	Falls, orthostatic hypotension, priapism
Mirtazapine	Antidepressant	20–40 hours	7.5–15 mg	Insomnia in context of depression, need to minimize risk of addiction	Weight gain
Doxepin	Antidepressant	8–24 hours	10–50 mg	Insomnia in context of depression or chronic pain	Constipation, dry mouth, orthostatic hypotension, cardiac conduction delays
Quetiapine	Atypical antipsychotic	6 hours	12.5–50 mg	Insomnia in context of bipolar disorder/ psychotic disorder; parasomnia (especially RBD in context of Lewy body dementia), minimize CD risk	Weight gain, metabolic syndrome, slight increase in stroke risk
Gabapentin	Anticonvulsant	5–7 hours	300–600 mg	Insomnia in context of RLS[24]/ chronic pain, hot flashes, minimize CD risk, coexisting seizures	

RBD, REM behavior disorder; RLS, restless legs syndrome; CD, chemical dependency.

way of addressing both insomnia and a coexisting mood disorder. The preferred agents have been mirtazapine, trazodone, and tricyclic antidepressants; however, the duration of sedation may be excessive. They also may have multiple side effects such as weight gain, depending on the particular agent selected. Unfortunately, these agents have not been carefully studied with respect to their benefits for sleep. Likewise, antipsychotic medications at times can be helpful, particularly quetiapine and olanzapine. Especially in the setting of serious psychiatric disorders such as bipolar disorder, schizophrenia, or dementia with psychosis, these agents have a role. In the absence of coexisting psychiatric disorders, however, the side effects of these medications need to be carefully weighed against the benefits. In particular, these agents may lead to weight gain and excessive daytime sleepiness.

Anticonvulsant medications have been used for a variety of sleep complaints. Clonazepam is a benzodiazepine that is also classified as an anticonvulsant. Despite its long half-life, it can be helpful for patients who have difficulty sleeping, especially for insomnia coexisting with a parasomnia such as REM sleep behavior disorder. The long half-life, however, also can lead to excessive daytime sleepiness. Some patients opt to obtain over-the-counter sleeping medications that contain diphenhydramine. These agents are widely used because they are available without a prescription. Tolerance quickly develops, however, and the usefulness of these agents is significantly limited as a result. Lastly, antihistamines can contribute to cognitive impairment.[20]

Behavioral therapies are often combined with medications. This approach is optimal, especially when using behavioral therapy in isolation, is not an option either because of the time lag in symptom improvement or lack of access to therapists. Relatively few studies have examined the value of combining these two approaches. Whether a patient may be as motivated to pursue behavioral therapy when medications are concurrently prescribed has been a matter of debate.[21] Nonetheless, in clinical practice this approach is commonplace. Patients often welcome the symptom relief they obtain from hypnotics. Ideally, patients can be persuaded also to look at the behaviors and attitudes that may have led to them developing insomnia or have perpetuated this condition.

REFERENCES

1. Morin CM, Culbert JP, Schwartz SM: Nonpharmacological interventions for insomnia: a meta analysis of treatment efficacy. Am J Psychiatry 151(8):1172–1180, 1994.

2. American Academy of Sleep Medicine: *International Classification of Sleep Disorders*, 2nd ed. Westchester, IL, American Academy of Sleep Medicine, 2005, p 3.

3. Angst J, Vollrath M, Koch R, Dobler-Mikola A: The Zurich Study. VII. Insomnia: symptoms, classification and prevalence. Eur Arch Psychiatry Neurol Sci 238(5–6):285–293, 1989.

4. American Academy of Sleep Medicine: *International Classification of Sleep Disorders*, 2nd ed. Westchester, IL, American Academy of Sleep Medicine, 2005, p 6.

5. Buysse DJ, Reynolds CF 3rd, Kupfer DJ, et al: Clinical diagnoses in 216 insomnia patients using the International Classification of Sleep Disorders (ICSD), DSM-IV and ICD-10 categories: a report from the APA/NIMH DSM-IV Field Trial. Sleep 17(7):630–637, 1994.

6. Salin-Pascual RJ, Roehrs TA, Merlotti LA, et al: Long-term study of the sleep of insomnia patients with sleep state misperception and other insomnia patients. Am J Psychiatry 149(7):904–908, 1999.

7. Edinger JD, Fins AI: The distribution and clinical significance of sleep time misperceptions among insomniacs. Sleep 18(4):232–239, 1995.

8. Reynolds CF 3rd, Kupfer DJ, Buysse DJ, et al: Subtyping DSM-III-R primary insomnia: a literature review by the DSM-IV Work Group on Sleep Disorders. Am J Psychiatry 148(4):432–438, 1999.

9. Nofzinger EA, Buysse DJ, Reynolds CF 3rd, Kupfer DJ: Sleep disorders related to another mental disorder (nonsubstance/primary): a DSM-IV literature review. J Clin Psychiatry 54(7):244–255; discussion 256–259, 1993.

10. Brown FC, Buboltz WC Jr, Soper B: Relationship of sleep hygiene awareness, sleep hygiene practices, and sleep quality in university students. Behav Med 28(1):33–38, 2002.

11. *International Classification of Sleep Disorders*, 2nd ed. Westchester, IL, American Academy of Sleep Medicine, 2005, p 18.

12. Gaylor EE, Goodlin-Jones BL, Anders TF: Classification of young children's sleep problems: a pilot study. J Am Acad Child Adolesc Psychiatry 40(1):61–67, 2001.

13. *International Classification of Sleep Disorders*, 2nd ed. Westchester, IL, American Academy of Sleep Medicine, 2005, p 26.

14. Morin CM, Culbert JP, Schwartz SM: Nonpharmacological interventions for insomnia: a meta-analysis of treatment efficacy. Am J Psychiatry 151(8):1172–1180, 1994.

15. Chesson AL Jr, Anderson WM, Littner M, et al: Practice parameters for the nonpharmacologic treatment of chronic insomnia. An American Academy of Sleep Medicine report. Standards of Practice Committee of the American Academy of Sleep Medicine. Sleep 22(8):1128–1133, 1999.

16. Smith MT, Huang MI, Manber R: Cognitive behavior therapy for chronic insomnia occurring within the context of medical and psychiatric disorders. Clin Psychol Rev 25(5):559–592, 2005.

17. Nowell PD, Mazumdar S, Buysse DJ, et al: Benzodiazepines and zolpidem for chronic insomnia: a meta-analysis of treatment efficacy. JAMA 278(24):2170–2177, 1997.

18. Scharf MB, Roth T, Vogel GW, Walsh JK: A multicenter, placebo-controlled study evaluating zolpidem in the treatment of chronic insomnia. J Clin Psychiatry 55(5):192–199, 1994.

19. Zammit G, Gillan JC, McNabb L, et al: Eszopiclone, a novel non-benzodiazepine. Sleep Abstract Supplement 26:A297, 2003.

20. Witek TJ Jr, Canestrari DA, Miller RD, et al: Characterization of daytime sleepiness and psychomotor performance following H1 receptor antagonists. Ann Allergy Asthma Immunol 74(5):419–426, 1995.

21. Hauri PJ: Can we mix behavioral therapy with hypnotics when treating insomniacs? Sleep 20(12):1111–1118, 1997.

22. Silber MH, Morganthaler TI, Krahn LE: *Sleep Medicine in Clinical Practice*. London, Taylor and Francis, 2004.

23. Silber MH: Clinical practice. Chronic insomnia. N Engl J Med 353(8):803–810, 2005.

24. Earley CJ: Clinical practice. Restless legs syndrome. N Engl J Med 348(21):2103–2109, 2003.

Introduction to Electroencephalography

DEREK J. CHONG ■ GREGORY L. SAHLEM ■ CARL W. BAZIL

INTRODUCTION TO ELECTROENCEPHALOGRAPHY (EEG)

EEG Basics

EEG is the study of the electrical activity of the brain over time. This is accomplished by comparing the difference in amount of electrical activity, or electrical potential, between two regions over time. Electrodes are attached directly to the scalp, recording microvoltages derived from the cerebral cortex. The signal is then filtered considerably to eliminate electrical noise and amplified to derive the EEG tracing. These electrical potentials are thought to arise from the extracellular currents generated from postsynaptic potentials (excitatory postsynaptic potentials [EPSPs] and inhibitory postsynaptic potentials [IPSPs]), primarily from pyramidal neurons of the cerebral cortex.[1]

There are limitations to scalp EEG. Information is lost when translating the three-dimensional structure of the brain into a two-dimensional array. Sulci and other cortical surface irregularities (including the insula, the mesial surfaces of the temporal lobes and the hemispheres, and the entire inferior surface of the brain) are electrically obscured as a result of tangential direction of electrical field, inability to place electrodes directly above these areas, physical distance, or excess intervening tissue. The electrical signal that is properly oriented for electrode recording and close to the skull is attenuated by the surrounding cerebrospinal fluid, meninges, skull, and scalp, leading to a small signal that is prone to artifact. The signal that is recorded at the scalp is thus a relatively crude aggregate of regional cortical activity, with an estimated 10^8 neurons contributing to the electrical field at a given electrode.[1] Despite these limitations, technological advances have helped the EEG improve, and currently the EEG supplies crucial and unique information about brain function over time that is helpful to epileptologists and sleep medicine experts and is not available by other tests.

Keep in mind that except where specified, information in this section refers to traditional EEG recordings, montages, settings, and speeds. Modern polysomnograms (PSGs) frequently have the capacity to use full EEG arrays when indicated; however, interpretation for the purposes of defining brain pathology (specifically epileptic potential) is usually done according to these settings rather than those used in scoring polysomnography.

EEG: Setup

The International 10–20 system is the standard EEG lead placement system in North America.[2] A minimum of 21 electrodes are placed on the head. The distance from the nasion to the inion is measured, and the first electrodes are 10%; the remaining are 20% of the distances (Figure 8-1). Similar measurements are made from both preauricular areas to determine the placements of the remaining electrodes. This allows standardization of placement across a wide variety of head sizes, from premature infants to individuals with hydrocephalus. By convention, left-sided electrodes are odd numbered, whereas those on the right are even numbered. The letters of the 10–20 system refer to frontalpolar (Fp), frontal (F), temporal (T), central (C), parietal (P), and occipital (O) regions. An electrical discharge from a region of the brain should be paralleled by a sensible field, meaning that the highest amplitude and clearest morphology are seen in one or a few adjacent electrodes, with gradual dropoff in surrounding electrodes. As such, brain activity is often compared to "ripples in a pond," growing fainter with distance from the source. This is true of most normal and abnormal discharges, whereas most artifacts (as from a faulty electrode) will have no effect on surrounding electrodes and thus no sensible field.

Electrodes can be affixed to the scalp in a number of different ways. The electrodes used most frequently in modern practice are disks of metal. They are commonly cup shaped to hold conducting paste or glue and are

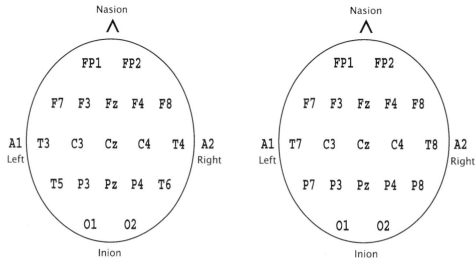

FIGURE 8-1 ■ The International 10–20 system of EEG electrode placement. By convention, left-sided electrodes are odd numbered, whereas those on the right are even numbered. The letters of the 10–20 system refer to frontal-polar (Fp), frontal (F), temporal (T), central (C), parietal (P), and occipital (O) regions. An electrode on the mastoid process (M) can replace the auricle (A). The Modified system substitutes T7/T8 for T3/T4 and P7/P8 for T5/T6, establishing a convention whereby larger numbers indicate a greater distance from midline. This becomes helpful when additional electrodes are used for epilepsy monitoring.

made of silver chloride or a similar substance. Recordings greater than 24 hours typically require the use of colodian, a type of biological glue that holds electrodes in place. A conductive paste is still required directly between the electrode and the scalp. Shorter recordings can use conductive paste between the scalp and electrodes, as well as act as the adhesive itself (our lab prefers 10–20 paste). There are marked advantages and disadvantages to each type of adhesive. Colodian has the advantage of holding electrodes more securely over time; however, colodian requires a significantly greater amount of preparatory time and effort. Beyond reduced time and labor, the use of 10–20 paste allows for replacement of dislodged electrodes during a recording by simply applying pressure; reapplying electrodes held in place by collodian is more difficult. Each option has its place in standard overnight recording, but practically speaking, 10–20 paste is sufficient for a standard PSG montage where the fewer leads can easily be replaced, whereas collodian becomes a better option when placing a full complement of EEG leads.

EEG: Technical Basics

Differential Amplification

Differential amplification is the principle of amplifying disklike signals while eliminating like signals. Each EEG channel is derived from the difference in the electrical input recorded from two different regions.

Signals that are identical throughout are likely to be either artifact (electrical activity is present constantly around us) or inconsequential and are thus rejected, termed *common mode rejection*. Only the difference between two sites is amplified. The channels are displayed in order; for instance, Fp1-F3 means that Fp1 is input 1 and F3 is input 2. By convention, an upward deflection on the EEG tracing indicates that input 1 is relatively negative compared with input 2, which could mean either a negative discharge at input 1 or a positive discharge at input 2.

Filters

The resulting signal can be "framed" by a series of filters so that only frequencies of interest are displayed. Filters modify the signal to attenuate frequencies based on a user-defined frequency cut-off point.

Low-frequency filters (LFF), or high-pass filters, exert their effect on slower waves (lower frequencies). If an LFF is set on 1 Hz, waves of 1 cycle per second and slower will be attenuated gradually, waves that are 1 Hz will be slightly attenuated (20–30%, depending on the machine), and increasingly slower waves will be increasingly attenuated. A 1-Hz LFF will still affect frequencies above 1 Hz, but to a much lesser degree, with the effect becoming negligible as frequencies increase.

High-frequency filters (HFF), known also as *low-pass filters*, work similarly. If an HFF is set to 70 Hz, waves of 70 cycles per second and faster will be attenuated. As the frequency of the wave increases, so does the attenuation. HFFs typically have even less effects below the cut-off point than LFFs have above the cut-off point.

The notch filter works differently in attempts to excise artifact produced by power line activity (60 Hz in North America). This filter is designed to have sharp cut-offs, eliminating signals with a frequency near 60 Hz. The notch filter should be used with caution because 60-Hz artifact in isolated leads may denote poor electrode contact (Figure 8-2). The lead should be repaired, as the information it provides can be extremely misleading.

Filters must be used carefully. Setting the HFF too low can make muscle artifact appear as normal brain waves (alpha or beta frequency) or as epileptiform activity (described later). An LFF that is set incorrectly can completely mask pathological slowing, or slow waves seen during normal sleep.

In a polysomnogram, the LFF should be set low enough to view clearly slow waves of 1 Hz (typically between 0.1 and 1 Hz). At the opposite end of the spectrum, cerebral activity on scalp EEG is typically no higher than 30 cycles per second. The HFF, however, should include faster waveforms (typically 70 Hz is sufficient) to avoid the distortion of higher frequencies to appear as possibly cerebral.

If electromyography (EMG) is the desired parameter, the filters would be changed in a way to specifically frame the relatively fast frequency. Muscle activity produces fast waveforms, and subsequently an LFF as high as 10 Hz can provide a view of all of the desired muscle activity while attenuating slow artifact such as body movement. In the case of EMG, it is desirable to view all fast frequencies, so the HFF can be set as high as 100 Hz or turned off.

Filters can be used to selectively reduce or eliminate artifact: Respiratory artifact can be removed from EEG channels by raising the LFF above the respiratory rate. Similarly, muscle artifact can be reduced using the HFF, but must be done so with recognition of the inherent risks.

Sensitivity

Sensitivity is the ratio of input voltage to the degree of signal displayed (or deflection), measured in microvolts per millimeter (μV/mm). A standard setting for EEG is 7 μV/mm, with a range of normal being 5–10 μV/mm. Amplitudes of waveforms can be calculated as the product of the sensitivity and the height of the waveform. The sensitivity can be modified based on the voltage of the signal. Waves with very small voltages require lower valued sensitivity settings to avoid overlooking subtleties.

Montages

As noted previously, each individual tracing in the EEG represents the difference in electrical potentials at two different regions; in fact, it is a direct subtraction of the second from the first. The electrodes themselves are affixed and immobile, but the comparisons between the electrodes are configured within the recording or displaying machine and are modifiable. Comparisons are set up in relatively standard arrangements, called *montages*. Just as a lung lesion can better be visualized by comparing different views on a chest radiograph, different montages are used to better detect, isolate, or otherwise visualize various types of cerebral potentials.

Bipolar Montages

Bipolar montages compare one electrode to other, often adjacent, electrodes arranged in straight lines, often referred to as *chains*.

- Longitudinal bipolar: The most commonly used montage, also known as the "double banana." The electrode comparisons are configured to create a parasagittal and a temporal "chain" (Figure 8-3A). For instance, Fp1-F3, F3-C3, C3-P3, and P3-O1 are four sequential electrode pair comparisons that comprise the left parasagittal chain. The temporal chain actually lies over the perisylvian fissure, just superior to the temporal lobe. An inferior temporal chain can be added when temporal lobe epilepsy is questioned.
- Transverse bipolar: The chains are arranged in a coronal fashion, taking left-to-right slices from anterior to posterior. One chain would consist of T7-C3, C3-Cz, Cz-C4, C4-T8. This montage accentuates activity at the midline; thus sleep architecture is well visualized.
- *Referential montages* compare each point to either a common point (e.g., common reference montage), or an average of all or many electrode potentials (e.g., common average montage). The reference can become contaminated, however, meaning that rather than being a relatively silent comparitor, one or more electrodes used in the reference have a waveform or artifact that is significant and may appear in all channels or in a select few.

Polysomnography typically uses a contralateral referential montage (Figure 8-3B). Large distances make for large amplitudes, but the ear/mastoid references can be contaminated by activity of the temporal regions.

Although the resulting tracing is dependent on the difference in electrical potentials, the amplitude is

Text continued on p. 110

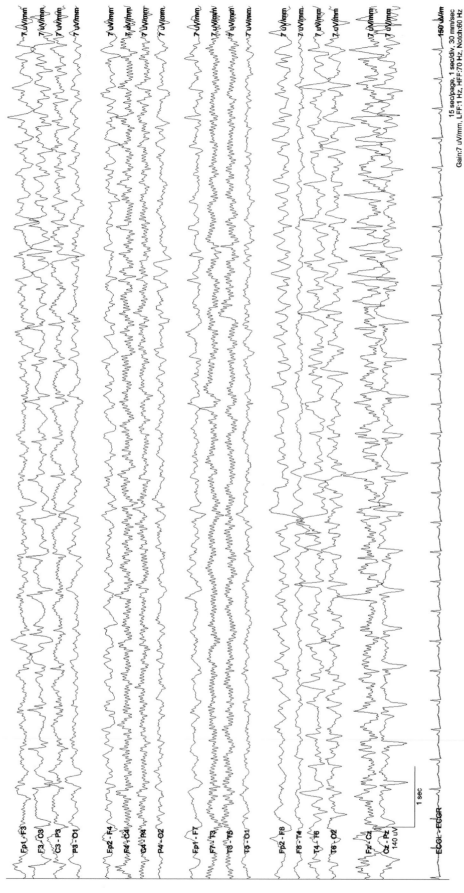

FIGURE 8-2 ■ Continued.

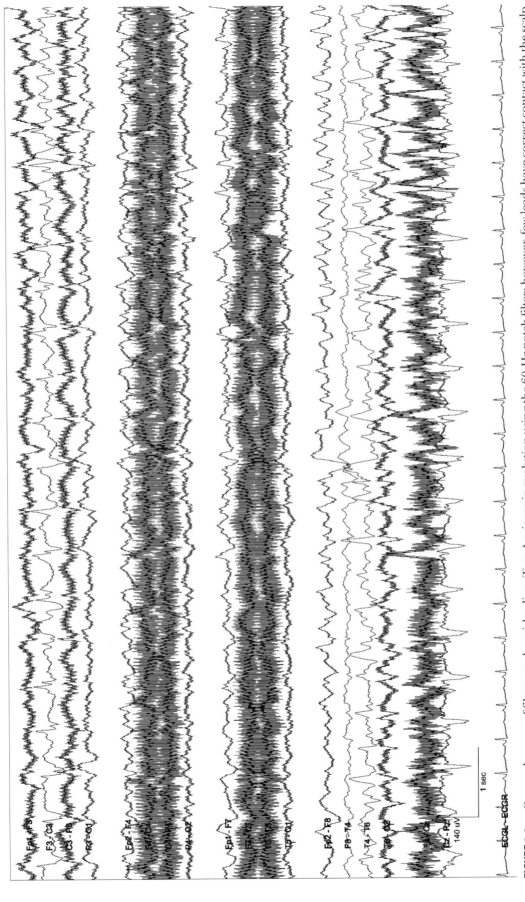

FIGURE 8-2 ■ Overzealous use of filters can be misleading. Top: A seizure in evolution using the 60-Hz notch filter; however, few leads have correct contact with the scalp. The notch filter removes the 60-Hz artifact but leaves behind an alpha wave tracing that appears believable, making for a seizure spread pattern that is difficult to understand. With the notch filter off, the pattern of spread is sensible because the leads with 60-Hz artifact can be ignored.

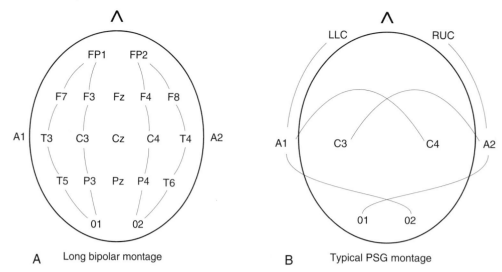

FIGURE 8-3 ■ A, Typical EEG montage, long bipolar or "double banana." B, Typical PSG montage.

dependent on the amount of brain involved in the discharge, the amount of tissue causing attenuation (i.e., skull thickness, or lack thereof), and the distance between the two points of comparison. Thus in a bipolar montage, if the electrodes are not arranged perfectly, amplitudes can appear erroneously larger or smaller in some channels, depending on exact distance between electrodes (larger distances tend to create larger amplitudes). A similar problem occurs when using a referential montage, for instance to Cz. There is a greater distance from Cz to the temporal chain as compared with the parasaggital chain. Activity below the central leads is most likely to be different from activity below those farther away; thus, the greater the distance between electrodes (determined to be up to 8 cm), the greater the disparity in the underlying potentials, and greater amplitudes will be displayed.

The Normal EEG

The essential aspects that every EEG report should contain include a description of the background activity in terms of frequency, amplitude, localization, quantity, organization, and variability, with abnormalities described in similar terms. These descriptors form the basis of interpretation. To make an interpretation, age and clinical state are clinically relevant. The electrical properties of the brain change with age. The resultant EEG changes dramatically from newborn to early childhood through adolescence; there are also some changes in older individuals. These changes are complex and beyond the scope of this book. The very basics of awake and sleep EEG through the ages are discussed here.

The standard electroencephalogram uses a paper speed of 30 mm/sec. In PSGs, a paper speed of 10 mm/

sec is used, compressing the study with respect to standard EEG. In digital systems, paper speed is a "virtual setting," and can be changed without difficulty, proving valuable when viewing a given recording for both sleep staging and epileptiform abnormalities.

Amplitude is measured in microvolts, measured from the low to high peak (not from the baseline) of waveforms, and is the product of the signal voltage and display sensitivity (or pen writer, if using paper EEG). Recall that the voltage is the potential difference between two points and does not have a direct relationship to the power of cerebral activity. Because small differences in electrode distances can show up as differences in amplitude, asymmetries in voltage need to be corroborated using either another bipolar montage perpendicular to the first or a referential montage. If all points of the brain have the same potential, it is termed *isoelectric* and indicates a lack of perceptible cortical activity.

The frequency of waveforms is measured in cycles per second, or Hertz. It can refer to how many turns of a wave actually occurred in one second, or how many of a single, nonrepeating wave would fit into 1 second. A standard definition of frequencies is as follows[3]:

Delta: <4 Hz
Theta: 4 to <8 Hz
Alpha: 8–13 Hz
Beta: >13 Hz–40 Hz
Gamma: >40 Hz

Distribution of Location of Waveforms

Frequencies and amplitudes vary from region to region in a normal brain. The location of waveforms of interest should be reported, referring to the frontal, temporal, parietal, or occipital region of the left or right side.

NORMAL AWAKE

In an awake adult, a normal EEG consists of low-voltage fast activity with little or no frequencies slower than 8 Hz. The record is frequently interrupted by eye movement artifact and EMG. Mild temporal slowing can be seen shifting between sides in individuals over age 60, particularly as drowsiness ensues, and while not technically normal, occurs in asymptomatic individuals.[4]

The background awake rhythms should be "organized" in an "anterior-to-posterior" gradient, meaning that there should be lower amplitude but faster frequencies at the front of the head, and higher amplitude rhythms at the back, with lower frequency. The posterior waveforms thus appear more prominently and are termed the *posterior dominant rhythm* (PDR), sometimes referred to as the *alpha*. As a general rule, it should be at least 6 Hz by the age of 1 year, 8 Hz by the age of 3, and 8.5–12 Hz in adolescence and adulthood. The PDR must be stereotyped and should become obliterated reliably (blocking) with eye opening or when the mind is occupied (i.e., concentrating on math questions). The PDR is best appreciated in a relaxed, awake patient with eyes closed. It is typically occipital but can be temporal or parietal. Clinically, the patient is fully aware of the environment, and muscle tone is high. Voltages most commonly seen are between 30 and 250 μV. The background in adults should be relatively symmetrical, referring to the amplitudes, frequencies, and morphologies of activity over analogous regions on both sides of the head. Adult EEG potentials are usually also synchronous, but this differs in neonates and infants.

Benign Waveforms of Wakefulness

Mu: Arch-shaped, 7–11 Hz trains of moderate voltage, seen best in the central regions, are called *mu*. They are blocked when moving the contralateral limb or even when planning the movement. They can be asynchronous and asymmetrical.

Lambda (Figure 8-4): Lambda waves are posterior, sharply contoured waveforms seen during visual scanning, particularly during reading. They are positive discharges at 01 and 02.

Excess beta: Beta activity, when diffuse, can be a sign of drowsiness or is seen during sleep, especially in the pediatric population. It is also a normal EEG reaction after administration of certain medications, namely benzodiazepines and barbiturates. Excess diffuse beta activity can obscure details of the normal background.

NORMAL SLEEP

Sleep is not a simple lack of awareness, but a complex series of distinct sleep phases, each of which has the potential for alterations that can be normal phenomenon, can represent a sleep disorder, or can be confused with epilepsy. Sleep staging is covered extensively elsewhere in this book and therefore is discussed only briefly here.

Sleep is divided into two general classes: REM sleep and non-REM (NREM) sleep.[5] Each stage is defined by a combination of electrophysiological parameters including EEG (Figure 8-5), respiration, eye movements, and EMG.

NREM sleep is divided into four stages, 1–4. Stage 1 is defined by onset of a low-voltage, intermixed pattern of frequencies on EEG and interruption of the posterior dominant rhythm. Vertex sharp waves may be present, as may positive occipital sharp transients of sleep (Figure 8-6). Bursts of high amplitude, diffuse, rhythmic delta activity can occur particularly in children and adolescents (hypnogogic hypersynchrony). Eye movements can be present, but these are slow and rolling compared with the sharp, predominantly vertical movements occurring with wakeful blinking. There is slight relaxation in musculature. Physiologically, this stage is *drowsiness*. Patients may have some continued awareness of their surroundings and can easily be aroused.

In stage 2, the low-voltage intermixed pattern continues; however, sleep spindles (bursts of 14–16 Hz vertex activity lasting at least 0.5 seconds) and/or K-complexes (high-amplitude biphasic discharges at the vertex) must be present. Arousal is slightly more difficult than from stage 1. In stage 3, between 20% and 50% of the record must be occupied by high-voltage delta activity. In stage 4, this increases to more than 50%. Throughout these NREM sleep stages, there is a further, progressive decrease in muscle tone. Stages 3 and 4 (also called *slow wave sleep*) are the most difficult to arouse from and can be associated with transient confusion on awakening.

REM sleep is a physiologic return to a low-voltage intermixed pattern. It differs from stage 1 by a profound reduction in muscle tone, rapid eye movements, irregular respiration, and occasionally, sawtooth waves on the PSG EEG. In this state, the most vivid dreams occur.

Text continued on p. 116

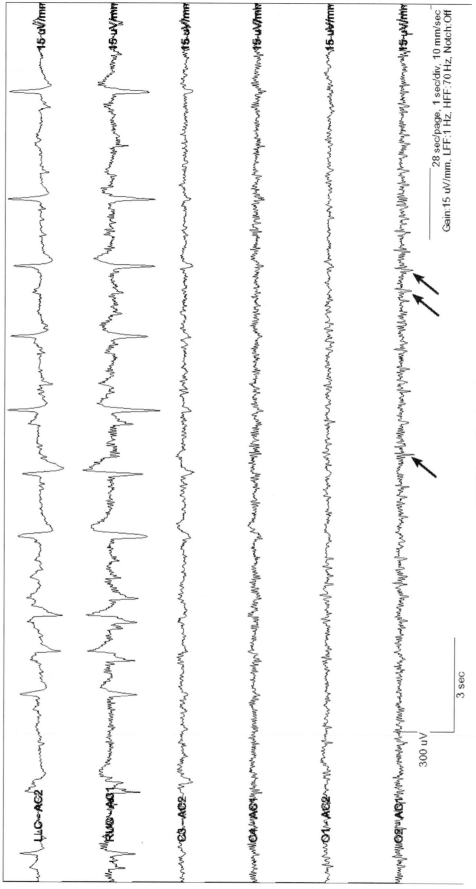

FIGURE 8-4 ■ Continued.

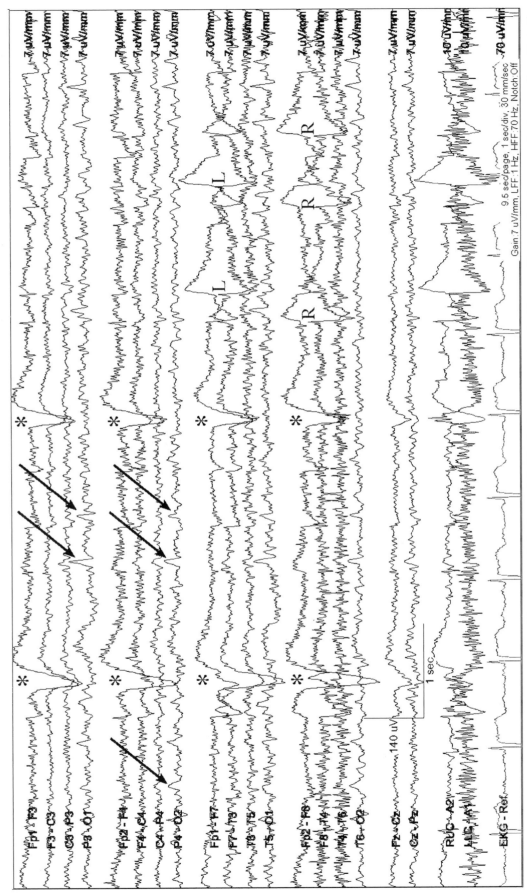

FIGURE 8-4 ■ Lambda waves (barbed arrows): Positive potentials in the occipital leads that are associated with saccadic pursuit, often seen during reading. Note the vertical (*) eye movements, likely related to blinks. Right (R) and left (L) lateral eye movements can be identified by ipsilateral lateral rectus muscle artifacts followed by a positivity from the cornea moving toward F8 or F7, respectively. Seen in typical PSG montage and reading speed (above) and EEG reading speed in long bipolar montage (below).

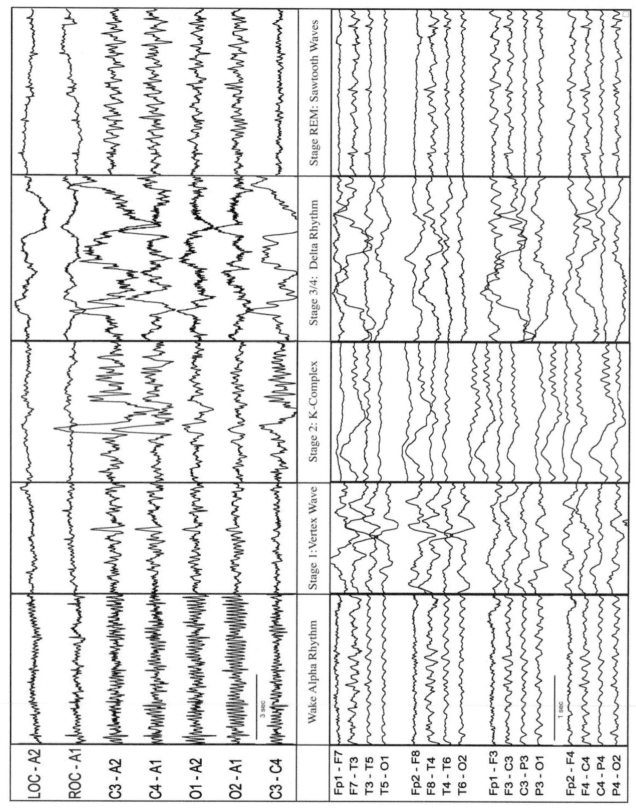

FIGURE 8-5 ■ A comparison of normal awake and asleep patterns in typical PSG and long bipolar EEG montages. Note differing paper speeds.

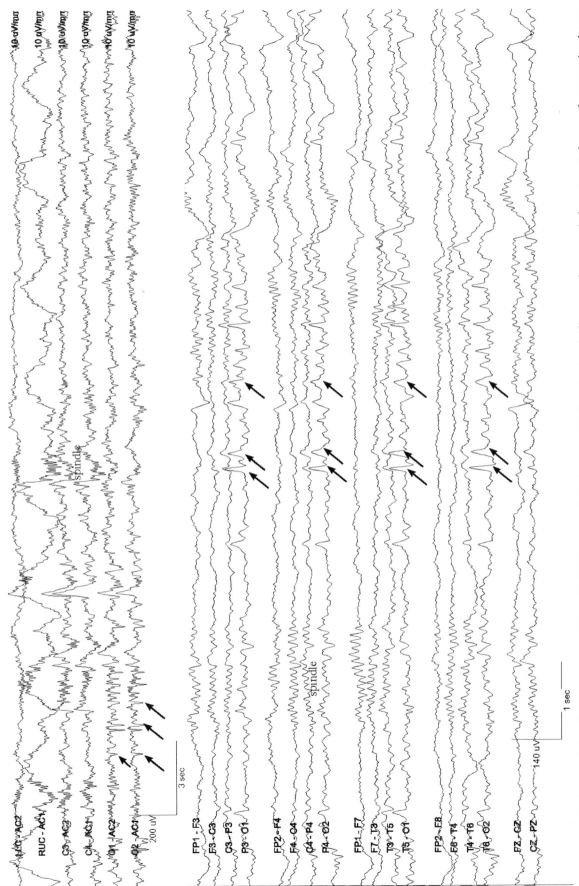

FIGURE 8-6 ■ Positive occipital sharp transients of sleep (POSTS) (arrows) during stage II sleep (note spindles) can also occur in late stage I sleep and are maximal over the posterior regions. They can be determined to be positive using a referential montage, as the downward deflection in O1/O2-AC (PSG, above). The large-amplitude upward deflection at P3-O1/P4-O2 (EEG, below) without clear phase reversal anteriorly also supports the idea that the discharge is positive and is situated more posteriorly (the other half of the deflection cannot be seen because it is at the end of the chain).

In normal patients, nocturnal sleep consists of a fairly stereotyped pattern of cycling through the various sleep stages. Patients descend through stages 1, 2, 3, and 4, followed by REM in a cycle lasting about 90 minutes. The cycle then repeats over the night, with progressively less time spent in slow wave sleep and more in REM sleep. In a normal young adult, stage 1 is less than 10% of the recording, stage 2 about 50%, and slow wave and REM about 25% each. Sleep efficiency (the time spent asleep divided by the total time in bed) should be well over 90%.

ABNORMALITIES OF BACKGROUND

Regional/Focal Findings (Figure 8-5)

Frequency

SLOWING

Focal slowing is generally considered to be due to regional subcortical dysfunction. Continuous slowing has been associated with underlying structural lesions (tumor, stroke, abscess), although intermittent slowing can be due to similar causes. In specific contexts (history of seizures), regional slowing can also be a marker of the focus of seizure origin. This is particularly true when it is temporal, intermittent, rhythmic delta activity (TIRDA)[6] (Figure 8-7). In PSG, continuous or intermittent slowing can make accurate determination of sleep stage more difficult.

FOCAL BETA ACTIVITY

Whereas diffuse beta activity is associated with medication effect or drowsiness/sleep, focal beta activity has been associated with structural or otherwise epileptogenic regions. Areas of dysplastic cerebral cortex have been implicated, although the sensitivity and specificity of the association has not been well documented.[6]

Voltage

ATTENUATION

Attenuation (decreased voltage) should always be determined relative to the background voltages. The terms *low* (<20 µV), *medium* (20–40 µV), and *high* (>50 µV) are used loosely to describe voltage. Cortical damage (owing to anoxic injury or stroke, for example) is associated with focal attenuation, particularly of faster frequency activity; however, this can also be seen where additional substances or fluid accumulates between the brain and the electrodes (such as the blood in a subdural hematoma).

Surprisingly, voltages often normalize with time following cerebral injuries. Focal or regional attenuation can also be artifactual, as a result of small differences in electrode distances, to electrical "bridging" between two electrodes with resulting apparent lack of potential differences, or be presumed as a result of increased voltage on the opposite side owing to "breach artifact" (see below).

INCREASED VOLTAGES

Focal high-voltage activity is unusual and often is due to breach artifact, which manifests as a regional increase in amplitude owing to decreased resistance, as seen with skull defects such as fractures (even hairline fractures), suture lines, craniotomy sites, or burr holes.

EPILEPTIFORM ABNORMALITIES AND SEIZURES

The Centers for Disease Control and Prevention (CDC) estimates that epilepsy affects 0.4–1.0% of the population, with a lifetime prevalence of 1.8–2.6%.[7] The prevalence of definite epilepsy (recurrent, unprovoked seizures) is estimated to be 6.5/1000 in the United States.[8] Most cases of epilepsy have an unknown etiology (Figure 8-8), with other various causes being vascular or congenital or resulting from neoplasm. Head trauma must be severe enough to cause loss of consciousness to carry appreciable risk of subsequent epilepsy. Epileptic conditions can be classified by seizure type or by etiology. With a history of probable epilepsy, the documentation of an unprovoked seizure during an EEG recording would make the diagnosis definite. A history of paroxysmal episodes along with epileptiform activity would be suspicious for an epileptic condition. Interictal (meaning "between seizures") epileptiform activity classically includes spikes and sharp waves and is either focal or generalized. Sleep and sleep deprivation are known to increase the occurrence of all of these discharges.[9,10] For focal discharges, the greatest frequency is in slow wave sleep, whereas REM has the opposite effect and a dramatic decrease of all discharges occurs.[11]

Focal spike (Figures 8-7 and 8-9): Transient potential, standing out from the background with duration of the base 20–70 ms. Spikes are typically negative in polarity, with a sensible electrical field, meaning that there is a region of maximal amplitude, with lesser amplitudes in neighboring electrodes, reflecting a discharge originating from a discrete region of cerebral cortex. These are often followed by a slow wave, again of negative polarity that disrupts the background.

Sharp wave (see Figure 8-7): As for spike, but 70–200 ms in duration.

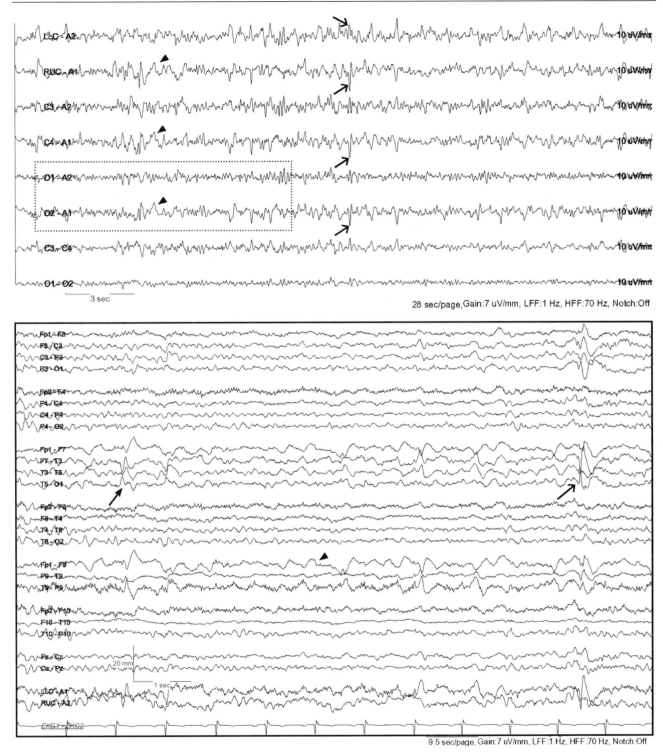

FIGURE 8-7 ■ Arrowhead showing left inferior temporal intermittent rhythmic delta activity (TIRDA), sharp wave (barbed arrow), and spikes (open arrow), all markers of temporal lobe epilepsy. On a basic PSG montage (above), the temporal activity is well recorded by the LLC and the A1 reference but is also broadly distributed over the left frontocentral regions. Thus the major asymmetry in channels (see dotted box) is between O2-A1 (in which O2 is inert but the A1 reference is involved) compared with O1-A2 (neither lead is involved, thus showing a normal posterior dominant rhythm). All other leads are involved to some extent. On the long bipolar montage with inferior temporal leads, the TIRDA is easily localized to the left inferior temporal region. Interspersed with the TIRDA are frequent spikes, maximal left temporal.

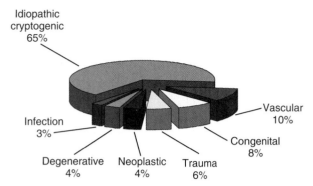

FIGURE 8-8 ■ Etiology of newly diagnosed epilepsy in Rochester, MN, 1935–1984. (Figure shown is composed of data extracted from Hauser WA, et al. Epilepsia 34(3):453–468, 1993).

Multifocal epileptiform discharges: Spikes and/or sharp waves with discrete origin in at least two locations on one hemisphere and one in the contralateral hemisphere are termed *multifocal*. For example, whereas F7 and T3 may denote one anterotemporal focality, a second focus at T5 and any on the right side would together denote multifocality, implying a more refractory epilepsy syndrome.

Generalized epileptiform discharges (Figure 8-10): These include generalized spike-wave and polyspike-wave discharges. Spike-wave activity can occur in runs and trains. Discharges typical of absence epilepsy repeat at frequencies approaching exactly 3 Hz, with faster frequencies being related to juvenile myoclonic epilepsy and slower frequencies being related to other primary generalized epilepsies.

Seizures: There is a wide variability of seizures. Most have both a clinical and EEG correlate. Others can be diagnosed on clinical grounds with no clear correlate on the EEG. The majority of seizures are characterized by rhythmic discharges that evolve in the frequency of the rhythmic pattern (speeds up, then slows down and abruptly ends), with spread of the electrical field and also usually increases in amplitude.

Nocturnal seizures: Both generalized and partial epilepsy syndromes can have a diurnal pattern. Many nocturnal paroxysmal events are not epileptic, with the EEG on overnight PSG potentially helpful in diagnosis. In addition, specific features can be elicited during a brief clinical evaluation, with a differential diagnosis of events and disorders listed in Table 8-1.

Primary Generalized Seizure Disorders

Primary (Idiopathic) Generalized Tonic-Clonic Seizures (Figure 8-11)

Generalized tonic-clonic seizures (GTCs) can be either primary (no known or suspected cause or location of onset) or secondarily generalized from an epileptogenic focus. In both, they can occur day or night. If exclusively nocturnal, the seizures are more likely to be idiopathic[12] and tend to occur during the onset or end of sleep and rarely out of REM. Onset should be bilateral and is typically maximal in the anterior regions, although a shifting asymmetry is sometimes seen. There may also be nothing apparent on the EEG at onset other than an arousal and a typical pattern of muscle artifact, which obscures the actual EEG and parallels the tonic (sustained contraction) and then clonic (rhythmic brief contractions) components of the seizure. Diffuse background slowing in the delta range is seen in the postictal phase.

Juvenile Myoclonic Epilepsy (Figure 8-10)

This is the most benign of the many myoclonic epileptic disorders, although still a lifelong condition.[12] Onset is frequently between 8 and 18 years, although presentation can be much later. There is a familial tendency, typically occurring in otherwise healthy individuals. Other clinical characteristics include myoclonic jerks or GTCs early or first thing in the morning. Myoclonic jerks can be very mild and relatively asymptomatic but can also consist of whole-body myoclonic activity. The highest-yield EEG occurs first thing in the morning, often recording spike-wave and polyspike-wave activity, sometimes repetitive at 4–6 Hz. Photic stimulation can activate EEG abnormalities and seizures.

Absence Epilepsy

Typical onset of the more benign childhood form is 3 to 12 years, with a peak at 6 to 7 years. The juvenile form starts later, and is more likely to be associated with GTCs and be treatment refractory.[12] Typical absence seizures occur in neurologically normal individuals, consisting of a brief (usually <15 seconds) behavioral arrest with rapid onset and offset. A 3-Hz generalized spike-and-wave complex (often appearing with maximal amplitude in the frontocentral region) is the typical EEG abnormality, but during sleep these often become fragmented and may appear more focal.

Localization-Related Epilepsy (Partial Epilepsy)

Partial seizures can arise from any area of the brain, but those arising from the frontal and temporal lobes are the most likely to have a diurnal pattern.

Text continued on p. 126

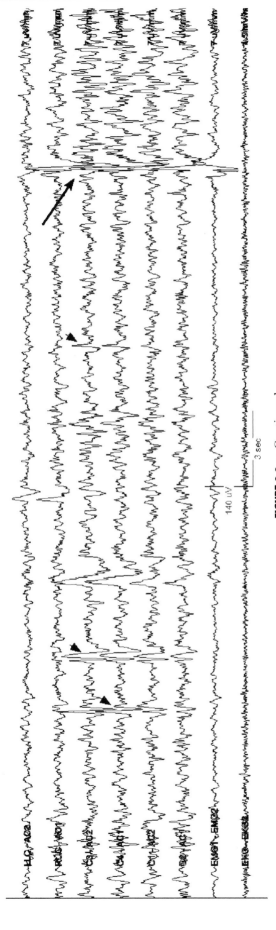

FIGURE 8-9 ■ Continued.

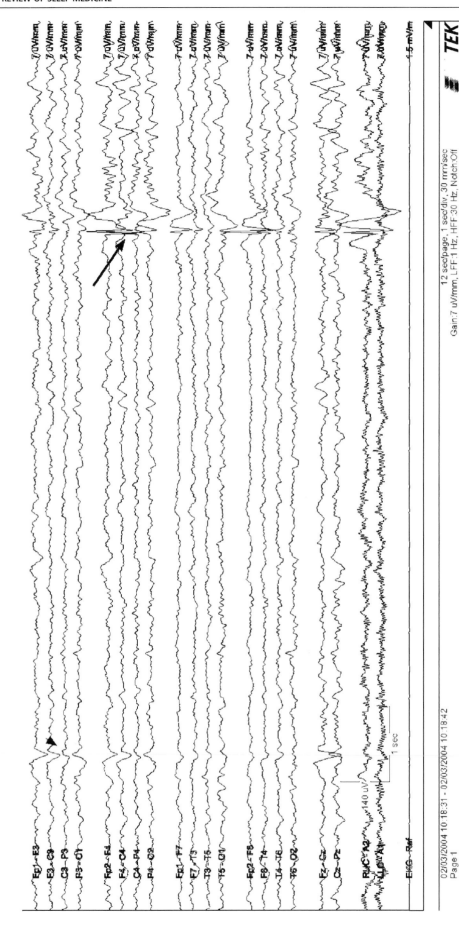

FIGURE 8-9 ■ Vertex waves (short arrows) and focal spike-wave (longer arrow) during the same recording, on both PSG (above) and EEG long bipolar (below) montages. Epileptiform activity is often activated during sleep, thus making differentiation of spikes from normal sleep architecture difficult but important. Identification is easier when using a full EEG montage.

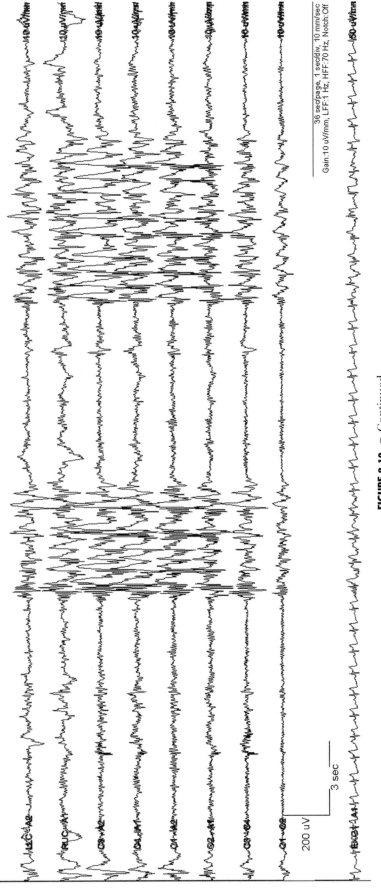

FIGURE 8-10 ■ Continued.

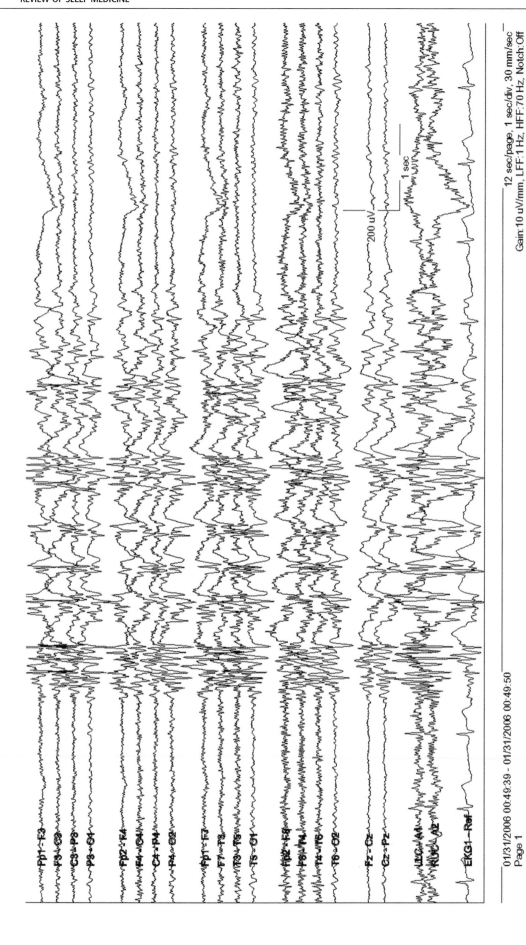

01/31/2006 00:49:39 - 01/31/2006 00:49:50
Page 1
12 sec/page, 1 sec/div, 30 mm/sec
Gain:10 uV/mm, LFF:1 Hz, HFF:70 Hz, Notch:Off

FIGURE 8-10 ■ Burst of generalized epileptiform activity, consisting of polyspikes, and polyspike-wave complexes. Seen in typical PSG montage and reading speed (above) and EEG reading speed in long biploar montage (below). Polyspike waves are typical of a generalized epilepsy syndrome, including juvenile myoclonic epilepsy.

TABLE 8-1 ■ Nocturnal Events: Differential Diagnosis

	Incontinence	Tongue Biting	Confusion	Tonic-Clonic Movement	Drooling	Amnesia	Occur While Awake
Seizure	+	+	+	+	+	+	+
Sleep drunkenness	−	−	+	−	−	+	−
Sleep terror	−	−	+	−	−	−	−
Somnambulism	−	−	+	−	−	+	−
Somniloquy	−	−	+	−	−	+	−
Sleep enuresis	+	−	−	−	−	−	−
PLMS/RLS	−	−	−	−	−	−	+
Nightmare	−	−	−	−	−	−	−
Cataplexy	−	−	−	−	−	−	+
Sleep paralysis	−	−	−	−	−	−	+
Hypnic hallucination	−	−	−	−	−	−	+
REM behavior disorder	−	−	+	−	−	−	−

PLMS, Periodic limb movements of sleep; RLS, restless legs syndrome.

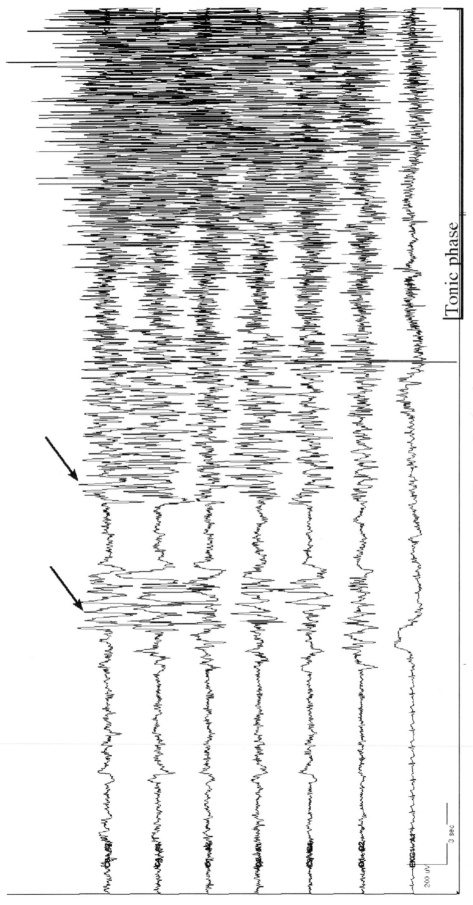

FIGURE 8-11 ■ Continued.

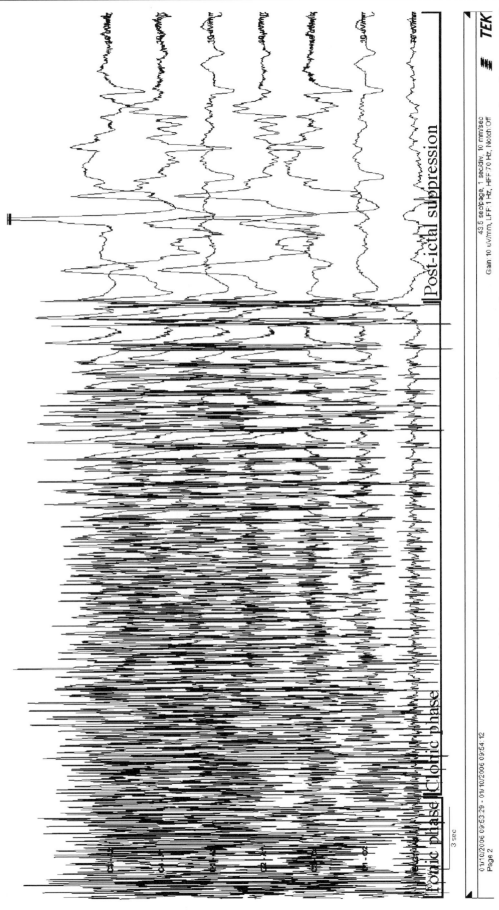

FIGURE 8-11 ■ Relatively short GTC using a typical PSG montage. Rapid clinical onset caused muscle artifact to obscure EEG evidence of the seizure, but the pattern of muscle artifact matches clinical phenomena. The densest muscle artifact occurs during the tonic phase of the seizure, with a progressively relenting on-off muscle pattern matching each clonic movement. The actual onset of the seizure may have been heralded by a number of myoclonic activity (arrows). This rapid onset may be due either to a primary generalized epilepsy syndrome or a rapidly secondarily generalized partial-onset seizure. These seizures can be overlooked as simple arousal and muscle artifact, with the only EEG correlate being postictal slowing and attenuation that is diffuse in this case but, if focal, may indicate partial onset.

Frontal Lobe Seizures (Figure 8-12A,B)

Frontal lobe seizures are clinically typified by an abrupt arousal with abnormal posturing of the body. The limbs can violently and chaotically flail in a ballistic manner, the legs may make bicycling motions, and there is often vocalization. Involvement of specific regions of the frontal lobe may give characteristic seizure semiology (clinical description), such as the supplementary motor area leading to tonic asymmetric posturing of the limbs. Self-injury can occur; patients often opt to sleep close to the floor. An abrupt onset of extremely fast beta with an apparent attenuation is classically associated with these seizures, although the EEG may not show a definite focus of onset, with muscle and movement artifact possibly obscuring the entire EEG tracing during the event. Generalization to tonic-clonic activity may occur but is not common. Patients have a very short postictal confusional stage, up to 1–2 minutes, and often rapidly return to sleep, amnestic to the event. Frontal lobe partial seizures commonly occur during sleep and are sometimes absent during wakefulness[13]; in this case they may be clinically unrecognized or confused with night terrors.

Temporal Lobe Seizures (Figure 8-13)

These seizures can occur during sleep or wakefulness, with or without secondary generalization to tonic-clonic activity.[13] Patients are often unaware of their partial seizures without generalization. Nocturnally, these seizures tend to cause arousal. They may secondarily generalize to a tonic-clonic seizure. Seizures involving the mesial temporal structures (hippocampus and amygdala) classically have a characteristic high-amplitude rhythmic discharge in the 7–8 Hz range, termed *rhythmic theta-alpha* (Figure 8-13B).

Rolandic Epilepsy (Figure 8-14)

Rolandic epilepsy is also known as *benign childhood epilepsy with centrotemporal spikes*. Age of onset is between 2 and 12 years of age, with seizures usually spontaneously remitting at ages 15 to 18 years. About 75% of seizures occur during sleep, which can be focal or generalized.[14] Seizures can consist of hemifacial twitching or hemiconvulsions, with characteristic seizures involving hypersalivation, gurgling, and speech arrest. Interictal EEG shows frequent central or temporal spikes with distinctive morphology that are unilateral in 70% of recordings but can vary in location from recording to recording. The spikes are often highly activated (more frequent) during drowsiness and sleep and are typified by a dipole, with a negativity focused centrotemporally and positivity maximally in the

bifrontal region. Sleep architecture is normal in these otherwise neurologically normal patients.

Epilepsy with Continuous Spike and Waves in Slow Wave Sleep (Electrical Status Epilepticus during Slow Wave Sleep [ESES])

This is a rare childhood syndrome with predominantly nocturnal seizures, either focal or generalized.[15] There is generalized epileptiform activity for at least 85% of recording during slow wave sleep. The EEG during wakefulness may show a combination of focal and generalized spikes. Although seizures tend to remit by age 20, intellectual deterioration is frequent.

Landau-Kleffner Syndrome

Landau-Kleffner syndrome is a rare form of childhood epilepsy characterized by a progressive and severe language disorder in addition to behavioral difficulties.[15] Abnormal electrical activity is recorded in one or both temporal lobes, often with multifocal EEG spikes. Sleep is very disturbed. Seizures are frequent initially with a tendency to lessen with time.

BENIGN VARIANTS AND ARTIFACT

The first step in interpretation of an EEG is to determine whether it is normal or whether there are abnormalities. Much of this process involves differentiation of benign variants and artifact from a real abnormality. Many benign variants can appear epileptiform, and many noncerebral events may create artifact that can appear rhythmic, epileptiform, or focal, leading to overcalling findings and potentially subjecting the individual to unnecessary long-term treatments.

Benign Variants

Rhythmic Midtemporal Theta of Drowsiness

Rhythmic midtemporal theta of drowsiness is also known as *rhythmic temporal theta bursts of drowsiness, rhythmic midtemporal discharges,* and *psychomotor variant.* Rhythmic, sharply contoured, short runs of theta-range activity occur maximally at T7 or T8. Asymmetrical, prolonged runs, especially when notched by faster frequencies, can be mistaken for a seizure, and fragments can be of higher amplitude than the background and be mistaken for a sharp wave. They are more commonly seen in young adults and in an awake, drowsy or light sleep state.

Text continued on p. 136

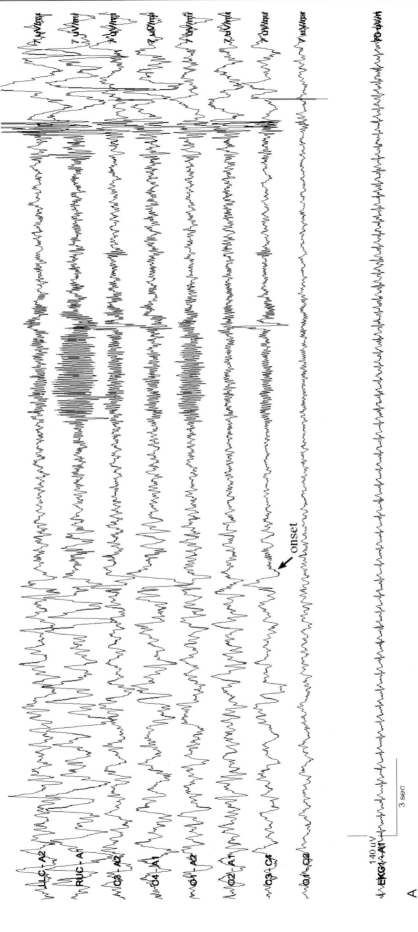

FIGURE 8-12 A,B ■ Continued.

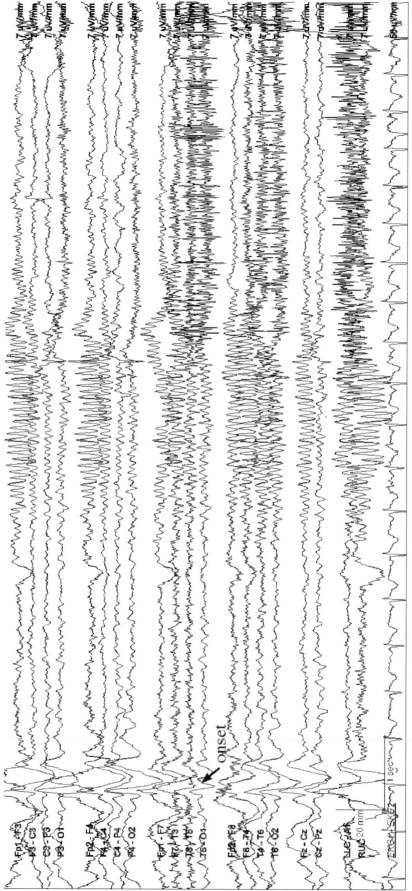

FIGURE 8-12 A,B ■ Continued.

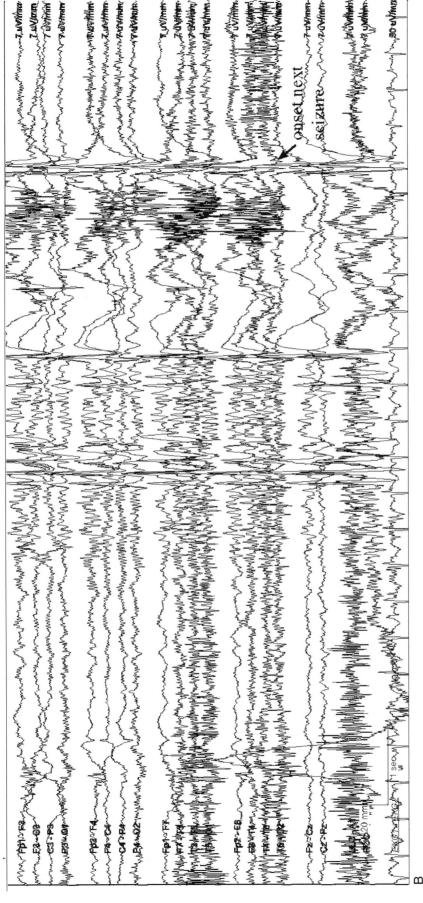

FIGURE 8-12 A,B ■ Frontal lobe seizure. The PSG (A) and EEG tracings (B) show a sudden change in background activity with a burst followed by diffuse attenuation (arrows) and then by a complex evolution of ictal activity: gradually increasing amplitude of fast activity, followed by another attenuation with fast beta activity following before a final abrupt diffuse attenuation and slowing. Utilizing referential montages (not shown), the seizures appeared to originate from the right frontal region. This patient had a tendency to cluster, with another seizure before and another ensuing directly afterward. During the seizures, the patient exhibited mild bicycling of the legs, thrashing of the limbs, and irritability. She was amnestic to the details of the events. She is developmentally normal otherwise.

FIGURE 8-13 A ■ Continued.

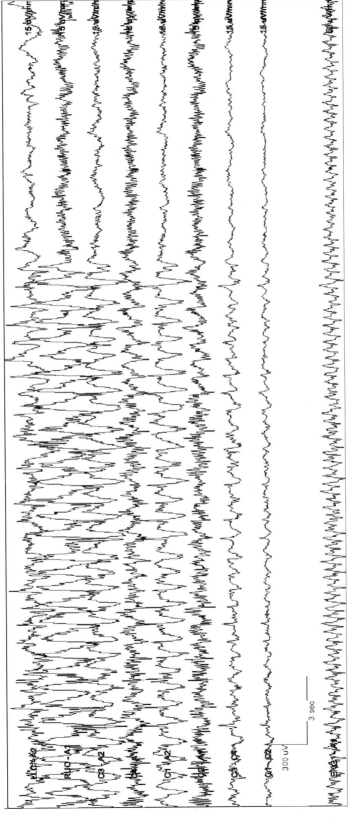

FIGURE 8-13 A ■ Right temporal seizure in typical PSG montage. Despite an absence of temporal coverage, the ear references (A1-A2) pick up temporal activity. Here, the rhythmic discharge contaminates the A2 reference; all channels referred to A2 (LLC-A2, C3-A2, O1-A2) demonstrate the seizure activity, potentially appearing left hemispheric. The same seizure is shown in Figure 8-13B, localizing to the right inferior temporal region. Note the evolution and abrupt offset of the rhythmic activity.

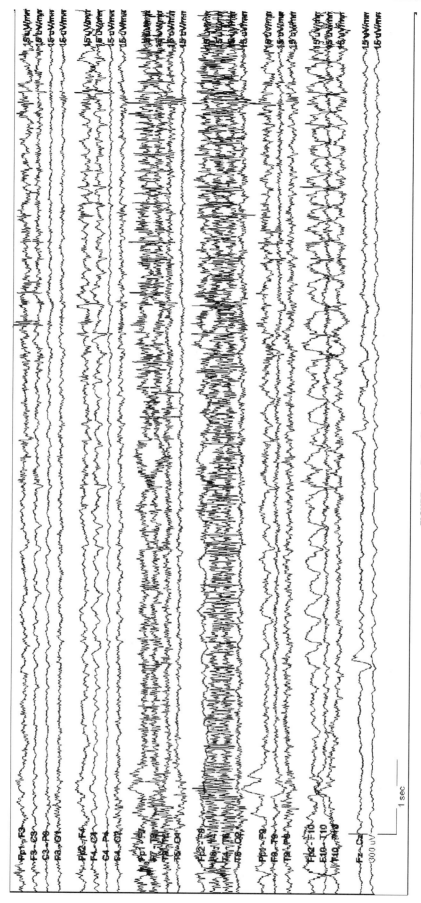

FIGURE 8-13 B ■ Continued.

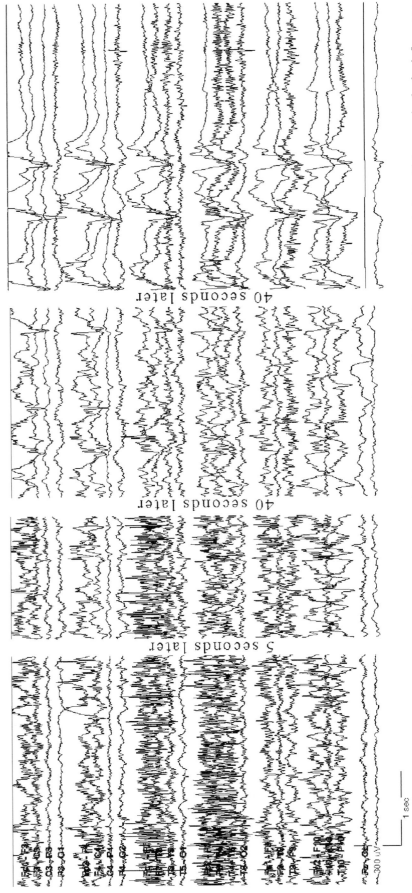

FIGURE 8-13 B ■ Right temporal seizure in long bipolar montage including inferior temporal chains. Note the electrographic evolution, with increase in rhythmic frequency up to 7 Hz, with spread in field (starting just in the inferior temporal leads, gradually spreading to involve all regions and increase in amplitude). The end of the seizure is shown, with large amplitude, rhythmic slow sharp-slow wave complexes followed by postictal diffuse attenuation and slowing. This patient had nocturnal awakenings without tonic-clonic activity, in addition to daytime staring spells with oromotor automatisms (lip smacking).

FIGURE 8-14 ■ Continued.

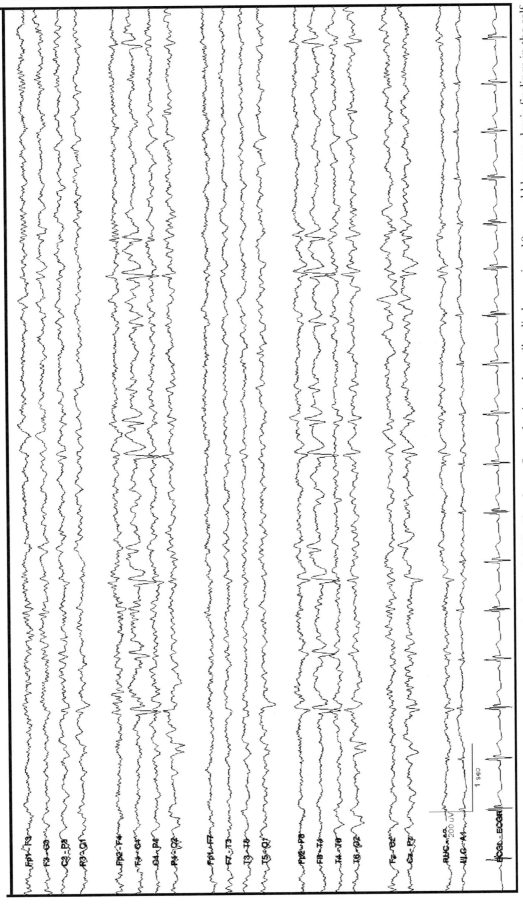

FIGURE 8-14 ■ Benign epileptiform centro-temporal spikes (BECTS). Simply configured, triangular spike discharges in a 10-year-old boy are classic findings in the self-limited Rolandic epilepsy syndrome. These are difficult to identify on PSG (above), but are clear on EEG montage (below).

Wickets

Wickets are monophasic negative discharges or trains of waves that are typically anterior or midtemporal and seen in older adults in a drowsy state. They are often arch shaped and should be considered benign but can be mistaken for an epileptiform discharge.

Benign Epileptiform Transients of Sleep, or Small Sharp Spikes (Figure 8-15)

These are small-amplitude spikes of very short duration and typically of broad field with no clinical significance. They can be numerous in one overnight recording.

Subclinical Rhythmic Electrographic Discharges of Adults

This is a rare, rhythmic, and sometimes evolving pattern, typically up to the theta range, and without postictal slowing or attenuation. The abrupt onset and offset have the appearance of a seizure, but it typically happens during wakefulness and without any clinical correlate. It is more common in older adults. Long-term follow-up has shown no clinical significance to the pattern.

Artifacts

Physiologic Artifacts

The most common artifacts are physiologic but not of cerebral origin.

BREACH ARTIFACT

Defects in the skull, either from fractures, unfused cranial sutures (from infancy) or prior cranial surgery will allow higher voltages to be recorded at the scalp. Typically, the effect is for higher frequencies; thus delta slowing in the same region for instance is usually due to underlying dysfunction and not the breach effect.

EYE MOVEMENTS

Movement of the eyes are recorded using eye channels during PSG, but their movements also cause changes in the EEG. The cornea is electropositive compared with the negatively charged retina. Whatever direction the eye looks, a large positivity is seen on EEG. On a longitudinal bipolar montage, vertical eye movements are best demonstrated in the frontopolar leads (Fp1, Fp2), whereas horizontal movements are seen best at F7 and F8 (Figure 8-4).

GLOSSOKINETIC ARTIFACT (FIGURE 8-16)

The tongue is also charged, with the tip being negative compared with the base. Movements of the tongue, seen during speech, for instance, can create the appearance of focal slowing in the temporal regions that can be quite difficult to distinguish from cerebral dysfunction.

MUSCLE ARTIFACT

Muscle within the scalp also causes electrical activity (EMG) but is usually easy to distinguish due to the typically sharper and higher frequency waveforms that are impossible for the brain to transmit to the scalp.

CHEWING AND BRUXISM (FIGURE 8-17)

Because the temporal chain resides over the temporalis muscles, activation of the muscle generates large-amplitude, very fast activity. During chewing it is very rhythmic, with bruxism classically producing a "checkerboard" pattern, with muscle artifact alternating side-to-side.

ELECTROCARDIOGRAPHIC (ECG) ARTIFACT

The EEG leads are often contaminated by electrical impulses from the heart. The degree of contamination can vary during a recording, depending on the position of the patient, presumably as the position of the heart shifts in comparison with the leads. The left ear or mastoid lead, A1/M1, has the tendency to record the greatest amount of artifact. If it becomes problematic, a bipolar montage or a different reference electrode should be used. It is also possible to "link the ears" to remove the artifact, by averaging the signals from A1 and A2 to "average out" the ECG signal. This can be accomplished either mechanically (using a wire bridge) or electronically (computerized).

PULSE ARTIFACT

Arteries and veins within the scalp can cause physical movement of a lead, which can appear as a periodic discharge, often as a delta wave. The field will typically be restricted to a single lead and should be temporally linked to the ECG recording.

CARDIOBALLISTIC ARTIFACT

Similar to pulse artifact, the movement of blood rushing to the head with each cardiac contraction can cause minute movements of the head or body, which will create the appearance of a periodic discharge, often in the leads on which the patient is resting.

Text continued on p. 140

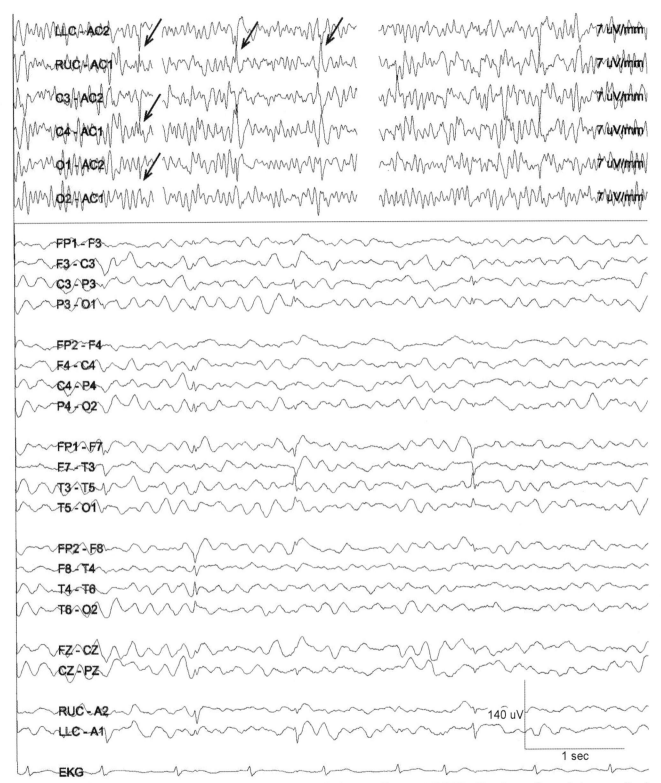

FIGURE 8-15 ■ Benign epileptiform transients of sleep/small sharp spikes (BETS/SSS). Simply configured, low-amplitude (typically <50 μV) waveforms with rapid up- and down-strokes that may meet formal duration criteria for spikes (20–70 μs) but are not considered epileptiform. They are often broadly distributed on either or both hemispheres and should only be seen during sleep.

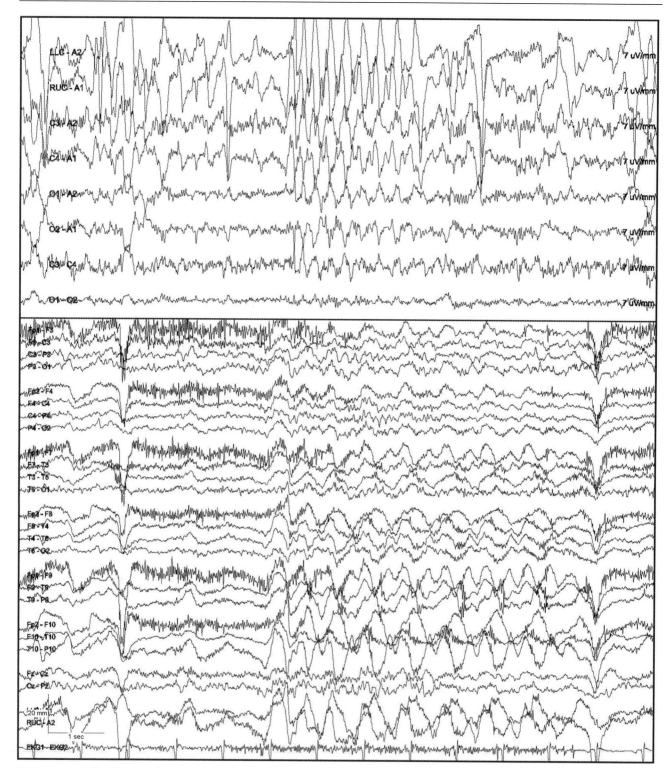

FIGURE 8-16 ■ Rhythmic activity, maximal over the temporal regions, resulting from artifact caused by drinking water. The tongue and oropharynx can cause rhythmic artifacts during talking, drinking, and snoring that can be mistaken for epileptiform activity. In this case, the rhythmic activity starts and stops abruptly, without evolution of the frequency of discharges, spread of electrical field, or increase in voltage, making this easier to identify as artifact.

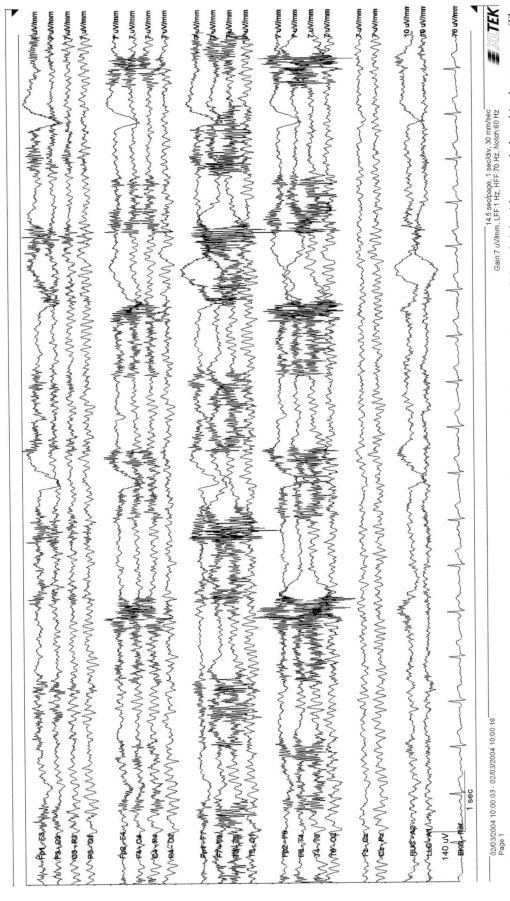

FIGURE 8-17 ■ Bruxism. This child exhibits the typical checkerboard pattern of muscle artifact alternating between left and right sides, seen in long bipolar montage. The pattern could not be identified using a typical PSG montage. Bruxism is typically seen during sleep; however, this child is awake (note eye blinks) but developmentally delayed.

RESPIRATORY ARTIFACT

Although not typically seen in healthy individuals, respiratory artifact can appear as large slow waves when electrodes are loosened by sweat. This effect is more common while viewing the recording in a PSG montage.

POSITIVE PRESSURE APPARATI

The machine itself may create artifact as a result of high-frequency oscillations of the breathing apparatus. Water trapped within the tubing can also vibrate with air flow, also causing a periodic high-frequency artifact, timed with respirations. This effect is seen more often in patients who are intubated than in patients undergoing noninvasive ventilation or continuous positive airway pressure.

Nonphysiologic Artifacts

MOVEMENT

Any movement of the wires can cause artifact; thus when the patient moves, there will often be a correlate on EEG that is not of cerebral origin.

LEAD IMPEDENCE/60 HZ (FIGURE 8-2)

The electrodes will record the signal with least resistance. With failing conductance between the scalp to electrode, signals from the surroundings are instead transmitted and then amplified. Power supplies in North America run on a 60-Hz cycle; a 60-Hz sinusoidal wave can be seen in those channels affected by poor electrical impedance, or in extreme situations (e.g., intensive care units). This artifact can overrun the entire recording. In the latter case, a notch filter can help eliminate this artifact.

POP

When an electrode intermittently loses proper contact with the scalp, relatively high amplitude deflections will be recorded, but only from channels that include that electrode.

REFERENCES

1. Ebersole JS: Cortical generators and EEG voltage fields. In Ebersole JS, Pedley TA (eds): *Current Practice of Clinical Electroencephalography*, 3rd ed. Philadelphia, Lippincott, Williams & Wilkins, 2003, pp 12–31.
2. Fisch BJ: *Fisch and Spehlmann's EEG Primer*, 3rd ed. Amsterdam, Elsevier, 1999.
3. Noachtar S, Binnie C, Ebersole J, et al: A glossary of terms most commonly used by clinical electroencephalographers and proposal for the report form for the EEG findings. The International Federation of Clinical Neurophysiology. Electroencephalogr Clin Neurophysiol Suppl 52:21–41, 1999.
4. Oken BS, Kaye JA: Electrophysiologic function in the healthy, extremely old. Neurology 42(3 Pt 1):519–526, 1992.
5. Rechtschaffen A, Kales A: *A Manual of Standardized Terminology, Techniques, and Scoring System for Sleep Stages of Human Subjects*. Los Angeles, UCLA Brain Information Service/Brain Research Institute, 1968.
6. Bazil CW, Herman ST, Pedley TA: Focal electroencephalographic abnormalities. In Ebersole JS, Pedley TA (eds): *Current Practice of Clinical Electroencephalography*, 3rd ed. Philadelphia, Lippincott, Williams & Wilkins, 2003, pp 303–347.
7. The Centers for Disease Control and Prevention: Prevalence of epilepsy and health-related quality of life and disability among adults with epilepsy—South Carolina, 2003 and 2004. MMWR Morbidity and Mortality Weekly Report 54:1080–1082, 2005. http://www.cdc.gov/mmwr/preview/mmwrhtml/mm5442a4.htm
8. Hauser WA, Annegers JF, Kurland LT: Incidence of epilepsy and unprovoked seizures in Rochester, Minnesota: 1935–1984. Epilepsia 34(3):453–468, 1993.
9. Malow BA, Selwa LM, Ross D, Aldrich MS: Lateralizing value of interictal spikes on overnight sleep-EEG studies in temporal lobe epilepsy. Epilepsia 40(11):1587–1592, 1999.
10. Fountain NB, Kim JS, Lee SI: Sleep deprivation activates epileptiform discharges independent of the activating effects of sleep. J Clin Neurophysiol 15(1):69–75, 1998.
11. Sammaritano M, Gigli GL, Gotman J: Interictal spiking during wakefulness and sleep and the localization of foci in temporal lobe epilepsy. Neurology 41(2 (Pt 1)):290–297, 1991.
12. Loddenkemper T, Benbadis SR, Serratosa JM, Berkovic SF: Idiopathic generalized epilepsy syndromes of childhood and adolescence. In Wyllie E (ed): *The Treatment of Epilepsy, Principles & Practice*. Philadelphia, Lippincott, Williams & Wilkins, 2006.
13. Herman ST, Walczak TS, Bazil CW: Distribution of partial seizures during the sleep-wake cycle: differences by seizure onset site. Neurology 56(11):1453–1459, 2001.
14. Mendez M, Radtke RA: Interactions between sleep and epilepsy. J Clin Neurophysiol 18(2):106–127, 2001.
15. Neville B, Cross JH: Continuous spike wave of slow sleep and Landau-Kleffner syndrome. In Wyllie E (ed): *The Treatment of Epilepsy, Principles & Practice*. Philadelphia, Lippincott, Williams & Wilkins, 2006.

An Overview of Polysomnography

SHARON A. KEENAN

INTRODUCTION

The term *polysomnography* (PSG) was proposed by Holland, Dement, and Raynal[1] in 1974 to describe the recording, analysis, and interpretation of multiple, simultaneous, physiologic parameters. As a tool, PSG is essential in the formulation of diagnoses for sleep disorder patients and in the enhancement of our understanding of both normal sleep and its disorders.[2–16] It is a complex procedure that should be performed by a trained technologist.[17] Today's sleep laboratory continues to undergo technological evolution, particularly in terms of the increased reliance on digital systems[18–20] and the collection of data outside of the traditional sleep laboratory setting.[21,22] This evolution requires sophisticated knowledge of equipment and procedures.

This chapter is a review of the technical and clinical aspects of PSG. The reader is directed to the references for current indications and standards of practice original sources.[17,21,23–38,67,68]

INDICATIONS FOR PSG

PSG is used to investigate the relationship between changes in physiology, impact on sleep, and consequences of waking function, performance, and behavior. Issues such as shift work, time zone change, or suspected advanced or delayed sleep phase syndrome should be considered when scheduling the study. The PSG should be conducted during the patient's usual major sleep period to avoid confounding circadian rhythm factors.

Questionnaires regarding sleep-wake history and a sleep diary that solicits information about major sleep periods and naps are useful adjuncts to PSG.[39,40] Questionnaires can be used to identify and triage patients before laboratory testing.[41–45]

A full medical and psychiatric history should be completed and made available to the technologist performing the study. Without this information, the technologist is at a loss to understand how aspects of the medical or psychiatric history may affect the study or to anticipate difficulties. Technologists must also understand what questions the study seeks to answer. This enhances the ability to make protocol adjustments when necessary and guarantees that the most pertinent data are collected.

PRESTUDY QUESTIONNAIRE

It is not uncommon for patients, particularly those with excessive sleepiness, to have a diminished capacity to evaluate their level of alertness.[46] In addition, many patients with difficulty initiating and maintaining sleep often report a subjective evaluation of their total sleep time and quality that is at odds with the objective data collected in the laboratory, referred to as *sleep state misperception*, an International Classification of Sleep Disorders (ICSD) diagnosis classification.[30,31] For these reasons it is recommended that subjective data be collected systematically, as part of the sleep laboratory evaluation.

The Stanford Sleepiness Scale (SSS) (Appendix 9-2)[47,48] is an instrument used to assess a patient's subjective evaluation of sleepiness before the PSG. The SSS is presented to the patient immediately before the beginning of the study. It offers a series of phrases describing states of arousal or sleepiness. Patients respond by selecting the set of adjectives that most closely corresponds with their current state of sleepiness or alertness. The scale is used extensively in both clinical and research environments; however, it has two noteworthy limitations: It is not suitable for children who have a limited vocabulary or for adults whose primary language is not English. In these situations a linear analog scale is recommended. One end of the scale represents extreme sleepiness, and the other end represents alertness. Patients mark the scale to describe their state just before testing (see Appendix 9-2).

This chapter is an updated version of the following: Keenan SA, Chokroverty S. In Chokroverty SA (ed): *Sleep Disorders Medicine, Basic Science, Technical Considerations and Clinical Aspects*, 2nd ed. Boston, Butterworth Heinemann, 1999, Ch 9, pp. 151–174. Reproduced with kind permission of the publishers.

Another instrument, the Epworth Sleepiness Scale,[40] lends information about chronic sleepiness. Patients are asked to report the likelihood of falling asleep in situations such as riding as a passenger in a car, watching TV, etc.

Patients are also asked about their medication history, smoking history, any unusual events during the course of the day, their last meal before the study, alcohol intake, and a sleep history for the last 24 hours, including naps. Involvement of the patient in providing this information usually translates into increased cooperation for the study. A technologist's complete awareness of specific patient idiosyncrasies, in the context of the questions to be addressed by the study, ensures a good foundation for the collection of high-quality data.

NAP STUDIES

A proposed alternative to PSG has been the nap study (to be distinguished from the Multiple Sleep Latency Test [MSLT]).[46,49,50] The rationale is that if a patient has a sleep disorder, it will be expressed during an afternoon nap, as well as during a more extensive PSG. The nap study approach has been used most frequently for the diagnosis of sleep-related breathing disorders and was proposed in an effort to reduce the cost of the sleep laboratory evaluation. The short study in the afternoon avoids the necessity of having a technologist present for an overnight study. There are serious limitations to the use of nap studies, however, including the possibility of false-negative results or the misinterpretation of the severity of sleep-related breathing disorders if the patient is sedated or sleep deprived before the study. When a nap study is performed, it should follow the guidelines as published by the American Thoracic Society[25]:

Although minimal systematic data exist on the value of nap recordings, nap studies of 2 to 4 hours' duration may be used to confirm the diagnosis of sleep apnea, provided that all routine polysomnographic variables are recorded, that both non-rapid eye movement (NREM) and REM sleep are sampled, and that the patient spends at least part of the time in the supine posture. Sleep deprivation or the use of drugs to induce a nap are contraindicated. Nap studies are inadequate to definitively exclude a diagnosis of sleep apnea.

DATA COLLECTION

Data are collected using a combination of alternating current (AC) channels and direct current (DC) channels.

Equipment for recording PSGs is produced by a number of manufacturers. Each instrument may have a distinctive appearance and some idiosyncratic features, but there is a remarkable similarity when the basic functioning of the instrument is examined.

Equipment preparation includes an understanding of how the filters and sensitivity of the amplifiers affect the data collected.

The amplifiers used to record physiologic data are very sensitive, so it is essential to eliminate unwanted signals from the recording. By using a combination of high- and low-frequency filters and appropriate sensitivity settings, we maximize the likelihood of recording and displaying the signals of interest and decrease the possibility of recording extraneous signals. Care must be taken when using the high- and low-frequency filters, however, to ensure that an appropriate window for recording specific frequencies is established and that the filters do not eliminate important data.

ALTERNATING CURRENT AMPLIFIERS

Differential AC amplifiers are used to record physiologic parameters of high frequency, such as the electroencephalogram (EEG), the electro-oculogram (EOG), the electromyogram (EMG), and the electrocardiogram (ECG). The AC amplifier has both high- and low-frequency filters. The presence of the low-frequency filter makes it possible to attenuate slow potentials not associated with the physiology of interest; these include galvanic skin response, DC electrode imbalance, and breathing reflected in an EMG, EEG, or EOG channel. Combinations of specific settings of the high- and low-frequency filters make it possible to focus on specific bandwidths associated with the signal of interest. For example, breathing is a very slow signal (roughly 12–18 breaths per minute) compared with the EMG signal, which has a much higher frequency (approximately 20–200 Hz or cycles per second).

DIRECT CURRENT AMPLIFIERS

In contrast to the AC amplifier, the DC amplifier does not have a low-frequency filter. DC amplifiers are typically used to record slower-moving potentials, such as output from the oximeter or pH meter, changes in pressure in positive airway pressure treatment, or output from transducers that record endoesophageal pressure changes or body temperature. Airflow and effort of breathing can be successfully recorded with either AC or DC amplifiers.

An understanding of the appropriate use of filters in clinical PSG is essential to proper recording technique.[18,20,50,51] Table 9-1 provides recommendations for filter settings for various physiologic parameters.

TABLE 9-1 ■ Recommendations for Filter and Sensitivity Settings for Various Physiologic Parameters

Channel[a]	Low-Frequency Filter (Hz)	Time Constant (s)	High-Frequency Filter (Hz)	Sensitivity
EEG	0.3	0.4	35	50 (μV/cm)
EOG	0.3	0.4	35	50 (μV/cm)
EMG	5[b]	0.03	90–120	20–50 (μV/cm)
ECG	1.0	0.12	15	1 MV/cm
Index of airflow	0.15[c]	5[b]	15	[†]
Index of effort	0.15[c]	5[b]	15	[†]

Modified from SA Keenan. Polysomnography: technical aspects in adolescents and adults. J Clin Neurophysiol 9:21, 1992.

EOG, Electro-oculography; EMG, electromyography; ECG, electrocardiography.

[a] EEG includes C3/A2, C4/A1, O1/A2, and O2/A1. EOG includes right outer canthus and left outer canthus referred to opposite reference.

[b] If shorter time constant or higher low-frequency filter is available, it should be used. This includes settings for all EMG channels including mentalis, submentalis, masseter, anterior tibialis, intercostal, and extensor digitorum.

[c] Because breathing has such a slow frequency (as compared with the other physiologic parameters), the longest time constant available, or the lowest setting on the low-frequency filter options, would provide the best signal. It is also possible to use a DC amplifier (with no low-frequency filter, time constant = infinity) to record these signals.

[†] It is common in clinical practice to index changes in airflow and effort to breathe by displaying qualitative changes in oral/nasal pressure, temperature, and chest and abdominal movement. It is well recognized that quantitative methods (such as endoesophageal pressure changes) provide a more sensitive and accurate measure of work of breathing. Ideally, a multimethod approach is used to increase confidence in detecting events of sleep-related breathing anomalies.

CALIBRATION OF THE EQUIPMENT

The PSG recording instrument must be calibrated to ensure adequate functioning of amplifiers and appropriate settings for the specific protocol. The first calibration is an all-channel calibration. During this calibration, all amplifiers are set to the same sensitivity and high- and low-frequency filter settings, and a known signal is sent through all amplifiers simultaneously. The proper functioning of all amplifiers is thus demonstrated, ensuring that all are functioning in an identical fashion (Figure 9-1A).

A second calibration is performed for the specific study protocol. During this calibration, amplifiers are set with the high- and low-frequency filter and sensitivity settings appropriate for each channel; the settings are dictated by the requirements of the specific physiologic parameter recorded on each channel (Table 9-1, Figure 9-1B). The protocol calibration ensures that all amplifiers are set to ideal conditions for recording the parameter of interest. Filter and sensitivity settings should be clearly documented for each channel.

DATA DISPLAY AND ANALYSIS

The process of sleep stage scoring and analysis of abnormalities is accomplished by an epoch-by-epoch review of the data.

Historically, a common paper speed for analog PSG was 10 mm/sec^{-1}, providing a 30-s epoch (another widely accepted paper speed was 15 mm/sec^{-1}, which gave a 20-sec epoch length). An expanded time base may be necessary to visualize EEG data, specifically the spike activity associated with epileptic discharges. Compressed displays of greater than 30-sec screen for EEG should be avoided because they compromise an adequate display of EEG data. Data such as oxygen saturation, respiratory signals, or changes in penile circumference, however, can be more easily visualized when display time is compressed to 2 to 5 minutes per screen. A major advantage of the digital systems lies in the ability to manipulate the display after data collection. A brief discussion of digital systems appears later in this chapter.

THE STUDY: ELECTRODE/MONITOR APPLICATION PROCESS

The quality of the tracing generated depends on the quality of the electrode application.[38,52] Before any electrode or monitor is applied, the patient should be instructed about the procedure and given an opportunity to ask questions. The first step in the electrode application process involves measurement of the patient's head. The International 10–20 System[53] of electrode placement is used to localize specific electrode sites (Figure 9-2). The following sections address the application process for EEG, EOG, EMG, and ECG electrodes.

ELECTROENCEPHALOGRAPHY

The EEG probably reflects local potential changes that occur on pyramidal cell soma and large apical dendrites of pyramidal cell neurons. The EEG is not likely the reflection of action potentials of the neurons.[54]

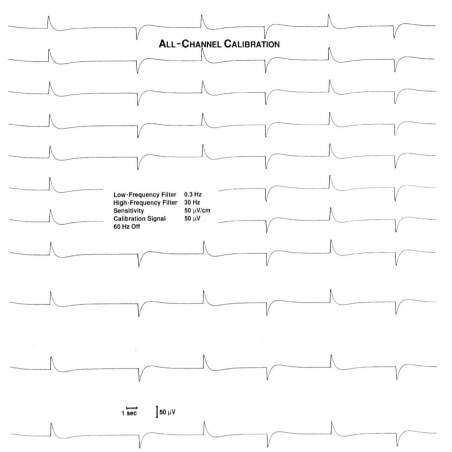

Low-Frequency Filter   0.3 Hz
High-Frequency Filter   30 Hz
Sensitivity   50 μV/cm
Calibration Signal   50 μV
60 Hz Off

1 sec   50 μV

FIGURE 9-1A ■ All-channel calibration is shown. All amplifiers have the same sensitivity and high- and low-frequency filter settings.

To record EEG, the standard electrode derivations for monitoring EEG activity during sleep are C3/A2 or C4/A1 and O1/A2 or O2/A1, but in many situations there may be a need for additional electrodes. For example, to rule out the possibility of epileptic seizures during sleep or the presence of any other sleep-related EEG abnormality, it may be necessary to apply the full complement of EEG electrodes according to the International 10–20 System (Appendix 9-3).

For recording EEG, a gold cup electrode with a hole in the center is commonly used. Silver-silver chloride electrodes are also useful to record EEG, although they may have limitations such as increased maintenance (evidenced by the need for repeated chloriding) and the inability to attach these electrodes to the scalp.

The placement of C3, C4, O1, and O2 are determined by the International 10–20 System of Electrode Placement. Reference electrodes are placed on the bony surface of the mastoid process. A description of the measurement procedure appears in Appendix 9-4.

A variety of methods are used to attach electrodes. The collodion technique[52,55] has long been an accepted and preferred method of application for EEG scalp and reference electrodes. This technique ensures a long-term placement and allows for correction of high (>5000 ohms) impedances after application. Other methods using electrode paste and conductive medium are acceptable and sometimes necessary in certain conditions.

ELECTRO-OCULOGRAPHY

The EOG is a reflection of the movement of the corneoretinal potential difference within the eye. The retina is negative with respect to the cornea. Thus the eye exists as the potential field within the head, which serves as the volume conductor for that field. It is important to recognize that EOG as described here does not measure eye muscle potentials changes.[54]

An electrode is typically applied at the outer canthus of the right eye (ROC) and is offset by 1 cm above the horizontal. Another electrode is applied to the outer canthus of the left eye (LOC) and is offset by 1 cm below the horizontal. The previously mentioned A1 and A2 reference electrodes are used as follows: ROC/A1 and LOC/A2. Additional electrodes can be applied

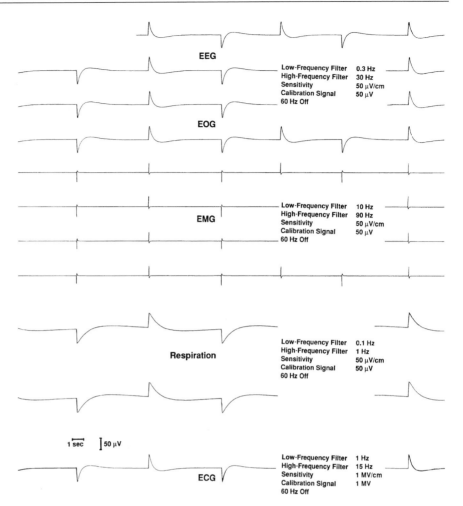

FIGURE 9-1B ■ The montage calibration shows changes in high- and low-frequency filter settings from the all-channel calibration to display a variety of physiologic signals for the polysomnograph. EOG, Electrooculogram; EMG, electromyogram; ECG, electrocardiogram.

infraorbitally and supraorbitally for either the right or left eye. The infraorbital and supraorbital electrodes enhance the ability to detect eye movements that occur in the vertical plane and can be particularly useful in the MSLT[5,11,56] (Figure 9-3).

EOG electrodes are typically applied to the surface of the skin with an adhesive collar.

ELECTROMYOGRAPHY

The EMG recording represents the summation of activity taking place on many individual motor endplates.[54]

A gold cup or a silver-silver chloride electrode attached with an adhesive collar is used to record EMG activity from the mentalis and submentalis muscles. At least three EMG electrodes are applied to allow for an alternative electrode, in the event that artifact develops in one of the others. The additional electrode can be placed over the masseter muscle to allow for detection of bursts of EMG activity associated with bruxism (Figure 9-4).

Additional bipolar EMG electrodes are placed on the surface of the anterior tibialis muscles to record periodic limb movements in sleep[57] and on the surface of the extensor digitorum muscles if REM sleep behavior disorder[58] is suspected.

ELECTROCARDIOGRAPHY

There are a variety of approaches for recording the ECG during PSG. The simplest approach involves use of standard gold cup electrodes; however, disposable electrodes are also available.

ECG electrodes are applied with an adhesive collar to the surface of the skin just beneath the right clavicle and on the left side at the level of the seventh rib. A stress loop is incorporated into the lead wire to ensure long-term placement.

MONITORING BREATHING DURING SLEEP

It is necessary to record airflow and effort to breathe, and it is with these two measures that breathing irregularities can be detected. There are many

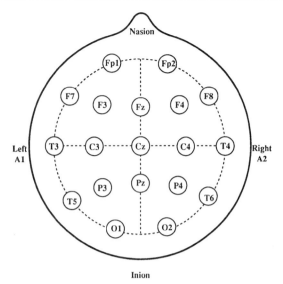

FIGURE 9-2 ■ The complete 10–20 system of electrode placement.

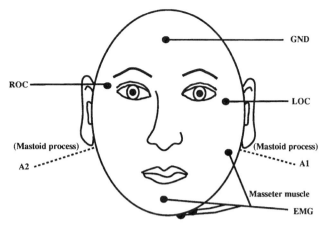

FIGURE 9-4 ■ Schematic diagram shows placement of the EMG electrodes to record activity from the mental, submental, and masseter muscles. ROC, LOC, Outer canthus of the right and left eye, respectively; GND, = ground (earth).

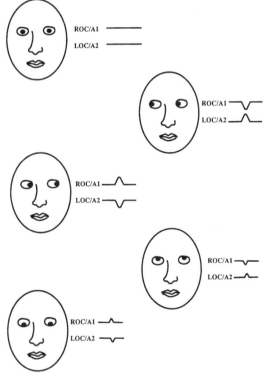

FIGURE 9-3 ■ The recording montage for a two-channel EOG demonstrates out-of-phase signal deflection in association with conjugate eye movements. Schematic diagram shows placement of the EMG electrodes to record activity from the mental, submental, and masseter muscles. ROC, LOC, Outer canthus of the right and left eye, respectively; GND, ground (earth).

sophisticated technical advances on the horizon, but the following describes common clinical practice.

It is well recognized that the pneumotachograph is the gold standard for measuring airflow. It is customary, however, for many clinical studies to rely on qualitative methods to index airflow during sleep. Historically, thermistors or thermocouples were used, whereas presently a more accepted practice is to record change in pressure to indicate airflow.[34]

Respiratory inductive plethysmography is often thought of as a reliable, noninvasive measure of work of breathing. If calibrated, it can give a measure of changes in tidal volume. There have been reports of difficulty maintaining calibration for the duration of the study. Piezo crystals embedded into adjustable belts worn around the chest and abdomen reflect changes in association with effort to breathe and are commonly used. There are numerous ways to index work of breathing, including but not limited to intercostal and/or diaphragmatic EMG and impedance pneumography.

A quantitative measure of work of breathing is endoesophageal manometry.[59] For greater reliability and validity, multiple methods of monitoring airflow and effort of breathing should be used.

Commercially available devices also allow for noninvasive blood gas monitoring during sleep. These measures are essential in assessment of the severity of the sleep-related breathing disorder.

GASTROESOPHAGEAL REFLUX STUDIES

It is common for PSG to include monitoring of endoesophageal pH when patients complain of reflux or waking with a choking sensation.[60] Commercially available devices allow for the recording of changes in pH at the level of the distal esophagus during sleep. Events of reflux and the "clearing time" or time necessary to return to normal acid levels can be demonstrated and correlated with other physiologic events or EEG arousals.

QUALITY CONTROL

Before recording, electrodes should be visually inspected to check the security of their placement, and an impedance check should be obtained and documented. Adjustment should be made to any EEG, EOG, ECG or chin EMG electrode with an impedance greater than 5000 ohms. Impedances of 20,000 ohms are acceptable for limb EMG recordings.[61]

PHYSIOLOGIC CALIBRATIONS

Physiologic calibrations are performed after the electrode and monitor application is complete. This calibration allows for documentation of proper functioning of the electrodes and other monitoring devices and provides baseline data for review and comparison when scoring the PSG. The specific instructions given to the patient for this calibration include:

- Eyes open, look straight ahead for 30 seconds.
- Eyes closed, look straight ahead for 30 seconds.
- Hold head still, look to left and right, up and down. Repeat.
- Hold head still, blink eyes slowly, five times.
- Grit teeth, clench jaw, or smile.
- Inhale and exhale.
- Hold breath for 10 seconds.
- Flex right foot, flex left foot.
- Flex right hand, flex left hand.

As these instructions are given to the patient, the technologist examines the tracing and documents the patient's responses. When the patient stares straight ahead for 30 seconds with the eyes open, the background EEG activity is examined. As the patient looks right and left, the tracing is examined for out-of-phase deflections of the signals associated with recording the EOG. Out-of-phase deflection occurs if the inputs to consecutive channels of the polygraph are ROC/A1 for the first EOG channel and LOC/A2 for the second. It is also important, when the patient closes the eyes, to observe the reactivity of the alpha rhythm seen most prominently in the occipital EEG (O1/A2 or O2/A1); usually alpha is best visualized when the patient's eyes are closed. The patient is also asked to blink five times.

The mentalis/submentalis EMG signal is checked by asking the patient to grit the teeth, clench the jaws, or yawn. The technologist documents proper functioning of the electrodes and amplifiers used to monitor anterior tibialis EMG activity by asking the patient to flex the right foot and the left foot in turn. If REM sleep behavior disorder is suspected, additional electrodes should be applied to the surface of the skin above the extensor digitorum muscles of each arm. Patients are asked to flex their wrists while the technologist examines the recording for the corresponding increase in amplitude of the EMG channel amplitude.

Inhalation and exhalation allow for examination of channels monitoring airflow and effort of breathing. A suggested convention is that inhalation causes an upward deflection of the signal, and exhalation causes a downward deflection. It is most important that the signals on all the channels monitoring breathing are in phase with each other to avoid confusion with paradoxical breathing. The technologist should observe a flattening of the trace for the duration of a voluntary apnea.

If the 60- or 50-Hz notch filter is in use, a brief examination (2–4 seconds) of portions of the tracing with the filter in the off position is essential. This allows for identification of any 60- or 50-Hz interference that may be masked by the filter. Care should be taken to eliminate any source of interference and to ensure that the 60- or 50-Hz notch filter is used only as a last resort. This is most important when recording patients suspected of having seizure activity, because the notch filter attenuates the amplitude of the spike activity seen in association with epileptogenic activity. If other monitors are used, the technologist should incorporate the necessary calibrations.

The physiologic calibrations enable the technologist to determine the quality of data before the PSG begins. If artifact is noted during the physiologic calibrations, it is imperative that every effort be made to correct the problem; the condition is likely to get worse through the remaining portions of the recording. The functioning of alternative (spare) electrodes should also be examined during this calibration.

When a satisfactory calibration procedure is completed and all other aspects of patient and equipment preparation are completed, data collection can begin. This is referred to as "lights-out," and the time should be clearly noted.

MONITORING RECORDING: DOCUMENTATION

Complete documentation for the PSG is essential. This includes patient identification (patient's full name and medical record number), date of recording, and a full description of the study. The names of the technologists performing the recording and any technologists involved in preparation of patient and equipment should be noted. The specific instrument used to generate the recording should be identified. This is particularly useful in the event that artifact is noted during the analysis portion (scoring) of the sleep study.

Specific parameters recorded on each channel should be clearly noted, as should a full description of sensitivity, filter, and calibration settings for each channel. The time of the beginning and end of the recording must be noted, as well as specific events that occur during the night. Usually a predetermined montage is available as a simple software selection. Any changes made to filter and sensitivity settings should be clearly noted.

The technologist is also responsible for providing a clinical description of unusual events. For example, if a patient experiences an epileptic seizure during the study, the clinical manifestations of the seizure must be detailed: deviation of eyes or head to one side or the other, movement of extremities, presence of vomiting or incontinence, duration of the seizure, and postical status. Similar information should be reported on any clinical event observed in the laboratory, such as somnambulism or clinical features of REM sleep behavior disorder. Physical complaints reported by the patient are also noted.

TROUBLESHOOTING/ARTIFACT RECOGNITION

In general, when difficulties arise during recording, the troubleshooting inquiry begins with the patient and follows the path of the signal to the recording device. More often than not, the problem can be identified as a difficulty with an electrode or other monitoring device. It is less likely that artifact is the result of a problem with an amplifier. If the artifact is generalized (i.e., on most channels), then the integrity of the ground electrode and the instrument cable should be checked. If the artifact is localized (i.e., on a limited number of channels), then the question should be "Which channels have this artifact in common, and what is common to the channels involved?" The artifact is probably the result of a problem located in an electrode or monitoring device that is common to both channels. If the artifact is isolated to a single channel, the source of artifact is limited to the inputs to the specific amplifier, the amplifier itself, or to the ink-writing system for the channel.

Figures 9-5 to 9-13 depict some frequently encountered artifacts seen during PSG.

ENDING THE STUDY

Clinical circumstances and laboratory protocol dictate whether the patient is awakened at a specific time or allowed to awaken spontaneously. After awakening, to end the study the patient should be asked to perform the physiologic calibrations to ensure that the electrodes and other monitoring devices are still functioning properly. The equipment should be calibrated at the settings used for the study, and finally, the amplifiers should be set to identical settings for high- and low-frequency filters and sensitivity, and an all-channel calibration should be performed. This is essentially the reverse of the calibration procedures mentioned for the beginning of the study.

A subjective evaluation is made by the patient. The patient is asked to estimate how long it took to fall asleep, the amount of time spent asleep, and if there were any disruptions during the sleep period. Patients should report on quality of sleep and the level of alertness upon arousal.

It is also worthwhile for the sleep laboratory staff to know how patients intend to leave the laboratory. A patient who has a severe sleep disorder should avoid driving. An arranged ride or public transportation should be used, particularly if the patient has withdrawn from stimulant medications for the purpose of the study.

THE FINAL REPORT

The interpretation of the PSG is a process involving review of clinical presentation and history, as well as parametric analysis of the PSG. The variables listed in Table 9-2 are most commonly used to inform the interpretation and create the final report.

DIGITAL SYSTEMS

Within the past 2 decades, digital systems have made it possible to manipulate data after recording and to permit extraction of otherwise inaccessible information. Digital systems provide flexibility in the manipulation of filter settings, sensitivities, and changes in the display of montages after collection. The first digital EEG systems became available in the late 1980s and caused a revolution in EEG and PSG.[18,20,38] This revolution has been primarily in making the static format of analog system data more flexible.

Significant advantages of digital systems include: autocorrection of amplifier gains, self-diagnostic tests

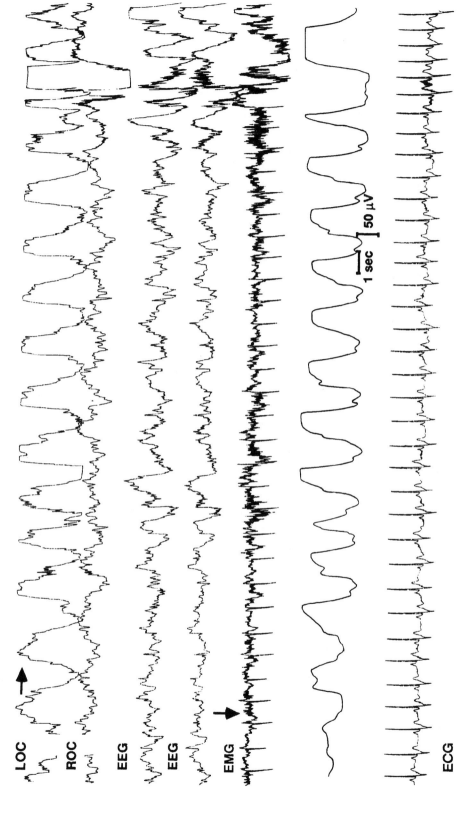

FIGURE 9-5 ■ Artifact in LOC channel (LOC/A1) can be localized to the LOC electrode. The EEG channels in the trace are C3/A2 and O2/A1. Because the artifact does not appear in the O2/A1 channel, the artifact is localized to the LOC electrode. The electrode placement may be insecure, or the patient may be lying on the electrode and producing movement of the LOC electrode in association with breathing. Additional artifact is noted in the EMG channel. This signal is contaminated with ECG artifact, and the intermittent slower activity as well as the wandering baseline are most likely due to a loose lead. The ECG channel also shows a pattern consistent with a loose electrode wire.

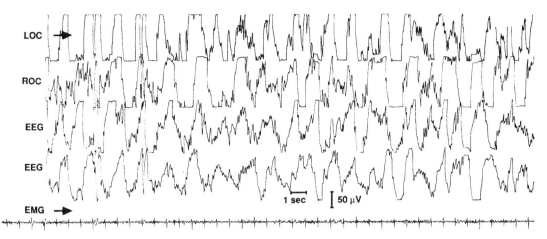

FIGURE 9-6 ■ This figure illustrates the blocking artifact seen with inappropriate sensitivity settings. This can be alleviated by decreasing sensitivity. If adjustments to sensitivity are made, they should be clearly noted and should be made on all channels displaying EEG data. It is common procedure to calibrate the equipment with decreased sensitivities (i.e., 100 μv/cm^{-1}) for children's studies or increasing sensitivity (i.e., 30 μv/cm^{-1}) for older patients. Typically, sensitivity settings are not changed frequently during the recording (as they may be in routine EEG). As a result, it is not uncommon to see this artifact when the patient enters slow wave sleep. This is not a common problem with digital systems because of the user's ability to manipulate sensitivity after collection.

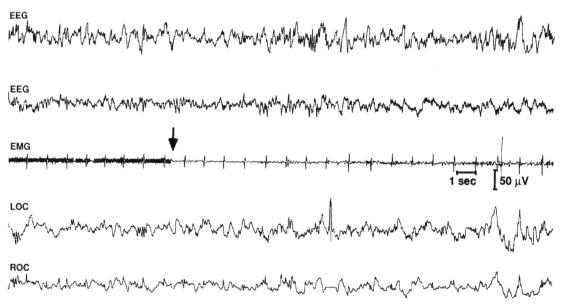

FIGURE 9-7 ■ A 60-Hz artifact exists in the EMG channel in this tracing. At the arrow the 60-Hz filter is turned on. There is continued evidence of difficulty with electrodes on this channel, however, as evidenced by the ECG artifact and occasional spikelike activity. Turning on the 60-Hz filter is not the correct response to eliminate the artifact. If possible, the technologist should switch to an alternative electrode or fix the one involved.

of amplifier functions, and the software-controlled, in-line impedance testing. The use of the computer has facilitated storage of data, manipulation of data after collection, and the presentation of different views of the data. Both analog and digital systems require electrodes and other sensors to be applied with the greatest of care. Ideally, calibration procedures should be performed to document and ensure the collection of high-quality data at the beginning and end of the recording. Knowledge of the specifics of the equipment and of the physiology of interest is important to ensure accurate signal processing.

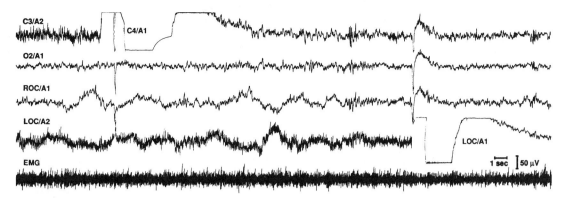

FIGURE 9-8 ■ The high-frequency (probably EMG) artifact noted in the C3/A2 and LOC/A2 channels can be localized to the A2 electrode. This problem can be solved by switching to the alternative reference (A1) electrode. A high-amplitude discharge is noted during the switch from C3/A2 to C4/A1 and LOC/A2 to LOC/A1. This can be avoided by placing the amplifier in standby mode while making the change.

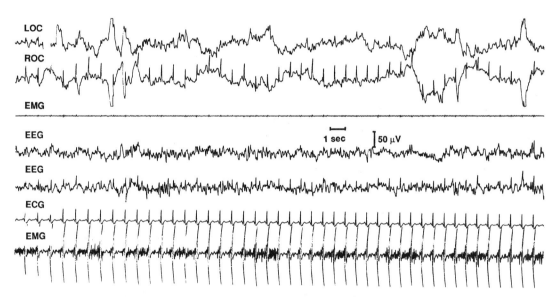

FIGURE 9-9 ■ The ROC channel (ROC/A1) and the second EEG (O2/A1) channels are contaminated with ECG artifact. The artifact can be identified by aligning the spikelike activity noted in channels with the R wave on the ECG channel. It is localized to the A1 electrode because it is seen in both ROC/A1 and O2/A1 channels and A1 is common to both channels. It should be noted that the high-amplitude ECG artifact, seen in the EMG channel below the ECG channel, is unavoidable. This artifact is due to the proximity of EMG electrodes to the heart, which creates a robust signal superimposed on the intercostal EMG signal.

In digital systems it is rare to encounter breakdown of any mechanical component; most frequently encountered problems have to do with the disk drives or cables. The most important things to avoid for trouble-free operation are mechanical shock, dust, or static electricity.

An important factor for understanding digital PSG systems is the concept of sampling rate. Sampling rate can be understood as the frequency with which the signal is reviewed (sampled) for conversion to a digital signal. The minimum acceptable sampling rate for EEG, EOG, and EMG in PSG is 100 Hz when using a 35-Hz filter. A 200-Hz sampling rate is required for a 70-Hz, high-filter setting.[62]

Another issue unique to digital systems is the accuracy or precision of recordings. The resolution of the signal is a function of the number of binary bits used to represent the digital values. Readers will recall that a bit is a value of 1 or 0. Eight bits is 2 to the 8th power, or 256. For example, if we assume an EEG voltage over 256 μV, from negative 128 μV to positive 128 μV, this would result in a resolution using an 8-bit system of 1 μV difference being represented in 1 bit of change. The 8-bit system is a system that represents the least

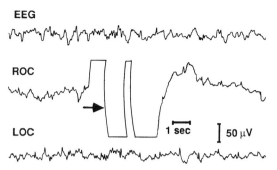

FIGURE 9-10 ■ The high-amplitude deflection in the ROC (ROC/A1) channel is associated with an electrode artifact, commonly referred to as an "electrode pop." This can be the result of a compromised electrode placement or insufficient electroconductive gel under the electrode. When this artifact is observed, the electrode involved should not be trusted to give reliable data.

amount of precision. A 12-bit system is the accepted minimum for sleep recording.[19] This provides a range of values between –2048 and –2047. The 12-bit successive digital values represent a 0.0625 μV change. The 12-bit representation is far more precise and reflects a smaller change in the signal. (It is interesting to note that the equivalent precision of paper-tracings is approximately 6 bits. The decreased precision for analog systems is a function of the limitation in the amount of paper available for one channel and pen thickness.)

Also to be considered is the display resolution, which is determined by the resolution of the monitor. The screen used for reviewing the data must be at least 20 inches in size and display a resolution of 1280 × 1024 pixels (flicker free; that is, 75-Hz monitor scan rate).[19]

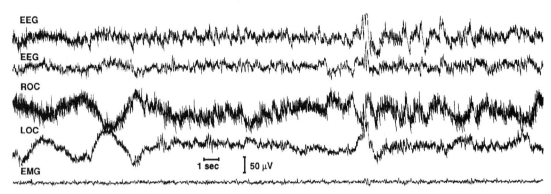

FIGURE 9-11 ■ There is a generalized, high-frequency activity superimposed on the EEG and EOG channels. This is most likely secondary to muscle activity. The EMG channel shows only artifact.

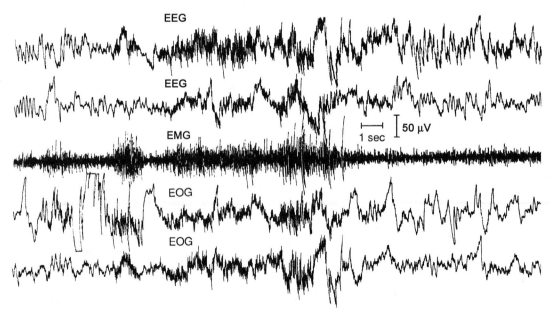

FIGURE 9-12 ■ This burst of high-frequency artifact, superimposed on the EEG and EOG channels, is due to a brief movement on the part of the subject. As in Figure 9-10, this is a superimposition of EMG activity on the EEG and EOG channels. It should also be noted that in the first EOG channel there is an electrode pop. The EMG channel in this tracing is of good quality and should be compared with Figure 9-10.

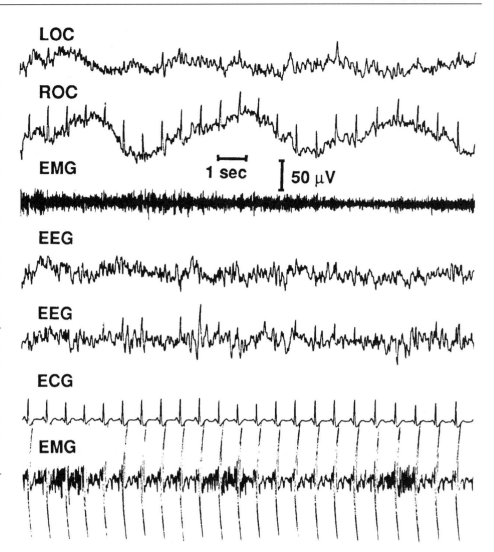

FIGURE 9-13 ▪ A high-amplitude, slow artifact is noted in the ROC (ROC/A1) channel. This is most likely associated with the patient's breathing and is secondary to a loose electrode or the patient lying on the right side and disturbing the electrode in synchrony with breathing. A relatively high-amplitude ECG artifact is also seen. The artifact can be localized to the ROC electrode. The EMG tracing noted at the bottom of this example is an intercostal EMG. The high-amplitude ECG spike in this channel is impossible to eliminate; however, the brief bursts of EMG activity can be noted in association with the artifact seen in the ROC/A1 channel. This lends further evidence that the artifact noted in the ROC electrode is probably associated with breathing in as much as the bursts of intercostal EMG activity are seen in association with the effort of breathing.

DIGITAL RECORDING SAMPLES

Figures 9-14 to 9-17 are examples of digital data used with permission of the author and publisher.[63]

SUMMARY

Throughout its evolution, PSG has proven a robust tool for enhancing understanding of sleep and its disorders. It is an essential diagnostic procedure.

PSG is complex and labor intensive. It requires specialized technical skills and knowledge of normal sleep and sleep disorders. Technologists need to be experts with equipment, competent in dealing with medically ill patients, and capable of dealing with emergencies that may be encountered in the sleep laboratory. They must also be skilled enough to work in many circumstances outside of the traditional laboratory setting.

Our field faces many challenges. Evaluation of sleep disorders must be made readily available to millions of sleep-disorder patients lacking diagnosis and treatment.[64–66] Cost effectiveness in sleep health care and maintenance of high-quality evaluation and treatment remain important challenges. Digital systems can facilitate data storage, manipulation, and analysis, provided that the user is knowledgeable of both instrumentation and the physiology of interest.

TABLE 9-2 ■ Polysomnography Variables

Variable	Units
Lights out	Time
Lights on	Time
Lights out to SO	Mins
SO	Time/epoch #
SO to S1	Mins
SO to S2	Mins
SO to SWS	Mins
SO to REM	Mins
TS1	Mins %TST
TS2	Mins %TST
TSWS	Mins %TST
TREM	Mins %TST
TMT	Mins %TST
TS1	Mins %TST
TRT	Mins
TWT	Mins
TST/TIB	Mins
WASO	Mins
WAFA	Mins
SE	%
TST	%
Events	
Average O_2 sat	%
Low O_2 sat	%
Total Events	
OSA	#
CSA	#
HYP	#
Indexes	
AHI	#
RDI	#
AI	#

SO, Sleep onset; S1, stage 1; S2, stage 2; SWS, slow wave sleep; TS1, total stage 1; TST, total sleep time; TS2, total stage 2; TSWS, total slow wave sleep; TREM, total REM; TMT, total movement time; TRT, total recording time; TWT, total wake time; TST/TIB, total sleep time/time in bed; WASO, wake after sleep onset; WAFA, wake after final wakening; SE, sleep efficiency; OSA, obstructive sleep apnea; CSA, central sleep apnea; HYP, hypopneas; AHI, apnea hypopnea index; RDI, respiratory disturbance index; AI, apnea index.

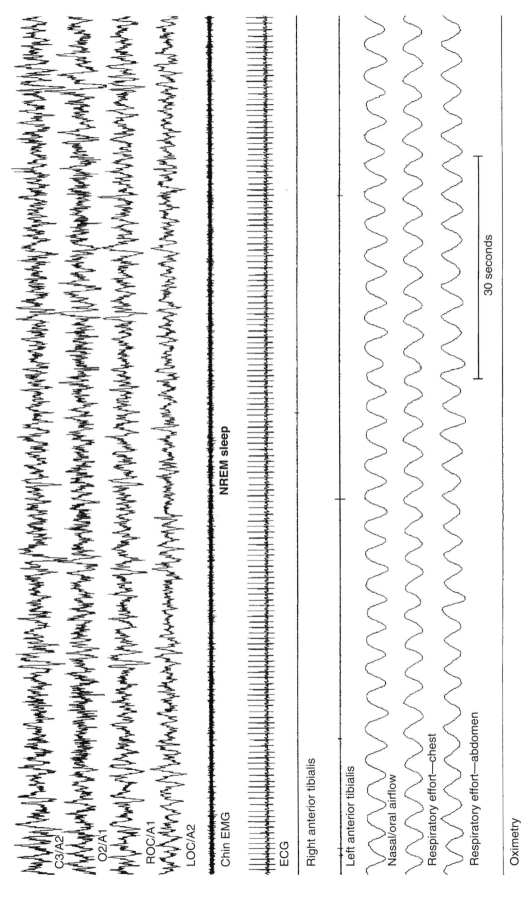

FIGURE 9-14 ■ Digital record sample of NREM sleep using time-scale compression. Digital data can be further compressed to display several epochs on a screen simultaneously. The previous sample and the recordings shown in Figures 9-15 to 9-17 have been compressed to accommodate four epochs of data (2 min) to a page. This type of display offers the scorer or interpreter a general overview of the sleep recording, as well as a practical method of counting any prominent sleep-related events such as obstructive apneas, hypopneas, or body movements. Resolution of the data is inadequate, however, for precise EEG evaluation or sleep-stage scoring. This sample shows a normal respiratory pattern during NREM sleep, without any apparent evidence of arousal, movement, or other form of sleep disturbance. ROC, LOC, Outer canthus of the right and left eye, respectively; EMG, electromyography; ECG, electrocardiography. (Reproduced with permission from Bukov N: *Atlas of Clinical Polysomnography*. Medford, OR, Synapse Media, 1996.)

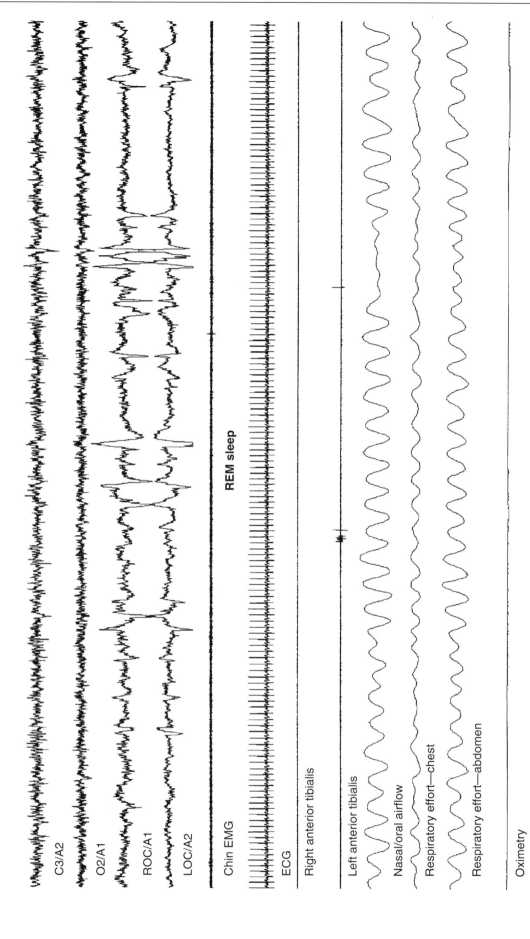

C3/A2

O2/A1

ROC/A1

LOC/A2

Chin EMG

REM sleep

ECG

Right anterior tibialis

Left anterior tibialis

Nasal/oral airflow

Respiratory effort—chest

Respiratory effort—abdomen

Oximetry

FIGURE 9-15 ■ Digital record sample of REM sleep. Although altered by time-scale compression, the sleep-stage pattern seen in this sample can readily be identified as REM. Note the mild respiratory irregularity, which is a normal variant of REM sleep physiology. ROC, LOC, Outer canthus of the right and left eye, respectively; EMG, electromyography. (Reproduced with permission from Butkov N: *Atlas of Clinical Polysomnography.* Medford, OR, Synapse Media, 1996.)

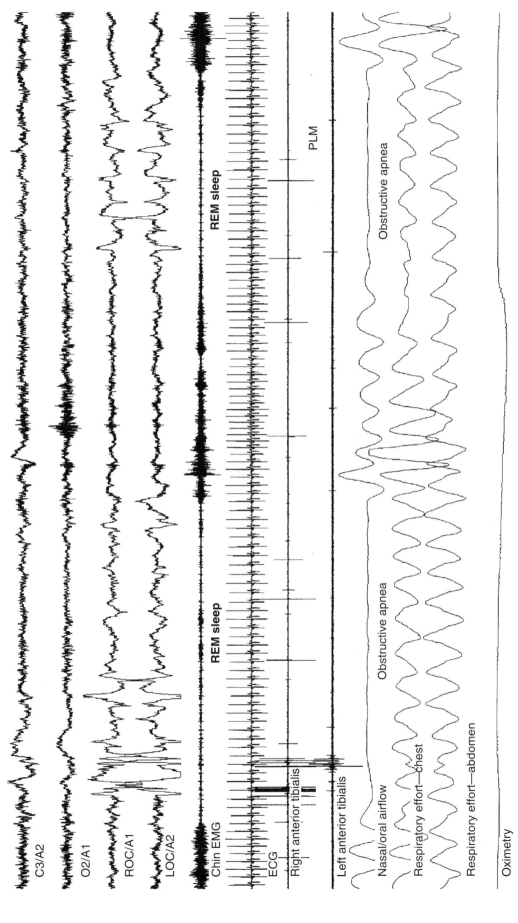

FIGURE 9-16 ■ Digital record sample of obstructive apneas. This sample shows a compressed display of repetitive obstructive apneas, occurring during REM sleep. As noted before, these represent the extreme end of the sleep-disordered breathing continuum. In the preceding example, all the features of classic obstructive sleep apnea are present, including distinct paradoxical (out-of-phase) respiratory effort, instances of complete cessation of airflow, subsequent EEG arousals, and cyclic O_2 desaturations. ROC, LOC, Outer canthus of the right and left eye, respectively; EMG, electromyography; ECG, electrocardiography. (Reproduced with permission from Butkov N: *Atlas of Clinical Polysomnography.* Medford, OR, Synapse Media, 1996.)

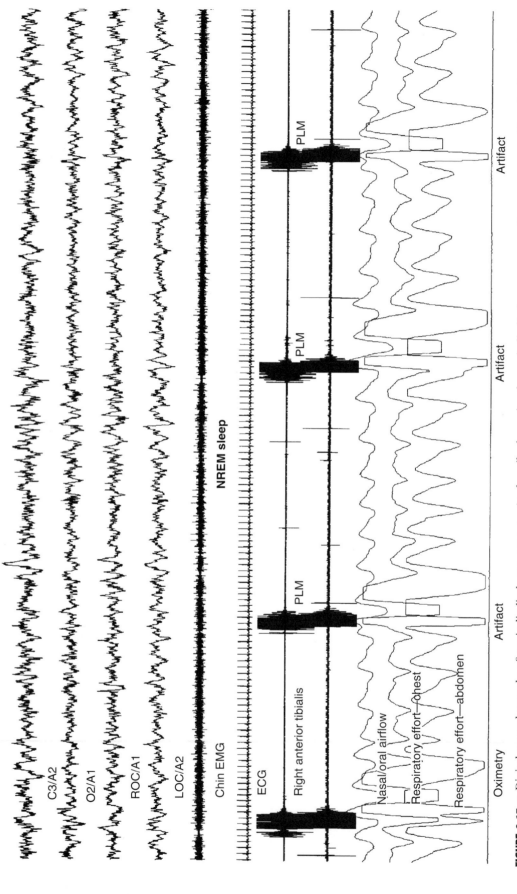

C3/A2

O2/A1

ROC/A1

LOC/A2

Chin EMG

NREM sleep

ECG

Right anterior tibialis

PLM

PLM

PLM

Nasal/oral airflow

Respiratory effort—chest

Respiratory effort—abdomen

Oximetry   Artifact   Artifact   Artifact

FIGURE 9-17 ■ Digital record sample of periodic limb movements. As described previously, periodic limb movements often generate artifacts in the respiratory channels that appear similar to cyclic hypopneas. This sample shows a compressed version of the characteristic pattern of periodic limb movement (PLM), recorded by the right and left anterior tibialis EMG. Note that the respiratory channel artifact appears almost identical to the cyclic hypopneas seen in the preceding sample. ROC, LOC, Outer canthus of the right and left eye, respectively; EMG, electromyography; ECG, electrocardiography. (Reproduced with permission from Butkov N: *Atlas of Clinical Polysomnography.* Medford, OR, Synapse Media, 1996.)

REFERENCES

1. Holland JV, Dement WC, Raynal DM: *Polysomnography: A Response to a Need for Improved Communication*. Presented at the 14th Annual Meeting of the Association for the Psychophysiological Study of Sleep, Jackson Hole, WY, 1974, p 121.
2. Dement WC, Kleitman N: Cyclic variation in EEG during sleep and their relation to eye movements, body motility and dreaming. Electroencephalogr Clin Neurophysiol 9:673–690, 1957.
3. Dement WC, Rechtschaffen A: Narcolepsy: polygraphic aspects, experimental and theoretical considerations. In Gastaut H, Lugaresi E, Berti Ceroni G (eds): *The Abnormalities of Sleep in Man*. Bologna, Italy, Aulo Gaggi Editore, 1968, pp 147–164.
4. Dement WC, Zarcone V, Guilleminault C, et al: Diagnostic sleep recording in narcoleptics and hypersomniacs. Electroencephalogr Clin Neurophysiol 35:220, 1973.
5. Raynal D: Polygraphic aspects of narcolepsy. In Guilleminault C (ed): *Narcolepsy*. Spectrum, New York, 1976, pp 669–684.
6. McGregor P, Weitzman ED, Pollack CP: Polysomnographic recording techniques used for diagnosis of sleep disorders in a sleep disorders center. Am J EEG Technol 18:107–132, 1978.
7. Weitzman ED, Pollack CP, McGregor P: The polysomnographic evaluation of sleep disorders in man. In Aminoff MJ (ed): *Electrodiagnosis in Clinical Neurology*. New York, Churchill Livingstone, 1980, pp 496–524.
8. Broughton RJ: Polysomnography: principles and applications in sleep and arousal disorders. In Niedermeyer E, Lopes da Silva F (eds): *Electroencephalography: Basic Principles, Clinical Applications, and Related Fields*, 2nd ed. Baltimore, Urban & Schwarzenberg, 1987, pp 687–724.
9. Guilleminault C: *Sleep Apnea in the Full-term Infant. Sleep and its Disorders in Children*. New York, Raven Press, 1987, pp 195–211.
10. Keenan SA: Polysomnography: technical aspects in adolescents and adults. J Clin Neurophysiol 9(1):21–31, 1992.
11. Keenan S: Polysomnographic technique: an overview. In Chokroverty S (ed): *Sleep Disorders Medicine: Basic Science, Technical Considerations and Clinical Aspects*, 2nd ed. Boston, Butterworth-Heinemann, pp 151–169, 1999.
12. Guilleminault C, Stoohs R, Clerk A, et al: A cause of excessive daytime sleepiness: the upper airway resistance syndrome. Chest 104(3):781–787, 1993.
13. Guilleminault C, Kim YD, Stoohs RA: Upper airway resistance syndrome. Oral Maxillofac Surg Clin North Am 7(2):243–256, 1995.
14. Springer EA, Kushida CA, Guilleminault C, et al: Upper airway resistance syndrome: polysomnographic characteristics. Sleep Res 25:373, 1996.
15. Butkov N: Polysomnography. In Lee-Chiong TL, Sateia M, Carskadon MA (eds): *Sleep Medicine*. Philadelphia, Hanley & Belfus, 2002, pp 605–638.
16. Carskadon M, Rechtschaffen A: Monitoring and staging human sleep. In Kryger MH, Roth T, Dement WC (eds): *Principles and Practice of Sleep Medicine*, 3rd ed. Philadelphia, Saunders, 2000, pp 197–215.
17. American Sleep Disorders Association: Role and Qualifications of Technologists Performing Polysomnography: Position Paper. *Adopted by the Executive Committee of the American Sleep Disorders Association*. April 1, 1998.
18. Wong PKH: *Digital EEG and Clinical Practice*. Philadelphia, Lippincott-Raven, 1996.
19. Hirshkowitz M, Moore CA: Computers in sleep medicine. In Kryger MH, Roth T, Dement WC (eds): *Principles and Practice of Sleep Medicine*, 3rd ed. Philadelphia, Saunders, 2000, pp 1302–1307.
20. Penzel T, Conradt R: Computer based sleep recording and analysis. Sleep Med Rev 4(2):131–148, 2000.
21. American Sleep Disorders Association: Practice parameters for the use of portable recording in the assessment of obstructive sleep apnea. ASDA Standards of Practice. Sleep 17(4):372–377, 1994.
22. Fry JM, Di Phillipo MA, Curran K, et al: Full polysomnography in the home. Sleep 21:635–642, 1998.
23. Block AJ, Cohn MA, Conway WA, et al: Indications and standards for cardiopulmonary sleep studies. Sleep 8(4): L371–L379, 1985.
24. Martin RJ, Block AJ, Cohn MA, et al: Indications and standards for cardiopulmonary sleep studies. Sleep 8(4):371–379, 1985.
25. American Thoracic Society: Indications and standards for cardiopulmonary sleep studies. Medical Section of the American Lung Association. Am Rev Respir Dis 139(2):559–568, 1989.
26. American Thoracic Society: Standards and indications for cardiopulmonary sleep studies in children. Am J Respir Crit Care Med 153(2):866–878, 1996.
27. American Electroencephalography Society. Guideline fifteen: guidelines for polygraphic assessment of sleep-related disorders. J Clin Neurophysiol 11:116–124, 1994.
28. American Sleep Disorders Association: Practice parameters for the use of actigraphy in the clinical assessment of sleep disorders. An American Sleep Disorder Association Report. Sleep 18(4):285–287, 1995.
29. American Sleep Disorders Association: Practice parameters for the use of polysomnography in the evaluation of insomnia. An American Sleep Disorders Association Report, Standards Practice Committee of the American Sleep Disorders Association. Sleep 18(1):55–57, 1995.
30. American Sleep Disorders Association: *ICSD: International Classification of Sleep Disorders, Revised: Diagnostic and Coding Manual*. Rochester, MN: American Sleep Disorders Association, 1997.
31. American Sleep Disorders Association: Practice parameters for the indications for polysomnography and related procedures. An American Sleep Disorders Association Report. Sleep 20(6):406–422, 1997.
32. AARC-APT. Polysomnography: AARC-APT (American Association of Respiratory Care—Association of Polysomnography Technologists) clinical practice guideline. Resp Care 40(12):1336–1343, 1995.
33. Reite M, Buysse D, Reynolds C, Mendelson W: The use of polysomnography in the evaluation of insomnia. An

American Sleep Disorders Association review. Sleep 18(1):58–70, 1995.

34. American Academy of Sleep Medicine: Sleep-related breathing disorders in adults: recommendations for syndrome definition and measurement techniques in clinical research. The report of an American Academy of Sleep Medicine Task Force. Sleep 22(5):667–689, 1999.

35. American Academy of Pediatrics, Policy Statement: Clinical practice guideline: diagnosis and management of childhood obstructive sleep apnea syndrome. Pediatrics 190(4):704–712, 2002.

36. American Academy of Sleep Medicine: *Accreditation Standards for Sleep Disorders Centers*. Rochester, MN, American Academy of Sleep Medicine, 2002.

37. Terzano MG, Parrino L, Chervin R, et al: Atlas, rules and recording techniques for the scoring of the cyclical alternating pattern—CAP—in human sleep. Sleep Med 2:537–554, 2001.

38. International Organization of Societies for Electrophysiological Technology: Guidelines for digital EEG. Am J Electroneurodiag Technol 39(4):278–288, 1999.

39. Douglas AB, Bornstein R, Nino-Murcia G, et al: Item test: reliability of the Sleep Disorders Questionnaire (SDQ). Sleep Res 19:215, 1990.

40. Johns MW: A new method for measuring daytime sleepiness: The Epworth Sleepiness Scale. Sleep 14(6):540–545, 1991.

41. Hoffstein V, Szalai JP: Predictive value of clinical features in diagnosing obstructive sleep apnea. Sleep 16(2):118–122, 1993.

42. Flemons WW, Whitelaw WA, Brant R, Remmers JE: Likelihood ratios for a sleep apnea clinical prediction rule. Am J Resp Crit Care Med 150:1279–1285, 1994.

43. Maislin G, Pack AI, Kribbs NB, et al: A survey screen for prediction of apnea. Sleep 8(3):158–166, 1995.

44. Alexander M, Ogilvie R, Simons I, et al: Predictive value of subsets of independent variables in the diagnosis of obstructive sleep apnea. Sleep Res 25:183, 1996.

45. Chervin RD, Hedger K, Dillon JE, Pituch KJ: Pediatric sleep questionnaire (PSQ): validity and reliability of scales for sleep-disordered breathing, snoring, sleepiness, and behavioral problems. Sleep Med 1:21–32, 2000.

46. Thorpy MJ: The clinical use of the multiple sleep latency test: the Standards of Practice Committee of the American Sleep Disorders Association. Sleep 15(3):268–276, 1992.

47. Hoddes E, Dement WC, Zarcone V: The development and use of the Stanford Sleepiness Scale (SSS). Psychophysiology 9:150, 1972.

48. Hoddes E, Zarcone V, Smythe H, et al: Quantification of sleepiness: a new approach. Psychophysiology 10:431–436, 1973.

49. Carskadon MA, Dement WC, Mitler MM, et al: Guidelines for the multiple sleep latency test (MSLT): a standard measure of sleepiness. Sleep 9(4):519–524, 1986.

50. Carskadon MA: Measuring daytime sleepiness. In Kryger MH, Roth T, Dement WC (eds): *Principles and Practice of Sleep Medicine*. Philadelphia, Saunders, 1989, pp 684–689.

51. Cooper R, Osselton JW, Shaw JC: *EEG Technology*, 2nd ed. London, Butterworths, 1974.

52. Tyner F, Knott JR, Mayer WB: *Fundamentals of EEG Technology, Volume 1: Basic Concepts and Methods*. New York, Raven Press, 1983.

53. Jasper HH: The ten/twenty electrode system of the International Federation. Electroencephalogr Clin Neurophysiol 10:371, 1958.

54. Walczak T, Chokroverty S. Electroenchephalography, electromyography, and electro-oculography: general principles and basic technology. In Chokroverty S (ed): *Sleep Disorders Medicine: Basic Science, Technical Considerations and Clinical Aspects*, 2nd ed. Boston, Butterworth-Heinemann, pp 151–169, 1999.

55. Cross C: Technical tips: patient specific electrode application techniques. Am J EEG Technol 32:86–92, 1992.

56. Mitler MM, Carskadon MA, Hirshkowitz M: Evaluating sleepiness. In Kryger MH, Roth T, Dement WC (eds): *Principles and Practice of Sleep Medicine*, 3rd ed. Philadelphia, Saunders, 2000, pp 1251–1257.

57. Coleman RM, Pollack C, Weitzman ED: Periodic movements in sleep (nocturnal myoclonus): relation to sleep-wake disorders. Ann Neurol 8:416–421, 1980.

58. Schenk CH, Bundlie SR, Ettinger MG, Mahowald MW: Chronic behavioral disorders of human REM sleep: a new category of parasomnia. Sleep 9:293–308, 1986.

59. German W, Vaughn BV: Techniques for monitoring intrathoracic pressure during overnight polysomnography. Am J End Technol 36:197–208, 1996.

60. Orr WC, Bollinger C, Stahl M: Measurement of gastroesophageal reflux during sleep by esophageal pH monitoring. In Guilleminault C (ed): *Sleeping and Waking Disorders: Indications and Techniques*. Menlo Park, NJ, Addison-Wesley, 1982, pp 331–343.

61. Bonnet M, Carley D, Carskadon M, et al: Recording and scoring leg movements (ASDA—The Atlas Task Force). Sleep 16(8):748–759, 1993.

62. American Electroencephalography Society: *Guidelines for Recording Clinical EEG on Digital Media*. Bloomsfield, CT, American EEG Society, 1991.

63. Butkov N: *Atlas of Clinical Polysomnography*. Medford, OR, Synapse Media, 1996.

64. Phillipson EA: Sleep apnea: a major public health problem. N Engl J Med 328(17):1271–1273, 1993.

65. Young T, Evans L, Finn L, Palta M: Estimation of the clinically diagnosed proportion of sleep apnea syndrome in middle-aged men and women. Sleep 20(9):705–706, 1997.

66. Young T, Palta M, Dempsey J, et al: The occurrence of sleep-disordered breathing among middle-aged adults. N Engl J Med 328(17):1230–1235, 1993.

67. American Sleep Disorders Association: Practice parameters for using polysomnography to evaluate insomnia: an update. An American Academy of Sleep Medicine Report, Standards Practice Committee of the American Academy of Sleep Medicine. Sleep 26(6):754–757, 2003.

68. American Thoracic Society: Cardiorespiratory sleep studies in children: establishment of normative data and polysomnographic predictors of morbidity. Am J Respir Crit Care Med 160:1381–1387, 1999.

Template for 24-Hour Sleep/Wake Log

This log should be completed by the patient for a period of 2 weeks before the study.

Date			Date			Date		
Time	Awake	Asleep	Time	Awake	Asleep	Time	Awake	Asleep
12:00			12:00			12:00		
13:00			13:00			13:00		
14:00			14:00			14:00		
15:00			15:00			15:00		
16:00			16:00			16:00		
17:00			17:00			17:00		
18:00			18:00			18:00		
19:00			19:00			19:00		
20:00			20:00			20:00		
21:00			21:00			21:00		
22:00			22:00			22:00		
23:00			23:00			23:00		
24:00			24:00			24:00		
01:00			01:00			01:00		
02:00			02:00			02:00		
03:00			03:00			03:00		
04:00			04:00			04:00		
05:00			05:00			05:00		
06:00			06:00			06:00		
07:00			07:00			07:00		
08:00			08:00			08:00		
09:00			09:00			09:00		
10:00			10:00			10:00		
11:00			11:00			11:00		
Exercise			Exercise			Exercise		
Treatment			Treatment			Treatment		
Sleep quality			Sleep quality			Sleep quality		
Medications			Medications			Medications		
Comments			Comments			Comments		

For each hour of the day:

- Indicate sleep or wake time with an (X) in the appropriate box(es).
- Indicate naps with an (N) in the appropriate box(es).
- Indicate periods of extreme sleepiness with an (S) in the appropriate box(es).

Subjective Evaluation of Sleepiness

STANFORD SLEEPINESS SCALE (16)

(1) Feeling active and vital; alert; wide awake.
(2) Functioning at a high level, but not at peak; able to concentrate.
(3) Relaxed; awake; not at full alertness; responsive.
(4) A little foggy; not at peak; let down.
(5) Fogginess; beginning to lose interest in remaining awake; slowed down.
(6) Sleepiness; prefer to be lying down; fighting sleep; woozy.
(7) Almost in reverie; sleep onset soon; lost struggle to remain awake.

LINEAR ANALOG SCALE

Ask patient to make a mark on the scale that corresponds with their state before testing.

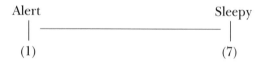

Alert   Sleepy

(1)   (7)

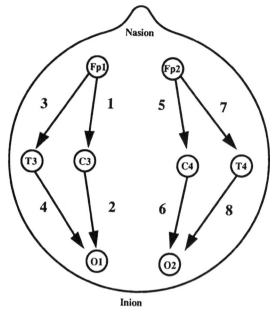

FIGURE 9-A2 ■ Suggested montage to be used to screen for possible seizure activity during sleep. Use of wide interelectrode distance affords for a global view of EEG activity and conserves the channels. To more adequately localize epileptogenic activity, a full complement of electrodes should be used. For a more comprehensive review of montages, the reader is referred to *Standard EEG Montages* as proposed by American EEG Society Guidelines 1980, No. 7, Grass Instruments.

Suggested Montages for Recording Sleep-Related Seizure Activity

Suggested montage for recording sleep-related seizure activity for a 12-channel study

(1) Fp1–C3
(2) C3–O1
(3) Fp1–T3
(4) T3–O1
(5) Fp2–C4
(6) C4–O2
(7) Fp2–T4
(8) T4–O2

(9) EMG–submentalis–mentalis
(10) Right outer canthus–left outer canthus
(11) Nasal/oral airflow
(12) ECG

Suggested montage for recording sleep-related seizure activity for a 21-channel study:

(1) Fp1–F3
(2) F3–C3
(3) C3–P3

(4) P3–O1
(5) Fp2–F4
(6) F4–C4
(7) C4–P4
(8) P4–O2
(9) Fp1–F7
(10) F7–T3
(11) T3–T5
(12) T5–O1
(13) Fp2–F8
(14) F8–T4
(15) T4–T6
(16) T6–O2
(17) EMG–submentalis–mentalis
(18) Right outer canthus/A1
(19) Left outer canthus/A2
(20) Nasal/oral airflow
(21) ECG

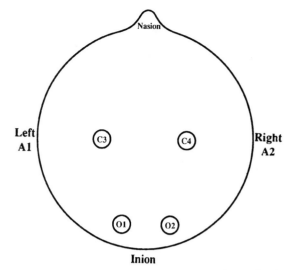

FIGURE 9-A3 ■ The International 10–20 EEG electrode placement for sleep recordings are shown.

Measuring the Head for C3, C4, O1, and O2

Before measuring the head, it is helpful to make an initial mark at the inion, the nasion, and the two preauricular points.

(1) Measure the distance from the nasion to inion along the midline through the vertex. Make a preliminary mark at the midpoint (Cz). An electrode will not be placed on this spot, but it will be used as a landmark.

(2) Center this point in the transverse plane by marking the halfway point between the left and right preauricular points. The intersection of marks from steps 1 and 2 give the precise location of Cz.

(3) Reposition the measuring tape at the midline through Cz and mark the points 10% up from the inion (0z) and nasion (Fpz).

(4) Reposition the measuring tape in the transverse plane, through Cz, and mark 10% (T3) and 30% (C3) up from the left preauricular point and 10% (T4) and 30% (C4) up from the right preauricular point.

(5) Position the tape around the head through Fpz, T3, Oz, and T4. Ten percent of this circumference distance is the distance between Fp1 and Fp2 and between O1 and O2. Mark these four locations on either side of the midline.

(6) The second marks for O1 and O2 are made by continuing the horizontal mark for Oz. Do this by holding the tape at T3 and T4 through Oz, and extend the horizontal mark to intersect the previous O1 and O2 marks.

(7) To establish the final mark for C3, place the tape from O1 to Fp1 and make a mark at the midpoint of this line. When extended, this mark will intersect the previous C3 mark. Repeat on the right side for C4.

Overview of the Clinical Use of the Multiple Sleep Latency Test (MSLT) and Maintenance of Wakefulness Test (MWT)

The MSLT and the MWT are laboratory-based clinical tools that allow for the characterization of excessive sleepiness (MSLT) and the assessment of the ability to stay awake (MWT). Both tests require integration of a thorough history and clinical judgment for proper assessment. Both tests suffer from the lack of large, multicenter, systematically collected repository of normative data across all age groups. The following is an overview of the indications and protocols for both tests.

MULTIPLE SLEEP LATENCY TEST

The MSLT provides an objective measure of sleepiness and is thought to measure the physiologic tendency to fall asleep in the absence of alerting factors. The expression of physiologic sleep tendency is demonstrated in the speed of falling asleep given appropriate conditions and instructions. The score for the test is the mean value of individual scores collected throughout the individual's habitual time of being awake.

The *MSLT is indicated* in suspected narcolepsy and to support a diagnosis of idiopathic hypersomnia.

The *MSLT is not routinely indicated* in initial evaluation of obstructive sleep apnea syndrome (OSAS), the assessment of treatment with continuous positive airway pressure (CPAP), or the evaluation of sleepiness in medical and neurological disorders (other than narcolepsy), insomnia, or circadian rhythm disorders.

The *MSLT protocol* consists of a series of four or five naps (or opportunities to fall asleep) at 2-hour intervals. The first nap is given 1.5 to 3 hours after final wake from a required polysomnogram (PSG). Each nap consists of a 20-minute opportunity to fall asleep. Each nap is ended after 20 minutes if no sleep occurs, or 15 minutes after sleep onset. MSLT *sleep onset* is defined as the first epoch of greater than 15 seconds of cumulative sleep in a 30-second epoch.

The *instructions* given to the patient before the test are: "Please lie quietly, assume a comfortable position, keep your eyes closed, and try to fall asleep."

The conventional *recording montage for the MSLT* includes central (C3-A2, C4-A1) and occipital (01-A2, 02-A1) electroencephalogram (EEG) derivations, left and right eye electrooculograms (EOG), mental/submental electromyogram (EMG), and electrocardiogram (ECG).

Most patients with narcolepsy have objective evidence of sleepiness associated with a mean sleep latency of 3.1 minutes (Table 9-A5). The presence of two or more sleep-onset REM periods (SOREMPs), defined as REM sleep at any time during the nap, was associated with a sensitivity of 0.78 and a specificity of 0.93. It is noted that other reasons for REM to appear (such as sleep deprivation, sleep fragmentation, medications, timing of the nap) should be considered before final diagnosis.

The reader should be aware that in the International Classification of Sleep Disorders (ICSD)[1] published by the American Academy of Sleep Medicine (AASM) in 2005, a mean sleep latency of less than 8 minutes on the MSLT is used to define *sleepiness* for diagnostic purposes. This value has been shown to be the best cut-off in the context of diagnosing narcolepsy, with approximately 90% of narcoleptic patients having a latency below this level.

MAINTENANCE OF WAKEFULNESS TEST

The MWT measures the ability to stay awake under nonstimulating conditions. The MWT is used primarily to assess effectiveness of treatment of a sleep disorder, particularly in situations of patient or public safety.

TABLE 9-A5 ■ Normative Values for MSLT and MWT

MSLT	"Normal/Control Values" Mean sleep latency ± SD (min)
4-nap protocol	10.4 ± 4.3
5-nap protocol	11.6 ± 5.2
(Patients with narcolepsy)	*(3.1 ± 2.9)*
MWT	
40-min protocol (latency to first epoch of sleep)	30.4 ± 11.20

Table 9-A5 summarizes normative data for the MSLT (4 and 5 naps) with a comparison to a group of patients with narcolepsy and MWT (40 minute). Establishing normative values for both the MSLT and MWT has been complicated and challenging. Studies reporting normative data frequently lack information regarding prior sleep time and sleep quality, operational definitions for sleep onset, nap termination, number of naps, and whether caffeine was allowed. In addition, although there has been standardization of the clinical protocol for the MSLT, at least four different protocols have been used for the MWT. These data represent the current evidence available and may only approximate data from large, well-controlled studies across all age groups. The data reported here are for ages 10 and older.

Data from American Academy of Sleep Medicine Standards of Practice Committee. Practice parameters for clinical use of the multiple sleep latency test and the maintenance of wakefulness test. Sleep 28(1):113–121, 2005.

The *MWT may be indicated* in the assessment of sleepiness that constitutes a safety issue, or in patients with narcolepsy or idiopathic hypersomnia to assess response to treatment.

For the *MWT protocol*, the use of MWT 40 (40-minute protocol) is recommended. MWT *sleep onset* is defined as the first epoch of greater than 15 seconds of cumulative sleep in a 30-second epoch. The trial is terminated after 40 minutes (if no sleep occurs), or after unequivocal sleep onset (3 continuous epochs of stage 1, or 1 epoch of any other stage of sleep).

The MWT protocol consists of four trials at 2-hour intervals. Unlike the MSLT, prior PSG is not required. The first test is performed at 1.5 to 3 hours after final wake.

The *instructions* given to the patient before the test are: "Please sit still and remain awake for as long as possible. Look directly ahead of you, and do not look directly at the light."

The conventional *recording montage for the MWT* includes central EEG (C3-A2, C4-A1) and occipital EEG (01-A2, 02-A1) derivations, left and right EOGs, mental/submental EMG, and ECG.

A mean sleep latency (arithmetic mean of 4 trials) (40-minute MWT) of less than 8 minutes is considered abnormal.

OTHER CONSIDERATIONS

Sleep logs may be used 1 week before the MSLT. No consensus has been reached for use of sleep logs with the MWT. Clinical judgment is recommended.

Room conditions for the MSLT should be dark and quiet, at a temperature comfortable for patients in bed ready for sleep. For the *MWT*, the room should be insulated from external light with the use of a 7.5-W night light for illumination. The patient should be seated in bed with the back and head supported. Room temperature should be determined by patient comfort.

Before each nap (MSLT) or trial (MWT), the patient should be instructed to use the restroom and asked about any other adjustments needed for comfort. Each recording should begin with biocalibrations (eyes open [30 sec], eyes closed [30 sec], look right and left, blink, grit teeth).

Regarding the *use of drugs and drug screens*, for the MSLT, the use of stimulants and REM-suppressing medications should be stopped 2 weeks before testing. The timing and administration of other medications should be considered to minimize any stimulating or sedating effect. Smoking should be stopped 30 minutes before the MSLT, and the patient must abstain from caffeine.

For the MWT, the use of tobacco, caffeine, and other medications by the patient before and during the MWT should be addressed and determined by the clinician.

Drug screening may be indicated during the MSLT or MWT. Timing and circumstance of drug screens are left to clinical judgment.

FINAL NOTES

The MSLT and MWT are useful clinical tools to generate objective data with regard to a patient's level of sleepiness (MSLT) or ability to stay awake (MWT). The recent Practice Parameters (Sleep 28[1], 2005) published by the AASM provide guidelines on appropriate clinical use of the MSLT and MWT and replace those published in 1992. These practice parameters were based on a rigorous review of the scientific literature. In cases where data were insufficient or inconclusive, however, expert opinion was used to support recommendation.

Both MSLT and MWT remain challenged by a lack of normative data across all age groups and across different patient groups. In addition, research is needed to correlate these objective measures of sleepiness and alertness with "real-life" circumstance.

(Primary Reference: American Academy of Sleep Medicine Standards of Practice Committee: Practice parameters for clinical use of the Multiple Sleep Latency Test and the Maintenance of Wakefulness Test. Sleep 28[1]:113–121, 2005.)

BIBLIOGRAPHY

1. American Academy of Sleep Medicine Standards of Practice Committee: Practice parameters for clinical use of the multiple sleep latency test and the maintenance of wakefulness test. Sleep 28(1):113–121, 2005.
2. Arand D, Bonnet M, Hurwitz T, et al: The clinical use of the MSLT and MWT. Sleep 28(1):123–144, 2005.
3. Carskadon MA, Dement WC, Mitler MM, et al: Association of Sleep Disorders Task Force on Daytime Sleepiness: Guidelines for the multiple sleep latency test (MSLT): a standard measure of sleepiness. Sleep 9(4):519–524, 1986.
4. Doghramji K, Mitler MM, Sangal RB, et al: A normative study of the maintenance of wakefulness test (MWT). Electroencephalogr Clin Neurophysiol 103(5):554–562, 1997.
5. Kryger MH, Roth T, Dement WC (eds): *Principles and Practice of Sleep Medicine*, 3rd ed. Philadelphia, Saunders, 2000.
6. Mitler MM, Gujavarty KS, Sampson MG, Browman CP: Multiple daytime nap approaches to evaluating the sleepy patient. Sleep 5:S119–S127, 1982.

Effects of Drugs on Sleep

PAULA K. SCHWEITZER

Disturbed sleep or impaired waking function may be a consequence of disease and/or the medications used to treat disease. Insomnia and sedation are commonly listed side effects of numerous drugs. Sedating drugs may improve sleep but can impair waking function if the sedating action carries over into waking hours or if the drugs are administered during waking hours. Conversely, drugs that disrupt sleep can lead to impaired waking function, while drugs that help promote alertness can negatively affect sleep. In addition, a number of drugs affect the architecture of sleep as evidenced by changes in the durations of various sleep stages or the frequency of stage transitions. This chapter briefly reviews effects of drugs on sleep and waking function. When available, polysomnographic (PSG) data are presented. Drugs that affect PSG-recorded total sleep time (TST), total wake time (TWT), wake after sleep onset (WASO), or number of awakenings are said to affect measures of sleep continuity. Thus improved sleep continuity would be reflected in increased TST and decreased TWT, WASO, and number of awakenings, and vice versa. The significance of drug effects on rapid eye movement (REM) sleep and slow wave sleep (SWS) is unclear, as the precise functions of these sleep stages are unknown. Increases in REM or rebound of REM after discontinuation of a drug that suppresses REM, however, can be associated with nightmares or vivid dreaming that may be bothersome to the patient. PSG data from well-designed and placebo-controlled studies exist for most drugs that have been evaluated as hypnotics, although data on long-term use are limited. For many other drugs with purported effects on sleep or waking function, conclusions regarding both PSG findings and subjective effects may be limited by a number of factors, including the population studied, lack of placebo control, dosage and duration of drug use, concomitant medications, and the disease process. Caution must also be used in interpreting what is meant when we say a drug is sedating or is associated with insomnia or nightmares. For example, although drugs such as hypnotics are clearly sedating for most individuals, other drugs that list sedation as a side effect may affect relatively few or many individuals and may vary in the degree of sedation caused.

Pharmacokinetic properties involved in drug-induced sleep-wake alterations include lipid solubility (which determines the degree of central nervous system [CNS] penetration), the receptor-binding profile, presence or absence of active metabolites, drug half-life, interactions with other drugs, and withdrawal effects. Many drugs that affect the CNS are hepatically metabolized by enzymes of the cytochrome P-450 (CYP) system; thus drug-drug interactions can occur that can enhance or reduce a drug's clinical effect. Sedation may be associated with a variety of pharmacological actions including activity at the gamma-aminobutyric acid (GABA) receptor, blockade of central histamine type 1 (H_1) receptors, antagonism at type 1 alpha-adrenergic (alpha$_1$) receptors, and antagonism of muscarinic cholinergic receptors.[1] Receptor mechanisms associated with sleep disruption are not fully understood but include stimulation of serotonin type 2-B (5-HT$_{2B}$) receptors and inhibition of dopamine reuptake.[2] The pharmacological mechanism for drug-induced nightmares is unknown; however, nightmares or dream alteration are most likely to occur with drugs that affect dopamine, norepinephrine, and serotonin but may also occur with drugs that affect acetylcholine or histamine and on withdrawal of drugs that affect GABA.[3,4] Other neurotransmitters involved with REM sleep regulation may also be important, but these effects are not well studied. Assessment of causality with nightmares is difficult, as nightmares cannot be directly measured and occur commonly in the healthy population. Table 10-1 summarizes mechanism of action, other receptor effects, effects on sleep architecture, and subjective effects for drugs reviewed in this chapter. Table 10-2 lists drugs associated with nightmares. More detailed information and additional references can be found in a number of review articles.[5–12] Drug metabolism is not discussed in this chapter, but the reader should be aware that clinically important drug interactions can occur when drugs metabolized by the CYP system are co-administered.

TABLE 10-1 ■ Effects of Drugs on Sleep and Wake

Drug Class/Drug	Mechanism of Action and Other Receptor Pharmacology	Sleep Latency	Sleep Continuity[1]	SWS	REM[2]	Subjective	Comments
ALCOHOL							
acute ingestion	Multiple receptor effects including GABA$_A$ agonism	↓	↑	↑	↓	Sedating	Impairs performance
withdrawal			↓	↓	↑	Fragments sleep; nightmares	
ANTIEPILEPTICS							
Established drugs							
Barbiturates (e.g., phenobarbital)	GABA agonism via increased duration of chloride channel opening, enzyme induction	↓	↑	↑↓	↓	Sedating; Very sedating	Most impair performance; High doses have direct action on chloride channel; ↑ spindle density; ↑ Spindle density
Benzodiazepines (e.g., diazepam, clonazepam)	GABA$_A$ agonism	↓	↑	↓	↓	Sedating	
Carbamazepine	NE agonism, partial adenosine agonism, enzyme induction	↓	↑	↓	↓	Sedating	↓ MSLT latency
Ethosuximide	Selective reduction of T-type calcium channel currents		↓	↓	↑↓; ↑	May be less sedating than other drugs	
Phenytoin	Decreased sodium flux, enzyme induction	↓	↓?	↑	↓	Sedating	
Valproic acid	GABA potentiation		?↑			May be less sedating than other drugs	
Newer drugs							
Felbamate	Unknown, glycine blockade, GABA potentiation					Sedating; Fatigue, insomnia	Interactions with other anticonvulsants, theophylline, warfarin
Gabapentin	Unknown, GABA potentiation	↑↓	↓	↑	↑↓	Mildly sedating	
Lamotrigine	Unknown, sodium channel inhibition			↑↓; ↓	↑↓	Rarely sedating in usual doses	Less likely to impair performance
Levetiracetam	Unknown, no affinity for GABA	↑↓	↓	↑↓	↓	Mildly sedating	No change in MSLT latency
Tiagabine	GABA reuptake inhibition	↑↓; ↓	↓	↓	↑↓	Sedating	
Topiramate	Unknown, excitatory amino acid receptor blockade, GABA potentiation			↑		Sedating	
Vigabatrin	Unknown, GABA reuptake inhibition	↑↓	↑↓	↑↓	↑↓	Mildly to moderately sedating	
Zonisamide	Unknown, sodium & calcium channel inhibition					Mildly sedating	

Drug	Mechanism of action	Sleep effects	Sedation	Comments
ANTIHISTAMINES				
First-generation H₁ antagonists	H_1 antagonism, significant CNS penetration; also cholinergic, adrenergic, & 5-HT antagonism		*Sedating*	*↓ MSLT latency, impair performance; Possible tolerance to sedation*
Diphenhydramine	H_1, cholinergic, adrenergic, 5-HT antagonism	↕ → ↕ ↑ ↕ →	Sedating	Primary ingredient in most OTC sleep aids
Doxylamine	H_1, cholinergic, adrenergic, 5-HT antagonism	↕ → ↕ ↑ ↕ →	Sedating	
Chlorpheniramine	H_1, cholinergic, adrenergic, 5-HT antagonism	↕ → ↕ ↑ ↕ →	Sedating	? Less sedating than others in this class
Hydroxyzine	H_1, cholinergic, adrenergic, 5-HT antagonism	↕ → ↕ ↑ ↕ →	Sedating	
Cyproheptadine	H_1, cholinergic, adrenergic, 5-HT antagonism		Sedating	
Second-generation H₁ antagonists	H_1 antagonism but little CNS penetration		*Nonsedating*	*No performance impairment*
Cetirizine	H_1 antagonism		Nonsedating	Nonsedating per MSLT; ? sedating in high doses
Loratadine	H_1 antagonism		Nonsedating	Nonsedating per MSLT
Terfenadine	H_1 antagonism		Nonsedating	Nonsedating per MSLT
H₂ antagonists	H_2 antagonism	↕ ↕ ↕ ↕		
Cimetidine	H_2 antagonism	↕ ↕ ↕ ↑?	Nonsedating	
Ranitidine	H_2 antagonism	↕ ↕ ↕	Nonsedating	
Famotidine	H_2 antagonism	↓? ↕ ↓	Nonsedating	
ANTIPARKINSONIAN DRUGS				
Levodopa	Precursor of DA & NE	↕ → ↕ ↑ ↕ ↓	Improved sleep at low doses; insomnia, nightmares at higher doses	↑ REM density at high doses; ↑ spindles; cognitive impairment
Bromocriptine	D_2 agonism; D_1 antagonism; ergot-derived	→	Sedating	
Pergolide	D_1 & D_2 agonism; ergot-derived	→ ←	Sedating	Decreases periodic limb movements
Pramipexole	DA agonism; ergot-derived	← →	Sedating; vivid dreams	Decreases periodic limb movements
Ropinirole	D_2 & D_3 agonism; non-ergot derived	→ ↕ ↕	Sedating	Decreases periodic limb movements

Continued

TABLE 10-1 ■ Effects of Drugs on Sleep and Wake—cont'd

Drug Class/Drug	Mechanism of Action and Other Receptor Pharmacology	Sleep Latency	Sleep Continuity[1]	SWS	REM[2]	Subjective	Comments
Selegiline	Selective MAO-B inhibition, partial metabolism to amphetamine		↓		↓	Insomnia	↓ SL in patient population
Amantadine	DA reuptake inhibition					Insomnia	Also used as an antiviral agent
Benztropine	Cholinergic & H₁ antagonism		↑↓	↑↓	↓		Cognitive impairment
Hyoscyamine	Cholinergic antagonism		↑↓	↑↓	↓		Cognitive impairment
CARDIOVASCULAR DRUGS							
Beta antagonists (listed from low to high lipid solubility)	*Beta adrenergic receptor blockade*						
Sotalol	Nonselective beta blockade						Insomnia less likely
Atenolol	Nonselective beta blockade						Insomnia less likely
Carvedilol	& High affinity for 5-HT receptors, alpha₁ blockade		↑↓			Fatigue, insomnia	
Nadolol	& High affinity for 5-HT receptors						
Bisoprolol	Selective for beta₁ receptors						
Metoprolol	Selective for beta₁ receptors		→		→	Fatigue, insomnia, nightmares	
Acebutolol	Selective for beta₁ receptors						
Pindolol	& High affinity for 5-HT receptors		→		→	Fatigue, insomnia, nightmares	
Timolol	& High affinity for 5-HT receptors						
Propranolol	& High affinity for 5-HT receptors		→		→	Fatigue, insomnia, nightmares	More disruptive of sleep than other beta blockers
Alpha₁ antagonists							
Prazosin	Alpha-adrenergic antagonism					Transient sedation	Used to treat nightmares in PTSD
Terazosin	Alpha-adrenergic antagonism					Transient sedation	

Drug	Mechanism					Sedation/effects	Comments
Alpha₂ agonists							
Clonidine	Alpha₂ agonism	↕	↑	↑	↓	Sedation, nightmares, insomnia	
Methyldopa	Alpha₂ agonism, NE depletion	↑	↔	↑	?	Sedation, nightmares	
ACE inhibitors (e.g., enalapril)	Angiotensin converting enzyme inhibition	↕	↕	↕	↕	Insomnia, nightmares	? OSA ↑
Other							
Reserpine	Catecholamine & serotonin depletion	↓	↓	↑	↓	Sedation, nightmares	
Hypolipidemic drugs	***HMG-CoA reductase inhibition***						
Atorvastatin		↕	↕			Insomnia?	
Lovastatin		↕	↕			Insomnia?	
Simvastatin						Insomnia?	
HYPNOTICS							
Benzodiazepines	***GABA_A agonism (nonselective binding)***					*Sedating*	*May ↑ spindles*
Estazolam	GABA_A agonism	→	←		→		
Flurazepam	GABA_A agonism	→	←		→		Carryover sedation most likely with flurazepam
Quazepam	GABA_A agonism	→	←		→		
Temazepam	GABA_A agonism	→	←	←	→		
Triazolam	GABA_A agonism	→	←	←	→		No residual sedation
Non-benzodiazepines	***GABA_A agonism***					*Sedating*	
Eszopiclone	GABA_A agonism (non-selective)	→	←	↕	↕		No residual sedation
Zaleplon	Selective binding to alpha₁ subunit of GABA_A receptor	→	←	↕	↑		No residual sedation
Zolpidem	Selective binding to alpha₁ subunit of GABA_A receptor	→	←	↓	→		No residual sedation
Indiplon	Selective binding to alpha₁ subunit of GABA_A receptor	→	↕	↕			Under development
Gaboxadol	Selective extrasynaptic GABA_A agonism	→	←	↕	↕		Under development
Other							
Ramelteon	Melatonin receptor agonism	→	↕	↕	↕	Nonsedating	Advances phase of circadian sleep-wake rhythm
PSYCHOTHERAPEUTIC DRUGS							
ANTIDEPRESSANTS							
Tricyclics	5-HT and NE reuptake inhibition; strong alpha₁, M₁, & H₁ antagonism	→	←	↕	↓	*Tertiary more sedating than secondary; may increase PLMs*	*↑ SWS during the first NREM period but not overall; may impair performance*

Continued

TABLE 10-1 ■ Effects of Drugs on Sleep and Wake—cont'd

Drug Class/Drug	Mechanism of Action and Other Receptor Pharmacology	Effects on Sleep Architecture				Subjective	Comments
		Sleep Latency	Sleep Continuity[1]	SWS	REM[2]		
Amitriptyline	5-HT reuptake inhibition > NE reuptake inhibition	→	←	↕	→	Very sedating	↑ REM density
Imipramine	5-HT reuptake inhibition > NE reuptake inhibition	→	←	↕	→	Very sedating	
Clomipramine	5-HT reuptake inhibition > NE reuptake inhibition	→	←	↕	↓↑	Not as sedating as other tertiary amines	↑ Eye movements in NREM
Trimipramine	No NE reuptake inhibition	→→	←←	↕↕	↕→	Sedating	Variable effects on REM
Doxepin	5-HT reuptake inhibition > NE reuptake inhibition					Sedating	↑ REM density
Desipramine	NE reuptake inhibition > 5-HT reuptake inhibition, no alpha$_2$ blockade	↕			→	Less sedating than tertiary amines	
Nortriptyline	NE reuptake inhibition > 5-HT reuptake inhibition		↕		→	Less sedating than tertiary amines	
Protriptyline	NE reuptake inhibition > 5-HT reuptake inhibition	↕	↕			Less sedating than tertiary amines	
SSRIs	*Primarily 5-HT reuptake inhibition*					*Insomnia more likely than sedation*	*Sleep continuity may improve with long-term use*
Fluoxetine	& NE reuptake inhibition, direct stimulation of 5-HT$_{2C}$		→	→	→	Vivid dreams	
Paroxetine	& NE reuptake inhibition, M$_1$ antagonism	←	→		→		May be more sedating than other SSRIs
Sertraline	& DA reuptake inhibition, weak NE reuptake inhibition	←	→	→	→	Vivid dreams	
Fluvoxamine Citalopram Escitalopram	Exclusive 5-HT reuptake inhibition Exclusive 5-HT reuptake inhibition Exclusive 5-HT reuptake inhibition		→	→	→→	Vivid dreams	
SNRIs	*5-HT & NE reuptake inhibition*					*Insomnia more likely than sedation*	
Venlafaxine	& weak DA reuptake inhibition		→	→	→		? Improvement in performance
Duloxetine	& weak DA reuptake inhibition		→		→		
Other							
Bupropion	NE and DA reuptake inhibition				↑?	Insomnia, nightmares	Limited data, may ↓ PLMs

Drug	Action					Subjective effect	Comments
Trazodone	5-HT$_2$ and alpha$_1$ antagonism, H$_1$ antagonism, 5-HT reuptake inhibition	↓	↔↑	↑	↔	Very sedating	May impair performance
Nefazodone	5-HT$_2$ and alpha$_1$ antagonism, 5-HT reuptake inhibition		↑	↔	↔	Sedating	Less likely to impair performance
Mirtazapine	Alpha$_2$, 5-HT, H$_1$, & alpha$_1$ antagonism	↓	↑	↔	↔	Sedating	
Phenelzine	Inhibition of MAO-A and MAO-B enzymes, thereby increasing NE, 5-HT, DA		↓		↓↓	Insomnia	
Tranylcypromine	Inhibition of MAO-A and MAO-B enzymes, thereby increasing NE, 5-HT, DA		↓		↓↓	Insomnia	
Moclobemide	Selective inhibition of MAO-A, reversible		↓		↔	Rare insomnia	Minimal effect on sleep; not available in United States
Selegiline transdermal	Selective inhibition of MAO-B		↑	↑←	↔↓	Little data	Nonselective at higher doses
Lithium	Unknown; 5-HT potentiation, 5-HT$_{1B}$ partial agonism		←	→	↔↑	Sedating	May impair performance
ANTIPSYCHOTICS *Traditional drugs*							*May impair performance*
Chlorpromazine	D$_2$, 5-HT$_2$, alpha$_1$, H$_1$, & cholinergic blockade		↓	↑	?	Moderately sedating	
Haloperidol	D$_2$, 5-HT$_2$, & alpha$_1$ blockade		←	←	?	Mildly sedating	
Thioridazine	D$_2$, 5-HT$_2$, alpha$_1$, D$_1$, H$_1$, cholinergic blockade		←	←	?	Very sedating	
Newer drugs Aripiprazole	D$_2$ and 5-HT$_{1A}$ partial agonism, 5-HT$_{2A}$ antagonism	↓	↓	↔→	↓?	Insomnia	Unlikely to impair performance
Clozapine	5-HT$_2$, alpha$_1$, H$_1$, cholinergic, D$_1$, D$_2$ blockade		↓	←	↓?	Markedly sedating	↑ REM density
Lamotrigine	Unknown; sodium channel inhibition, weak 5-HT$_3$ inhibition			←	↓?	Mildly sedating	Less likely to impair performance
Olanzapine	D$_2$, 5-HT$_{2A}$, M$_1$, H$_1$, alpha$_1$, D$_1$ antagonism	↔→	↓	↑	↔→	Markedly sedating	May impair performance

Continued

TABLE 10-1 ■ Effects of Drugs on Sleep and Wake—cont'd

Drug Class/Drug	Mechanism of Action and Other Receptor Pharmacology	Effects on Sleep Architecture				Subjective	Comments
		Sleep Latency	Sleep Continuity[1]	SWS	REM[2]		
Quetiapine	H₁, alpha₁, alpha₂, 5-HT₂ₐ, D₂ antagonism		↑	↔	→	Moderately sedating	May impair performance
Risperidone	D₂, 5-HT₂, alpha₁ blockade		↑	↑	→	Mildly sedating	
Sertindole	5-HT₂, alpha₁, D₂, blockade					Mildly sedating	Less sedating than others in this class
Ziprasidone	D₂, 5-HT₂, alpha₁, D₁ blockade					Mildly sedating	
ANXIOLYTICS							
Benzodiazepines	*GABAₐ agonism*						
Alprazolam	GABAₐ agonism	→	←	→	→	Sedating	
Lorazepam	GABAₐ agonism	→	←	→	→	Sedating	
Buspirone	5-HT₁ₐ partial agonism, D₂ antagonism	↔	↔	↔	↔	Nonsedating	No effect on MSLT
STIMULANTS							
Amphetamine, Methamphetamine	DA & NE (& 5-HT at higher doses) release & reuptake inhibition	←	→	↔	→	Increased alertness, insomnia	↑ MSLT latency
Methylphenidate	DA & NE release & reuptake inhibition	←	→	↔	→	Increased alertness, insomnia	↑ MSLT latency
Pemoline	Unknown	←	→			Mildly increased alertness	Withdrawn from market in 2005
Modafinil	Unknown		→			Increased alertness	↑ MSLT latency
Caffeine	Adenosine receptor antagonism	←	→			Increased alertness, insomnia	↑ MSLT latency
Theophylline	Adenosine receptor antagonism		→	↓		Insomnia	May improve sleep as asthma symptoms are treated
Nicotine	Cholinergic agonism	←	→		→	Insomnia	Insomnia on withdrawal
OTHER DRUGS							
Corticosteroids			→	↔	→	*Insomnia*	*Results inconsistent*

Drug	Mechanism					Effect / Comment
Dexamathesone						
Hydrocortisone						
Prednisone				→		Insomnia
NSAIDs	*Prostaglandin inhibition*					
Aspirin		→	↔			No effect
Acetaminophen						No effect
Ibuprofen		→	↔			No effect
Opioids						
Morphine	Opioid receptor stimulation	↔→	→	→	↓	Acutely sedating, insomnia with chronic use. Causes respiratory depression; impairs performance; tolerance may develop; withdrawal ↑ sleep disturbance
Tramadol	Opioid receptor stimulation; weak reuptake inhibition of NE & 5-HT		→	→	→	Sedating. Synthetic opioid
Other						
Atomoxetine	NE reuptake inhibition		→			Nonsedating
Chloral hydrate	Barbiturate-like effect on GABA		←	→	→	Sedating
Gamma-hydroxybutyrate (GHB)	Unknown; possibly a direct neurotransmitter, increases DA		←	→	→	Sedating
Pseudoephedrine			→			Insomnia
Phenylpropanolamine						Insomnia
Melatonin	Endogenous hormone		↔↑ ↔↓	↔↑ ↔↓	↔→ ↔↑	May affect circadian phase
Valerian	Unknown; may inhibit GABA, affect 5-HT, inhibit adenosine	↔→	↔↑ ↔↓		↔↑ ↔↓	Sedating

5-HT, 5-hydroxytryptamine (serotonin); D or DA, dopamine; NE, norepinephrine; NREM, non-REM; OTC, over-the-counter; PTSD, post-traumatic stress disorder; REM, rapid eye movement; SNRI, serotonin and norepinephrine reuptake inhibitor; SSRI, selective serotonin reuptake inhibitor; SWS, slow wave sleep; ↑, increase; ↓, decrease; ↔, no change.

[1] Sleep continuity refers to the proportion of sleep relative to wake, as reflected by sleep efficiency. Thus, ↑ indicates improvement in sleep continuity as would be reflected by increased sleep efficiency or decreased wake.

[2] Decreased REM is typically accompanied by increased REM latency, and vice versa.

TABLE 10-2 ■ Drugs Reported to Cause Vivid Dreams or Nightmares in Clinical Studies or Case Reports			
Drug Class	**Example**	**Possible Mechanism for Inducing Nightmares**	**Comments**
Alcohol		REM rebound	With acute use and withdrawal
Amphetamine		Norepinephrine, dopamine	With chronic use and withdrawal
Antibiotics/antivirals		Sleep-related immunologic response?	
	Erythromycin		
	Ciprofloxacin		
	Amantadine		
	Ganciclovir		
Antidepressants			
Tricyclics		Norepinephrine, serotonin	With use and withdrawal
	Amitriptyline		
	Clomipramine		
	Desipramine		
	Doxepin		
	Imipramine		
	Nortriptyline		
SSRIs		Serotonin	Suppress dream recall frequency but increase dream intensity and bizarreness
	Escitalopram		
	Fluoxetine		
	Fluvoxamine		
	paroxetine		
	Fluvoxamine		
	Paroxetine		Nightmares possibly more common than with other SSRIs
	Sertraline		
Other			
	Bupropion	Dopamine	Nightmares more common than with other antidepressants
	Nefazodone	Serotonin	
	Venlafaxine	Norepinephrine, serotonin	
Antiepileptics	Gabapentin	GABA	
	Ethosuximide		
	Lamotrigine		
	Tiagabine	GABA	
	Valproic acid	GABA	
	Zonisamide		
Antipsychotics		Unknown	
	Chlorpromazine		
	Clozapine		
	Risperidone		
	Thioridazine		
	Thiothixene		
Barbiturates		REM rebound	Upon withdrawal
Benzodiazepines	Triazolam	GABA, REM rebound	
Cardiovascular drugs			
ACE inhibitors		Norepinephrine?	
	Captopril		
	Enalapril		
	Losartan		
	Quinapril		
Beta antagonists		Norepinephrine	Nightmares common in this class of drugs
	Atenolol		
	Labetalol		
	Metoprolol		
	Propranolol		
Other			
	Clonidine	Norepinephrine	
	Methyldopa	Norepinephrine	
	Digoxin	Unknown	

Continued

TABLE 10-2 ■ Drugs Reported to Cause Vivid Dreams or Nightmares in Clinical Studies or Case Reports—cont'd

Drug Class	Example	Possible Mechanism for Inducing Nightmares	Comments
Cholinergic agonists		Acetylcholine	
	Rivastigmine		
	Tacrine		
Dopamine agonists		Dopamine	With chronic use
	Amantadine		
	Levodopa		
	Ropinirole		
	Selegiline		
Other			
	GHB	GABA	
	Chlorpheniramine	Histamine?	
	Naproxen	Unknown	
	Tramadol	Unknown	
	Zopiclone	GABA	

GABA, Gamma aminobutyric acid; REM, rapid eye movement; SSRI, selective serotonin reuptake inhibitor.

ALCOHOL

Alcohol is commonly used as a sleep aid in the general population. In nonalcoholics, when ingested acutely, alcohol decreases sleep latency (SL) and REM while increasing TST and SWS during the first part of the night.[13] Because alcohol is relatively rapidly metabolized, however, withdrawal occurs during the latter portion of the night, leading to increased sleep fragmentation, increased REM, and decreased SWS. With continued use, tolerance to these effects develops in as little as 3 nights. In alcoholics during periods of heavy drinking, TST and REM are decreased, and sleep is highly fragmented, especially during the second half of the night. Acute withdrawal of alcohol in alcoholics results in increased wake, increased REM, and decreased SWS, which may return to baseline levels over time. Alcohol may be initially stimulating at low to moderate doses as alcohol concentration increases, but it is sedating at higher doses and as alcohol concentration plateaus and decreases. Thus daytime sleepiness as measured by the multiple sleep latency test (MSLT) is increased. This sleepiness is potentiated by prior sleep loss and use of sedating drugs such as benzodiazepines.

ANTIEPILEPTIC DRUGS

Established antiepileptic drugs include barbiturates (e.g., phenobarbital), benzodiazepines (e.g., clonazepam, diazepam), carbamazepine, ethosuximide, phenytoin, primidone, and valproic acid. Most of these drugs are GABA$_A$ agonists. All of these medications cause sedation both subjectively and objectively, as well as performance impairment. PSG data generally show decreased SL, increased sleep continuity, and decreased REM.[12,14] Barbiturates are similar to the benzodiazepines in that they have anticonvulsant, anxiolytic, myorelaxant, and hypnotic properties. They are rarely used as hypnotics because of their greater toxicity and liability for dependence and abuse compared with the other drugs now available for treatment of insomnia. Barbiturates increase GABA transmission by increasing the duration of the opening of the chloride ion channel and, in high doses, have a direct effect on the chloride channel even if GABA is not present. Clonazepam is similar to other benzodiazepines, causing decreased SL, REM, and SWS and increased sleep continuity. Both barbiturates and benzodiazepines can increase sleep spindle density. Carbamazepine and phenytoin may increase SWS, whereas ethosuximide appears to decrease SWS. Valproic acid does not appear to affect sleep architecture.[12]

The newer antiepileptic drugs (felbamate, gabapentin, lamotrigine, levetiracetam, tiagabine, topiramate, vigabatrin, and zonisamide) have multiple mechanisms of action that have led to their evaluation and use in other neurological and psychiatric conditions and in insomnia. Most of these drugs are sedating but not to the degree seen in the older antiepileptic drugs.[15,16] Exceptions may be gabapentin and tiagabine, which have been used as hypnotics. Both drugs increase TST and SWS; gabapentin may also increase REM.[8,12] Gabapentin has also been used to treat chronic pain and restless legs syndrome. Lamotrigine may increase REM.[12]

ANTIHISTAMINES

The first-generation H$_1$ antagonists (diphenhydramine, doxylamine, chlorpheniramine, hydroxyzine, meclizine, promethazine, cyproheptadine) are lipophilic and easily penetrate the CNS. These drugs also have antagonistic action at cholinergic, adrenergic, and serotonergic receptors. They cause sedation, decreased alertness, and decrements in performance as measured both subjectively and objectively.[5] Sedation may lessen with chronic use, however. Because of their sedating effects, these drugs (in particular, diphenhydramine and doxylamine) are widely used as over-the-counter hypnotics. Subjectively, these drugs decrease sleep latency and increase sleep continuity. Limited PSG data indicate that SL and TST may be unaffected or slightly improved and that REM is decreased. MSLT latency is decreased with acute administration.

The second-generation H_1 antihistamines (cetirizine, loratadine, terfenadine) are hydrophilic and have few CNS effects. Controlled studies evaluating performance and alertness indicate no daytime impairment with these drugs,[5] although cetirizine may cause sedation at very high doses. Effects on sleep architecture are not known.

Histamine type 2 receptor antagonists (cimetidine, ranitidine, famotidine) generally have no effect on sleep or waking function, but one study of cimetidine showed increased SWS and one study of famotidine showed decreased SL. These drugs are metabolized by the CYP system, however, which may result in increased plasma concentration and increased sedation of co-administered sedative-hypnotics such as diazepam.

ANTIPARKINSONIAN DRUGS

Low doses of levodopa improve sleep, and higher doses disrupt sleep. PSG studies show mixed effects on REM and SWS, but increased REM density is noted and may account for reports of vivid dreams and nightmares.[5] Levodopa, pergolide (an ergot derivative dopamine agonist), and pramipexole and ropinirole (both non-ergot dopamine agonists) have shown efficacy for treatment of restless legs syndrome. These drugs produce subjective improvement in sleep, but PSG data are limited. Ropinirole decreases SL and improves sleep continuity.[17] In patients with Parkinson's disease, the dopamine agonists have been associated with increased daytime sleepiness, but this appears to be related to total dopaminergic dose or to disease pathology rather than to specific drugs. Ropinirole and pergolide decrease periodic limb movements and are effective in treating restless legs symptoms.[17] Selegiline, a monoamine oxidase (MAO)-B inhibitor used as adjunctive therapy in Parkinson's disease, partially metabolizes to amphetamine and methamphetamine and has been associated with insomnia. Of interest, PSG studies show increased wake and decreased REM in healthy subjects but decreased SL in patients.[5] Amantadine, also used as an antiviral agent, reportedly causes insomnia, but there are no PSG studies. Anticholinergic drugs such as benztropine and hyoscyamine may be sedating, but high doses can cause agitation.

CARDIOVASCULAR DRUGS

CNS side effects reported with beta antagonists include fatigue, insomnia, nightmares, mental confusion, and psychomotor impairment.[5,9] These symptoms appear to be more common with the more lipophilic drugs and those drugs that have higher affinity for 5-HT receptors. Among these drugs, propranolol, which has high lipid solubility and high 5-HT affinity, is most commonly associated with disturbed sleep. Although lipid solubility is low for carvedilol, 5-HT affinity is high and alpha$_1$ blockade is noted. Beta blockers with vasodilating properties, such as carvedilol and labetalol, have been associated with fatigue. PSG studies of lipophilic drugs with high 5-HT affinity demonstrate decreased sleep continuity; REM may be decreased with moderate to high clinical doses. Daytime sedation and cognitive impairment are reported with beta blockers, but objective data are limited. The mechanism for these effects is unclear but may involve central beta receptors involved in vigilance or effects on other receptors such as 5-HT.

Sedation, nightmares, and decreased concentration have been reported with the alpha$_2$ agonists clonidine and methyldopa, but sedation may diminish with time.[5,9] Insomnia has also been reported with clonidine. Clonidine decreases REM and increases SWS, and methyldopa decreases SWS.

Alpha$_1$ antagonists such as prazosin do not appear to have significant effects on sleep, although transient sedation is sometimes reported clinically. Prazosin has been reported to improve sleep and decrease nightmares in patients with post-traumatic stress disorder.[18] Angiotensin-converting enzyme inhibitors have been associated with insomnia and nightmares, and there are case reports of increased sleep apnea in susceptible individuals who develop cough with these drugs.[19] Reserpine, which depletes stores of catecholamines and serotonin, increases REM and decreases SWS. Drowsiness, lethargy, and nightmares have been reported.

Subjectively, a number of hypolipidemic drugs (most notably atorvastatin and lovastatin) have been associated with insomnia, but controlled clinical trials and limited PSG data have not confirmed sleep disturbance.[5] Antiarrhythmic drugs have been associated with fatigue, but there are no studies evaluating effects on sleep or waking function.

HYPNOTICS

Drugs with a Food and Drug Administration (FDA) indication for treatment of insomnia include a number of benzodiazepine agonists and ramelteon, a melatonin receptor agonist. Drug characteristics are listed in Table 10-3. Other drugs used as hypnotics but

TABLE 10-3 ■ Characteristics of Drugs Used to Treat Insomnia

Drug	Chemical Class	Half-life (hr)
Benzodiazepines		
Estazolam	Benzodiazepine	8–24
Flurazepam	Benzodiazepine	48–120
Quazepam	Benzodiazepine	48–120
Temazepam	Benzodiazepine	8–20
Triazolam	Benzodiazepine	2–6
Nonbenzodiazepines		
Eszopiclone	Cyclopyrrolone	5–7
Indiplon	Pyrazolopyrimidine	1–1.5
Zaleplon	Pyrazolopyrimidine	1
Zolpidem	Imidazopyridine	1.5–2.4
Sedating antidepressants used as hypnotics		
Amitriptyline	Tricyclic	5–45
Doxepin	Tricyclic	10–30
Trimipramine	Tricyclic	15–40
Trazodone	Phenylpiperazine	3–14
Nefazodone	Phenylpiperazine	2–4 (6–18 for active metabolites)
Mirtazapine	Noradrenergic and specific serotoninergic antidepressant	13–40
Other drugs used as hypnotics		
Chloral hydrate	Two-carbon molecule	5–10
Diphenhydramine	Antihistamine	4–8
Gabapentin	Anticonvulsant	5–9
Gammahydroxybutyrate (GHB)	Four-carbon molecule	20–70 minutes
Olanzapine	Thienobenzodiazepine antipsychotic	20–54
Tiagabine	Anticonvulsant	8
Valerian	Plant extract	Uncertain

without FDA indication for insomnia are also listed in Table 10-3. Because these latter drugs are nonscheduled, they may be perceived as being safer than the benzodiazepine receptor agonists; however, their efficacy in treating insomnia has not been established and their side effects can be clinically significant.

Benzodiazepine receptor agonists include the benzodiazepines estazolam, flurazepam, quazepam, temazepam, and triazolam and the newer nonbenzodiazepines zaleplon, zolpidem, eszopiclone, and indiplon (under development). Both classes bind to the GABA$_A$ receptor; however, the nonbenzodiazepines bind more selectively to GABA$_A$ receptors containing alpha$_1$ subunits. Elimination half-life of these drugs varies widely (Table 10-3). Accumulation of longer half-life compounds (e.g., flurazepam) may result in daytime sedation. In general, these drugs decrease sleep latency and increase TST.[10,20] The exception is zaleplon, which may not increase TST because of its very short half-life; however, this drug may be taken in the middle of the night with minimal risk for residual daytime sedation. The benzodiazepines also decrease REM and SWS, but the nonbenzodiazepines tend to preserve sleep architecture.[20] Benzodiazepines may worsen sleep apnea, but the nonbenzodiazepines do not appear to have a deleterious effect on breathing during sleep. Abrupt withdrawal from benzodiazepines, particularly the shorter-acting compounds, may lead to rebound of REM (and resultant nightmares), as well as rebound insomnia (temporary worsening of insomnia beyond pretreatment level). Rebound insomnia and psychomotor impairment are unlikely with the nonbenzodiazepines.

Ramelteon, which has no affinity for the GABA$_A$ receptor, is a melatonin receptor agonist that is selective for the MT$_1$ and MT$_2$ receptor subtypes, which appear to be involved with the regulation of sleep and circadian rhythms. Ramelteon has a half-life of 1 to 2.6 hours and produces significant decreases in PSG-recorded SL.[21] The increase in TST seen with this drug is accounted for primarily by the decrease in SL. Sleep architecture is unaffected. Patients have not consistently reported shortened sleep onset, possibly because the drug does not have the same feeling of sedation as drugs that act at the GABA receptor. Ramelteon produces a phase advance in the circadian sleep-wake rhythm, which may explain its ability to decrease SL.[22]

PSYCHOTHERAPEUTIC DRUGS

Antidepressants

Most antidepressants decrease REM sleep and increase REM latency (exceptions include trazodone, nefazodone, and mirtazapine).[5,8,23,24] Abrupt discontinuation of these REM-suppressant medications results in REM rebound and reports of nightmares. Antidepressants that are sedating most likely have antagonist effects at H$_1$, 5-HT$_2$, and/or alpha$_1$-adrenergic receptors, whereas antidepressants that decrease sleep continuity are likely to have agonistic effects at 5-HT$_2$ receptors. REM sleep suppression is probably mediated by 5-HT$_{1A}$ stimulation. Antidepressants are metabolized by the CYP system and can thus interact with some sedative-hypnotic medications.

The tricyclic antidepressants are well absorbed, have long half-lives (12–50 hours), are strongly lipophilic and thus widely distributed throughout the body, and have multiple mechanisms of action including 5-HT and norepinephrine reuptake inhibition as well as alpha$_1$, cholinergic, and H$_1$ blockade. The tertiary amines (amitriptyline, doxepin, trimipramine, imipramine) are more sedating than the secondary amines (desipramine, nortriptyline, protriptyline) and have significant effects on sleep and sleep architecture. Clomipramine is an exception, although as a tertiary amine, it is not as sedating as amitriptyline, imipramine, or doxepin and may be activating in some individuals. Tricyclic antidepressants decrease REM and increase phasic REM activity; they also decrease SL and increase TST. These drugs tend to increase SWS during the first non-REM (NREM) period but do not increase the overall amount of SWS.[5,23] Increases in the frequency of periodic limb movements and slow eye movements during NREM sleep have also been observed. These drugs do not appear to worsen sleep apnea. Daytime sedation and performance impairment have been demonstrated, although it is possible that these effects may lessen with time.

Selective reuptake inhibitors have more selective mechanisms of action but rarely act exclusively at one receptor site. Selective serotonin reuptake inhibitors (SSRIs) act primarily on the serotonin system, a complex system with at least seven identified receptor classes. These drugs (fluoxetine, paroxetine, sertraline, fluvoxamine, citalopram, and escitalopram) are more likely to be associated with insomnia than with sedation, at least acutely, but daytime sedation may be noted with higher doses. SSRIs typically decrease TST and REM.[5,23] The sleep-fragmenting effect of these drugs is likely associated with agonistic activity at 5-HT$_{2B}$ receptors. Sleep continuity may improve with long-term use. Periodic limb movements and prominent slow eye movements in NREM sleep have been noted with fluoxetine and may occur with other drugs in this class.

The selective serotonin and norepinephrine reuptake inhibitors venlafaxine and duloxetine also decrease TST and REM.[5,23] These drugs also weakly inhibit dopamine reuptake. Bupropion, a norepinephrine and dopamine reuptake inhibitor, has been associated with both insomnia and vivid dreams or nightmares. Unlike most antidepressants, this drug may increase REM. In addition it may decrease PLMs, possibly because of its effect on dopamine reuptake.

Trazodone and nefazodone are both 5-HT$_2$ receptor antagonists. Trazodone also inhibits 5-HT$_{1A}$, 5-HT$_{1C}$, alpha$_1$, and H$_1$ receptors. It is a weak 5-HT reuptake inhibitor. Nefazodone is a weak inhibitor of both 5-HT and norepinephrine reuptake but has little affinity for 5-HT$_1$, H$_1$, or alpha-adrenergic receptors. Sedation is reported in more than 40% of patients taking trazodone. This drug is rarely prescribed for depression but is commonly used to treat insomnia. In fact, trazodone is prescribed for insomnia more than any other drug, including the benzodiazepine receptor agonists, despite the limited availability of data

regarding efficacy.[25] Trazodone decreases SL and increases TST and SWS without affecting REM sleep, at least with short-term use.[5,8,23] Nefazodone is not as sedating as trazodone but has shown increased sleep efficiency and mixed effects on REM and SWS.[5,8]

Mirtazapine blocks alpha$_2$ autoreceptors, 5-HT$_2$ receptors, and H$_1$ receptors, which likely accounts for its sedating effect. Mirtazapine decreases SL and increases TST but has no effect on REM or SWS.[8]

Monoamine oxidase inhibitors (MAOIs) inhibit the action of MAO enzymes, which metabolize serotonin, norepinephrine, and dopamine. The classic MAOIs (isocarboxazid, phenelzine, tranylcypromine) inhibit both MAO-A and MAO-B enzymes, profoundly decrease REM, and increase wake while decreasing TST.[5] Moclobemide (not available in the United States) selectively inhibits MAO-A and is much less likely to cause insomnia or changes in sleep architecture than other MAOIs.

Lithium is subjectively associated with improved nocturnal sleep and increased daytime sleepiness, at least initially. It increases TST; REM may be unaffected or decreased, and SWS may be unaffected or increased.[6,26]

Antipsychotics

Sedation is a common effect of both traditional and newer antipsychotics, with the degree of sedation related to dose as well as affinity for H$_1$ receptors, although antagonistic action at alpha$_1$-adrenergic receptors may also contribute.[27,28] Among the traditional drugs, chlorpromazine and thioridazine tend to be more sedating than haloperidol. These drugs increase TST, but effects on REM and SWS are unclear. Clinically, clozapine is the most sedating of all antipsychotics. Limited PSG data on olanzapine show increased TST and SWS along with decreased REM. Olanzapine and quetiapine have been investigated as hypnotics, but there are no published PSG data on quetiapine.[8]

Anxiolytics

Benzodiazepines used for anxiety (e.g., alprazolam, lorazepam) have similar effects on sleep and waking function as benzodiazepines used for insomnia. Because these drugs may be taken during the day as well as at night, sedation and performance impairment are of concern. SSRIs and other antidepressants used for anxiety are discussed in the antidepressant section. Buspirone is a 5-HT$_{1A}$ partial agonist and dopamine D$_2$ antagonist, and metabolizes to an alpha$_2$ receptor antagonist. It does not have the hypnotic, anticonvulsant, or myorelaxant properties of the benzodiazepines and does not affect sleep, sleepiness, or daytime performance.

STIMULANTS

The alerting effects of amphetamine and amphetamine-like stimulants such as methylphenidate and pemoline (removed from the market by the manufacturer in 2005) are mediated by increased dopaminergic transmission via stimulating dopamine release or blocking dopamine reuptake. These drugs increase SL, decrease TST, and decrease REM.[11] They may also decrease SWS. At higher doses daytime administration can result in impairment of sleep. The mechanism of action of modafinil, a chemically unique compound, is unclear but may involve both noradrenergic and dopaminergic systems. Modafinil has fewer side effects and less abuse potential than amphetamine stimulants. It increases SL on both MSLT and MWT, but its alerting effects do not appear to carry over to the main sleep period unless dosing occurs too close to bedtime.[11]

Caffeine, a methylxanthine, causes wakefulness by antagonizing adenosine receptors. When taken near bedtime or in the afternoon in susceptible individuals, caffeine prolongs SL and decreases sleep continuity. Effects on REM are variable. Theophylline, which is structurally similar to caffeine, has frequently been reported to cause sleep disturbance. PSG studies in normal individuals, patients with asthma, and children with cystic fibrosis confirm decreased sleep continuity.[5] In some cases of asthma, however, improved sleep continuity may result as asthma symptoms are treated. Nicotine (including transdermal nicotine delivery) increases SL and decreases sleep continuity and REM.[13] Sleep disruption may be a wake-promoting effect or a withdrawal effect.

OTHER DRUGS

Corticosteroids (dexamethasone, hydrocortisone, prednisone) are frequently associated with sleep disturbance, but objective studies show inconsistent results. The most common PSG finding is a significant decrease in REM sleep, although increased wake may also occur.[29]

Nonsteroidal anti-inflammatory drugs (NSAIDs) may affect sleep by decreasing the synthesis of prostaglandin D2, suppressing the normal surge in melatonin synthesis at night, and affecting body temperature. Aspirin and ibuprofen, when acutely administered, decrease sleep efficiency and increase wake. Nightmares have been reported with naproxen. There are no PSG studies on the newer NSAIDs.

Opioids impair performance and decrease SL, SWS, and REM when acutely administered.[5,13] Insomnia may develop with chronic use. Tolerance to the sedating and performance-impairing effects is believed to develop with chronic use, but there are no well-controlled studies to support this claim. These drugs also suppress respiratory drive and interact additively with other CNS depressants. Tramadol, a synthetic opioid, decreases SWS and REM.[30]

Chloral hydrate decreases SL and improves sleep continuity without other sleep architecture effects. It is not indicated for treatment of insomnia but is used as a sedative in children undergoing clinical procedures.

Gamma-hydroxybutyrate (GHB), approved for treatment of narcolepsy, increases sleep efficiency and SWS and decreases REM latency in both healthy individuals and narcolepsy patients.[8] The mechanism of action is unknown, but it appears to increase dopamine and is metabolized to a limited extent to GABA. It is highly sedating and can cause coma in high doses. Onset of action is rapid, and its half-life is exceedingly short (<1 hour); thus patients typically take a middle-of-the-night dose in addition to a bedtime dose. Recreational users of GHB typically ingest the drug in high doses and may experience insomnia and anxiety on withdrawal.

Pseudoephedrine and phenylpropanolamine are similar pharmacologically to ephedrine but are much less lipophilic and thus have less potent CNS effects. These drugs have been associated with insomnia.[5] A single PSG study of pseudoephedrine showed increased wake when the drug was taken at bedtime.

Melatonin is a lipid-soluble endogoneous hormone, normally secreted at night (even in night-active species) and suppressed by light. Its effects on sleep are variable. It appears to be more likely to induce sleep during the day, when homeostatic sleep drive is low, than at night, when sleep drive is high.[31]

Valerian preparations typically contain unknown proportions of a number of chemicals with CNS activity. Thus the mechanism of action is unknown but may involve inhibition of GABA metabolism, antagonism of adenosine receptors, or activity at serotonin receptors. Valerian extracts reportedly improve sleep subjectively. PSG studies indicate increased SWS and decreased stage 1 but mixed effects on SL and sleep continuity.[8]

CONCLUSIONS

Numerous drugs affect sleep and waking function. Disturbed sleep, daytime sleepiness, and decreased cognitive functioning can be caused by illness or the medications used for treatment. Effects on waking function can be caused by a drug's direct action (e.g., carryover sedation from a long-acting sedating compound) or indirect action (e.g., daytime fatigue from a drug that disrupts sleep). Similarly, effects on sleep can be a direct drug effect (e.g., improved sleep continuity via GABA agonism from a hypnotic) or an indirect effect (e.g., improved sleep resulting from drug treatment of depression). Knowledge of pharmacokinetics and receptor mechanisms of these drugs can assist the clinician in predicting which drugs will improve or disrupt sleep and which drugs will affect daytime function.

REFERENCES

1. Bourin M, Briley M: Sedation, an unpleasant, undesirable and potentially dangerous side effect of many psychotropic drugs. Hum Psychopharmacol 19:135–139, 2003.

2. Boutrel B, Koob G: What keeps us awake: the neuropharmacology of stimulants and wakefulness-promoting medications. Sleep 27:1181–1194, 2004.

3. Thompson DF, Pierce DR: Drug-induced nightmares. Ann Pharmacother 33:93–98, 1999.

4. Pagel JF, Helfter P: Drug induced nightmares: an etiology based review. Hum Psychopharmacol 18:59–67, 2003.

5. Schweitzer PK: Drugs that disturb sleep and wakefulness. In Kryger MH, Roth T, Dement WC (eds): *Principles and Practice of Sleep Medicine*, 4th ed. Philadelphia, Saunders, 2005, pp 499–518.

6. Buysse DJ: Drugs affecting sleep, sleepiness and performance. In Monk T (ed): *Sleep, Sleepiness and Performance*. Hoboken, NJ, John Wiley & Sons, Ltd., 1991, pp 249–306.

7. Obermeyer WH, Benca RM: Effects of drugs on sleep. Neurol Clin 14:827–840, 1996.

8. Buysse DJ, Schweitzer PK, Moul DE: Clinical pharmacology of other drugs used as hypnotics. In Kryger MH, Roth T, Dement WC (eds): *Principles and Practice of Sleep Medicine*, 4th ed. Philadelphia, Saunders, 2005, pp 452–467.

9. Novak M, Shapiro C: Drug-induced sleep disturbances. Focus on nonpsychotropic medications. Drug Safety 16:133–149, 1997.

10. Mendelson WB: Hypnotic medications: mechanisms of action and pharmacologic effects. In Kryger MH, Roth T, Dement WC (eds): *Principles and Practice of Sleep Medicine*, 4th ed. Philadelphia, Saunders, 2005, pp 444–451.

11. Nishino S, Mignot E: Wake-promoting medications: basic mechanisms and pharmacology. In Kryger MH, Roth T, Dement WC (eds): *Principles and Practice of Sleep Medicine*, 4th ed. Philadelphia, Saunders, 2005, pp 468–483.

12. Walter TJ, Golish JA: Psychotropic and neurologic medications. In Lee-Chiong TL, Sateia MJ, Carskadon MA (eds): *Sleep Medicine*. Philadelphia, Hanley & Belfus, Inc., 2002, pp 587–599.

13. Gillin J, Drummond S, Clark C, Moore P: Medication and substance abuse. In Kryger MH, Roth T, Dement WC (eds): *Principles and Practice of Sleep Medicine*, 4th ed. Philadelphia, Saunders, 2005, pp 1345–1358.

14. Sammaritano M, Sherwin A: Effect of anticonvulsants on sleep. Neurology 54:S16–S24, 2000.

15. Blum DE: New drugs for persons with epilepsy. In French J, Leppik I, Dichter MA (eds): *Antiepileptic Drug Development (Advances in Neurology,* vol 76). Philadelphia, Lippincott, Williams & Wilkins, 1998, pp 57–87.

16. Bazil CW: Effects of antiepileptic drugs on sleep structure: are all drugs equal? CNS Drugs 17:719–728, 2003.

17. Allen R, Becker PM, Bogan R, et al: Ropinirole decreases periodic leg movements and improves sleep parameters in patients with restless legs syndrome. Sleep 27:907–914, 2004.

18. Raskind MA, Peskind ER, Kanter ED, et al: Reduction of nightmares and other PTSD symptoms in combat veterans by prazosin: a placebo-controlled study. Am J Psychiatry 160:371–373, 2003.

19. Cicolin A, Mangiardi L, Mutani R, Bucca C: Angiotensin-converting enzyme inhibitors and obstructive sleep apnea. Mayo Clin Proc 81:53–55, 2006.

20. Walsh JK, Roehrs T, Roth T: Pharmacologic treatment of primary insomnia. In Kryger MH, Roth T, Dement WC (eds): *Principles and Practice of Sleep Medicine*, 4th ed. Philadelphia, Saunders, 2005, pp 749–760.

21. Erman M, Seiden D, Zammit G, et al: An efficacy, safety, and dose-response study of ramelteon in patients with chronic primary insomnia. Sleep Med 7:17–24, 2006.

22. Richardson G, Zammit G, Rodriguez L, Zhang J: Evaluation of circadian phase-shifting effects of ramelteon in healthy subjects. In *Proceedings of International Congress of Applied Chronobiology & Chronomedicine* June 1–5, 2005, Antalya, Turkey.

23. Wilson S, Argyropoulos S: Antidepressants and sleep. A qualitative review of the literature. Drugs 65:927–47, 2005.

24. Mann JJ: The medical management of depression. N Engl J Med 353:1819–34, 2005.

25. Walsh JK, Schweitzer PK: Ten-year trends in the pharmacological treatment of insomnia. Sleep 22:371–75, 1999.

26. Friston KJ, Sharpley AL, Solomon RA, et al: Lithium increases slow wave sleep: possible mediation by brain 5-HT2 receptors. Psychopharmacology 98:139–140, 1989.

27. Leucht S, Wahlbeck K, Hamann J, et al: New generation antipsychotics versus low-potency conventional antipsychotics. A systematic review and meta-analysis. Lancet 361:1581–1589, 2003.

28. Gerlach J, Peacock L: New antipsychotics: the present status. Int Clin Psychopharmacol 10(suppl 3):39–48, 1995.

29. Born J, Zwick A, Roth G, et al: Differential effects of hydrocortisone, fluocortolone, and aldosterone on nocturnal sleep in humans. Acta Endocrinol 116:129–137, 1987.

30. Walder B, Tramer M, Blois R: The effects of two single doses of tramadol on sleep: a randomized, cross-over trial in healthy volunteers. Eur J Anaesthesiol 18:36–42, 2001.

31. Scheer FA, Cajochen C, Turek F, Czeisler CA: Melatonin in the regulation of sleep and circadian rhythms. In Kryger MH, Roth T, Dement WC (eds): *Principles and Practice of Sleep Medicine*, 4th ed. Philadelphia, Saunders, 2005, pp 395–404.

Pediatric Sleep-Wake Disorders

SURESH KOTAGAL

HISTORICAL ASPECTS

In 1929, Hans Berger[1] recorded electrical activity from the exposed surface of the cerebral cortex in a patient who had a piece of skull removed. In 1937, Loomis and colleagues[2] reported their findings on all-night sleep studies of humans. They observed that sleep consisted of alternating stages that could be differentiated by their electroencephalographic (EEG) pattern. In 1953, Aserinsky and Kleitman[3] identified a novel EEG pattern consisting of low-voltage, fast activity that occurred in conjunction with bursts of rapid eye movements. Dement and Kleitman[4] then recognized that this state was associated with dreaming. They coined the term *rapid eye movement (REM) sleep.*

In 1966, Roffwarg, Muzio, and Dement[5] reported on the maturation of human sleep from a developmental perspective. In 1970, Dreyfus-Brisac[6] observed that active (REM) sleep could be identified on polygraphic tracings by 32 weeks of gestation owing to the presence of frequent bodily movements, irregular respiration, and REM while the eyes were closed. In 1972, Parmelee and Stern[7] recognized quiet or non-REM sleep after 36 weeks of gestation and characterized it by the presence of closed eyes with no eye movements, no bodily movements, and very regular respiration. The relationship of non-rapid eye movement (NREM) sleep to growth hormone release was reported by Shaywitz and colleagues[8] in 1972. Clinical sleep disorders in childhood remained largely obscure until the pioneering studies of Christian Guilleminault et al[9] in the late 1970s and early 1980s, who documented obstructive sleep apnea in children. In 1982, Elliott Weitzman et al[10] described the first case of delayed sleep phase syndrome in a medical student at the Montefiore Hospital in New York, thereby ushering in the era of understanding circadian rhythm sleep disorders. In 1992, the American Academy of Pediatrics initiated the "Back to Sleep" campaign, which recommended supine sleep in all infants when they are placed in bed in an effort to prevent sudden infant death syndrome (SIDS).[11] The relationship between prone sleeping, rebreathing of exhaled air, and SIDS was also elucidated by Kemp et al.[12] The usage of home apnea monitors, which had flourished dramatically in the 1980s when these devices were prescribed routinely to siblings of SIDS babies and to infants with recurrent apnea, fell dramatically in the late 1990s after the "Back to Sleep" recommendations of the American Academy of Pediatrics.

The Anders manual for the scoring of sleep in newborns was first developed by Anders et al[13] in 1971. Shortly thereafter, Guilleminault and Soquet[14] published a manual on the scoring of sleep and respiration during infancy. The past decade and a half have ushered in technological advances in the laboratory assessment of childhood sleep-wake disorders, with nasal thermocouples and thermistors giving way to nasal pressure transducers as the gold standard of monitoring nasal respiration; respiratory inductance plethysmography has replaced mercury-filled strain gauges in the measurement of thoracic and abdominal respiratory effort. Analog polygraphs have been largely replaced by digital systems.

The molecular biologic and genetic era of sleep medicine was ushered in by observations such as those of de Lecea et al[15] who in 1988 recognized the hypocretin system in the central nervous system and its alerting effects. Subsequently, Lin et al[16] demonstrated that canine narcolepsy was associated with mutations in the hypocretin-2 receptor gene. Nishino et al[17] demonstrated a deficiency of hypocretin-1 in the cerebrospinal fluid in human narcolepsy. Thanickal and colleagues[18] demonstrated a reduced number of hypocretin neurons postmortem in the hypothalamus of humans with narcolepsy. The increasing recognition of the neurobehavioral aspects of sleep disturbance by Beebe and Gozal[19] and colleagues has further broadened the field of pediatric sleep medicine. This chapter addresses some key sleep-wake issues in infancy, childhood, and adolescence.

NORMAL SLEEP AND BREATHING DURING INFANCY

EEG activity can be clearly recorded from the fetus by 24 weeks of gestation. Wakefulness can be differentiated from sleep by 27 to 28 weeks postconceptional age. By 30 to 32 weeks postconception, the low voltage and irregular EEG pattern of active (REM) sleep can be clearly distinguished from the high voltage and slow wave EEG pattern of quiet (NREM) sleep (Figures 11-1 and 11-2). At this age, close to 80% of the total sleep time is spent in active sleep. By full term or 40 weeks postconception, the proportion of time spent in active sleep decreases to approximately 55–65% of total sleep time, with a corresponding increase with quiet sleep.[20] Active sleep is associated with higher values of cerebral blood flow and metabolic rate as compared with quiet sleep. Respiration during active sleep is irregular, with intermittent inhibition of the striated muscle of the upper airway and the rib cage; however, diaphragmatic activity remains relatively unaltered. The incoordination between the intercostal muscles and the diaphragm during active sleep predisposes to paradoxical chest and abdominal wall motion, inefficient breathing, and oxygen desaturation. The paradoxical chest and abdominal wall movement pattern is most prominent during active sleep of premature infants, gradually subsides over the first 5 to 6 months of life, and disappears by age 3 years. By contrast, respiration during quiet or NREM sleep is deep and regular. The responsiveness of the brainstem chemoreceptors to hypercapnia is blunted during active sleep as compared with quiet sleep.[21]

The carotid body contains receptors that contain oxygen-sensitive K^+ channels.[22] The carotid sinus nerve carries hypoxia-mediated afferent impulses from the carotid body to the petrosal sinus, thence via the glossopharyngeal nerve to the nucleus of the tractus solitarius in the medulla.[23] Exposure to high levels of nicotine prenatally or to perinatal hyperoxia reduces the size of the carotid body, with possible blunting of the compensatory responses to hypoxia,[24] thus underscoring the critical role of the peripheral chemoreceptors of the carotid body in terminating apnea and initiating normal breathing. The role of an exaggerated laryngeal chemoreflex in the pathogenesis of apnea in preterm infants should also be emphasized.[25] This reflex is characterized by central apnea, glottic closure, and bradycardia in response to instillation of water, saline, or milk into the pharynx. This vagally mediated laryngeal reflex may become more prominent during upper respiratory infections. It is most prominent during the neonatal period and gradually subsides during infancy.

Adults and most infants prefer to breathe through the nose, but infants do have the ability to switch to mouth breathing if necessary, although this switching ability is not fully developed in the preterm infant. Periodic breathing is a normal variant that is defined as three or more apnea episodes of 3 seconds or more with an intervening period of 20 seconds or less. It is most prevalent during active sleep in preterm infants and gradually resolves during infancy. Prolonged periodic breathing may be associated with oxygen desaturation.

Patterns of apnea vary with the age of the infant; premature infants are more likely to exhibit mixed or obstructive apneas, whereas term infants are more likely to have central apneas. Only central apneas of more than 20 seconds are considered significant in infants. In preterm infants, the frequency of apneic pauses decreases by more than 80% between 40 and 52 weeks postconception and ultimately matches that of infants born at full term.

THE PEDIATRIC SLEEP CONSULTATION

Consultation requests must be triaged in advance to gauge the nature and the urgency of the sleep complaint and also to facilitate scheduling of diagnostic procedures. A questionnaire concerning the patient's sleep-wake function should be completed by the family members before the visit. Key elements of the sleep history are listed in Table 11-1, and important aspects of the sleep-related examination are shown in Table 11-2. A provisional diagnosis should be established on completion of the history and examination. A plan for investigations is drawn up, and the studies are completed, subsequent to which the patient returns for discussion of test results and for formulation of the final management plan, which includes patient and family education.

APNEA OF PREMATURITY

This disorder of respiratory control affects between 70% and 90% of premature infants of less than 1500 g birth weight or <28 weeks of gestation. It is characterized by prolonged apneas of 20 or more seconds in association with bradycardia (heart rate <80–100/min). There is a lingering concern that recurrent events may affect brainstem neural structures that regulate respiration. Also of concern is the possible occurrence of long-term cognitive and behavioral disturbances.[26]

Patients may exhibit central, obstructive, or mixed apneas, or a combination thereof. There may be recurrent episodes of periodic breathing, oxygen desaturation, and bradycardia.[27] Periodic breathing is the alteration between 5- and 10-second periods of apnea and regular breathing. It is most often observed

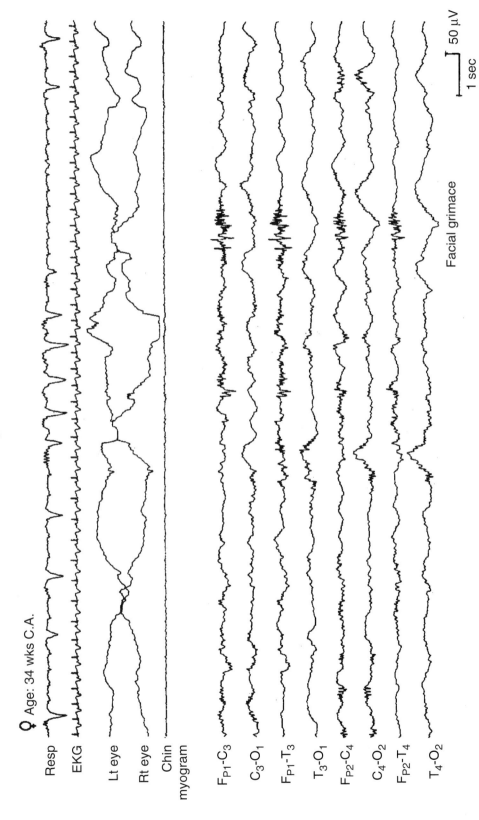

Active Sleep in a Normal Premature Infant

♀ Age: 34 wks C.A.

Resp

EKG

Lt eye

Rt eye

Chin
myogram

F_{P1}-C_3

C_3-O_1

F_{P1}-T_3

T_3-O_1

F_{P2}-C_4

C_4-O_2

F_{P2}-T_4

T_4-O_2

Facial grimace

50 μV

1 sec

FIGURE 11-1 ■ EEG in a 36-week-old preterm infant during active sleep, showing a low-voltage, mixed-frequency pattern.

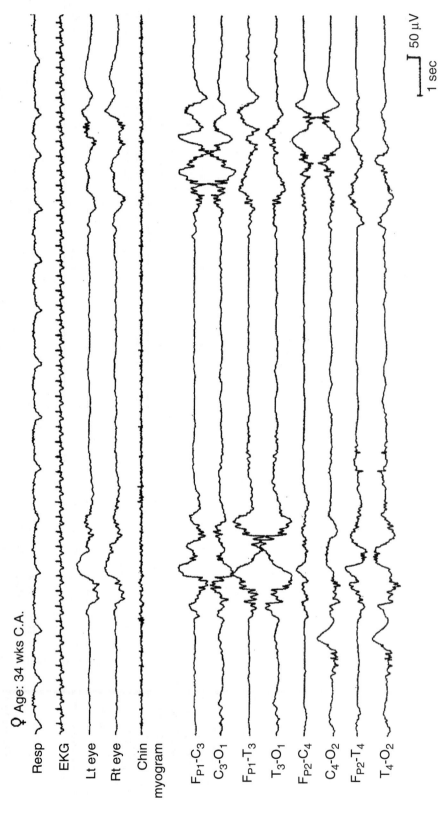

FIGURE 11-2 ■ EEG in a 36-week preterm infant showing a trace alternans pattern during quiet sleep—periods of high-voltage cortical activity alternate with low-amplitude periods.

TABLE 11-1 ■ Pediatric Sleep History

Evening/Nighttime Function	Daytime Function
Nature and duration of sleep complaint	Final morning awakening time (weekdays and weekends)
Evening and bedtime issues	Does the child feel refreshed or tired on awakening?
Rituals around bedtime, (e.g., rocking, patting, reading in bed, etc.)	School start time
Bed onset time (weekdays and weekends)	Days of school missed due to sleepiness during current academic year
Any sensation of restlessness in the legs before sleep onset	Daytime sleepiness, voluntary and involuntary naps; their duration
Estimated sleep onset time	Dreamlike feelings during these daytime naps
Sleeping position (prone/supine, etc.)	Impaired concentration, mood swings, and declining grades
Habitual snoring, mouth breathing, observed apnea, excessive sweating	Episodes suggestive of cataplexy or sleep paralysis
Dysphagia, salivary drooling	Afternoon and evening activities, including after-school employment
Restless sleep	A review of other systems
Estimated number and length of nighttime awakenings, and behavior during these awakenings	Medications used
Nocturnal enuresis	Allergies
Parasomnias/seizure-like behavior	

TABLE 11-2 ■ Essential Elements of the Pediatric Sleep-Related Examination

- Pulse, blood pressure, body mass index, head circumference
- Craniofacial abnormalities, tonsil size, mouth breathing, inflammation and narrowing of the anterior nasal passages, deviated nasal passages, enlargement of the tongue base, soft palate mobility
- Neck and submandibular lymph node enlargement, thyromegaly
- Lungs and heart auscultation
- Musculoskeletal: kyphoscoliosis
- Abdomen palpation for mass or tenderness
- Higher cortical functions: digit span (for attention span), recall of recent information, mood, memory, speech comprehension and expressive ability, involuntary movements, hypotonia, weakness, abnormal tendon reflexes, and gait

during active sleep and may predispose to oxygen desaturation and longer episodes of apnea.

Pathophysiology

The pathophysiology is complex and multifactorial. Passive collapse of the hypotonic upper airway of the premature infant predisposes to obstructive apnea. Furthermore, preterm infants of 30 to 32 weeks postconceptional age spend close to 80% of their total sleep time in active (REM) sleep and thus encounter an increased likelihood of hypotonic collapse of the upper airway when asleep. The central control of ventilation is immature, being characterized by a blunted central ventilatory response to the accumulation of carbon dioxide.[27] There is also immaturity of the excitatory, N-methyl-D-aspartate (NMDA) receptors located in the nucleus of the tractus solitarius in the medulla. These receptors increase ventilation in response to recurrent hypoxia.[28] Also, exposure to hypoxia usually increases ventilation via enhanced expression in the brainstem of neuronal nitric oxide synthase activity. This compensatory mechanism may be insufficiently developed in the preterm infant and may predispose to recurrent central apneic spells. Another important causative factor is that preterm infants respond by decreasing ventilation when challenged with hypoxia. This is most likely a consequence of suppression of the central ventilatory drive by hypoxia. Adenosine plays a likely role in mediating this inhibition.[29] Caffeine (used frequently to treat apnea of prematurity) is an inhibitor of adenosine metabolism. Paradoxical chest and abdominal wall motion is common during the active sleep of premature infants, and this may further exacerbate inefficient breathing. Yet another contributing factor might be immaturity of the Hering-Breur reflex; small increases in lung volume may thus trigger apnea.[30] Gastroesophageal reflux disease is a factor in some patients. Poets[31] has reported that although cardiorespiratory events and gastroesophageal reflux are common in preterm infants, they are not causally related. Perhaps they are dual manifestations of central autonomic nervous system immaturity.

The diagnostic workup usually includes an EEG to exclude the possibility of a seizure disorder, esophageal pH study if gastroesophageal reflux (GER) is suspected, otolaryngology consultation to exclude structural airway lesions such as partial choanal atresia, and a chest radiograph to exclude cardiomegaly or chronic pulmonary disease. Laryngoscopy might reveal a "cobblestone" appearance of the mucosa secondary to GER.

The respiratory stimulant doxapram appears to have some immediate and short-lived efficacy, but long-term benefit has not been established.[32] Theophylline has also been used. Owing to the prolonged half-life

(~30 hours) and nonlinear pharmacokinetics, theophylline should be used carefully, with close monitoring of serum levels. Toxic effects of theophylline include jitteriness, tachycardia, vomiting, and seizures. If medical therapy fails, consideration can be given to the use of continuous positive airway pressure breathing or nasal intermittent positive pressure breathing. Levo-carnitine has also been tried, but without proven benefit.[33] Apneic events subside spontaneously and resolve after 46 to 48 weeks postconceptional age. The benefits of home apnea monitoring are uncertain, but monitoring can be provided to cover the risk period.

SUDDEN INFANT DEATH SYNDROME

SIDS is defined as the sudden death of an infant of less than 1 year of age that remains unexplained after a complete clinical review, autopsy, and death scene investigation.[34] Since the introduction of the "Back to Sleep" campaign in the early 1990s, there has been a significant decline in the incidence of SIDS in the United States. It is currently estimated at 0.8/1000 live births. This decline has leveled off despite widespread adoption of the supine sleeping position for babies, suggesting that SIDS is multifactorial in etiology, with persistence of congenital or additional, undetermined environmental risk factors.[35]

Pathophysiology

A total of 90% of SIDS cases occur between birth and 4 months of age, suggesting that this is the most vulnerable period. Major epidemiological risk factors for SIDS are maternal anemia, maternal illicit drug use during pregnancy, maternal smoking, prematurity, and blunting of central arousal mechanisms by an overheated environment.[36–39] Prone sleeping position is a major contributor, as infants younger than 2–2.5

months are unable to sufficiently change body position to overcome suffocation from being placed prone on a soft mattress. This predisposes to rebreathing, hypercapnia, and consequent depression of the central ventilatory drive. Systemic infections may also alter the arousal threshold.[40] Filiano and Kinney[41] have proposed a triple-risk model that considers epidemiological, physiologic, and autopsy data. This model proposes that SIDS is likely to occur only when *exogenous stressors* affect *homeostatic control* in a *vulnerable infant* (Figure 11-3). They have established that the critical region for ventilatory control is the arcuate nucleus, which is derived from the caudal raphe system and located over the ventromedial aspect of the medulla. Using tissue autoradiography, they have also demonstrated decreased binding of ^{3}H-lysergide to serotonergic receptors 5-hydroxytryptamine$_{1A-D}$ and 5-hydroxytryptamine$_{2A}$ in the arcuate nuclei of SIDS patients compared with that of age-matched controls.[42] Furthermore, the application of a 5-HT$_{1A}$ serotonin agonist 8-hydroxy-2 (di-n-propylamino) tetralin (8-OHDPAT) to the ventral surface of the cat medulla increases the respiratory rate,[42] which confirms the role of medullary serotonergic network in the control of breathing. These findings might ultimately lead to an understanding of molecular factors that regulate the proliferation, migration, and maturation of cells from the caudal raphe system to the medullary arcuate nucleus.

A small percentage of SIDS cases are of cardiac etiology. At the Mayo Clinic, Ackerman et al[43] studied postmortem cardiac tissue from 93 SIDS patients, as well as 400 control subjects, and found two distinct mutant alleles in 2 of 93 subjects in the cardiac sodium channel gene, SCN5A, which predisposed to prolongation of the QT interval on electrocardiograms. Furthermore, when the mutant alleles were introduced *in vitro* into wild-type human cardiac sodium channels, voltage-clamp studies showed that the rates of voltage conductance were significantly slowed.

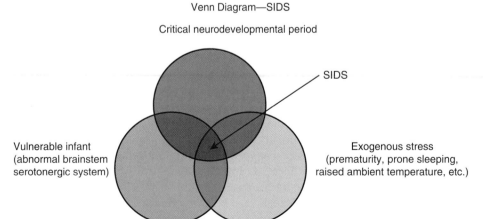

Venn Diagram—SIDS

Critical neurodevelopmental period

SIDS

Vulnerable infant
(abnormal brainstem
serotonergic system)

Exogenous stress
(prematurity, prone sleeping,
raised ambient temperature, etc.)

FIGURE 11-3 ■ Venn diagram describing the pathogenesis of SIDS. (Reprinted with permission from Filiano JJ, Kinney HC: A perspective on neuropathological findings in victims of the sudden infant death syndrome: the triple-risk model. Biol Neonate 65:194–197, 1994.)

Prevention

The management strategy for SIDS prevention will continue to be risk reduction, with emphasis on preventing prenatal exposure to nicotine, education of underserved and low socioeconomic populations about the dangers of prone sleeping position in infants, and avoiding excessive swaddling and overheating.

CONGENITAL CENTRAL HYPOVENTILATION SYNDROME (CCHS)

CCHS is characterized by defective automatic control of breathing during sleep. Patients generally become symptomatic at birth or shortly thereafter, but a late-onset childhood form has also been reported.[44]

Etiology

The primary form of CCHS is linked to mutations in the homeobox gene *Phox2B*, which maps to chromosome 4p12 and is transmitted in an autosomal dominant manner.[45] The gene encodes a highly conserved transcription factor. Approximately 92% of primary CCHS patients carry this mutation.[46] Approximately 20% of CCHS patients have coexisting Hirschprung's disease, a disorder of bowel motility resulting from a defect in development of autonomic ganglia of the wall of a segment of the large bowel. This combination of CCHS and Hirschprung's disease is called the *Haddad syndrome*. There is also an association between CCHS and neural crest tumors such as ganglioglioma and neuroblastoma, which are seen in 5–10% of CCHS cases. Frameshift and missense *Phox2b* mutations predispose to neuroblastoma. It has been postulated that CCHS is a neural crest disorder in which there is defective fetal development as brainstem neurons that regulate chemosensitivity are derived from the neural crest.

Secondary forms of central hypoventilation, although infrequent, may be related to subtle or overt developmental malformations of the brainstem, head injury, bulbar poliomyelitis, syringobulbia, Arnold Chiari type II malformation, Zellweger syndrome, and mitochondrial disorders such as Leigh syndrome. In some instances, no specific etiology is identifiable. The report of a mother-to-daughter transmission of the disorder suggests an autosomal dominant transmission in some families.[47]

Pathology

Common sites of hypoplasia or neurodegeneration include the arcuate nucleus of the medulla (regulates chemosensitivity), ventrolateral nucleus of the tractus solitarius, nucleus ambiguous or nucleus retroambigualis, and nucleus parabrachialis in the dorsolateral pons.

Clinical Features

The respiratory rate and depth are initially normal during wakefulness, but shallow and infrequent breathing, hypercarbia, and oxygen desaturation appear initially during NREM sleep and then during REM sleep. The $PaCO_2$ is >60 mm during sleep despite absence of pulmonary, neuromuscular, or cardiac disease. Ventilatory challenge with inhalation of a mixture of 5% CO_2 and 95% O_2 during NREM sleep fails to evoke the physiologic, threefold to fivefold increase in minute volume.

Management

There is no definitive and satisfactory treatment, although acetazolamide and theophylline may enhance chemoreceptivity of the brainstem respiratory neurons to a modest degree. Diaphragmatic pacing and home ventilation via tracheostomy are other therapeutic modalities. Patients may die in infancy or early childhood.

APPARENT LIFE-THREATENING EVENT (ALTE)

Introduction

The National Institutes of Health Consensus Development Conference on Infantile Apnea defined an ALTE as an episode that is frightening to the observer and characterized by a combination of apnea, skin color change, marked changes in muscle tone, choking, and gagging.[48] The disorder is most prevalent during the first 6 months of life (in the 2–6-month age range as compared with the 0–3-month range for SIDS). The incidence is about half that of SIDS (i.e., approximately 0.46/1000 live births).[49] ALTEs are about 14 times more common in preterm infants than in full-term infants.

Etiology

ALTEs are of diverse etiology, as shown in Table 11-3. Events occurring during wakefulness are often linked to gastroesophageal reflux. No definite etiology is found in close to 40–50% of cases.[50] This is especially likely in those manifesting only isolated episodes, whereas those with recurrent episodes frequently have gastroesophageal reflux, obstructive sleep apnea, sleep-related epilepsy, cardiac arrhythmias, congenital

TABLE 11-3 ■ Etiology of Apparent Life-Threatening Events

Category	Disorder
Respiratory	Upper airway infections (e.g., respiratory syncytial virus)
	Upper airway obstruction: retrognathia, adenoidal hypertrophy
	Lower airway closure or obstruction-tracheomalacia
	Intrapulmonary shunting: cyanotic breath holding spells
Neurological	Partial seizures with orbitofrontal onset
	Intracranial hemorrhage: shaken infant syndrome
	Central hypoventilation: congenital, drug-mediated
	Neuromuscular disease: botulism
Infective	Sepsis
	Meningoencephalitis
Autonomic	Vasovagal
	Gastroesophageal reflux disease
Cardiac	Wolff-Parkinson-White syndrome; long QT syndrome
	Congenital heart disease
Inborn errors of metabolism	Medium and long-chain acyl CoA dehydrogenase deficiency

heart disease, or congenital central hypoventilation syndrome. Partial seizures originating over the orbital surface of the frontal lobe or over the mesiotemporal region can also be characterized by an inspiratory whoop, followed by apnea. Aspiration of pharyngeal or gastric secretions might be another mechanism for apnea during seizures.

Clinical Assessment

As with any episodic disturbance of bodily function, a detailed history is the cornerstone of evaluation. The body position in which the infant was placed to sleep (supine versus prone), the position in which the infant was found by the parent/guardian, the state of the infant just before the event (awake or asleep), presence of head segment automatisms such as lip smacking or eyelid fluttering, and tachycardia that are suggestive of seizures, duration of the event, whether resuscitation measures were used and of what type, constipation, nonreactive pupils and weakness (suggestive of infantile botulism), history of gastroesophageal reflux, family history of SIDS, fever and lethargy (suggestive of sepsis), feeding, thermoregulation and sweating abnormalities (suggestive of dysautonomia), habitual snoring, and mouth breathing (suggestive of upper airway obstruction) should be subjects of inquiry.

Special attention should be paid during the examination to pulse, blood pressure, cardiac and respiratory examination, craniofacial abnormalities, mouth breathing, tonsillar hypertrophy, hypotonia, pupil size and reactivity, and motor activity and tendon reflexes.

Investigations

Instead of using a "shotgun" approach, investigations should be directed toward the most probable etiologies, based on clues gathered from the history and examination. The most commonly obtained studies are EEG, magnetic resonance imaging of the head, electrocardiogram (ECG), echocardiogram, urinary organic acid assay and serum carnitine levels (to rule out medium-chain acyl CoA dehydrogenase deficiency), and esophageal pH monitoring (to evaluate for gastroesophageal reflux). Nocturnal polysomnography and video-EEG telemetry are of limited utility in isolated apneic episodes but may be informative in those with recurrent spells. When indicated, the polysomnogram is complemented by laryngoscopy and lateral soft tissue radiographs of the neck. Hospitalization during this evaluation process is indicated, as it affords the family members time to ask questions of the medical team, learn cardiopulmonary resuscitation techniques, and collaborate with the health professionals in the discharge planning process.

Outcome and Management

The recurrence rate for severe ALTEs may be as high as 60%, with the second event generally occurring within a few days of the initial event. There is an active and unresolved debate about whether infants should be sent home on apnea–heart rate monitors. Opponents of apnea monitors state that they do not prevent SIDS—patients have died while still wearing these devices—and that they are not cost effective.[51] Proponents may counter that an estimated 13% of ALTE subjects can go on to develop SIDS[52]; thus monitoring is vital. The bias of this author is toward monitoring for 2 to 3 months after the initial event. Monitoring should be discontinued by the age of 6 months, which is well past the age of occurrence of SIDS. Parents should be familiar with cardiopulmonary resuscitation and may also need refresher courses.

RESTLESS LEGS SYNDROME

History

In 1994, Walters et al[53] described restless legs syndrome (RLS) in a mother and her three children, ages 6, 4, and 1 year, as well as in a 16-year-old from an unrelated family. The disorder exhibited autosomal transmission. The patients experienced leg discomfort and nocturnal motor restlessness, with temporary relief by voluntary movement. They also observed that on nocturnal polysomnography, children with RLS tended to show periodic limb movements during sleep (PLMS), which are defined as a series of four or more limb electromyographic discharges of 0.5- to 5-second duration that are separated by intervals of 4–90 seconds. The presence of PLMS is not essential to the diagnosis of RLS, although close to 80% of RLS patients have PLMS on nocturnal polysomnography. Owing to the subjective nature of RLS, it may be difficult to accurately diagnose RLS in young or nonverbal children. The recognition of childhood RLS has been greatly facilitated by the recently published diagnostic criteria that were established at a Consensus Conference at the National Institutes of Health[54] (Table 11-4).

TABLE 11-4 ■ Diagnostic Criteria for Adult and Childhood Restless Legs Syndrome[54]

Essential Diagnostic Criteria (Adults)

1. An urge to move the legs, usually accompanied or caused by uncomfortable and unpleasant sensations in the legs
2. The urge to move or unpleasant sensations begin or worsen during periods of rest or inactivity such as lying down or sitting
3. The urge to move or unpleasant sensations are partially or totally relieved by movement, such as walking or stretching, at as long as the activity continues
4. The urge to move or unpleasant sensations are worse in the evening or night than during the day, or only occur during the evening or night

Definite Childhood Restless Legs Syndrome (RLS)

1. The child meets all four essential adult criteria, **and**
2. The child relates a description in his or her own words that is consistent with leg discomfort

or

1. The child meets all four essential adult criteria, and two of three of the following:
   a. Sleep disturbance for age
   b. A biologic parent or sibling has definite RLS
   c. The child has polysomnographically documented periodic limb movement index of 5 or more per hour of sleep

Probable Childhood Restless Legs Syndrome (RLS)

1. The child meets all four essential adult criteria for RLS except criterion #4 (the urge to move or sensations are worse in the evening or at night than during the day), **and**
2. The child has a biologic parent or sibling with definite RLS

or

1. The child is observed to have behavior manifestations of lower extremity discomfort when sitting or lying, accompanied by motor movement of the affected limbs; the discomfort has characteristics of adult criteria 2, 3, and 4, **and**
2. The child has a biologic parent or sibling with definite RLS

Clinical Features

Children may describe a "creepy" or "crawling" feeling in their limbs that appears late in the evening or at night. There is an irresistible urge to move the legs. This sensorimotor disturbance shows a circadian variation, being most prominent in the evenings and at night. It is relieved by movement and exacerbated by rest. Although childhood RLS is now subclassified into *probable* and *definite* categories (Table 11-2), both groups seem to be likely defining the same underlying disorder,[55] as inheritance patterns, periodic limb movement index (PLMI), levels of serum ferritin, and clinical response to pharmacotherapeutic agents are similar.[55] The increased sleep fragmentation from RLS may provoke disorders of partial arousal such as confusional arousals or sleep walking. The child may be tired and unrefreshed on awakening in the morning. Attention deficit hyperactivity disorder (ADHD; a disorder characterized by inattentiveness, hyperactivity, and impulsivity) and RLS are comorbidities, as between 25% and 30% of patients with ADHD have coexisting RLS.[56]

Pathogenesis

A positive family history for RLS is present in close to three fourths of children with RLS.[55] Children most likely develop RLS when the genetic predisposition interacts with environmental factors, which have yet to be fully established. Applying complex segregational analysis on predominantly adult RLS patients and their relatives, Winkelmann et al[57] found that patients with onset of symptoms before age 30 years showed single gene, autosomal dominant transmission, with a multifactorial component. Periodic limb movement disorder appears to be linked to systemic iron deficiency.[58] In a prospective study of 39 children with a mean age of 7.5 years (standard deviation [SD] 3.1 years) they found that patients with serum ferritin levels of less than 50 μg/dL showed significantly higher PLMI as compared with those with serum iron levels >50 μg/dL (42.8 ± 18.3 versus 23.1 ± 10.1; $p = 0.02$). Furthermore, the PLMI was reduced following oral iron replacement therapy. Iron is a cofactor for tyrosine hydroxylase synthesis, which is the rate-limiting step in the synthesis of dopamine. The end result of iron deficiency appears to be a relative/absolute lowering of levels of central nervous system dopamine concentrations.

The term *growing pains* is applied to a conglomeration of symptoms of discomfort in the limbs that are seen in children, usually at night, that may be secondary to arthritic or nonarthritic conditions. Rajaram and Walters[59] have pointed out the heterogeneous nature of growing pains and that a subset of children with growing pains might actually have RLS.

Diagnosis

As in adults, childhood RLS is a clinical diagnosis that is based on sleep history and family history. One ends up resorting to polysomnography more often than in adults simply because children are at times unable to provide reliable history and because a PLMI >5 is one of the supportive diagnostic criteria under the present classification. An inexpensive and useful diagnostic aid is a videotape of the child's sleep in the home environment, which may show periodic limb movements. Serum ferritin levels should be checked to ensure that they are not below 50 µg/L. ADHD may be an important comorbidity necessitating neuropsychological assessment.

Treatment

Large, prospective studies on the treatment of childhood RLS are lacking. Drugs commonly used to treat adults with RLS have been prescribed for children as well on an off-label basis, with a generally favorable response. Agents that can potentially be prescribed include levodopa-carbidopa; dopamine receptor agonists such as pergolide, pramipexole, and ropinorole; benzodiazepines such as clonazepam; and anticonvulsants such as gabapentin.[60] Walters et al[61] described the response of six children with ADHD and RLS to treatment with levodopa-carbidopa or pergolide. All six subjects showed subjective improvement in their sleep, as well as significantly reduced PLMI and arousals from sleep. The daytime behavior also improved; three of six patients no longer met the diagnostic criteria for ADHD. Also, a welcome development was the resolution of associated oppositional defiant disorder, as verified on the Connors subscale and the Oppositional Defiant Disorder Scale. This author has used the dopamine receptor agonist, pramipexole, with a favorable response.[55] The dose is 0.125–0.375, generally administered about an hour before bedtime. Potential side effects are tremor, confusion, and augmentation (reappearance of RLS symptoms earlier in the evening). Gabapentin in a dose of 100–300 mg at bedtime might also be helpful in children with RLS, especially in those with a superimposed element of pain.[62]

Iron replacement therapy may ameliorate RLS symptoms over time, as observed by Kryger et al.[63] It should be stressed to the patient and family that improvement of RLS after oral iron therapy is gradual (over months), lest they develop unrealistic expectations about a prompt response. Combining oral iron with a dopamine agonist is a reasonable option for providing quick symptomatic relief and attempting full recovery over time. The long-term outcome of childhood RLS is unknown, especially in terms of characteristics that predict its resolution/persistence over time.

SLEEP-RELATED BREATHING DISTURBANCES (SRBD)

Obstructive sleep apnea (OSA) is characterized by prolonged partial upper airway obstruction, intermittent complete or partial obstruction (obstructive apnea or hypopnea), or both prolonged and intermittent obstruction that disrupts normal ventilation during sleep, normal sleep patterns, or both.[64] OSA has a prevalence rate of 2–4%[65] and is more common in those born prematurely and in those of African-American or Hispanic ethnicity.[66] It is equally prevalent in boys and girls. The most common etiological factors are adenotonsillar hypertrophy, neuromuscular disorders, and craniofacial syndromes that are associated anomalies, such as mid-face hypoplasia, retrognathia, and macroglossia. Obesity accompanies childhood OSA less often than in adults, although it is now starting to become a significant risk factor in adolescents given the significant rise of obesity in this age group. Childhood OSA also differs from adult OSA because of a greater likelihood of partial airway obstructions rather than frank apneas. Also, the duration of obstructive events is generally 5 to 10 seconds rather than 10 seconds or longer.

Primary snoring is characterized by habitual snoring that is not accompanied by sleep-wake complaints. It has now also been linked to neurobehavioral disturbances.[67] Childhood sleep-related breathing disturbances are a spectrum, ranging from primary snoring to OSA. An intermediate form of SRBD between primary snoring and OSA is the *upper airway resistance syndrome* (UARS). It is characterized by habitual snoring, increased negative intrathoracic pressure on esophageal manometry, and increased respiratory event–related arousals (RERAs) (Figure 11-4). The mean critical pressure at which the upper airway collapses (Pcrit) is higher at 1 cm H_2O (standard deviation 3) in children with OSAS compared with that in children with primary snoring (Pcrit of –20 cm H_2O, standard deviation 9).[68]

Clinical Features

The nocturnal features of OSA include habitual snoring, mouth breathing, periods of observed apnea, restless sleep, and urinary incontinence. There is no correlation between how loudly a child snores and the presence or severity of sleep-disordered breathing. Infants with OSA may show significant gastroesophageal reflux, which may predispose to chronic

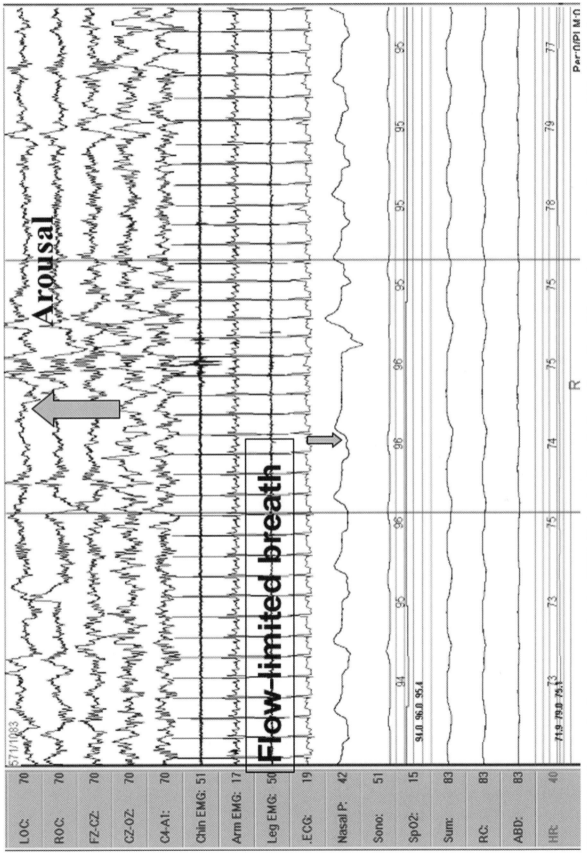

FIGURE 11-4 ■ Nocturnal polysomnogram showing UARS. Notice the change in the configuration of the nasal pressure transducer tracing, which shows a flow-limited breath (down arrow) that is followed by an EEG arousal (up arrow) and acceleration of heart rate.

upper airway inflammation. Hypoventilation may accompany obstructive sleep apnea in those who are obese, those having neuromuscular disorders, or those with Down syndrome. It is most reliably documented by measuring end tidal CO_2 levels during polysomnography that exceed 50 mm. Early morning headaches may accompany OSA, developing either as a consequence of sleep fragmentation and fluctuating blood flow velocities or owing to hypercarbia resulting from hypoventilation. The daytime features of childhood OSA include waking up feeling unrefreshed, mood swings, hyperactivity, inattentiveness, and (infrequently) hypersomnolence. Some children may be mistakenly diagnosed as having an attention deficit disorder. It is thus important to take a detailed sleep-wake history in every patient presenting for evaluation of inattentiveness. The neurobehavioral abnormalities in children with OSA are due to frontal lobe dysfunction, which may lead to hyperactivity, inattentiveness, and impaired executive function.[69] A history should also be taken of exposure to second-hand smoke in the home environment and any family history of sleep apnea.

Failure to thrive and poor weight gain are now observed less often than in the past, perhaps owing to increased awareness and earlier diagnosis of childhood OSA. Height, weight, and blood pressure should be recorded, and the body mass index calculated. The examination should also focus on determining the presence of craniofacial abnormalities such as retrognathia or dental malocclusion, enlarged tongue size, swelling of the uvula, crowded oropharynx, mouth breathing and inflamed nasal mucous membranes, polyps, deviated nasal septum, and thyroid gland enlargement. Tonsillar size (hypertrophy) should be graded on a 0 to IV grade.

Diagnosis

Oximetry

When there is severe tonsillar hypertrophy and a history that is classic for OSA, the documentation of recurrent episodes of oxygen desaturation on an overnight oximetry study is sufficient to establish the diagnosis. A "normal" overnight oximetry study, however, does not rule out mild or moderate OSA, and, based on the history, one might still need to resort to a nocturnal polysomnogram.

Nocturnal Polysomnography

This is the gold standard for diagnosing SRBD, as it can detect and quantify respiratory events accurately. Ideally, respiration is sampled using nasal pressure transducers, thoracic and abdominal respiratory inductance plethysmography, pulse oximetry, and end tidal CO_2. Infants and toddlers do not always tolerate nasal pressure cannulae, and one may have to substitute with an oronasal thermocouple. Obstructive events need to be longer than 5 seconds, rather than 10 seconds as established in adults. The threshold of oxygen desaturation that should be applied for scoring respiratory events is 3–4%. Nasal thermistors and thermocouples are not sensitive enough to detect UARS. It is thus critical to use nasal pressure transducers, which will show a pattern of flow limitation immediately preceding the EEG arousal (Figure 11-4). Normative values for pediatric polysomnography are shown in Table 11-5.[70]

The EEG manifestations of OSA consist of decreased sleep efficiency, suppression in the proportion of time spent in REM and slow wave sleep, and an increase in the number of RERAs to more than 10–12% of the total arousal index.

Cardiopulmonary Assessment

Sinus arrhythmia and a tachy-bradycardia pattern may accompany OSA. If uncorrected, the recurrent episodes of oxygen desaturation may lead to significant pulmonary vasoconstriction, right ventricular hypertrophy, and cor pulmonale. Patients with severe OSA (apnea-hypopnea index >10, oxygen saturation nadir below 80%) may therefore need a chest radiograph, electrocardiogram, and echocardiogram to evaluate for right heart failure consequent to pulmonary hypertension.

Evaluation of Autonomic Disturbance

Apneic events provoke oxygen desaturation, as well as shifts in the frequency of the EEG waveforms, and these are denoted as RERAs. The traditional polysomnographic method of visual analysis and scoring of

TABLE 11-5 ■ Reference Values for Pediatric Polysomnography[70] N=151, Ages 3.4 to 8.3, Mean Age 6.2 Years

Variable	Value	Standard Deviation
Total sleep time	7.8 hours	0.9 hours
Sleep latency	26.6 minutes	26.6 minutes
REM latency	109 minutes	51.9 minutes
Sleep efficiency	88.9%	7.6%
Arousal index	9	3.6
Respiratory event–related arousals	0.8	1.5
Apnea hypopnea index	0.7	0.7
Mean oxygen saturation	97.7%	0.9%
Oxygen saturation nadir	93%	3.6
Periodic limb movement index	2.5	3.7

respiratory events, however, is not sensitive enough. Using spectral array EEG analysis, Bandla and Gozal[71] have detected changes during apnea suggestive of arousal that could not be picked up on the routine scalp EEG.

Neuropsychological Assessment

Although not routinely indicated, neuropsychological assessment should be considered on a case-by-case basis. The neuropsychological sequelae of classic childhood OSA are presumed to be secondary to sleep fragmentation. O'Brien et al[72] reported on 35 children with OSA (mean age 6.7 years) and an equal number of closely matched control subjects. Those with OSA had significant deficits in attention span, executive function, phonological processing, visual attention, and general conceptual ability compared with control subjects. Also worrisome is that phonological processing is a basic building block in learning to read.

Management

Adenotonsillectomy is generally the first step in management. Although this procedure is widely applied as initial therapy, its benefit has not been firmly established through evidence-based research. About one fifth of patients below the age of 36 months develop dangerous postoperative airway edema after this procedure. All children below age 36 months or those with severe OSA, craniofacial anomalies, and neuromuscular disorders should undergo close postoperative observation for at least 24 hours in an intensive care unit setting equipped to manage airway compromise from edema.

About 10–15% of patients fail to show complete resolution of SRBD after adenotonsillectomy. If the patient has a residual UARS, consideration may be given to providing a nasal corticosteroid spray to shrink the mucous membrane lining of the nasal passages, or to using a leukotriene-receptor antagonist. This group that does not show complete resolution of SRBD includes patients with obesity, Down syndrome, neuromuscular problems, and craniofacial abnormalities such as Crouzon syndrome. In these patients, repeat nocturnal polysomnography is helpful in establishing the degree of resolution and also whether residual SRBD can be relieved by positive pressure breathing, which works by splinting the upper airway and thus keeping it patent. Although not approved by the Food and Drug Administration (FDA) for use in children, continuous positive airway pressure (CPAP) breathing or bilevel positive airway pressure (BiPAP) can be applied and titrated during the sleep study to determine the optimal degree of improvement. Side effects of positive pressure breathing include dryness of the nose and mouth.

SLEEP IN CENTRAL NERVOUS SYSTEM DISORDERS

Alterations in sleep-wake function vary depending on the anatomical location of the neurological lesion. For example, patients with Arnold Chiari malformation type II are likely to exhibit an SRBD as a result of altered development of the medulla, whereas those with mental retardation may exhibit cortical dysfunction in the form of excessive awakening and daytime or nighttime seizures. The severity of alterations in sleep-wake function also depends on the extent of the lesion and whether it is static or progressive. Medications used to treat neurological disorders may also impact sleep architecture (e.g., benzodiazepines and barbiturates used in the treatment of seizures) may suppress REM sleep. Fragmentation of sleep is in general quite common in children with neurological disorders. Treatment of the sleep-wake disorder may enhance the quality of life in these children.

Cerebral Palsy

Cerebral palsy is defined as a static insult to the developing central nervous system, which may have been acquired prenatally, perinatally, or during early infancy. The incidence of cerebral palsy is approximately 1.2 per 1000 live births. Risk factor for its development include birth weight less than 2500 g, maternal mental retardation, breech presentation, and multiple congenital anomalies. The disorder leads to abnormalities of muscle tone, resting posture, muscle coordination, and joints. Cerebral palsy may be of the spastic, dyskinetic, or hypotonic types. Spastic cerebral palsy can be further subcategorized into the hemiplegic, diplegic, or quadriplegic types.

Although their exact incidence has not been established, sleep-related breathing problems are commonly encountered in cerebral palsy. The upper airway may collapse as a consequence of neuromuscular incoordination, associated craniofacial abnormalities, or adenotonsillar hypertrophy. Children with spastic cerebral palsy may exhibit daytime irritability, fragmented sleep with frequent nighttime awakenings, and nocturnal oxygen desaturation.[73] The inability to compensate for the disordered breathing by changes in body position makes obstructive sleep apnea an especially dangerous condition in this group of patients. Patients may also be at risk for gastroesophageal reflux and aspiration pneumonia. Periodic change of body position at night by the caretaker might be indicated. Coexisting seizures also tend to increase the fragmentation of night sleep. Treating epilepsy with phenytoin should perhaps be avoided in children with cerebral palsy owing to its tendency to cause adenotonsillar hypertrophy from lymphoid hyperplasia. Circadian rhythm abnormalities and sleep-related epilepsy (see later) might also complicate sleep-wake function in cerebral palsy.

Patients with severe brain damage in the perinatal period can show highly disorganized or undifferentiated sleep with absence of sleep spindles and lack of a clear distinction between REM and NREM sleep or, for that matter, between sleep and wakefulness. This is presumably related to severe dysfunction of the brainstem, thalamic, and forebrain structures that regulate REM and NREM sleep.

Mental Retardation

Patients with severe mental retardation may show a prolonged initial REM latency and suppression in the proportion of time spent in REM sleep. Decreased REMs and spindle density, as well as the presence of "undifferentiated" sleep, correlate with low levels of intelligence. Piazza et al[74] used a momentary time-sampling observational method to study sleep in 51 young people of 3–21 years of age in an inpatient unit. When compared with control subjects, they found delays in sleep onset, reduced total sleep time, excessive night awakenings, and early awakenings. Depression may coexist with mild mental retardation, in which case it may lead to early morning awakenings. Physical problems such as obstructive sleep apnea and seizures may also coexist. It is imperative to exclude these problems before attempting cognitive and behavioral treatments such as ignoring the child, use of reward systems,[75] or short-term hypnotics therapy.

Down Syndrome

Patients with Down syndrome have very complicated sleep problems. First, they may develop obstructive sleep apnea as a consequence of macroglossia, midface hypoplasia, and hypotonic upper airway musculature.[76] Obesity may coexist. Superimposed on this may be an element of chronic hypoventilation from hypotonic intercostal and diaphragmatic musculature that leads to CO_2 retention. Sleep architecture is frequently abnormal, with decreased sleep efficiency, increased arousals, and suppression of slow wave and REM sleep. Behavioral problems in Down syndrome may in part be linked to these abnormalities of respiratory function. Central sleep apnea has also been observed in Down syndrome. Once nocturnal polysomnography has confirmed obstructive sleep apnea or obstructive hypoventilation, a stepwise management approach is recommended; adenotonsilectomy is usually the first step, followed a few weeks later by repeat clinical and polysomnographic assessment and a trial of CPAP or BiPAP pressure device for any residual obstructive sleep apnea. Behavioral conditioning techniques may be needed for facilitating patient compliance with the mask and positive pressure ventilation.

Autistic Spectrum Disorders

Autism, Asperger syndrome, and pervasive developmental disorder not otherwise specified are categorized under the broad term *autistic spectrum disorders* (ASD). About two thirds of children with ASD have sleep-wake problems.[77] In a sleep diary study, Richdale and Prior[78] found that those with higher intelligence quotient had more severe sleep problems. Anxiety and obsessive compulsive behaviors frequent children with ASD and may underlie at least some of the sleep initiation and maintenance difficulties in this population. Polygraphic studies have shown prolonged initial sleep latency, decreased sleep efficiency, and low early morning awakening–spontaneous arousal thresholds.

Rett Syndrome

Rett syndrome is an X-linked dominant neurodegenerative disorder that occurs exclusively in girls and is characterized by progressive speech and cognitive regression during early childhood in association with stereotypical hand-wringing movement and gait apraxia that seem to develop after apparent normal psychomotor development during the first 6–18 months of life. In about 80% of cases of Rett syndrome, there is a mutation in the methyl-CpG-binding protein 2 gene, which regulates transcriptional silencing and epigenetic control of methylated deoxyribose nucleic acid. It is located on Xq28. The Rett trait is lethal to males. Sekul and Percy[79] have reported that more than 80% of children with Rett syndrome develop sleep problems, with irregular sleep-wake rhythms being the most common. Nighttime screaming, crying, and episodes of laughter have also been reported.[80] As a group, patients with Rett syndrome may show less sleep at night and increased sleep fragmentation, combined with carryover sleepiness into the daytime. There have been anecdotal reports of the success of melatonin in ameliorating this sleep disruption, but a recent meta-analysis did not find any significant improvement in sleep latency in insomnia secondary to neurological disorders (including Rett syndrome).[81] Melatonin is not regulated by the FDA. Bioequivalence between various preparations has therefore not been established. The hypnotic dose is generally 0.5–5 mg around bedtime. Side effects are usually minor, consisting of headache, dizziness, or nausea. Patients with Rett syndrome also display episodic hyperventilation during wakefulness, but respiratory rate and rhythm remain unaffected during sleep. About 50% of patients manifest partial or generalized seizures, some of which may include apnea as an ictal manifestation.

Prader Willi Syndrome (PWS)

This syndrome of congenital hypotonia, hypogonadism, and cognitive dysfunction is linked to microdeletion of the paternally contributed region of chromosome 15q11.2-q13. During the neonatal period and infancy, patients manifest severe hypotonia, anorexia, and feeding difficulties to the point of requiring nasogastric tube feedings. Around early childhood, however, there is an increase in appetite to the point that it becomes almost voracious and may become associated with morbid obesity. Patients with PWS have elevated *ghrelin* levels that might contribute to their hyperphagia.[82] Although it was not evaluated systematically, mild to moderate daytime sleepiness is common in PWS, affecting perhaps half the subjects. It may be associated with sleep-onset REM periods on the multiple sleep latency test (MSLT).[83] Results of nocturnal polysomnography are highly variable. Sleep apnea seems to be relatively infrequent,[83] however, and does not contribute to the daytime sleepiness, which appears to be a consequence of hypothalamic dysfunction. In support of this is the finding of low levels of cerebrospinal fluid (CSF) hypocretin-1 in a patient with combined PWS and Kleine Levin syndrome who was tested at the time of increased sleepiness.[84]

Lately, it has been recognized that treatment of PWS with growth hormone promotes an increase in muscle mass and motor development. The long-term impact of growth hormone therapy on PWS has not been clearly established. These patients need to be monitored closely in a multidisciplinary setting for the development of obstructive apnea secondary to growth hormone therapy, as deaths have occurred in patients receiving growth hormone, although the exact underlying mechanism has not been established.[85]

Blindness

Blindness associated with loss of light perception resulting from lesions of the eye or the optic nerves and chiasm can disrupt circadian rhythms and neuroendocrine functions. The resultant "free running" sleep-wake cycles are longer than 24.2 hours and tend to shift toward progressively later times around the clock.[86] The basis for the free running cycles seems to be dysregulation of the secretion of melatonin, which is a light-sensitive hormone secreted by the pineal gland and dependent on an intact retinohypothalamic pathway. In sighted individuals, melatonin has low secretion during the daytime, but its plasma levels rise immediately before bedtime and during the night. It has important sleep induction and maintenance properties. Children with severe retinopathy of prematurity, congenital bilateral glaucoma, septo-optic dysplasia, or severe bilateral optic neuritis may show "free running" or non–24-hour sleep-wake cycles owing to lack of light perception. In a questionnaire survey of 77 blind children ranging in age from 3 to 18 years and sighted control subjects, Leger et al[87] found that 17% of blind children reported sleeping less than 7 hours at night compared with 2.6% of control subjects, with blind children awakening much earlier in the morning and also exhibiting increased daytime sleepiness. In turn, daytime sleepiness may affect attention, concentration, and the behavior of blind children. The presence of multiple associated physical and neurological handicaps can further complicate management. Administration of 0.5–5 mg of melatonin 1 hour before bedtime seems to facilitate sleep onset, increase total sleep time, and reduce awake time at night.[86] Manipulation of nonphotic *zeitgebers* such as food, music, physical activity, and exercise might also be of some value in establishing sleep-wake schedules when circadian rhythms are disrupted in blind children.

Arnold Chiari Malformations

Myelomeningocele is invariably associated with Arnold Chiari malformation type II, in which a segment of the medulla and the fourth ventricle is congenitally located below the foramen magnum (generally in the cervical spine 1–2 level), along with hydrocephalus. About two thirds of children with myelomeningocele and Chiari type II malformation give a history of breathing disturbance, one third of whom also have moderate to severe abnormalities. Mechanisms underlying the sleep-related breathing disturbance in these patients include developmental malformations involving brainstem respiratory areas, mechanical compression of the brainstem from a small posterior fossa combined with hydrocephalus, unilateral or bilateral vocal cord paralysis, obstructive apnea from adenotonsillar hypertrophy, or collapse of the hypotonic upper airway, as well as hypoventilation from obesity and intercostal muscle paralysis. A combination of multiple factors might also be operative. Those who have cervicomedullary junction compression from the tonsillar descent through the foramen magnum need urgent surgical decompression of the posterior fossa. Patients with thoracic or thoracolumbar myelomeningocele and those with pulmonary function abnormalities from kyphoscoliosis can show persistent sleep-related breathing abnormalities such as obstructive sleep apnea, obstructive hypoventilation, and central sleep apnea. Respiratory abnormalities in these patients are generally more severe during REM sleep than during NREM sleep. The management is complicated and at times discouraging. Adenotonsillectomy is the initial step in managing obstructive sleep apnea, but patients may ultimately end up needing CPAP or BiPAP breathing devices. Counseling of pre-teens about the importance of avoiding obesity at the time of adolescence is also recommended.

Combined obstructive and central sleep apnea may also be infrequently seen in Chiari type I malformation, characterized by descent of the cerebellar tonsils below the plane of the foramen magnum, with a normally positioned fourth ventricle and no hydrocephalus. There have been isolated case reports of obstructive sleep apnea in such patients responding successfully to posterior fossa decompression.[88]

The Relationship Between Sleep and Epilepsy

The onset of sleep may be associated with increased interictal spiking, as well as an increased propensity to clinical seizures.[89] Frontal and temporal lobe seizures are especially prone to occur during sleep and to exhibit secondary generalization. In some children with new onset of seizures, interictal epileptiform discharges are observed only during sleep. Nocturnal seizures are most likely to occur during stage II, followed by stage I, stage III, and stage IV of NREM sleep, in that order, and are least likely to occur during REM sleep. The syndrome of *electrical status epilepticus during slow wave sleep* is characterized by continuous spike and wave discharges during 85% or more of nocturnal NREM sleep, along with cognitive and behavioral regression. *Landau Kleffner syndrome* is characterized by regression in language function (auditory verbal agnosia) in association with continuous epileptiform activity during both REM and NREM sleep. Sleep deprivation itself is associated with activation of seizures. Patterns of epileptiform abnormality are influenced considerably by sleep. For example, the 3 per second spike and wave complexes of absence seizures are replaced by single spike and waves or by polyspike and wave complexes in sleep. The hypsarrhythmia of infantile spasms is replaced during sleep by brief periods of generalized voltage attenuation. Patients with Lennox Gastaut syndrome may manifest long runs of generalized spike and wave discharges.

Conversely, seizures also suppress REM sleep, with a corresponding increase in slow wave sleep. This effect may persist for as long as 24 hours after the seizure event. Frequent nocturnal seizures tend to disrupt sleep, with an increased number of arousals. Patients with Lennox Gastaut syndrome may exhibit tonic seizures during sleep. Sleep disorders can also adversely affect seizure control. Patients with obstructive sleep apnea may manifest poor seizure control, which is improved after obstructive sleep apnea is corrected.[90] In some instances, daytime somnolence is mistaken for being a side effect of antiepileptic therapy when in fact it may be the consequence of an underlying sleep disorder.

Antiepileptic drugs in general lead to stabilization of sleep, with a decrease in the amount of sleep fragmentation. Phenobarbital therapy is associated with suppression in the proportion of time spent in REM sleep and increased stage III and IV NREM sleep (slow wave sleep). Phenytoin and carbamazepine increase slow wave sleep at the expense of stage I–II NREM sleep. Benzodiazepines increase slow wave sleep at the expense of stage REM sleep. Lamotrigine therapy is associated with an increase in the proportion of time spent in REM sleep, with fewer sleep stage shifts. Felbamate is associated with insomnia in about 9% of subjects.

DAYTIME SLEEPINESS: GENERAL COMMENTS

Excessive daytime sleepiness is a common, disabling, and frequently under-recognized symptom of diverse etiology.[91] Many of the underlying disorders are treatable. Questionnaire surveys indicate a prevalence of 4–14%. Most teenagers are chronically sleep deprived and report sleep lengths of 6.5–7.5 hours in contrast to the optimum amount of sleep necessary to maintain adequate daytime alertness of around 8.5–9.5 hours.

Consequences

Teenagers are sleep deprived for a variety of reasons: there is a physiologic delay in onset of sleep to 10:30 or 11:00 P.M., coupled with social pressures to stay up late. When this is juxtaposed with the early high school start times of 7:25–7:40 A.M., it is easy to understand why teenagers are chronically in a state of sleep debt. Sleepiness interferes with the consolidation of short-term memory into long-term memory. It also leads to loss of "affect control" as a result of disinhibition of the prefrontal cortex, with resultant mood swings, inattentiveness, and impulsivity. Motor speed and judgment also become impaired, resulting in an increased propensity for accidents. Common etiologies for daytime sleepiness are listed in Table 11-6. Multiple factors may sometimes coexist.

TABLE 11-6 ■ Common Etiologies for Daytime Sleepiness in Childhood

Insufficient sleep at night (e.g., from abnormal sleep hygiene)

Delayed sleep phase syndrome

Drugs (over-the-counter/prescription; hypnotics and sedatives/ psychostimulants)

Depression

Obstructive hypoventilation

Upper airway resistance syndrome

Narcolepsy

Idiopathic hypersomnia

Kleine-Levin syndrome

Restless legs syndrome

Post-traumatic hypersomnia

Assessment

The sleep history, sleep logs, wrist actigraphy, and nocturnal polysomnography, which may or may not be followed by the multiple sleep latency test, are the most commonly administered tests. The laboratory tests are tailored to the specific underlying problem. Psychological assessment and child psychiatry consultation are also helpful when there are emotional and behavioral issues. Histocompatibility antigen typing and CSF hypocretin analysis may be indicated in selected patients with narcolepsy-cataplexy. Narcolepsy is characterized by relatively early appearance of REM sleep on the nocturnal polysomnogram, sleep fragmentation, periodic leg movements, marked shortening of the daytime mean sleep latency on the MSLT (<5 minutes in contrast to a normal value of 16–18 minutes), and associated two or more sleep-onset REM periods.

PERIODIC HYPERSOMNIA

Also termed *Kleine-Levin syndrome*, periodic hypersomnia is generally seen in adolescents. It has a male predominance. Patients develop periods of hypersomnolence lasting 1–2 weeks, during which they may sleep 18–20 hours a day and also manifest cognitive and mood disturbances in association with compulsive hyperphagia and hypersexual behavior, with intervening 2–4 months of normal alertness and behavior.[92] Incomplete forms of the syndrome have also been recognized. The hyperphagia may be in the form of binge eating and can actually be associated with a 2- to 5-kg increase in body weight. Nocturnal polysomnography during the sleepy periods shows decreased sleep efficiency, shortened REM latency, and decreased percentage of time spent in stages III–IV of NREM sleep and in REM sleep. The MSLT shows moderately shortened mean sleep latency in the 5- to 10-minute range, but without the two or more sleep onset REM periods (SOREMPs) that are typical for narcolepsy. The periodic hypersomnia gradually subsides over 2–3 years or evolves into classic depression, thus raising the issue of whether the disorder is a variant of depression. A disturbance of hypothalamic-thalamic function has been hypothesized but not established. The association of Kleine-Levin syndrome with histocompatibility antigen DQB1*0201, the occasional precipitation following systemic infections, and the relapsing and remitting nature also raise the possibility of an underlying autoimmune disturbance.[93] There is no satisfactory treatment, although lithium has been reported to be effective in case reports.

NARCOLEPSY

Chronic daytime sleepiness, fragmented night sleep, and superimposition of REM sleep phenomena onto wakefulness in the form of hypnagogic hallucinations (vivid dreams at sleep onset), sleep paralysis, and cataplexy (sudden loss of skeletal muscle tone in response to emotional triggers such as laughter, fright, or surprise) are the characteristic clinical features of narcolepsy. The incidence in the United States is 1.37 per 100,000 persons per year (1.72 for men and 1.05 for women).[94] It is highest in the second and third decades, followed by a gradual decline thereafter. The prevalence is approximately 56 persons per 100,000 persons.[93] Although the age of onset is generally in the latter half of the first or second decade, rare cases with onset of extreme sleepiness and cataplexy in early childhood have also been reported.[95] The daytime sleepiness may be overlooked by parents, school teachers, and physicians alike. Sleepy children may be mistaken for being "lazy" and frequently also exhibit mood swings and inattentiveness. Cataplexy is present in about two thirds of patients. Cataplexy attacks generally last for a few minutes and are characterized by muscle atonia, or absence of muscle stretch reflexes in the face of fully preserved consciousness. Because cataplexy can be subtle, the examiner might need to ask leading questions about sudden muscle weakness in the lower extremities, neck, or trunk that are triggered by laughter, fright, excitement, or anger. Children below the age of 7 or 8 years are unable to provide a reliable history of hypnagogic hallucinations or sleep paralysis. Narcolepsy may be variably associated with a periodic limb movement disorder.[96] Patients exhibit less circadian drive–dependent alertness during the daytime and also less sleepiness at night.[97] In rare instances *secondary narcolepsy* may develop in patients after closed head injury, primary brain tumors, lymphomas, and encephalitis.[98]

The presence of the histocompatibility antigen DQB1*0602 in close to 100% of persons with narcolepsy, compared with a 12–32% prevalence in the general population, indicates a genetic susceptibility, which per se, however, is insufficient to precipitate the clinical syndrome; monozygotic twins have remained discordant for the development of narcolepsy.[99] In genetically susceptible individuals, however, acquired life stresses such as minor head injury, systemic illnesses such as infectious mononucleosis, and bereavement may trigger narcolepsy and have been reported to occur in about two thirds of subjects—the *"two-hit"* hypothesis.

The key pathophysiological event in narcolepsy-cataplexy is *hypocretin* deficiency.[100] Hypocretin (orexin) is a peptide that is produced by neurons of the dorsolateral hypothalamus. Hypocretins 1 and 2 (synonymous with orexins A and B) are peptides that are synthesized from preprohypocretin. Although the hypocretin type 1 receptor has affinity for only hypocretin 1, the hypocretin type 2 receptor has affinity for both type 1 and 2 ligands. Hypocretin neurons have widespread projections to the forebrain and brainstem. Hypocretin promotes alertness and increases motor activity and basal metabolic rate. Of significance is the autopsy finding in human narcolepsy by Thannickal et al[101] of an 85–95% reduction in the number of hypocretin neurons in the hypothalamus, whereas melanin-concentrating hormone neurons that are intermingled with hypocretin neurons remained unaffected, thus suggesting a targeted neurodegenerative process. It is hypothesized that degeneration of the hypocretin-producing cells of the hypothalamus (perhaps linked to HLA DQB1*0602 by mechanisms yet unknown) provokes a decrease in forebrain noradrenergic activation, which in turn decreases alertness. A corresponding decrease of noradrenergic activity in the brainstem leads to disinhibition of brainstem cholinergic systems, thus triggering cataplexy and other phenomena of REM sleep such as hypnagogic hallucinations and sleep paralysis.

The decrease in hypocretin secretion-1 that is characteristic of human narcolepsy-cataplexy is reflected in the CSF. Using a radioimmunoassay, Nishino et al[100] found that the mean level of hypocretin 1 in healthy control subjects was 280.3 ± 33.0 pg/mL; in neurological control subjects, 260.5 ± 37.1 pg/mL, whereas in those with narcolepsy, hypocretin 1 was either undetectable or below 100 pg/mL. Low to absent levels were found in 32 of 38 narcolepsy patients, who were all also HLA DQB10*0602–positive. Narcolepsy patients who were HLA DQB1*0602 antigen–negative tended to have normal to high CSF hypocretin 1 levels. In another study of narcolepsy with cataplexy, narcolepsy without cataplexy, and idiopathic hypersomnia, Kanbayashi et al[102] found that their

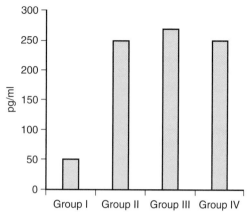

FIGURE 11-5 ■ A comparison of CSF hypocretin 1 levels in HLA DQB1*0602–positive narcolepsy-cataplexy (group I) with narcolepsy-cataplexy that is HLA DQB1*0602 negative (group II), narcolepsy without cataplexy (group III), and idiopathic hypersomnia (group IV). (Data adapted from Kanbayashi T, Inoue Y, Chiba S, et al: CSF hypocretin-1 (Orexin A) concentrations in narcolepsy with and without cataplexy and idiopathic hypersomnia. J Sleep Res 11:91–93, 2002.)

9 CSF hypocretin- deficient patients were all HLA DQB1*0602–positive, including 3 preadolescents. In contrast, patients with narcolepsy *without* cataplexy and idiopathic hypersomnia showed normal CSF hypocretin levels (Figure 11-5). The application of CSF hypocretin-1 assays in the diagnosis of narcolepsy-cataplexy is an important development. It is most useful when a HLA DQB1*0602–positive patient with suspected narcolepsy-cataplexy is already receiving central nervous stimulants on initial presentation, and when discontinuation of these medications for the purpose of obtaining polysomnography and a MSLT is inconvenient or impractical.

A combined battery of nocturnal polysomnogram and MSLT is still the most widely used method to diagnose narcolepsy. The nocturnal polysomnogram shows increased arousals, decreased initial REM latency of less than 70 minutes (time from sleep onset to onset of the first REM sleep epoch; normal value in teenagers is around 140 minutes), and absence of any other significant sleep pathology such as obstructive sleep apnea. The MSLT, which is obtained on the day after the nocturnal polysomnogram, shows sleep onset on each of the four nap opportunities within 5 minutes of "lights out," whereas the reference value is approximately 16–18 minutes. Sleep-onset REM periods are also seen during at least 2 of 4 nap opportunities. Because narcolepsy is a lifelong condition, the diagnostic test results need to be clear and unambiguous.

Management requires a combination of lifestyle changes and pharmacotherapy.[103] A planned

TABLE 11-7 ■ Pharmacotherapy of Childhood Narcolepsy

Target Symptom	Drug	Dose Range
Sleepiness	Methylphenidate, regular or extended release	20–60 mg/day in two divided doses
	Dextroamphetamine, regular or extended release	10–30 mg/day in two divided doses
	Modafinil	100–400 mg in two divided doses
Cataplexy	Protriptyline	5–10 mg in two divided doses
	Chlorimipramine	25–50 mg once a day
	Sodium oxybate	3–6 g at night, in two divided doses given 2–3 hours apart
Emotional/behavioral problems	Fluoxetine	10–30 mg /day
	Sertraline	25–50 mg/day
Periodic limb movement disorder/restless legs syndrome	Clonazepam	0.5–1.0 mg at bedtime
	Pramipexole	0.125–0.25 mg at bedtime
	Ropinirole	0.25–0.5 mg at bedtime

daytime nap of 20 to 30 minutes at school and another one in the afternoon after returning home may enhance alertness. The patient should observe regular sleep onset and morning wake-up times, avoid alcohol, and exercise regularly. To minimize the risk of accidents, the patient should stay away from sharp, moving objects. Driving should be avoided until daytime alertness has been brought into the normal or near-normal range. Drugs commonly used in the management of narcolepsy are listed in Table 11-7. Besides the use of selective serotonin reuptake inhibitors, emotional and behavioral problems that commonly accompany childhood narcolepsy may require supportive psychotherapy.

DELAYED SLEEP PHASE SYNDROME

This is a circadian rhythm disturbance related to dysfunction of the suprachiasmatic nucleus, which serves as the circadian timekeeper. The disorder typically has onset in adolescence, with a male predominance. Patients have a constitutional difficulty in preponing (phase advancing) sleep and can only fall asleep at progressively later times at night (Figure 11-6). They are frequently misdiagnosed as having severe insomnia. Sleep onset time may be delayed past midnight into the early morning hours.[104] Once asleep and if allowed to sleep uninterrupted, patients show normal sleep quantity and quality. Most patients are generally obligated to wake up by 6:30 or 7:00 A.M. to attend school, which results in chronic sleep deprivation and sleep "drunkenness" on awakening, along with variable degrees of depression and personality changes. In an unsuccessful attempt to regulate their sleep-wake function, delayed sleep phase syndrome (DSPS) patients may abuse stimulants during the daytime and hypnotics at night. Polymorphisms in the Per3 gene and the HLA DR$_1$ allele have been

associated with increased predisposition to DSPS. There is increased clustering of DSPS within some families. DSPS must be differentiated from school avoidance seen in adolescents with delinquent and antisocial behavior, as these individuals may be able to fall asleep at an earlier hour at night in the controlled sleep laboratory setting. Maintenance of sleep logs and wrist actigraphy for 1–2 weeks is helpful in establishing the diagnosis of DSPS.

"Bright light" therapy is helpful in advancing the sleep onset time. It consists of the provision of 8000–10,000 lux of bright light via a "light box" for 20–30 minutes immediately on awakening in the morning. The light box is kept at a distance of 18–24 inches from the face. It leads to a gradual advancement (shifting back) of the sleep onset time at night. Bright light therapy may be combined with administration of melatonin about 5–5.5 hours before the required bedtime in a dose of 0.5–1 mg. Diminished exposure to light in the evening such as by using sunglasses may facilitate earlier sleep onset at night. The other therapeutic option is one of gradually *delaying* bedtimes by 3–4 hours per day until it becomes synchronized with socially acceptable sleep-wake times, and then adhering to this schedule (chronotherapy). Over time, however, all DSPS patients are at risk for drifting forward to progressively later bedtimes. Daytime stimulants such as modafinil (100–400 mg/day in two divided doses) may also improve the level of daytime alertness. The physician may also need to write a letter to the school, requesting a late mid-morning school start time on medical grounds.

IRREGULAR SLEEP-WAKE RHYTHMS

Patients with this disorder have a hard trying to fall asleep at a scheduled time of the night and may manifest three or more major periods of sleep over 24 hours.

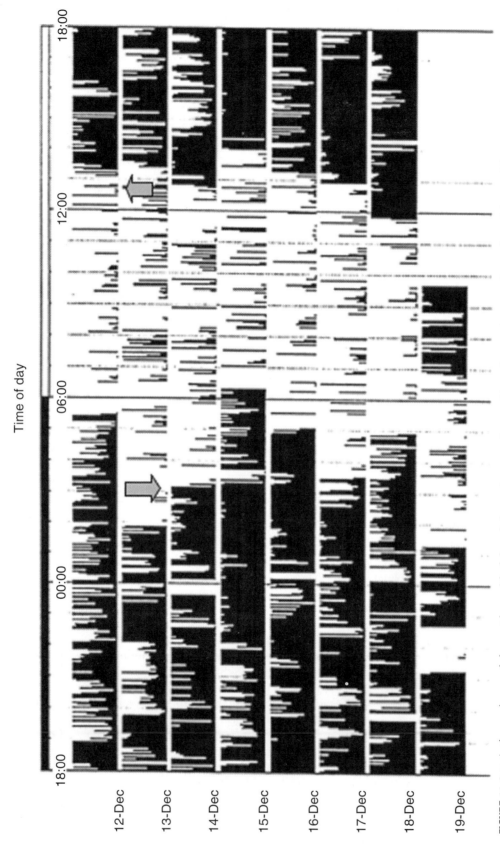

FIGURE 11-6 ■ Actigram in an adolescent boy with delayed sleep phase syndrome. Note the persistence of muscle activity until late at night, correlating with remaining awake. Sleep onset time is indicated by the down arrow. The early afternoon waking up time is indicated by the up arrow (Data from Kotagal S. Sleep disorders in childhood. Neurol Clin 21:1–21, 2003.)

Total sleep time over the 24-hour period, however, is essentially within normal limits. A lack of exposure to orienting light (sunlight) during the daytime may play a causative role. The diagnosis can be established on the basis of sleep logs and actigraphy, with the latter demonstrating multiple irregular periods of sleep onset. Treatment consists of providing a consistent bedtime and morning wakeup time and exposure to bright light immediately on awakening.

PARASOMNIAS

Events that occur at the sleep-wake interface or during sleep without altering sleep quality and quantity are termed *parasomnias*. Common sleep-wake transition disorders include hypnic starts and rhythmic movement disorder (head banging, head rolling, or body rocking).

Common NREM sleep parasomnias include confusional arousals, sleep terrors, and sleep walking.[105] NREM parasomnias are characteristically due to an attempted partial arousal from stage III and IV of NREM sleep and are thus likely to occur in the first third of night sleep. Sleep deprivation, fever, underlying obstructive sleep apnea, periodic limb movement disorder, or RLS may increase susceptibility to NREM parasomnias by enhancing arousal. There is often a strong familial predisposition to NREM parasomnias. In contrast to sleep walking and sleep terrors, patients with confusional arousals exhibit little in the way of motor and autonomic activity. Sweating, flushing of the face, and agitation, however, are quite common in sleep terrors and sleep walking. The duration of NREM parasomnias may be anywhere from 5 to 30 minutes. Although the sleep of the entire family is disrupted by severe NREM parasomnias, the patient generally has no recollection of these events on awaking the following morning.

Nightmares, terrifying hypnagogic hallucinations, and REM sleep behavior disorder are common parasomnias of REM sleep. By virtue of being a REM sleep phenomenon, they are generally likely to occur in the early morning hours.

Sleep enuresis is a parasomnia that may occur in all stages of sleep. It is categorized as primary when the patient has not achieved bladder control during sleep for 6 or more months, and secondary when the patient has relapse of bedwetting after having achieved bladder control for 6 months or more. Primary enuresis is present in about 30% of 4-year-olds, 10% of 6-year-olds, 5% of 10-year-olds, and 1–2% of 18-year-olds.[106] Primary enuresis may be associated with ADHD, living in disorganized families, insufficient rise in nocturnal vasopressin secretion, elevated arousal threshold, relatively uninhibited detrusor muscle contractility, or a decreased bladder capacity. Secondary enuresis may accompany a significant psychosocial stress, chronic constipation, severe obstructive sleep apnea, and urinary tract infections. Sleep enuresis is in general more common in boys than girls by a 3:2 ratio. There is a high incidence of other family members with a similar disturbance in the case of primary nocturnal enuresis. The management of sleep enuresis consists of correcting the underlying disturbance if possible, limiting fluid intake after dinner time, use of alarm-conditioning devices applied to the skin that sense moisture in the underwear and trigger arousal, or use of medications. Imipramine, 10–25 mg at bedtime, may decrease detrusor muscle contractility, but there may be relapse of enuresis after an initial favorable response. The vasopressin analog, desmopressin given in a dose of 0.1 to 0.2 mg at bedtime, is also effective.

The history is of key importance in diagnosing parasomnias. A home videotape that has captured the event can also be very helpful. Nocturnal polysomnography with synchronized video monitoring and a 16-channel EEG montage may be needed if the diagnosis cannot be established on the basis of history. Nocturnal seizures can sometimes be mistaken for parasomnias, but seizures tend to occur most often during stages I and II of NREM sleep and are thus distributed randomly through the night sleep. They are also much shorter than parasomnias, typically 30 seconds to 5 minutes, and may occur on multiple occasions during the same night. In contrast to parasomnias, patients with seizures are often tired on awakening in the morning.

Most parasomnias are benign events and do not warrant specific therapy. Environmental safety issues such as placing deadbolts on the doors and removing sharp objects from the customary path should be considered for sleep walking. Underlying obstructive sleep apnea and RLS should be treated when they are suspected as triggers for NREM parasomnias. The technique of "anticipatory awakening" has been tried in patients with NREM parasomnias with mixed results. The parent awakens the child about 15–20 minutes before the usual time of occurrence of the NREM parasomnia, generally by wiping the face with a wet washcloth in an effort to shift the patient into a lighter stage of sleep and thus abort the event. Parents prefer this technique because it is nonpharmacological. Its effectiveness, however, remains questionable and has not been evaluated in a large series of subjects. Clonazepam, 0.05–0.1 mg at bedtime, is effective in preventing most parasomnias, probably by virtue of consolidating sleep.

(Adapted in part with permission from Kotagal S: Sleep disorders in children. Neurol Clin 21[4]:961–981, 2003.)

REFERENCES

1. Berger H: Uber das Elektroenkephalogram des Menschen. J Psychol Neurol (Lpz) 40:160–179, 1930.
2. Loomis A, Harvey EN, Hobart GA: Cerebral states during sleep as studied by human brain potentials. J Exp Psychol 21:127, 1937.
3. Aserinsky E, Kleitman N: Regularly occurring periods of eye motility and concomitant phenomena during sleep. Science 118:273–274, 1953.
4. Dement WC, Kleitman N: Cyclic variations of EEG during sleep and their relation to eye movements, body motility and dreaming. Electroencephlaogr Clin Neurophysiol 9:67390, 1957.
5. Roffwarg H, Muzio J, Dement WC: Ontogenetic development of the human sleep-dream cycle. Science 152:604, 1966.
6. Dreyfus-Brisac C: Ontogenesis of sleep in human prematures after 32 weeks of conceptional age. Dev Psychobiol 3:91–121, 1970.
7. Parmelee AH, Stern E: Development of states in infants. In Clemente CD, Purpura DP, Mayer FE (eds): *Sleep and the Maturing Nervous System*. New York, Academic Press, 1972, pp 199–215.
8. Shaywitz BA, Finkelstein J, Hellman L, et al: Growth hormone in newborn infants during sleep-wake periods. Pediatrics 48:103–109, 1971.
9. Guilleminault C, Eldridge FL, Simmons FB, et al: Sleep apnea in eight children. Pediatrics 58:23–30, 1976.
10. Weitzman ED, Czeisler CA, Coleman RM, et al: Delayed sleep phase syndrome. A chronobiological disorder with sleep-onset insomnia. Arch Gen Psychiatry 38:737–746, 1981.
11. American Academy of Pediatrics: Task Force on Infant Sleep Position and SIDS. Pediatrics 89:1120–1126, 1992.
12. Kemp JS, Kowalski RM, Burch PM, et al: Unintentional suffocation by rebreathing: a death scene and physiologic investigation of a possible cause of sudden infant death. J Pediatr 122:874–880, 1993.
13. Anders TF, Emde R, Parmelee AH: *A Manual of Standardized Terminology, Techniques and Criteria for Scoring the States of Sleep and Wakefulness in Newborn Infants*. Los Angeles, Brain Information Service, UCLA, 1971.
14. Guilleminault C, Soquet M: Sleep states and related pathology. In Guilleminault C, Korobkin R (eds): *Advances in Neonatal Neurology, Volume I*. New York, Spectrum Publications, 1979, pp 225–247.
15. de Lecea L, Kilduff TS, Peyron C, et al: The hypocretins: hypothalamus-specific peptides with neuroexcitatory activity. Proc Natl Acad Sci 95:322–327, 1998.
16. Lin L, Faraco J, Li R, et al: The sleep disorder, canine narcolepsy, is caused by a mutation in the hypocretin (orexin) receptor 2 gene. Cell 98:365–376, 1999.
17. Nishino S, Ripley B, Overeem S, et al: Hypocretin (orexin) deficiency in human narcolepsy. Lancet 355:39–40, 2000.
18. Thannickal TC, Moore RY, Nienhuis R, et al: Reduced number of hypocretin neurons in human narcolepsy. Neuron 27:469–474, 2000.
19. Beebe DW, Gozal D: Obstructive sleep apnea and the prefrontal cortex: towards a comprehensive model linking nocturnal upper airway obstruction to daytime cognitive and behavioral deficits. J Sleep Res 11:1–16, 2002.
20. Curzi-Dascalova L: Development of the sleep and autonomic control in premature and full-term newborn infants (French). Arch Pediatr 2:255–262, 1995.
21. Moriette G, Van Reempts P, Moore M, et al: The effect of rebreathing CO_2 on ventilation and diaphragmatic electromyography in newborn infants. Resp Physiol 62:387–397, 1985.
22. Peers C: Hypoxic regulation of ion channel function and expression. Exp Physiol 87:413–422, 2002.
23. Tankersley CG, Haxhiu MA, Gauda EB: Differential CO_2 induced c-fos gene expression in the nucleus tractus solitarii of inbred mouse strains. J Appl Physiol 92:1277–1284, 2001.
24. Lahiri S: Carotid body chemoreception: mechanisms and dynamic protection against apnea. Biol Neonate 65:134–139, 1994.
25. Wennergren G, Hertzberg T, Milerad J, et al: Hypoxia reinforces laryngeal reflex bradycardia in infants. Acta Pediatr Scand 78:11–17, 1989.
26. Cheung P, Barrington KJ, Finer NN, et al: Early childhood neurodevelopment in very low birth weight infants with pre-discharge apnea. Pediatr Pulmonol 27:14–20, 1999.
27. Rigato H: Breathing and sleep in preterm infants. In Loughlin GM, Carrol JL, Marcus CL (eds): *Sleep and Breathing in Children. A Developmental Approach*. New York, Marcel Dekker, 2000, pp 495–523.
28. Ohtake PJ, Simakajornboon N, Fehniger MD, et al: D-aspartate receptor expression in the tractus solatarii and maturation of hypoxic ventilatory response in the rat. Am J Respir Crit Care 162:1140–1147, 2000.
29. Phillis JW, Scislo TJ, O'Leary DS: Purines and the nucleus tractus solitarius: effects on cardiovascular and respiratory functions. Clin Exp Pharmacol Physiol 24:738–742, 1997.
30. Hannam S, Ingram DM, Milner AD: A possible role for the Hering-Breuer deflation reflex in apnea of prematurity. J Pediatr 132:35–39, 1998.
31. Poets CF: Gastroesophageal reflux: a critical review of its role in preterm infants. Pediatrics 113:e128–e132, 2004.
32. Henderson-Smart D, Steer P: Doxapram treatment for apnea in preterm infants. Cochrane Database Sys Rev 18(4):CD 00007, 2004.
33. O'Donnell J, Finer NN, Rich W, et al: Role of L-carnitine in apnea of prematurity: a randomized, controlled trial. Pediatrics 109:622–626, 2002.
34. Willinger M, James LS, Catz C: Defining the sudden infant death syndrome (SIDS): deliberations of an expert panel convened by the National Institute of Child Health and Human Development. Pediatr Pathol 11:677–684, 1991.
35. McCullogh K, Dahl S, Johnson S, et al: Prevalence of SIDS risk factors: before and after the "Back To Sleep" campaign in North Dakota Caucasian and American Indian infants. Clin Pediatr 39:403–410, 2000.

36. McMartin KI, Platt MS, Hackman R, et al: Lung tissue concentrations of nicotine in sudden infant death syndrome (SIDS). J Pediatr 140:205–209, 2002.

37. Hafstrom O, Milerad J, Sundell HW: Prenatal nicotine exposure blunts the cardiorespiratory response to hypoxia in lambs. Am J Respir Crit Care Med 166:1544–1549, 2002.

38. Schoendorf KC, Kiely JL: Relationship of sudden infant death syndrome to maternal smoking during and after pregnancy. Pediatrics 90:905–908, 1992.

39. Anderson HR, Cooke DG: Passive smoking and the sudden infant death syndrome: review of the epidemiologic evidence. Thorax 52:1003–1009, 1997.

40. Horne RS, Osborne A, Vitkovic J, et al: Arousal from sleep is impaired following an infection. Early Hum Dev 66:89–100, 2002.

41. Filiano JJ, Kinney HC: A perspective on neuropathological findings in victims of the sudden infant death syndrome: the triple-risk model. Biol Neonate 65:194–197, 1994.

42. Kinney HC, Filiano JJ, White WF: Medullary serotonergic network deficiency in the sudden infant death syndrome: review of a 15-year study of a single dataset. J Neuropathol Exp Neurol 60:228–247, 2001.

43. Ackerman MJ, Siu BL, Sturner WQ, et al: Postmortem molecular analysis of SCN5A defects in SIDS. JAMA 286:2264–2269, 2001.

44. Katz ES, McGrath S, Marcus CL: Late-onset central hypoventilation with hypothalamic dysfunction: a distinct clinical syndrome. Pediatr Pulmonol 29:63–68, 2000.

45. Weese-Mayer DE, Berry-Kravis EM, Marazita ML: In pursuit (and discovery) of a genetic basis for congenital central hypoventilation syndrome. Respir Physiol Neurobiol 149:73–82, 2005.

46. Trochet D, Hong SJ, Lim JK, et al: Molecular consequences of PHOX2B frameshift and alanine expansion mutations leading to autonomic dysfunction. Hum Mol Genet 14:3697–3708, 2005.

47. Sritippayawan S, Hamutcu R, Kun SS, et al: Mother-daughter transmission of congenital central hypoventilation syndrome. Crit Care Med 16:367–369, 2002.

48. National Institutes of Health: Infantile Apnea and Home Monitoring. Report of a consensus development conference, 1987. NIH Publication No. 87-2905. Washington, DC, US Department of Health and Human Services, Public Health Service, 1987.

49. Wennergren G, Milerad J, Lagercrantz H, et al: The epidemiology of sudden infant death syndrome and attacks of lifelessness in Sweden. Acta Pediatr Scand 76:898–906, 1987.

50. Samuels MP: Apparent life-threatening events. Pathogenesis and management. In Loughlin GM, Carroll JL, Marcus CL (eds): *Sleep and Breathing in Children. A Developmental Approach.* New York, Marcel Dekker, 2000, pp 423–441.

51. Wolf SM: Negative outcomes of infant home apnea monitoring. JAMA 286:304, 2001.

52. Oren J, Kelly D, Shannon DC: Identification of a high risk group for sudden infant death syndrome among infants who were resuscitated for sleep apnea. Pediatrics 77:495–499, 1986.

53. Walters AS, Pichhietti DL, Ehrenberg DL, et al: Restless legs syndrome in childhood and adolescence. Pediatr Neurol 11:241–245, 1994.

54. Allen RP, Pichhietti D, Hening WA, et al: Restless legs syndrome: diagnostic criteria, special considerations, and epidemiology. A report from the restless legs syndrome diagnosis and epidemiology workshop at the National Institutes of Health. Sleep Med 4:101–119, 2003.

55. Kotagal S, Silber MH: Childhood-onset restless legs syndrome. Ann Neurol 56:803–807, 2004.

56. Chervin RD, Dillon JE, Basetti C, et al: Symptoms of sleep disorders, inattention and hyperactivity in children. Sleep 20:1185–1192, 1997.

57. Winkelmann J, Muller-Myhsok B, Wittchen HU, et al: Complex segregation analysis of restless legs syndrome provides evidence for an autosomal dominant mode of inheritance in early age at onset families. Ann Neurol 52:297–302, 2002.

58. Simakajornboon N, Gozal D, Vlasic V, et al: Periodic limb movements and iron status in children. Sleep 26:735–738, 2003.

59. Rajaram SS, Walters AS, England SJ, et al: Some children with growing pains may actually have restless legs syndrome. Sleep 27:767–773, 2004.

60. Tan E-K, Ondo W: Restless legs syndrome: clinical features and treatment. Am J Med Sci 319:397–403, 2000.

61. Walters AS, Mandelbaum DE, Lewin DS, et al: Dopaminergic therapy in children with restless legs/periodic limb movements in sleep and ADHD. Pediatr Neurol 22:182–186, 2000.

62. Garcia-Borreguero D, Larossa O, de la Llave Y, et al: Treatment of restless legs syndrome with gabapentin. A double-blind, cross-over study. Neurology 59:1573–1579, 2002.

63. Kryger MH, Otake K, Foerester J: Low body stores of iron and restless legs syndrome: a correctable cause of insomnia in adolescents and teenagers. Sleep Med 3:127–132, 2002.

64. American Academy of Sleep Medicine. *International Classification of Sleep Disorders, Diagnostic and Coding Manual,* 2nd ed. Westchester, IL, American Academy of Sleep Medicine, 2005, pp 56–59.

65. Goodwin JL, Babar SI, Kaemingk KL, et al: Symptoms related to sleep disordered breathing in White and Hispanic children. The Tucson Children's Assessment of Sleep Apnea Study. Chest 124:196–203, 2003.

66. Rosen CL, Larkin EK, Kirchner L, et al: Prevalence and risk factors for sleep disordered breathing in 8 to 11 year old children: association with race and prematurity. J Pediatr 142:383–389, 2003.

67. O'Brien LM, Mervis CB, Holbrook CR, et al: Neurobehavioral implications of habitual snoring in children. Pediatrics 114:44–49, 2004.

68. Marcus CL, McColley SA, Carroll JL, et al: Upper airway collapsibility in children with obstructive sleep apnea syndrome. J Applied Physiol 77:918–924, 1994.

69. Beebe DW, Wells CT, Jeffries J, et al: Neuropsychological effects of pediatric obstructive sleep apnea. J Int Neuropsychol Soc 10:962–975, 2004.

70. O'Brien L, et al: Normal values for pediatric polysomnography. Sleep 27:A97, 2004.

71. Bandla HPR, Gozal D: Dynamic changes in EEG spectra during obstructive apnea in children. Pediatric Pulmonol 29:359–365, 2000.

72. O'Brien LM, Mervis CB, Holbrook CR, et al: Neurobehavioral correlates of sleep disordered breathing in children. J Sleep Res 13:165–172, 2004.

73. Kotagal S: Sleep abnormalities and cerebral palsy. In Stores G, Wiggs L (eds): *Sleep Disturbance in Children and Adolescents with Disorders of Development: Its Significance and Management.* London, Mac Keith Press, 2001, pp 107–110.

74. Piazza CC, Miller WW, Kahng SW: Sleep patterns in children and young adults with mental retardation and severe behavior disorders. Dev Med Child Neurol 38:335–344, 1996.

75. Owens JL, France KG, Wiggs L: Behavioral and cognitive-behavioral interventions for sleep disorders in infants and children: a review. Sleep Med Rev 3:281–302, 1999.

76. de Miguel-Diez J, Villa-Asensi JR, Alvarez Sala JL: Prevalence of sleep disordered breathing in children with Down syndrome: polygraphic findings in 108 children. Sleep 26:1006–1009, 2003.

77. Wiggs L, Stores G: Sleep patterns and sleep disorders in children with autistic spectrum disorders: insights using parent report and actigraphy. Dev Med Child Neurol 46:372–380, 2004.

78. Richdale AL, Prior MR: The sleep/wake rhythm in children with autism. Eur Child Adolesc Psychiatry 4:175–186, 1995.

79. Sekul E, Percy A: Rett syndrome: clinical features, genetic considerations, and the search for a biological marker. Curr Neurol 12:173–200, 1992.

80. Roane HS, Piazza CC: Sleep disorders and Rett syndrome. In Stores G, Wiggs L (eds): *Sleep Disturbance in Children and Adolescents with Disorders of Development: Its Significance and Management.* London, Mac Keith Press, 2001, pp 83–86.

81. Buscemi N, Vandermeer B, Hooton N, et al: Efficacy and safety of exogenous melatonin for secondary sleep disorders and sleep disorders accompanying sleep restriction: meta-analysis. BMJ 332:385–393, 2006.

82. Haqq AM, Stadler DD, Rosenfeld RG, et al: Circulating ghrelin levels are suppressed by meals and octreotide therapy in children with Prader-Willi syndrome. J Clin Endocrinol Metab 88:3573–3576, 2003.

83. Manni R, Politini L, Nobili L, et al: Hypersomnia in the Prader Willi syndrome: clinical-electrophysiological features and underlying factors. Clin Neurophysiol 112:800–805, 2001.

84. Dauvilliers Y, Baumann CR, Carlander B, et al: CSF hypocretin-1 levels in narcolepsy, Kleine-Levin syndrome, and other hypersomnias and neurological conditions. J Neurol Neurosurg Psychiatry 74:1667–1673, 2003.

85. Eiholzer U: Deaths in children with Prader-Willi syndrome. A contribution to the debate about the safety of growth hormone treatment in children with PWS. Horm Res 63:33–39, 2005.

86. Sack RL, Brandes RW, Kendall AR, et al: Entrainment of free-running circadian rhythms by melatonin in blind people. N Engl J Med 343:1070–1077, 2000.

87. Leger D, Prevot E, Philip P, et al: Sleep disorders in children with blindness. Ann Neurol 46:648–651, 1999.

88. Zolty P, Sanders M, Pollack IF: Chiari malformation and sleep-disordered breathing: a review of diagnostic and management issues. Sleep 23:637–643, 2000.

89. Dinner DS: Effect of sleep n epilepsy. J Clin Neurophysiol 19:504–513, 2002.

90. Malow BA, Weatherwax KJ, Chervin RD, et al: Identification and treatment of obstructive sleep apnea in adults and children with epilepsy: a prospective pilot study. Sleep Med 4:509–515, 2003.

91. Millman RP: Excessive sleepiness in adolescents and young adults: causes, consequences, and treatment strategies. Pediatrics 115:1774–1786, 2005.

92. Papacostas SS, Hadjivasilis V: The Kleine Levin syndrome. Report of a case and review of the literature. Eur Psychiatry 15:231–235, 2000.

93. Dauvilliers Y, Mayer G, Lecendreux M, et al: Kleine Levin syndrome. An autoimmune hypothesis based on clinical and genetic analyses. Neurology 59:1739–1745, 2002.

94. Silber MH, Krahn LE, Olson EJ, et al: Epidemiology of narcolepsy in Olmstead County, Minnesota. Sleep 25:197–202, 2002.

95. Challamel MJ, Mazzola ME, Nevsimalova S, et al: Narcolepsy in children. Sleep 17(suppl 1):17S:17–20, 1994.

96. Wittig R, Zorri F, Roehrs T, et al: Narcolepsy in a 7 year old. J Pediatr 102:725–727, 1983.

97. Broughton R, Krupa S, Boucher B, et al: Impaired circadian waking arousal in narcolepsy-cataplexy. Sleep Res Online 1:159–165, 1998.

98. Autret A, Lucas F, Henry-Lebras F, de Toffol B: Symptomatic narcolepsies. Sleep 17(suppl 1):21–24, 1994.

99. Lin L, Hungs M, Mignot E: Narcolepsy and the HLA region. J Neuroimmunol 117:9–20, 2001.

100. Nishino S, Ripley B, Overeem S, et al: Low cerebrospinal fluid hypocretin (orexin) and altered energy homeostasis in human narcolepsy. Ann Neurol 50:381–388, 2001.

101. Thannickal TC, Moore RY, Nienhuis R, et al: Reduced number of hypocretin neurons in human narcolepsy. Neuron 27:469–474, 2000.

102. Kanbayashi T, Inoue Y, Chiba S, et al: CSF hypocretin-1 (Orexin A) concentrations in narcolepsy with and without cataplexy and idiopathic hypersomnia. J Sleep Res 11:91–93, 2002.

103. Littner M, Johnson SF, McCall WV, et al: Practice parameters for the treatment of narcolepsy: an update for 2000. Sleep 24:451–466, 2001.

104. Wyatt JK: Delayed sleep phase syndrome: pathophysiology and treatment options. Sleep 27:1195–1203, 2004.

105. Sheldon SH: Parasomnias in childhood. Pediatr Clin North Am 51:69–88, 2004.

106. Sleep enuresis. In *American Academy of Sleep Medicine.* International Classification of Sleep Disorders. *Diagnostic and Coding Manual*, 2nd ed. American Academy of Sleep Medicine, Westchester, IL, 2005, pp 162–164.

Practice Exams for the Adventurous

Normal Sleep Patterns

VLAD DIMITRIU ▪ TERI J. BARKOUKIS

Questions

1. Sleep deprivation has been shown to induce significant changes in various metabolic and endocrine functions. Which of the following alterations frequently accompanies sleep restriction?
   A. Increased plasma levels of leptin
   B. Increased plasma levels of ghrelin
   C. Increased cortisol level in the early morning
   D. Increased appetite for protein-rich foods

2. Sleep loss causes a wide array of physiologic changes. Among them are neurological changes, sometimes subtle enough that they can be detected only by an electroencephalogram (EEG). The EEG changes commonly associated with sleep loss are:
   A. Increase in alpha waves, proportionally with sleep loss duration
   B. Decrease in beta activity
   C. Increase in delta and theta patterns in a waking EEG
   D. Delta waves are present only during sleep.

3. Sleep research has shown that there are differences in sleep behavior between males and females. Which of the following is true regarding the gender differences in sleep patterns?
   A. During infancy there is less sleep and more awakenings in boys than in girls.
   B. During childhood there are more severe sleep problems in girls than in boys.
   C. During adolescence there are earlier wake-up times in boys than in girls on weekdays.
   D. During adulthood there are more awakenings in women than in men.

4. A complex phenomenon, the menstrual cycle involves not only rhythmic changes in the female reproductive hormone levels but also sleep and behavioral alterations that are reflected in subtle physiologic processes. Which of the following statements are true regarding the influence of the menstrual cycle on sleep and circadian rhythm?

A. There is an increase in REM duration and in REM latency in the luteal phase.
B. Subjective sleep disturbances are maximal during the mid-follicular phase.
C. Sleep onset latency and sleep efficiency are profoundly affected by the phases of the menstrual cycle.
D. Young women complain more about sleep disturbances around menses than at any other time.

5. Changes in body metabolism observed during sleep reflect more than a mere decrease in muscular and digestive activities. They are rather the result of a complex interaction between environmental stimuli and innate physiologic mechanisms. Which one of the following statements is true?
   A. The mean drop in metabolism between sleep and wakefulness is 50%.
   B. Metabolic differences between waking and sleep increase at lower temperatures.
   C. There is an increase in metabolism in stages 3 and 4 compared with stage REM.
   D. The brain metabolism decreases during stage REM compared with NREM sleep.

6. Different types of infections can interfere with sleep, altering the concentrations of various sleep stages. The effects of a viral infection on sleep are best described by:
   A. Great stimulation of REM sleep and inhibition of NREM sleep
   B. The molecule through which viruses influence sleep is double-stranded RNA.
   C. Large loads of influenza virus are required to induce sleep modification.
   D. High doses of interferon-α (IFN-α) inhibit both stage REM and NREM sleep.

7. The preoptic area of the central nervous system (CNS) has a pivotal role in sleep promotion and is involved in integration of the thermoregulatory responses during sleep. How do the warm-sensitive

neurons (WSN) of the preoptic area influence sleep architecture?
A. They increase REM sleep in sustained sleep.
B. They decrease delta activity in sleep.
C. They suppress the arousal-promoting neurons.
D. They inhibit sleep onset.

8. Chronic sleep deprivation induces numerous physiologic, neurocognitive, and behavioral changes. Which of the following has been found to be true in normal humans when they are chronically sleep deprived?
A. The alpha activity decreases proportionally with sleep loss.
B. Antibody production is increased by sleep deprivation.
C. Mortality risk from cardiovascular causes increase, as predicted by a decrease in C-reactive protein.
D. Sleeping less than 9 hours per night increases the risk for coronary events.

9. Recovery sleep is needed to reverse the effects of sleep deprivation and to normalize the EEG changes that occur after sleep loss. Human studies in this field have shown that:
A. An amount of sleep equal to the sleep loss duration is required to recover.
B. Young adults recover faster from sleep loss on the initial recovery night compared with their older counterparts.
C. On the first recovery night there is a large decrease in slow wave sleep.
D. Older subjects have daytime multiple sleep latency test (MSLT) values at baseline after one night of sleep loss and a single night of recovery sleep.

10. The interaction between bacteria and a host induces predictable sleep responses. These responses are mediated by an amplification of the physiologic sleep-regulatory biochemical cascade. Regarding the sleep effects induced by bacterial challenge, it is true that:
A. The timing of sleep responses is independent of the type of bacteria involved.
B. Reduction of the bacterial population in the intestine is associated with an increase in sleep.
C. Bacterial replication inside the host is not necessary for the sleep effects to occur.
D. Muramyl peptides are somnogenic only at toxic doses.

11. Cardiac rhythm is locally generated but is influenced by the neurohumoral activity of the CNS.

Dynamic fluctuations in blood pressure, heart rate, and coronary blood flow occur during various stages of sleep. How are these parameters affected by the sleep stages?
A. During NREM sleep, absence of intrinsic variability of the heart rate heralds an underlying heart condition.
B. The blood pressure surges commonly observed during NREM sleep predispose to coronary events.
C. In tonic REM sleep there are abrupt accelerations in heart rate, preceded by a drop in arterial blood pressure.
D. A gradual decrease in blood pressure and heart rate has been noted during phasic REM sleep.

12. Breathing is mostly an automatic process, controlled by neurological centers situated in the brainstem. Knowing the localization of the breathing centers is important not only for understanding breathing control during sleep but also for designing and conducting the most needed future research in the field. Regarding the respiratory centers of the pons and medulla, it is true that:
A. The pneumotaxic center is located in the caudal region of the pons.
B. The apneustic center is located in the dorsolateral area of the pons.
C. The nucleus tractus solitaris is located in the ventral respiratory group of the medulla and controls both inhalation and exhalation.
D. The dorsal respiratory group of the medulla contains the nucleus parabrachial and Kölliker-Fuse nuclei.

13. The relationship between the immune system and sleep is bidirectional. On one hand, sleep stages are accompanied by specific changes in immune cell populations and by increased secretions of certain cytokines. On the other hand, various interleukins can promote or inhibit sleep. The cytokines that have been found to decrease NREM sleep are:
A. IL-1, TNF-α, and IFN-α
B. IL-2, IL-6, and IL-1β
C. IL-8, IL-18, and IFN-α
D. IL-10, IL-13, and TGF-β

14. Studies have shown that sleep is able to heighten prior learning. Motor and perceptual skills, word associations, and emotional memories can all be enhanced by sleep. Which association between sleep and improvement of a specific skill is accurate?

A. Paired word associate learning correlates with late-night sleep.

B. Emotionally declarative memory improvement depends on early-night sleep.

C. Visual perception task improvement correlates with late-night REM and early-night, slow wave sleep.

D. Improvement in motor skills is associated with amounts of late-night REM sleep and early-night, slow wave sleep.

15. The circulation in peripheral vascular beds during sleep is regulated by a combination of autonomic and local stimuli. The following statement is true about the effect of sleep stages on blood flow and vasomotor tone in peripheral organs:

A. There is a significant decrease in splanchnic circulation during sleep.

B. In skeletal muscles, the blood flow in red fibers increases during REM sleep and decreases in NREM sleep.

C. The renal blood flow is strongly stage dependent, decreasing in NREM sleep.

D. Coronary blood flow decreases significantly in NREM sleep and increases in REM sleep.

16. By integrating reports about dreams with sleep stages recorded simultaneously, researchers have been able to correlate specific dream traits with different stages and to better define the role of each stage in enhancing memory during sleep. It is true that:

A. REM sleep has been implicated in simple memorization of word pair lists.

B. REM sleep helps facilitate consolidation of perceptual and emotional memories.

C. In NREM sleep, dreams are more narrative and have frequent fictive movements.

D. In NREM sleep, dreams are more hallucinatory and emotional.

17. As the name states, REM sleep was initially identified by its characteristic movements of the eyes during sleep. Since then, many other particularities of REM sleep have been defined, both in humans and animals. Can you identify the correct statement among the following?

A. There are periods of irregularity in respiratory and heart rates during phasic REM.

B. During tonic REM the skeletal muscles contract in phase with the eye muscles.

C. Thermoregulation increases in REM sleep, mostly during the tonic phase of REM sleep.

D. Dreams rarely occur during REM sleep, and they are rarely remembered after awakening.

18. Control of the sleep-wake cycle involves diverse CNS structures and multiple neurotransmitters. The role of some of the neural formations and neurotransmitters has been established in animal models by electrophysiological and neuroanatomical studies. It is true that:

A. The predominant neurotransmitter in the reticular activating system is glycine.

B. Sleep-inducing neurons are concentrated in the lower brainstem reticular formation.

C. Lesions of the preoptic area of the forebrain will induce a state of continuous sleep.

D. Loss of sleep can be produced by destroying the posterior hypothalamus.

19. The relationship between gastrointestinal motility and sleep is one of interdependence. Not only does the state of sleep affect the gastrointestinal motor and secretory functions, but also stimuli originating in the digestive system can influence various aspects of sleep physiology. From animal and human experiments it is known that:

A. Administration of cholecytokinin decreases REM sleep.

B. Low levels of intestinal stimulation decrease both NREM and REM sleep duration.

C. A solid meal before bedtime can decrease sleep onset latency more than a liquid meal.

D. Electrical stimulation of the stomach will stimulate neurons in the auditory cortex.

20. Studies in normal rats have shown that total sleep deprivation produced a progressively fatal syndrome, with multiple physiologic components. Which of the following statements regarding changes in rats under these circumstances is true?

A. Some rats died while others adapted by decreasing their energy expenditure.

B. The body temperature decreased constantly during the experiment.

C. The animals lost weight in proportion with their decrease in food intake.

D. A decrease in plasma thyroxine and an increase in plasma norepinephrine were recorded.

21. The sleep architecture can be influenced by many exogenous substances, which interact with receptors from the CNS, either directly or through their metabolites. One well-known effect of such a substance is:

A. Ingestion of alcohol right before sleep increases stage REM early in the night.

B. Benzodiazepine ingestion dramatically decreases REM sleep.

C. Tricyclic antidepressant ingestion can suppress REM sleep.

D. Regular marijuana users have a long-term suppression of stage REM.

22. Control of breathing during the waking state is dually controlled via automatic and behavioral mechanisms, both voluntary and reflexive. The voluntary control of breathing, such as singing or speaking, and reflexive control, such as sneezing or coughing, is known to originate in the cerebral cortex. Automatic control of breathing predominates during sleep and originates in the respiratory neurons of the brainstem. The center for generation of respiratory rhythm is the:
A. Pneumotaxic center in the dorsal lateral pons
B. Ventrolateral area of the nucleus of the tractus solitarius
C. Motor cortex projections through the descending corticospinal tract.
D. All respiratory neurons in the pons and medulla generate respiratory rhythm.
E. Bilateral ventral respiratory group of the medulla.

23. A 22-year-old healthy college student is part of a sleep deprivation study. He has stayed up for about 72 hours and is really struggling with sleepiness. He is finally reconnected to the EEG and told that he may sleep for his initial sleep period. On this first recovery night of sleep, which change would you expect in his sleep architecture?
A. Normal sleep architecture should occur regardless of sleep deprivation because he is healthy.
B. Slow wave sleep will be increased over baseline values.
C. REM sleep will be increased because of preferential REM recovery.
D. Stage 1 will be increased because of an increase in NREM sleep.
E. Stage 2 will be increased over baseline values.

24. Figure 12-1 is an epoch from a recent polysomnogram that the technologist brought for your review. This particular stage of sleep is known to occur in which one of the following situations?
A. Within the first 20 minutes of sleep in a 5-year-old child
B. The predominant sleep stage on the first recovery night after 72 hours of sleep loss
C. Usually seen at the onset of sleep on two naps during an MSLT in recurrent hypersomnia

D. Can be seen during a 20-minute nap at 11 A.M. in a traveler seven time zones eastward

25. Healthy normal subjects have been known to increase gastric acid secretion with meal stimulation during the wake period. There is a basal gastric acid secretion with an underlying circadian-linked rhythm that tends to peak during which 4-hour segment of a 24-hour day?
A. Between 6 A.M. and 10 A.M.
B. Between 10 P.M. and 2 A.M.
C. Between 12 P.M. and 4 P.M.
D. Between 4 P.M. and 8 P.M.

26. The epoch in Figure 12-2 was taken from a patient during a polysomnogram. The next two epochs are similar in appearance. The previous epoch showed about 80% alpha patterns seen in the four EEG leads. Lights were out at 10:30 P.M. A new technologist is currently being trained in scoring and has a question about this particular patient's sleep latency. You explain:
A. This patient only had a microsleep followed by a snoring-related awakening that cannot be used to define this patient's sleep latency.
B. This patient has alpha waves and cannot be scored as the sleep latency until the first of three consecutive epochs show no alpha waves.
C. This patient has 30% concentration of alpha waves yet there cannot be more than 20% on three consecutive epochs and is not this patient's sleep latency.
D. This is the first of three consecutive epochs of <50% alpha waves and defines this patient's sleep latency.

27. Minute ventilation has been shown to change from wake to sleep. This subsequent change in the normal sleeping individual results in:
A. No change in PaO_2
B. Elevation in $PaCO_2$
C. Elevation in PaO_2
D. Elevation in oxygen saturation

28. Growth hormone (GH) has been shown to be secreted by the pituitary after stimulation of hypothalamic growth hormone-releasing hormone (GHRH). The secretory patterns show slight differences between men and women, with men having the largest pulse soon after sleep onset, whereas women have both daytime and sleep-related growth hormone pulses. In addition to GHRH, growth hormone pulses are stimulated by one of the following:

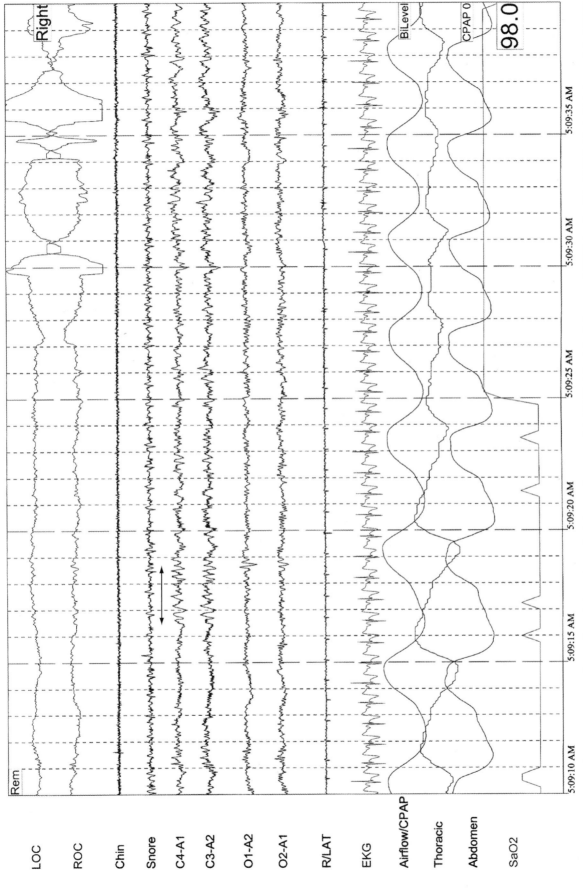

FIGURE 12-1 ■ Question 24. 30-second epoch. LOC/ROC, Left/right oculogram; C4-A1/C3-A2, right/left central EEG leads; O1-A2/O2-A1, left/right occipital EEG leads; R/LAT, right/left leg EMG; "Airflow/CPAP" is only an airflow channel with no continuous positive airway pressure (CPAP) on this patient.

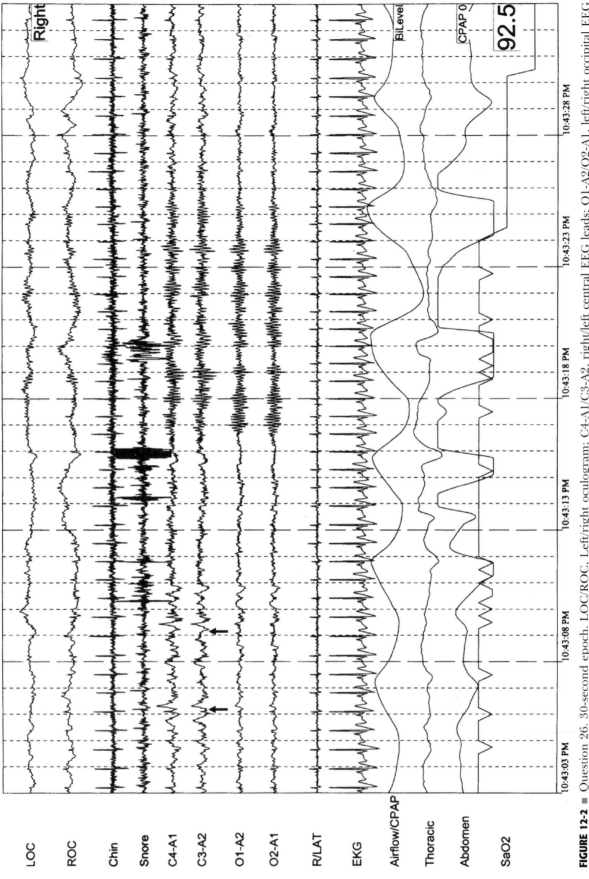

FIGURE 12-2 ■ Question 26. 30-second epoch. LOC/ROC, Left/right oculogram; C4-A1/C3-A2, right/left central EEG leads; O1-A2/O2-A1, left/right occipital EEG leads; R/LAT, right/left leg EMG; "Airflow/CPAP" is only an airflow channel with no CPAP on this patient.

A. The acylated form of the peptide, ghrelin
B. Acute total sleep deprivation
C. During work in a night-shift worker
D. Somatostatin

29. The stage of sleep shown in Figure 12-3 in this 65-year-old individual is known to:
    A. Decline significantly with age equally in men and women
    B. Increase with age in men more than women
    C. Not change with the aging process in men or women
    D. Show no significant decline in elderly women compared with men

30. One of your office staff is a 27-year-old man who is an athlete with experience in triathlons. His most recent interest has been in learning how to climb. He has been working with a local sport enthusiast who is an experienced climber and has trained well. He is physically fit and has always been a normal sleeper at his sea-level home. He leaves for his first mountain climbing experience next week to 4500 meters at the summit. What could he expect during initial sleep at this elevation?
    A. Decreased slow wave sleep, decreased total sleep time, and no periodic breathing
    B. Decreased stage 1 sleep, normal total sleep time, and increased stage REM sleep
    C. Decreased slow wave sleep, increased sleep fragmentation, and probable periodic breathing
    D. Increased stage 2 sleep, increased sleep fragmentation, and normal total sleep time

31. The suprachiasmatic nucleus is known to regulate sleep-wake rhythms in mammals and is the location of the CLOCK gene, which regulates the mammal's intrinsic circadian rhythm. Necessary for photic entrainment of the circadian pacemaker is the retinohypothalamic tract (RHT). RHT terminals release which of the following?
    A. Neurotransmitter: glutamate and two co-transmitters: substance P and pituitary adenyl-cyclase-activating peptide (PACAP)
    B. Neurotransmitter: glycine and one co-transmitter: substance P
    C. Neurotransmitter: histamine and one co-transmitter: PACAP
    D. Neurotransmitter: aspartate and two co-transmitters: substance P and PACAP

32. You plan to study the circadian rhythm of subjects over an imposed 28-hour day that includes one sleep-wake cycle to study the underlying circadian rhythm over 7 days. As a research tool, you will use the *forced desynchrony protocol* and would expect:
    A. 6 sleep-wake cycles; 6 body-temperature circadian cycles
    B. 7 sleep-wake cycles; 7 body-temperature circadian cycles
    C. 6 sleep-wake cycles, 7 body-temperature circadian cycles
    D. 6 sleep-wake cycles, 5 body-temperature circadian cycles

33. In a healthy patient with a normal sleep-wake cycle, prolactin is secreted according to which one of the following?
    A. Levels are maximal at 4:00 P.M. and increase only modestly in the second half of sleep.
    B. No levels are detected during the waking period and only secrete evenly throughout sleep.
    C. Levels have a diurnal variation at sleep onset and on morning awakening.
    D. Levels are minimal at noon and increase dramatically soon after sleep onset.

34. A 20-year-old patient was being evaluated as part of a research study and used as a normal control. The epochs in Figures 12-4 and 12-5 represent two segments of 30 seconds each of his sleep time. This particular stage of sleep is known to occur in this age group at what percentage of the normal sleep time?
    A. 10–20%
    B. 45–55%
    C. 65–75%
    D. 25–35%

35. In the healthy elderly subject, the aging effect on sleep is known to:
    A. Cause a phase delay
    B. Develop more awakenings from sleep
    C. Markedly reduce stage REM
    D. Increase delta wave amplitude

36. Understanding sleep regulation, you know that a 35-year-old subject who purposely stays awake for 30 hours will:
    A. Have a buildup of the homeostatic process (process S)
    B. Demonstrate a reduction of waking theta wave activity
    C. Have a circadian rhythm (process C) that is dependent on the length of this wake period
    D. Have no effect on either process C or process S

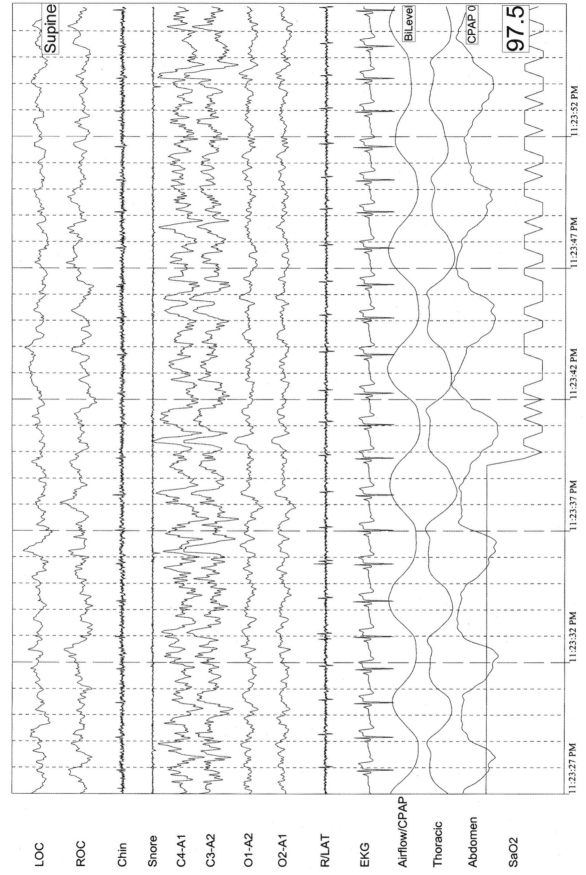

FIGURE 12-3 ■ Question 29. 30-second epoch. LOC/ROC, Left/right oculogram; C4-A1/C3-A2, right/left cetral EEG leads; O1-A2/O2-A1, left/right occipital EEG leads; R/LAT, right/left leg EMG; "Airflow/CPAP" is only an airflow channel with no CPAP on this patient.

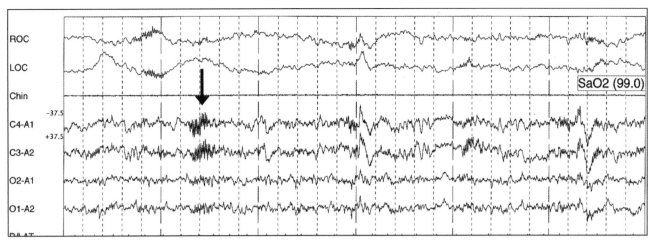

FIGURE 12-4 ■ Question 34. 30-second epoch. LOC/ROC, Left/right oculogram; C4-A1/C3-A2, right/left central EEG leads; O1-A2/O2-A1, left/right occipital EEG leads; each vertical dotted line represents 1 second.

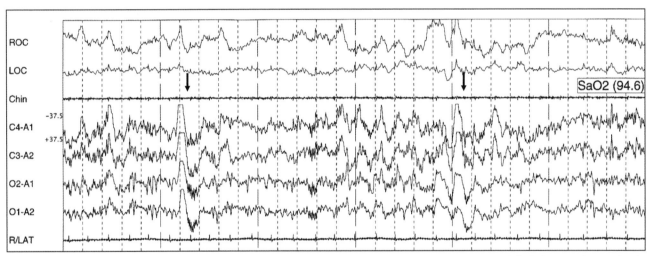

FIGURE 12-5 ■ Question 34. 30-second epoch. LOC/ROC, Left/right oculogram; C4-A1/C3-A2, right/left central EEG leads; O1-A2/O2-A1, left/right occipital EEG leads (C4-A1; C3-A2; O2-A1; O1-A2); left ocular; 30-second epoch; each vertical dotted line represents 1 second.

37. In the normal sleeping individual, the upper airway dilator group of muscles has been described to:
   A. Contribute to upper airway resistance only during NREM sleep
   B. Contribute to upper airway resistance in both NREM and REM sleep, which increases in REM sleep
   C. Have no effect on upper airway resistance in normal control subjects but only sleep apnea patients
   D. Contribute to upper airway resistance only during REM sleep

38. A 23-year-old college student curbsides you after your sleep lecture about concerns over an exacerbation in the last semester of sudden "whole body jerks" at sleep onset that has occurred occasionally in class, which has caused some embarrassment. Over the last semester there has been a huge load of classes with an erratic sleep pattern and insufficient sleep. This student has always been healthy, and this has never occurred before. Your advice is to:
   A. Be evaluated in a 24-hour video monitoring EEG laboratory
   B. Be evaluated for calcium, magnesium, and phosphorous
   C. Be evaluated by the campus counseling department for stress management
   D. Reassure the student that this is not pathological given the circumstances and no further evaluation is necessary

39. Upper airway motor neurons have been studied extensively to evaluate and better understand the pathophysiological mechanisms of obstructive sleep apnea syndrome. Normal mechanisms of the upper airway motor neurons have which primary receptors mediating the excitatory effects of 5-hydroxytryptamine (5-HT) and norepinephrine (NE)?
    A. Type alpha$_1$β-adrenergic and type 5-HT$_2$α receptors
    B. Type adenosine α$_1$ and type 5-HT$_3$ receptors
    C. Type 5-HT$_2$α receptors and type HCRT2 receptors
    D. Type adenosine A$_1$ and type HCRT1 receptors

40. Thyroid-stimulating hormone (TSH) is known to:
    A. Rise during stage 1 sleep with a secondary peak in stage 3 sleep
    B. Have a diurnal rhythm with sleep inhibition
    C. Be suppressed during the wake period in a sleep-deprived state
    D. Peak just before sleep onset with a rapid drop on morning awakening

41. The anterior pituitary secretes adrenocorticotropic hormone (ACTH), which triggers cortisol secretion from the adrenocortex. In normal human physiology, cortisol has been discovered to:
    A. Have the first nocturnal pulse between 10:00 and 11:00 P.M.
    B. Have the first nocturnal pulse between 2:00 and 3:00 A.M.
    C. Have the first nocturnal pulse between 12:00 and 1:00 A.M.
    D. There are no nocturnal but only daytime pulses of cortisol.

42. Hypocretins (orexins) are synthesized in the hypothalamus, modulate glutamate release along with other amino acid transmitters, and are released at high levels during:
    A. The late-afternoon waking period and not during sleep
    B. Both NREM and REM sleep
    C. Both the waking period and stage REM sleep
    D. The early-morning waking period and NREM sleep

43. Chronobiology research over many years has led to the development of terminology that needs to be understood. All of the following terms are correctly defined *except:*
    A. *Phase shift* means the displacement forward or backward in time of the intrinsic circadian rhythm of an organism as a result of heat that is 5 degrees centigrade above the core body temperature.
    B. *Entrainment* means behavior timed by circadian clocks that adjust their periods each cycle to conform to the difference between the organism's intrinsic day and the environmental day and become synchronized to daily phases.
    C. *Zeitgeber* means environmental time cues such as sunlight, alarm clocks, or social interaction that helps trigger an organism to entrainment to a 24-hour cycle.
    D. *Phase response curve* (PRC) for light is a graphical representation of the entrainment process whereby a plot is made of the magnitude of the phase shift that occurs versus the circadian phase or time of light presentation.

44. Sleep spindles characteristic of stage 2 sleep are cyclical oscillations generated from which one of the following?
    A. Thalamic reticular nucleus
    B. Parabrachial nucleus
    C. Ventral medulla
    D. Solitary tract nucleus

45. Physiology of normal sleep and breathing has been extensively studied to help in the understanding of sleep breathing disorders. There are multiple neurotransmitters that have certain functions involved in breathing regulation. Which of the following statements is true?
    A. Glycine inhibits the hyperpolarization of lumbar motoneurons that leads to intercostal muscle atonia in REM sleep.
    B. Serotonin (5-HT) acts as a ventilatory inhibitor.
    C. Inhibitors of catecholamines increase respiratory activity.
    D. Gamma-aminobutyric acid (GABA) causes ventilatory stimulation.

46. Melatonin is a circadian-linked hormone secreted by the pineal gland. After release into the circulation, the maximal plasma levels tend to occur around:
    A. 3:00 to 4:00 A.M.
    B. 3:00 to 4:00 P.M.
    C. 9:00 to 10:00 P.M.
    D. 9:00 to 10:00 A.M.

47. Early research studied the electrical activity of the brain during sleep versus the awake state. A section of the lower medulla called the *encèphale isolè* was known to:
    A. Show a deep sleep EEG pattern without wakefulness
    B. Allow the study of cortical electrical activity affected by visual and olfactory impulses

C. Show a waking pattern on the EEG without any sleep periods

D. Allow the study of cortical electrical activity affected by vestibular, visual, auditory, olfactory, and musculocutaneous impulses

48. Sleep regulation has been studied extensively in animals. One interesting facet of mammal and bird research has been the discovery of unihemispheric sleep. It is now known that:

A. Birds will sleep in stage 1 with one eye open on the hemisphere associated with sleep.

B. The eye contralateral to the sleeping hemisphere in the white whale is open.

C. Bottle-nose dolphins have no evidence of unihemispheric sleep when in captivity.

D. In birds, REM sleep occurs only bihemispherically.

49. Genetic studies in normal sleep are continually being explored. The EEG has been used to study the waking and sleeping pattern in many small twin studies. Preliminary evidence has shown that:

A. There is a higher concordance rate for REM sleep percentage in monozygotic than in dizygotic twins.

B. Although there is a concordance between monozygotic twins in the waking EEG, none exists in the EEG during sleep.

C. There is a greater concordance of sleep spindle density in dizygotic twins than in monozygotic twins.

D. Both monozygotic and dizygotic twins are similar for a striking concordance of EEG similarities of sleep architecture for all sleep stages.

50. Melatonin (*N*-acetyl-5-methoxytryptamine) is a hormone synthesized from serotonin and secreted by the pineal gland. Which of the following is also true about endogenous melatonin or its receptors?

A. Melatonin is a weak free radical scavenger, much less potent than vitamin E.

B. There is close correlation between the plasma melatonin nadir and minimum core temperature.

C. The MT2 receptor mRNA in human brain and retina is responsible for circadian rhythm entrainment in the suprachiasmatic nuclei of the hypothalamus.

D. Melatonin decreases the levels of superoxide dismutase and glutathione reductase.

Answers

1. B. Increased plasma levels of ghrelin

The connection between sleep deprivation and the development of obesity has been shown to be mediated by alterations in the neuroendocrine regulation of appetite and food intake. Human and animal studies have shown that plasma levels of ghrelin, a peptide produced mostly by the stomach, increase during partial sleep deprivation, concomitantly with a decrease in the levels of leptin. The net effect of this combined alteration is an increase in appetite and in the subjective sensation of hunger.

The cortisol level is also influenced by sleep deprivation, with an elevation of the plasma level occurring in the afternoon and early evening hours. Although the appetite is generally augmented by sleep deprivation, the specific appetite for protein-rich foods is not increased.

2. C. Increase in delta and theta patterns in a waking EEG

EEG analysis in extensive sleep deprivation studies has shown a consistent decrease in alpha activity. This decrease is directly proportional to the extent of sleep deprivation. In some cases, no alpha activity is seen after more than 115 hours of sleep loss, even with eye closure of subjects. The same subjects also demonstrate an increase in both delta and theta wave concentration in the waking EEG. In some studies, beta waves were found to be unchanged and in others to be increased; however, a decrease in beta activity was not observed with sleep deprivation. Sleep deprivation can induce the presence of delta waves even during wakefulness.

3. A. During infancy there is less sleep and more awakenings in boys than in girls.

Despite a certain degree of controversy regarding the influence of gender on the development of sleep patterns, studies have shown statistically significant differences between males and females. In a study by Bach et al (J Sleep Res 9:249, 2000), infant boys were found to have less total sleep and more frequent awakenings than infant girls. They also had more active sleep and less quiet sleep than girls. Quine (Child Care Health Dev 27[3]:201, 2001) found that in children ages 4–12 years, boys were twice as likely as girls to wake before 5 a.m. several times per week and also had more daytime sleepiness, more head-banging behavior, and more bed-wetting than girls. In adolescence, Lee and collaborators (Sleep 23[7]:877, 2000) found that girls reported an earlier wake-up time on weekdays, with the reverse being found on weekend days. Girls have more daytime sleepiness and more difficulty falling asleep at bedtime.

Multiple studies have shown that men have a lower sleep efficiency, more stage 1 sleep, and more awakenings. Interestingly, although polysomnographic data indicate more fragmented sleep in men, the subjective perception of poor sleep is more prevalent in women.

4. D. Young women complain more about sleep disturbances around menses than at any other time.

The 1998 National Sleep Foundation's poll found that a majority of young women (71%) complain more about sleep problems around their menses than at any other time. This interval starts 1 week before and continues in the first few days of menstruation, when the most common symptoms are bloating and tender breasts; however, the sleep disturbances occur during this period irrespective of the presence of the premenstrual symptoms. Amid all the menstrual and sleep disturbance symptoms, the sleep latency and sleep efficiency remain unchanged during different phases of the menstrual cycle, as shown by Baker et al (Pflugers Arch 442:729, 2001). Polysomnographic studies have shown that both REM-onset latency and the concentration of REM are decreased during the luteal phase. Furthermore, this change is more pronounced in the case of an ovulatory cycle versus an anovulatory cycle. This finding suggests that either the concentration of the ovarian hormones or the increase in the core body temperature is related directly to the onset of REM sleep.

5. B. Metabolic differences between waking and sleep increase at lower temperatures.

The more the temperature falls below thermoneutrality, the larger the drop in metabolism between waking and sleep. Up to a 40% decrease in oxygen consumption was observed when human subjects slept at 21° C versus 27° C, in a study by Palca and co-workers (J Appl Physiol 61:940, 1986). In humans as well as in animals, there is an overall decline in the metabolic rate from the awake to the sleeping state. The decrease was observed to range from 5% to 17% in various studies and was in proportion to the decrease in minute ventilation between the two states.

Unlike in animals, where a decreased metabolic rate during REM sleep has been observed, human studies have shown that metabolism during REM sleep is equal or even increased compared with NREM sleep. A larger contribution of the brain to the total metabolism in humans is possibly the explanation. Cerebral blood flow and metabolism both increase during the transition between NREM and REM sleep, as shown by Braun et al (Brain 120:1173, 1997).

6. B. The molecule through which viruses influence sleep is double-stranded RNA.

Double-stranded RNA (dsRNA) seems to be the key molecule in triggering sleep responses in the infected host. dsRNA is formed during viral replication. Therefore to produce sleep alterations, a virus needs to replicate inside the host. The same responses can be obtained by injecting experimental animals with live viruses, dsRNA extracted from lungs of infected animals, or synthetic dsRNA (poly I:C) as shown by Krueger et al (Am J Physiol 255:R748–R755, 1988). Conversely, administering the corresponding single strands of RNA (poly I and poly C) does not induce alteration in sleep patterns.

Both viral and bacterial infections have been shown to induce an initial increase in NREM combined with a decrease in stage REM concentration. The course of the sleep response depends on the nature of the infectious agent, the route of inoculation, and the time of day when the infection is acquired. Low viral loads of influenza are sufficient to cause excess sleep and cognitive dysfunction, even at concentrations that will not induce other classic symptoms of infection, such as fever.

IFN-α is produced with other cytokines by the host in response to the infectious challenge and has important antiviral activities. Sleep alterations similar to those caused by viruses can be obtained by injecting IFN-α in healthy humans. High doses will stimulate NREM sleep while increasing REM latency and total time spent in REM sleep.

7. C. They suppress the arousal-promoting neurons.

The preoptic area (POA) of the hypothalamus has been identified as the thermoregulatory control site. The area contains both warm-sensitive and cold-sensitive neurons, which can be differentiated by measuring neuronal firing after locally applied thermal stimuli. Warming of the POA induces NREM sleep or slow wave activity in laboratory animals. Delta waves are increasingly observed on the EEG during sustained NREM sleep, further suggesting that the sleep drive is influenced by POA thermosensitive neurons. These neurons send afferents to the posterior hypothalamus, midbrain, raphe nuclei, and lateral hypothalamus, suppressing the discharge in arousal-related neurons.

8. A. The alpha activity decreases proportionally with sleep loss.

The EEG of individuals with chronic sleep deprivation shows a consistent decrease in alpha activity. The more extensively the subjects are sleep deprived, the less alpha activity is observed. When the sleep loss goes beyond 115 hours, no alpha activity is seen, even with the eyes closed. The same subjects have an increase in delta and theta concentration in the waking EEG and, at the same time, beta concentration is unchanged.

Most studies of sleep-deprived subjects have found a reduction in natural killer cells and their activity, plus a decrease in lymphocytes and granulocytes in response to antigens. The antibody production was also reduced, and a 50% reduction was found 10 days after immunization with influenza vaccine in people whose sleep was restricted to 4 hours per night. Three to four weeks after vaccination, however, the antibody titer was the same in this group compared with control subjects.

C-reactive protein (CRP) is increased in both sleep-deprived normal humans and in obstructive sleep apnea patients, and its elevation is associated with an increased risk for cardiovascular disease.

The finding of increased risk of mortality with sleep deprivation (<6.5 hours) may not be very surprising, given the previous knowledge that total sleep deprivation in animals causes death in a few weeks. More intriguing is the discovery that people who reported more than 7.4 hours of sleep per night also show an increase in mortality risk in a study by Kripke and co-workers (Arch Gen Psychiatry 59:137–138, 2002). The Nurses Health Study also found an increase in risk for coronary events in subjects reporting more than 9 hours per night versus those with 8 hours per night of sleep.

9. D. Older subjects have daytime MSLT values at baseline after sleep loss and a single night of recovery sleep.

A study by Carskadon and Dement (Sleep 8:207–221, 1985) of 10 elderly volunteers assessed sleep performance and sleepiness before, during, and after 38 hours of sleep loss. After only 1 night of recovery sleep, the MSLT scores on these subjects showed no significant difference at any time of the day versus baseline. These results contrast with those found in younger subjects, in whom sleep latency test scores return to normal only gradually over the course of the first recovery day.

Numerous studies have shown that recovery from sleep loss can be rather rapid. One to three nights of sleep may be enough to negate the effects of up to 10 nights of sleep deprivation; however, different age groups required different times to recover from sleep loss. Young adults' reaction time was significantly slower after 1 recovery night compared with older subjects, and this pattern extended into the second recovery night.

After extended days of total sleep deprivation (up to 200 hours of sleep loss), the first recovery night is marked by a predominance of slow wave sleep,

TABLE 12-1 ■ First Night Recovery Sleep Architecture After Acute Sleep Deprivation

	Young Adults	Elderly Adults
Sleep latency	Reduced	Reduced
Stage 1 sleep	Reduced	Reduced
Stage 2 sleep	Reduced	No change or increased
Slow wave sleep (stages 3 & 4)	Increased	Increased slightly
REM latency	Increased	Decreased
Stage REM sleep	Decreased	Little change

more so in younger than in older adults. Therefore the older adults have a lesser slow wave rebound than their younger counterparts. The architecture of sleep in the first recovery night is summarized in Table 12-1.

10. C. Bacterial replication inside the host is not necessary for the sleep effects to occur.

The initial effects seen after a bacterial challenge are large increases in NREM sleep duration and intensity, with an increase in the slow wave amplitude, followed by an even more prolonged phase of a decrease in duration of NREM sleep and decreased slow wave amplitude. At the same time, REM sleep is inhibited.

In contrast with viral infection, bacteria do not need to replicate inside the host to induce sleep alterations. When injected into a host, killed bacteria or purified cell walls induce the same effects as the live pathogen. The mechanism involves phagocytosis of the live organism by the macrophages and subsequent expression of the cell wall–derived substances in the intercellular environment. Among the somnogenic molecules are muramyl peptides and endotoxin (lipopolysaccharide) derived from the bacterial wall. These two molecules have somewhat different properties regarding sleep alteration. The muramyl peptides are relatively non-toxic and are capable of inducing sleep even at very high concentrations. Endotoxin, on the other hand, is somnogenic only at lower doses, higher concentrations being responsible for inducing shock. Other cytokines with somnogenic properties are TNF, IFN-α, and acidic fibroblast growth factor.

Although the sleep responses to a bacterial challenge follow the same pattern of increasing NREM and decreasing REM sleep, the timing of these changes is dependent on the type of bacteria involved and the route of inoculation.

The immune system comes in permanent contact with bacteria present naturally inside the intestines. There seems to be an effect of this continuous interaction on the amount of sleep, as suggested by a few interesting studies showing that reduction of the intestinal bacterial population is associated with a reduction in sleep.

11. A. During NREM sleep, absence of intrinsic variability of the heart rate heralds an underlying heart condition.

Normal cardiovascular changes take place during sleep, with variations depending on the specific stage. NREM sleep is defined by autonomic stability, under parasympathetic activity dominance. The heart rate increases during inspiration, stimulated physiologically by the increased venous return, and returns to baseline during expiration. This variability is normal and is generally considered to reflect a state of cardiovascular health. Conversely, its absence has been associated with cardiac pathology.

Blood pressure falls by 5–14% during NREM sleep, tends to fluctuate during REM sleep, and will suddenly surge with any arousal from sleep. Heart rate slows during NREM sleep and tends to fluctuate during REM sleep. Bradycardia can occur during NREM sleep because of unopposed vagal activity and drop slower during REM sleep as a result of the additional effect of sympathetic inhibition in tonic REM sleep. Because phasic REM is marked by a reverse of this autonomic activity, the blood pressure and heart rate can transiently increase. Overall, stage REM sleep is marked by fluctuations in both blood pressure and heart rate.

Cardiac output falls during sleep regardless of the stage, with the greatest drop during the last REM cycle of the night. Because adverse effects tend to cluster during these same early-morning hours, this drop in cardiac output may be contributory.

Systemic vascular resistance (SVR) is affected by the vasodilation that occurs in stage REM sleep and therefore decreases. SVR is relatively unchanged or diminishes slightly in NREM sleep.

12. B. The apneustic center is located in the dorsolateral area of the pons.

Automatic control of ventilation is centered in the pons and medulla, which controls breathing regardless of whether the subject is awake or asleep. Animal studies have shown that the pons pneumotaxic center is at the rostral pons in the area of the nucleus parabrachial and Kölliker-Fuse nuclei. The dorsolateral area of the lower pons has been referred to as the *apneustic center*, which may be the location of the inspiratory "off-switch" to medullary inspiratory neurons. The medulla control is centered in two basic areas: (1) the dorsal respiratory group (DRG) and the (2) ventral respiratory group (VRG). The medullary responses for inhalation are principally controlled by the DRG in the nucleus tractus solitarius (NTS). Both inhalation and exhalation are controlled in the medulla ventral respiratory center in the nucleus ambiguus and retroambigualis. The VRG is believed to be the center of intrinsic respiratory rhythm generation at the pre-Bötzinger complex. The neurotransmitter crucial in respiratory rhythm generation interacting principally at the non-*N*-methyl-D-aspartate (NMDA) receptors is *glutamate*, which also connects the transmission of this rhythm to the phrenic motoneurons. Orexin, expressed by pre-Bötzinger neurons and phrenic nuclei, may also be involved in respiratory regulation.

13. D. IL-10, IL-13, and TGF-β

The current general opinion is that sleep is essential for the normal function of the immune system. This statement is very broad and might not be easy to prove in every aspect, but there is now enough evidence accumulated from animal and human studies to support it.

Sleep deprivation affects the immune responses to vaccines, hepatitis A, and influenza, for example. In both cases, substantial decreases in antibody responses were noted in sleep-deprived subjects. Sleep also influences the cellular immunity with shifts in the T helper 1/T helper 2 ratios being recorded during different stages of sleep.

Sleep deprivation increases IL-1, TNF-α, and interferon levels. IL-6 elevations are noted during stages 1, 2, and REM sleep. Cytokines play key roles in inflammatory responses and host defense, and IL-6 also has a potent stimulatory effect on the hypothalamic-pituitary axis. IL-1, IL-2, IL-6, IL-8, IL-18, and TNF-α promote NREM sleep; IL-4, IL-10, IL-13, and TGF-β inhibit NREM sleep.

14. C. Visual perception tasks improvement correlates with late-night REM and early-night slow wave sleep.

The meaning of sleep stages and the many changes that occur in the brain during sleep have not ceased to puzzle researchers. No integrative explanation of brain changes during sleep has been uniformly accepted yet by the scientific community, but more and more pieces of information are emerging from the numerous studies in the field.

Sleep has been shown to enhance prior learning of various skills and emotions. It has been found that consolidation of different skills requires involvement of different portions of sleep.

Gais and co-workers (Neurosci 3[12]:1335–1359, 2000) have shown that in laboratory rats, late-night REM and early-night slow wave sleep correlated with improvements in visual texture discrimination (Stickgold, J Cogn Neurosci 12[2]:246, 2000. Humans were trained to recognize differences in orientation of certain arrays) and that this improvement was superior when compared with the same amount of time spent in the awake state. Other studies showed improvement in motor skills in correlation with late-night NREM sleep. 11 (Walker, Neuron 35:205–211, 2002. Humans trained to perform finger tapping patterns), paired word associate learning enhanced by early night sleep (Philal, Psychoneuroendocrinology 24:313–331, 1999. Recall of a paired associate list), and emotional declarative memory improved by late-night sleep (Wagner, Learn Mem 8:112–119, 2001. Memory retention of emotional versus neutral text material).

15. D. Coronary blood flow decreases significantly in NREM sleep and increases in REM sleep.

The coronary blood flow decreases between wakefulness and NREM sleep, and it increases in REM sleep. The increase observed in REM sleep can be triggered by local metabolic factors and sympathetic discharge (when accompanied by tachycardia) or by cholinergic vasodilation (with no corresponding surge in heart rate).

Animal and human studies have shown that the circulation in peripheral organs (other than brain) changes during sleep and is further influenced by autonomic activity and local metabolic factors. The resultant changes are dependent on the sleep stages and may not follow the "physiological logic" of the organs, and as a result they may disrupt the homeostasis of the respective systems; for example, loss of thermoregulation during REM sleep.

There is no significant variation of the blood flow in the splanchnic circulation compared with wakefulness. Finely tuned local regulatory mechanisms control the flow of blood in both portal and arterial vascular beds.

In muscles, the blood flow does not change between wakefulness and NREM sleep. In REM sleep, however, it decreases in the red fibers, but in the white fibers, the changes vary among the different species that have been studied.

Although the renal vascular tone can respond to changes in temperature, animal studies have found that the blood flow in the kidney is not sleep-stage dependent.

16. B. REM sleep helps facilitate consolidation of perceptual and emotional memories.

Studies have shown that humans dream different types of dreams depending on the stage of sleep. A parallel can be drawn between the characteristic of the dreams and the memory each stage of sleep seems to facilitate.

In REM sleep, dreams are hallucinatory, emotional, narrative, and with frequent fictive movements. Stage REM is also thought to facilitate consolidation of visual perceptual and emotional memories. In NREM sleep, dreams are less hallucinatory and more thought-like. NREM sleep, on the other hand, has been implicated in simple memorization of word pair lists.

17. A. There are periods of irregularity in respiratory and heart rates during phasic REM.

Stage REM is characterized by intermittent rapid eye movements and muscle atonia. Dreams are also associated with stage REM sleep. The sleeping cat brain was extensively studied in the early days of sleep research. The principal electrical signs of REM sleep initially described include a reduction in EEG amplitude, particularly of its lower-frequency components (Chow KL, Dement WC, Mitchell SA Jr, Electroencephalogr Clin Neurophysiol Suppl 11:107, 1959) and *ponto-geniculo-occipital* (PGO) spikes, large-amplitude, isolated potentials that appear 30 seconds before REM's onset, which can be recorded in the lateral geniculate nucleus. The same waves may be present in human REM sleep but cannot be measured by current standard EEG techniques.

The tonic type of REM is stage REM without electro-oculographic evidence of rapid eye movement that is still scored as stage REM. During the phasic type of REM, the PGO potentials trigger the characteristic rapid eye movements. In humans, these movements are associated with contractions of the muscles in the middle ear and of other muscles, which briefly interrupt the tonic muscle atonia of REM sleep.

The muscle activity in REM sleep is characterized by atonia, readily identified on EMG by a dramatic decrease in chin muscle tone, which reaches the lowest level of the entire PSG recording. Other changes of the tonic phase include pupilary constriction, penile erections, and clitorial enlargements. Thermoregulation ceases, and body temperature is mostly influenced by environmental temperature.

REM sleep is also characterized by periods of marked heart and respiratory rate irregularities, which lack their coordinated, periodic nature of the NREM sleep. Dreams that occur during REM sleep are more vivid, more story-like, and are easier to recall compared with NREM sleep.

18. B. Sleep-inducing neurons are concentrated in the lower brainstem reticular formation.

The role of the brainstem in the physiology of sleep has been described more than half a century ago, starting with the work of Moruzzi and Magoun (Electroencephalogr Clin Neurophysiol 1:455–473, 1949). In 1949, they published their findings regarding the transition from sleep to wakefulness by describing the EEG waveforms originating from the brainstem reticular formation. Ten years later, Batini, Moruzzi, and co-workers (Arch Ital Biol 97:1, 1959) found that by transecting the brainstem behind the oral pontine tegmentum, they created a state of total insomnia in laboratory animals. This discovery pointed at the lower brainstem as the structure containing essential sleep-generating structures, capable of antagonizing the ascending activating system in the upper brainstem.

Glutamate (not glycine) is one of the main excitatory neurotransmitters in the brain. It is found in high concentrations in the neurons of the reticular formation in the brainstem. Its agonists can induce seizures, and ketamine, a glutamate antagonist, is an efficient anesthetic. Glycine, on the other hand, has been described to inhibit the motoneurons in the ventral horn and hypoglossal nuclei during REM atonia.

Lesions of the preoptic area and basal forebrain that involve GABAergic neurons produce loss of natural sleep, whereas lesions of the oral pontine, midbrain tegmentum, posterior hypothalamus, or basal forebrain that involve cholinergic neurons can result in complete loss of wakefulness.

19. C. A solid meal before bedtime can decrease sleep onset latency more than a liquid meal.

The fact that drowsiness follows a meal is a common observation both in humans and other mammals. To determine if the meal composition influences postprandial sleepiness, Orr and co-workers (Orr WC, Physiol Behav 62:709–712, 1997) administered different test meals to 10 normal men. Results indicate that in contrast to a liquid meal, a solid meal produces a decrease in sleep latency when compared with an equivalent volume of water. The meal constituents did not seem to affect sleep latency in the immediately following period.

In experimental studies of viscerosensory evoked potentials during sleep in cats, Juhasz (Act Nerv Super [Praha] 19:212–214, 1977) found that stimulating the intestinal mucosa triggers different responses in the visual cortex of animals, depending on the stage of the sleep-wake cycle they were in. The largest effect was observed in slow wave sleep, and the smallest during the wake state. Interestingly, the low-voltage stimuli triggered larger changes in evoked potentials than strong ones. The same type of stimulation increased the duration of NREM sleep and the number of REM sleep episodes.

Multiple studies have tried to find if cholecystokinin or other intestinal hormones affect sleep. The results so far are inconclusive. Increases in NREM sleep and stage REM or no change in sleep architecture was noted after intraperitoneal, intraduodenal, or intravenous injection of cholecystokinin in animal models. No decrease in stage REM was also reported.

20. D. A decrease in plasma thyroxine and an increase in plasma norepinephrine were recorded.

In 1989, a series of related experiments about sleep deprivation in rats was published by a group coordinated by Rechtschaffen (Sleep 12:68–87, 1989). They showed that all rats totally deprived of sleep died in 2–3 weeks. Numerous other changes were described, including an increase in norepinephrine and reduction in thyroxine plasma levels. The rats showed progressive debilitation, with brownish, disheveled fur, with severe ulcerative and hyperkeratotic skin lesions localized to the tails and to the plantar surface of the paws. The animals lost weight despite an increase in food intake of about 80–100% above baseline. The energy expenditure more than doubled compared with baseline. The body temperature decreased in the second half of the survival period, preceded by a transitory increase in the first half of the same interval.

The significance of these changes has not been fully elucidated, but failure of host defense, changes in brain structure and chemistry, deficiencies of temperature regulation and impaired metabolism, or most likely a combination of these factors has been thought to be important determinants of the outcome.

21. C. Tricyclic antidepressant ingestion can suppress REM sleep.

Good knowledge of the effects that commonly used drugs (prescribed or illicit) have on the CNS, and especially on sleep stages, is essential for sleep researchers and practitioners. On one hand, some of these substances possess the ability of interacting with receptors naturally found in important structures that control sleep and can be used to study sleep physiology and pathophysiology. On the other hand, for the practitioner reading polysomnograms, such knowledge is invaluable in making a differential diagnosis, if one of the alterations that these drugs can bring about is encountered.

The tricyclic antidepressants (TCAs) and some selective serotonin reuptake inhibitors (SSRIs) tend to suppress REM sleep and at the same time can increase the level of motor activity during sleep. The result is a pattern of reduction in REM sleep concentration. Subjects may also have an increased incidence of periodic limb movements during sleep (PLMS). Among SSRIs, fluoxetine is associated with rapid eye movements across all stages, a phenomenon commonly referred to as *Prozac eyes*. Benzodiazepines have no major effect on REM sleep but can suppress slow wave sleep. Ingestion of alcohol just before sleep

increases slow wave sleep and suppresses REM sleep in the first part of the night, with stage REM rebound in the second part of the night. When used chronically, marijuana can suppress slow wave sleep for a long time. The acute usage of marijuana slightly reduces REM sleep, but no significant sleep disruption occurs.

22. E. Bilateral ventral respiratory group of the medulla

The center for generating the rhythm of respiration is in the bilateral ventral respiratory group (VRG) of the medulla. Other structures of the medulla, including the dorsal respiratory group (DRG) of the medulla, are not necessary for the generation of respiratory rhythm. Within the VRG itself there is some controversy as to the specific group of neurons responsible for generation of the respiratory rhythm including the pre-Bötzinger area or rostral to this area in the rostroventrolateral medulla.

The pneumotaxic center in the dorsal lateral pons contains neurons that modulate respiratory frequency but is not necessary for respiratory rhythm generation. The ventrolateral area of the nucleus of the tractus solitarius contains neurons of the DRG of the medulla primarily responsible for the inhalation portion of the respiratory cycle and provides rhythmic drive to phrenic motoneurons. Motor cortex projections through the descending corticospinal tract are involved in the voluntary control of breathing and not the generation of the rhythm of respiration.

23. B. Slow wave sleep will be increased over baseline values.

Studies in acute sleep deprivation in the young adult have shown that the first night of recovery sleep has a change in sleep architecture over baseline values. There is a predominance of slow wave sleep recovery that results in the reduction of other sleep stages. Sleep latency is reduced, and wake after sleep onset is also reduced. Owing to the rebound of slow wave sleep, stages 1, 2, and REM are all decreased. REM latency tends to be prolonged in the young adult; however, in the older adult, REM latency is reduced. Insomniacs and elderly normal sleepers have less slow wave sleep rebound with little change in stage 2. On the second night of recovery sleep in the young adult, REM sleep concentration tends to increase as slow wave sleep approaches baseline values. Please see Table 12-1 for a summary chart of sleep architecture changes in recovery sleep after acute sleep deprivation.

24. D. Can be seen during a 20-minute nap at 11 A.M. in a traveler seven time zones eastward

The polysomnogram (PSG) epoch shown in Figure 12-1 represents stage REM or rapid eye movement sleep. Stage REM sleep is characterized by rapid eye movements at the same time that the chin EMG is at the lowest level of the entire recording. The EEG is a low-voltage, mixed-frequency pattern that is generally 1 to 2 cps (cycles per second) slower than stage 1. Sleep spindles and K-complexes stop while the EEG pattern becomes activated and desynchronized. Saw-tooth waves of theta frequency are characteristic of stage REM sleep (seen at the arrow in Figure 12-1) and, if present, are more prominent over the frontal and vertex regions, with the vertex showing the highest amplitude.

Characteristically stage REM is at an increased concentration during the second half of night, which correlates with the intrinsic circadian rhythm of an individual. If the home time zone is 4 A.M. during the time of this increased REM pressure, then traveling seven time zones eastward would put the individual at 11 A.M. during the intrinsic circadian pressure to have stage REM. In this situation, and until the traveler adapts to the new time zone cues, sleep-onset stage REM is likely to occur.

Stage REM at sleep onset is normal in newborn babies but not a 5-year-old child. Sleep onset begins to change from REM to NREM sleep by age 3 months but can occur up to age 6 months. The first recovery night after total sleep deprivation has a predominance of slow wave sleep recovery. Narcolepsy has two or more sleep-onset REM periods on an MSLT. Recurrent hypersomnia (Kleine-Levin syndrome or menstrual-related hypersomnia) does not have characteristic findings on an MSLT.

25. B. Between 10 P.M. and 2 A.M.

Unstimulated gastric acid secretion has a circadian periodicity that peaks between 10 P.M. and 2 A.M. in normal individuals. Moore and Englert (Nature 226:1261, 1970) studied 45 people with 24-hour gastric acid collections. They discovered a circadian pattern of secretion with great consistency, with the greatest secretion rate in the evening and the lowest in the morning between 5 A.M. and 11 A.M. This was later substantiated by other research studies. Despite its circadian rhythm, there also tends to be a drop in gastric acid secretion with sleep compared with the waking state. There are different study results regarding variation in this endogenous gastric acid secretion with sleep stage changes, but overall gastric acid is not affected by a particular sleep stage. Gastric acid output tends to increase on arousal or awakening from sleep. Vagal stimulation is likely the regulator of this circadian periodicity, as patients who have undergone a vagotomy have lost this circadian rhythm. Plasma gastrin levels, on the other hand, do not have circadian rhythm.

26. D. This is the first of three consecutive epochs of <50% alpha waves and defines this patient's sleep latency.

The 30-second epoch shown in Figure 12-2 shows less than 15 seconds (or 50%) of alpha waves. For polysomnography, the definition of sleep latency is from lights out until the first of three consecutive epochs, at which point the EEG changes from clear rhythmic alpha waves to a relatively low-voltage, mixed-frequency for >50% of the epoch for at least three consecutive epochs. The sleep latency for this patient is 13 minutes from lights out at 10:30 P.M. until this epoch, which is 10:43 P.M. The actual onset of sleep in polysomnography is at least three consecutive epochs of stage 1 sleep or one epoch of stage 2 sleep. Stage 1 sleep on an EEG is a background of low-voltage, mixed-frequency waves. Alpha waves, seen best in the occipital leads, comprise <50% of each epoch. Stage 1 may also be accompanied by vertex sharp waves, seen best in the central leads shown at the arrows in Figure 12-2.

Option A is correct in mentioning a snoring-related arousal; however, this is still the first of three consecutive epochs with less than 50% alpha waves and fits the definition of sleep latency on polysomnography. Options B and C are incorrect by the definition of sleep latency explained here.

27. B. Elevation in PCO_2

When sleep is entered, both NREM and REM sleep have a reduction in minute ventilation by about 0.5–1.5 L/min as compared with the waking state. This effective sleep hypoventilation subsequently causes a slight increase in PCO_2 by about 2–3 mm Hg (2–3 additional mm Hg in REM), a reduction in PO_2 by 3–10 mm Hg and a decrease in oxygen saturation by 0–2%. In the transition from wake to the lighter stages of sleep, especially when an individual is transitioning between wake and stage 1 sleep, episodes of periodic breathing can occur. If the PCO_2 drops below the PCO_2 threshold, this relative hypocapnea is sensed chiefly at the medullary chemoreceptor level with subsequent hypoventilation or an apneic response until the PCO_2 rises again to trigger resumption of minute ventilation. Breathing stabilizes in the deeper stages of stage 2 and stages 3 and 4 sleep, with the most regular minute ventilation of any stage of sleep, although still at a slightly reduced minute ventilation compared with the waking state.

28. A. The acylated form of the peptide, ghrelin

The peptide, ghrelin, originates from the endocrine cells of the stomach and has been shown to stimulate growth hormone (GH) secretion by binding to the growth-hormone-secretogue receptor, a different receptor than the GHRH receptor. Ghrelin has also been shown to enhance slow wave sleep.

GH is secreted with a major pulse of activity during the first half of sleep. Studies have shown that GH is secreted only during about one third of slow wave sleep and can even be secreted without slow wave sleep occurring. GH secretion has also been detected in the evening just before sleep onset. In general, however, there is a linear association between GH secretion and slow wave sleep. Awakening from sleep suppresses GH secretion. Sleep fragmentation suppresses nocturnal GH secretion as well. Although GH has been detected outside of slow wave sleep, its primary secretion is linked to slow wave sleep. Any pharmacological agent that suppresses or enhances slow wave sleep can thus suppress or enhance GH concentration. An example is gamma hydroxybutyrate (GHB), a metabolite of GABA that has been shown to stimulate slow wave sleep and enhanced GH secretion. Ritanserin, a selective 5-HT receptor antagonist, can also increase slow wave sleep and subsequent GH secretion.

Response B, acute total sleep deprivation, suppresses GH secretion with a large pulse of secretion upon recovery sleep. Chronic partial sleep deprivation, on the other hand, has been associated with a GH pulse just before sleep onset, with the larger pulse still noted soon after sleep onset in a biphasic pattern. Night-shift workers (response C) still have suppression of GH during the waking period compared with sleep and experience the characteristic GH pulse after sleep regardless of the fact that this is during the day. Somatostatin (response D) inhibits GH secretion in the pituitary but can also inhibit GHRHergic neurons in the hypothalamus.

29. D. Show no significant decline in elderly women compared with men

This stage of sleep in Figure 12-3 is representative of stage 3 sleep with at least 20% of this epoch showing delta waves that also reflect into the ocular channels. Slow wave sleep is a combination of stages 3 and 4 sleep, also known as *delta sleep*. Stage 3 sleep is defined by at least 20–50% of an epoch consisting of delta waves defined by ≤2 cps in frequency and >75 μV in amplitude. Wave amplitude is peak to the trough and not peak to the isoelectric baseline. Stage 4 is >50% delta waves. Chin EMG continues to show tone, but less tone with deepening sleep.

Slow wave sleep has its highest percentage of total sleep in young children and decreases with age with an initial rapid decline in the second decade. There is a greater loss of slow wave sleep as men age, whereas women tend to have a relative preservation of this

stage of sleep. One study (Redline S. et al., Arch Intern Med 164:406, 2004) reported women ages 61 to 70 as having a mean of 16.7% of slow wave sleep compared with a mean of 6.7% in this same age group.

30. C. Decreased slow wave sleep, increased sleep fragmentation, and probable periodic breathing

Sleep at altitude has been studied by multiple researchers. In general, there is an increase in stage 1 sleep. Sleep becomes more fragmented with increased wake-after-sleep periods. Despite this sleep disruption, total sleep time remains relatively preserved. Stage 2 is decreased, and there is a significant reduction in slow wave sleep. It is not yet clear whether REM has a significant change.

Above 4000 meters, periodic breathing is common during sleep, with sleep fragmentation marked by frequent arousals from sleep during the hyperpnea phase. Periodic breathing is described as episodes of hypopneas or central apneas cycling with hyperpneas. Recurrent desaturations regularly occur. Oxygen may blunt or abolish periodic breathing; however, sleep quality may not be improved. It is interesting to note that periodic breathing tends to predominate in NREM sleep with resumption of normal breathing in stage REM, with the exception of altitudes greater than 4300 meters. Acetazolamide, a carbonic anhydrase inhibitor, has been successfully used to reduce periodic breathing, improve hypoxemia, and may secondarily improve sleep quality because of sedative side effects. This drug blocks the enzymatic hydration of CO_2 to carbonic acid leading to bicarbonate diuresis and metabolic acidosis, and thus stimulating ventilation. Over time (just a few days), the mountain climber usually becomes "acclimatized" with a reduction or resolution of periodic breathing, except in climbers at altitudes >4500 meters.

31. A. Neurotransmitter: glutamate and two cotransmitters: substance P and PACAP

Glutamate is an excitatory neurotransmitter released by the RHT as a result of photic stimulation. Glutamate acts through NMDA and non-NMDA receptors, with intracellular signaling molecules and early-response genes leading to *Per1* and *Per2* clock gene expression. This leads to a series of events that likely involve other clock genes and their protein products involved in phase shifting. RHT terminals also release two co-transmitters: substance P and PACAP. Substance P, in conjunction with glutamate, can lead to phase shifting. PACAP, on the other hand, in high doses, blocks glutamate action at night and triggers phase advance by day. In low doses, PACAP can also work in conjunction with glutamate to stimulate the suprachiasmatic nucleus (SCN). The RHT and the geniculohypothalamic tract are the main pathways by which light reaches the SCN in the hypothalamus of the brain that affects circadian rhythms. Nonphotic input to the SCN is transmitted via the midbrain raphe nuclei.

Light is an important cause of circadian rhythm shifts. When healthy young adults with normal sleep patterns and body temperatures were studied, they had a core body temperature minimum that occurred about 2 hours before the habitual wake time, at around 4 to 5 A.M. If light therapy is given before this minimal core body temperature, then the circadian rhythm will phase delay or shift to a later clock time. If light therapy is given after this minimal core body temperature, however, then the circadian rhythm will phase advance or shift to an earlier clock time. For example, if a patient's core body temperature occurred around 5 A.M. and the patient is consistently exposed to light therapy around 7 A.M., then the circadian rhythm will shift to an earlier clock time. This becomes useful if someone with a tendency toward a phase delay rhythm or who is a "night owl" is having a difficult time fitting into a day job. Morning light therapy can help to phase advance the person's circadian rhythm and eventually improve the ability to get up in the morning with a decrease in morning sleepiness.

32. C. 6 sleep-wake cycles, 7 body temperature circadian cycles

There are 168 hours in a week and if the patient's subjective day is 28 hours, then there will be six actual sleep-wake cycles during that time frame. Professor Nathaniel Kleitman from the University of Chicago conducted experiments in 1938 in Mammouth Cave, Kentucky to control for environmental factors while studying circadian temperature rhythms on a forced 28-hour cycle. This was compared with a 24-hour cycle on the surface. This led to the discovery that there were seven cycles of body temperature rhythms during the same time period of 1 week regardless of the six sleep-wake cave cycles versus the typical seven on the 24-hour surface. The imposed separation of the synchronized homeostatic sleep-wake cycle and the circadian temperature cycle occurred by imposing a forced sleep-wake schedule in a controlled cue-free environment. This later became known as the *forced desynchrony protocol* and paved the way for understanding that there was a near 24-hour circadian cycle regardless of the sleep-wake cycle.

Core body temperature is constantly measured during these types of experiments. Body temperature is circadian driven, with a characteristic nadir during the last half of the usual nocturnal sleep period. This circadian periodicity continues regardless of whether the subject is awake or asleep. Sleep itself has also been known to lead to a drop in body temperature, and when sleep coincides with the circadian rhythm, there is a further reduction in body temperature.

33. D. Levels are minimal at noon and increase dramatically soon after sleep onset.

Prolactin levels are minimal at approximately noon, increase slightly in the afternoon, and are maximal just after sleep onset. This pattern is also seen in night shift workers who sleep during the day and in subjects who take a daytime nap. Prolactin secretion is sleep-linked and triggered by sleep onset regardless of the time of day. The largest sleep-related surge tends to be associated with slow wave sleep. Any awakenings or arousals from sleep suppress prolactin secretion. Benzodiazepines and zolpidem cause an increase in prolactin secretion during sleep compared with a placebo. Although prolactin secretion is very strongly sleep-linked, there is also an underlying circadian component with a gradual elevation in levels in the evening that is more pronounced in women than in men.

34. B. 45–55%

Figures 12-4 and 12-5 represent stage 2 sleep. Figure 12-4 shows stage 2 sleep, with a sleep spindle seen at the arrow in the EEG most prominent in the central leads (C4-A1; C3-A2). Figure 12-5 shows stage 2 sleep with a K-complex around 6 seconds into this epoch and an overlapping sleep spindle seen at the end of the wave form in the EEG channels. The K-complex (arrows) also reflects through the top two eye channels as well.

The defining feature of stage 2 sleep is either a K-complex or sleep spindle that must be seen within 3 minutes to continue scoring as stage 2. If 3 minutes or more elapse with continued low-voltage, mixed-frequency waves and no evidence of K-complexes or sleep spindles, then this is scored as stage 1. This is what is called the *3-minute rule* of stage 2 sleep. A K-complex is an initial sharp negative deflection with a slower positive downward wave for which the entire complex is at least 0.5 seconds (arrows in Figure 12-5). A sleep spindle is a 12- to 14-cps burst of waves lasting between 0.5 and 1.5 seconds (arrow in Figure 12-4) and can overlap a K-complex. Eyes show little motion, and K-complexes do reflect within the EOG leads. Chin EMG continues to show tone but does generally diminish as sleep progresses.

The normal adult patient falls asleep initially in NREM sleep. Sleep consists of NREM and REM that alternate approximately every 90 to 110 minutes. Whereas slow wave sleep is predominant in the first half of sleep, REM sleep is concentrated within the second half of sleep and is circadian-linked. Stage 2 sleep averages about 45–55% of sleep, whereas slow wave sleep averages about 15–25% of total sleep time. Stage REM sleep is generally about 20–25% of total sleep time.

35. B. Develop more awakenings from sleep

Awakenings and arousals during sleep increase with age. Thus sleep efficiency, as defined by total sleep time divided by total time in bed, has a reduction in the elderly with greater sleep fragmentation. Along with this greater wake after sleep onset, stage 1 tends to increase. Interestingly enough, the REM concentration tends to be relatively preserved, and therefore option C is incorrect. Slow wave sleep, as already pointed out, tends to decrease to a greater extent in aging women than in men.

Although elderly subjects tend to go to bed earlier and awaken earlier in the morning, recent studies have suggested that this pattern cannot be explained by a phase advance in the circadian rhythm. Option A is incorrect because the aging individual does not develop a phase delay. Delta wave amplitude decreases and does not increase with age, and therefore option D is incorrect.

36. A. Have a buildup of the homeostatic process (process S)

Process S is a term used to describe the homeostatic cycle. *Process C* is a term used to describe the circadian rhythm. This has been described as a two-process model by Borbely and Achermann of sleep-wake regulation because process C and process S work in concert to determine when sleep onset and offset will ultimately take place. Process S increases sleep pressure need the longer one is awake and declines with sleep. Therefore A is correct; there is a buildup of process S with increased waking time. Option B is incorrect, owing to EEG demonstration that theta activity rises with an increase in the wake time in conjunction with the increased need to sleep. The more sleep deprived a person becomes, the greater the slow wave activity, an indicator of sleep homeostasis in NREM sleep, during the subsequent sleep period. The circadian process (process C) is independent of the length of the wake period (or sleep), and therefore option C is incorrect.

37. B. Contribute to upper airway resistance in both NREM and REM sleep, which increases in REM sleep

There are a group of upper airway muscles that work in concert to maintain a patent airway. Many of these have been studied, most notably the genioglossus, as well as the geniohyoid, tensor palatini, and others. These airway dilator muscles show a reduction in electromyography (EMG) tone during NREM sleep with a further reduction in stage REM. Subsequently, airway resistance rises and minute ventilation decreases relative to this increased airway resistance. Hypotonia of the airway dilator group of muscles, as well as the intercostal muscles of breathing, occur during NREM sleep. With arousals from sleep, airway dilator muscle tone abruptly increases, with a reduction in upper airway resistance. This is part of normal physiology and is not exclusive to the patient with sleep apnea.

38. D. Reassure the student that this is not pathological given the circumstances and no further evaluation is necessary.

Hypnic myoclonia or "sleep starts" are either generalized or localized sudden muscle contractions that may also be associated with vivid imagery. These sudden jerks occur just after the transition to sleep onset. A common example is the sleepy student in a class who unexpectedly drifts off to sleep and suddenly jerks, much to his or her embarrassment. Many times there is a sensation of falling associated with the jerk. This is a benign disorder that is often part of the normal transition to sleep onset with unclear mechanisms. This tends to start or worsen with schedule changes or stress that can trigger a greater frequency of hypnic myoclonia. This is considered part of a normal wake to sleep transition and should not be confused with a seizure disorder, especially in a healthy subject with no medical history in conjunction with this type of circumstance. The mechanism of hypnic myoclonia is unclear but may represent a brief dissociation of the imagery portion of stage REM.

39. A. Type alpha1β-adrenergic and type 5-HT2α receptors

Animal studies have shown that NE, a modulator of brainstem motoneurons, is released at higher levels during wakefulness than sleep. One of the receptors mediating the postsynaptic effect of NE to XII motoneurons (hypoglossal) is the type alpha1β-adrenergic receptor. In addition, Fenik and Veasey (Am J Respir Crit Care Med 167[4]:563, 2003) studied rats and concluded that "serotonin 2A is the predominant excitatory serotonin receptor subtype at the hypoglossal motor neurons." Both these two receptors, type alpha1β-adrenergic and type 5-HT2α, appear to be the main receptors involved in the excitatory effects of 5-HT and NE in the hypoglossal motor neuron. The activity of both NE and 5-HT neurons in the brainstem have reduced activity in sleep with a greater suppression during REM sleep that ultimately supplies output to hypoglossal innervation of upper airway dilator muscles. This causes increased upper airway resistance over wakefulness in the normal physiology of sleep that is more pronounced in patients with sleep breathing disorders in combination with other factors.

The other answers listed are involved in the following: (1) adenosine A1 receptor interacts with adenosine involved in wakefulness, and caffeine blocks this receptor; (2) type HCRT1 and HCRT2 receptors are hypocretin receptors that are also involved in wakefulness, as a deficiency can cause narcolepsy symptoms. Although recent research has shown that orexin (hypocretin) may be involved in stimulating respiration via activation within the phrenic nucleus and pre-Bötzinger region and may be involved in hypoglossal motoneurons that affect the airway dilator muscles via the HCRT-1 receptors.

40. B. Have a diurnal rhythm with sleep inhibition

TSH secretion is inhibited by sleep. There is a low level during the daytime with a progressive increase in levels toward evening, reaching a maximum just before sleep onset and into the initial onset of sleep. TSH appears to have the greatest inhibition during nocturnal slow wave sleep. If a subject is awakened from sleep, there is a transient TSH elevation. Daytime sleepers do not have much of an inhibition below typical daytime levels. Sleep deprivation has led to an increase in TSH levels to about double what they normally are. There is also a continued diurnal pattern of secretion, suggesting a circadian influence on secretion. Bright light therapy in the evening can cause a phase delay of TSH secretion.

41. B. Have the first nocturnal pulse between 2:00 and 3:00 A.M.

ACTH triggered cortisol secretion reaches the lowest levels during the evening and on into the first part of sleep. During the night, however, cortisol starts to secrete in pulses, with the first nocturnal pulse between 2:00 and 3:00 A.M. and later reaching an early morning maximum between 4:00 and 8:00 A.M. Regardless of sleep timing, corticotropic activity has a circadian-linked periodicity that is marked by elevated morning plasma ACTH and cortisol levels. ACTH and cortisol plasma levels decline throughout the day to the lowest measured levels in the early evening and early part of the nocturnal sleep period. Although corticotropic activity shows a circadian pattern regardless of sleep patterns, sleep can serve to modulate its activity. Sleep onset has been shown to have an inhibitory effect on cortisol secretion that may be linked to

slow wave sleep activity. Awakenings from sleep have been associated with an increase in cortisol levels.

42. C. Both the waking period and stage REM sleep

The hypocretins (orexins) are neuropeptides that have been shown to be released at high levels during the waking period, with greater levels during increased motor activity than during quiet wakefulness. REM sleep has shown to be associated with high levels of hypocretins compared with NREM sleep and, in fact, NREM sleep is associated with the lowest levels.

43. A. *Phase shift* means the displacement forward or backward in time of the intrinsic circadian rhythm of an organism as a result of heat that is 5 degrees centigrade above the core body temperature. The correct definition is: *Phase shift* means the displacement forward or backward in time of the intrinsic circadian rhythm of an organism as a result of light affecting the circadian clock to accelerate or slow to cause entrainment. The other three definitions for responses B through D are listed as correct.

44. A. Thalamic reticular nucleus

Sleep spindles are generated from the region of the thalamus. The thalamus and cerebral cortex can produce cyclical oscillations of neuronal cells. Sleep spindles are generated by repetitious bursts from thalamic reticular cells at a frequency of approximately 12–14 Hz. These recurrent bursts of spindle activity are preceded by prolonged hyperpolarizing potentials in intracellular recordings of thalamic reticular neurons. During polysomnography, they are best visualized over the vertex and thus the central leads show more predominant spindle activity than the occipital leads. Neuronal cells of the ventral medulla, parabrachial nucleus, and solitary tract nucleus do not generate sleep spindles.

45. B. Serotonin (5-HT) acts as a ventilatory inhibitor

Serotonin (5-hydroxytryptamine or 5-HT) acts as a ventilatory inhibitor. Studies on blocking 5-HT synthesis have shown an increase in respiratory frequency, minute ventilation, and hypercapnic ventilatory response. Response A is incorrect, as glycine actually triggers hyperpolarization of lumbar motoneurons and is involved centrally as part of the final respiratory output to spinal respiratory motoneurons. For response B, catecholamine inhibitors have been shown to reduce respiratory activity. Finally, in response D, GABA actually has a strong inhibitory action on ventilation. In fact, both GABA and glycine are released into the motoneurons during REM sleep, leading to muscle atonia. In contrast, neuroepinephrine and 5-HT release into motoneurons are both decreased during this period.

46. A. 3:00 to 4:00 A.M.

Melatonin is a lipid-soluble hormone released from the pineal gland that has sleep-promoting effects. The pineal gland secretes melatonin (*N*-acetyl-5-methoxytryptamine) in a circadian rhythmic cycle with increased levels at night and suppression of secretion in the daytime. Although secreted the majority of the night, maximal plasma levels usually peak at 3:00 to 4:00 A.M. Light inhibits melatonin synthesis via output from the RHT. The circulating amino acid precursor, tryptophan is converted to serotonin (5-HT) in the pineal gland that is then converted to melatonin by further enzymatic reactions. Eventually, the liver deactivates it. Melatonin taken in the early morning to noon can cause a phase delay, and taken in the late afternoon or early evening, a phase advance. For this reason, melatonin is referred to as a *chronobiotic* because it is a substance that can induce phase shifts and entrain the circadian clock. Melatonin production tends to decrease with age.

47. D. Allow the study of cortical electrical activity affected by vestibular, visual, auditory, olfactory, and musculocutaneous impulses

In 1935 and 1936, Dr. Frederick Bremer reported on his research findings of the electrical rhythms in the cat brain. He had developed two different cat brain sections for his experiments. The *encéphale isolè* was a section in the lower part of the medulla that was used in the study of cortical electrical rhythms responsive to the visual, auditory, olfactory, vestibular, and musculocutaneous impulses. The *cerveau isolè* was made by cutting behind the origin of the oculomotor nerves in the midbrain that served to isolate the study of the olfactory and visual impulses. The EEG of the *encéphale isolè* demonstrated an alternating pattern between the waking and sleeping state. The EEG of the *cerveau isolè* demonstrated a sleeping state that led to the realization that this brain section effectively suppresses nerve impulses necessary for the waking state of the telencephalon. In this brain section the eyeballs turned downward with a progressive miosis along with EEG evidence of a sleeping pattern. This led to the conclusion that sleep is a reversible deafferentation of the cerebral cortex.

48. D. In birds, REM sleep occurs only bihemispherically.

Certain birds and aquatic mammals have been discovered to have unihemispheric sleep, defined by EEG evidence of sleep in one hemisphere simultaneous with a waking pattern in the opposite hemisphere. Certain flying birds such as the common swift have been thought to sleep while in flight owing to evidence of unihemispheric slow wave sleep occurring in one hemisphere, and the eye connected to the awake hemisphere remains open. REM sleep, on the other hand, occurs only bihemispherically.

Cetaceans have had the greatest amount of studies done on unihemispheric sleep. Dolphins, eared seals, manatees, and white whales have all displayed unihemispheric sleep of one hemisphere consistent with delta sleep at the same time that the opposite hemisphere shows EEG evidence of a waking pattern. One study (Lyamin et al., Behav Brain Res 129:125, 2002) showed that the contralateral eye to the sleeping hemisphere was closed in the white whale. For both aquatic mammals and birds, unihemispheric sleep serves as a protective feature to allow the mammal or bird to monitor the environment and remain vigilant for safety. In the aquatic mammal, it also serves to permit surfacing to breathe.

49. A. There is a higher concordance rate for REM sleep percentage in monozygotic than in dizygotic twins.

There are several small twin studies regarding sleep architecture; however, they show consistent results of a higher concordance rate for REM sleep percentage in monozygotic than in dizygotic twins. In fact, sleep architecture seems to show similarity in all-night sleep patterns of monozygotic twins. It is interesting that even awake EEG patterns show similar waking alpha rhythms between monozygotic twins. EEG studies have even showed identical EEG patterns in up to 85% of monozygotic twins but only 5% of dizygotic twins during waking studies.

For the sleep EEG studies, there are also similarities in monozygotic twins with a greater concordance than dizygotic twins, with a higher monozygotic concordance for REM amounts, sleep latency, stage changes, and sleep spindle density.

50. C. The MT2 receptor mRNA in human brain and retina is responsible for circadian rhythm entrainment in the suprachiasmatic nuclei of the hypothalamus.

There are two subtypes of melatonin receptors, the MT1 and MT2. The MT2 receptor mRNA in human brain and retina is responsible for circadian rhythm entrainment in the suprachiasmatic nuclei of the hypothalamus. Mouse studies have shown that melatonin, acting through MT1 receptors, regulate rhythmicity in hypophyseal pars tuberalis (PT) cells and clock gene expression by determining availability of mPER1, mPER2, and mCRY1 (circadian proteins). Variations of MT1 and MT2 in humans may be linked to certain sleep disorders.

In commenting on the other answer choices, melatonin is a potent free radical scavenger, greater than vitamin E. There is close correlation between the plasma melatonin peak (not nadir) and minimum core temperature. Finally, melatonin has antioxidative features and increases (not decreases) the levels of superoxide dismutase, glutathione reductase, and glutathione peroxidase (antioxidative enymes).

REFERENCES

1. Armitage R, Baker FC, Parry BL: The menstrual cycle and circadian rhythm. In Kryger MH, Roth T, Dement WC (eds): *Principles and Practice of Sleep Medicine*, 4th ed. Philadelphia, Elsevier Saunders, 2005, pp 1266–1269.

2. Bach V, Telliez F, Leke A, et al: Gender-related sleep differences in neonates in thermoneutral and cool environments. J Sleep Res 9:249–254, 2000.

3. Baker FC, Mitchell D, Driver HS: Oral contraceptives alter sleep and raise body temperature in young women. Pflugers Arch 442(5):729–737, 2001.

4. Berger AJ, Mitchell RA, Severinghaus JW: Regulation of respiration (second of three parts). N Engl J Med 297(3):138–143, 1977.

5. Bliwise DL: Normal aging. In Kryger MH, Roth T, Dement WC (eds): *Principles and Practice of Sleep Medicine*, 4th ed. Philadelphia, Elsevier Saunders, 2005, pp 24–38.

6. Bolton CF, Chen R, Wijdicks EFM, Zifko UA: Anatomy and physiology of the nervous system control of respiration. In Bolton CF, Chen R, Wijdicks EFM, Zifko UA (eds): *Neurology of Breathing*. Philadelphia, Butterworth Heinemann Elsevier, 2004, pp 19–36.

7. Bonnet MH: Acute sleep deprivation. In Kryger MH, Roth T, Dement WC (eds): *Principles and Practice of Sleep Medicine*, 4th ed. Philadelphia, Elsevier Saunders, 2005, pp 51–66.

8. Borbely AA, Achermann P: Sleep homeostasis and models of sleep regulation. In Kryger MH, Roth T, Dement WC (eds): *Principles and Practice of Sleep Medicine*, 4th ed. Philadelphia, Elsevier Saunders, 2005, pp 405–417.

9. Boselli M, Parrino L, Smerieri A, Terzano MG: Effect of age on EEG arousals in normal sleep. Sleep 21(4):351–357, 1998.

10. Braun AR, Balkin TJ, Wesensten NJ: Regional cerebral flow throughout the sleep-wake cycle. Brain 120:1173–1197, 1997.

11. Carskadon MA, Dement WC: Normal human sleep: an overview. In Kryger MH, Roth T, Dement WC (eds): *Principles and Practice of Sleep Medicine*, 4th ed. Philadelphia, Elsevier Saunders, 2005, pp 13–23.

12. Carskadon MA, Dement WC: Sleep loss in elderly volunteers. Sleep 8:207–221, 1985.

13. Chokroverty S: Physiologic changes in sleep. In Chokroverty S (ed): *Sleep Disorders Medicine: Basic Science, Technical Considerations, and Clinical Aspects*, 2nd ed. Boston, Butterworth-Heinemann, 1999, pp 5–126.

14. Chow KL, Dement WC, Mitchell SA Jr: Effects of lesions of the rostral thalamus on brain waves and behavior in cats. Electroencephalog Clin Neurophysiol Suppl 959: 11(7):107–120, 1959.

15. Claustrat B, Brun J, Chazot G: The basic physiology and pathophysiology of melatonin. Sleep Med Rev 9(1):11–24, 2005.

16. Copinski G: Metabolic and endocrine effects of sleep deprivation. Essent Psychopharmacol 6(6):341–347, 2005.

17. Czeisler CA, Buxton OM, Khalsa SBS: The human circadian timing system and sleep-wake regulation. In Kryger MH, Roth T, Dement WC (eds): *Principles and Practice of Sleep Medicine*, 4th ed. Philadelphia, Elsevier Saunders, 2005, pp 375–394.

18. Dauvilliers Y, Maret S, Tafti M: Genetics of normal and pathological sleep in humans. Sleep Med Rev 9(2):91–100, 2005.

19. Dement WC: History of sleep physiology and medicine. In Kryger MH, Roth T, Dement WC (eds): *Principles and Practice of Sleep Medicine*, 4th ed. Philadelphia, Elsevier Saunders, 2005, pp 1–12.

20. Dimitrov S, Lange T, Tieken S, et al: Sleep associated regulation of T helper1/T helper 2 cytokine balance in humans. Brain Behav Immunity 18(4):341–348, 2004.

21. Fenik P, Veasey SC: Pharmacological characterization of serotonergic receptor activity in the hypoglossal nucleus. Am J Respir Crit Care Med 167(4):563–569, 2003.

22. Franzini C: Cardiovascular physiology: the peripheral circulation. In Kryger MH, Roth T, Dement WC (eds): *Principles and Practice of Sleep Medicine*, 4th ed. Philadephia, Elsevier Saunders, 2005, pp 203–212.

23. Fuentealba P, Timofeev I, Steriade M: Prolonged hyperpolarizing potentials precede spindle oscillations in the thalamic reticular nucleus. Proc Natl Acad Sci 101(26):9816–9821, 2004.

24. Gais S: Early sleep triggers memory for early visual discrimination skills. Nat Neurosci 3(12):1335–1339, 2000.

25. Jilg A, Moek J, Weaver DR, et al: Rhythms in clock proteins in the mouse pars tuberalis depend on MT1 melatonin receptor signalling. Eur J Neurosci 22(11):2845–2854, 2005.

26. Jones BE: Basic mechanisms of sleep-wake states. In Kryger MH, Roth T, Dement WC (eds): *Principles and Practice of Sleep Medicine*, 4th ed. Philadephia, Elsevier Saunders, 2005, pp 136–153.

27. Joseph V, Pequignot JM, Van Reeth O: Neurochemical perspectives on the control of breathing during sleep. Respir Physiol Neurobiol 130(3):253–262, 2002.

28. Juhasz G, Kukorelli T: Modifications of visceral evoked potentials during sleep in cats. Act Nerv Super (Praha) 19:212–214, 1977.

29. Krimsky WR, Leiter JC: Physiology of breathing and respiratory control during sleep. Semin Respir Crit Care Med 26(1):5–12, 2005.

30. Kripke DF, Garfinkel L, Wingard DL, et al: Mortality associated with sleep duration and insomnia. Arch Gen Psychiatry 59(2):137–138, 2002.

31. Krueger JM, Majde JA, Blatteis CM, et al: Polyribonosinic acid (poly I:C) enhances rabbit slow-wave sleep. Am J Physiol 255:R748–R755, 1988.

32. Krueger JM, Majde JA: Host defense. In Kryger MH, Roth T, Dement WC (eds): *Principles and Practice of Sleep Medicine*, 4th ed. Philadelphia, Elsevier Saunders, 2005, pp 256–265.

33. Krueger JM, Majde JA: Microbial products and cytokines in sleep and fever regulation. Crit Rev Immunol 14:355–379, 1994.

34. Lee KA, McEnany G, Zaffke ME: REM sleep and mood state in childbearing women: sleepy or weepy? Sleep 23:877–885, 2000.

35. Lyamin OI, Mukhametov LM, Siegel JM, et al: Unihemispheric slow wave sleep and the state of the eyes in a white whale. Behav Brain Res 129(1–2):125–129, 2002.

36. Meier-Ewert HK, Ridker PM, Rifai N, et al: Effect of sleep loss on C-reactive protein, an inflammatory marker of cardiovascular risk. J Am Coll Cardiol 43:678–683, 2004.

37. Moore JG, Englert E Jr: Circadian rhythm of gastric acid secretion in man. Nature 226(252):1261–1262, 1970.

38. Moore JG, Halberg F: Circadian rhythm of gastric acid secretion in active duodenal ulcer: chronobiological statistical characteristics and comparison of acid secretory and plasma gastrin patterns with healthy subjects and postvagotomy and pyloroplasty patients. Chronobiol Int 4(1):101–110, 1987.

39. Moruzzi G, Magoun H: Brainstem reticular formation and activation of the EEG. Electroencephalogr Clin Neurophysiol 1:455–473, 1949.

40. Obal F Jr, Krueger JM: GHRH and sleep. Sleep Med Rev 8(5):367–377, 2004.

41. Orr WC, Shadid G, Harnish MJ, Elsenbruch S: Meal composition and its effect on postprandial sleepiness. Physiol Behav 62(4):709–712, 1997.

42. Orthmann J, Rogers NL, Price NJ, et al: Changes in plasma growth hormone levels following chronic sleep restrictions. Sleep 24:A248–A249, 2001.

43. Palca JW, Walker JM, Berger RJ: Thermoregulation, metabolism, and stages of sleep in cold exposed men. J Appl Physiol 61:940–947, 1986.

44. Philal W, Pietrowsky R, Born J: Dexamethasone blocks sleep induced improvement of declarative memory. Psychoneuroendocrinology 24:313–331, 1999.

45. Quine L: Sleep problems in primary school children: comparison between mainstream and special school children. Child Care Health Develop 27(3):201, 2001.

46. Rattenborg NC: Do birds sleep in flight? Naturwissenschaften 93(9):413–425, 2006 (Epub ahead of print).

47. Rechtschaffen A, Kales A: *A Manual of Standardized Terminology, Techniques, and Scoring System for Sleep Stages of Human Subjects*. Los Angeles, UCLA Brain Information Service/BRI Publications, 1968.

48. Rechtschaffen A, Bergmann BM, Everson CA, et al: Sleep deprivation in the rat: X. Integration and discussion of the findings. Sleep 12(1):68–87, 1989.

49. Redline S, Kirchner HL, Quan SF, et al: The effects of age, sex, ethnicity, and sleep-disordered breathing on sleep architecture. Arch Intern Med 164(4):406–418, 2004.

50. Sakakibara S, Kohsaka M, Kobayashi R, et al: Gender differences in self-evaluated sleep quality and activity of middle-aged and aged subjects. Psychiatry Clin Neurosci 52:184–186, 1998.

51. Sheldon SH: Polysomnography in infants and children. In Sheldon SH, Ferber R, Kryger MH (eds): *Principles and Practice of Pediatric Sleep Medicine*, 4th ed. Philadelphia, Elsevier Saunders, 2005, pp 49–71.

52. Siegel JM: Hypocretin (orexin): role in normal behavior and neuropathology. Annu Rev Psychol 55:125–148, 2004.

53. Spath-Schwalbe E, Lange T, Perras P, et al: Interferon-α acutely impairs sleep in healthy humans. Cytokine 2:518–521, 2000.

54. Spiegel JM: REM Sleep. In Kryger MH, Roth T, Dement WC (eds): *Principles and Practice of Sleep Medicine*, 4th ed. Philadelphia, Saunders, 2005, pp 120–135.

55. Spiegel K, Leproult R, Colecchia EF, et al: Adaptation of the 24-h growth hormone profile to a state of sleep debt. Am J Physiol Regul Integr Comp Physiol 279(3):R874–R883, 2000.

56. Spiegel K, Sheridan JF, Van Cauter E: Effect of sleep deprivation on response to immunization. JAMA 288:1471–1472, 2002.

57. Stickgold R: Why we dream. In Kryger MH, Roth T, Dement WC (eds): *Principles and Practice of Sleep Medicine*, 4th ed. Philadelphia, Saunders, 2005, pp 579–588.

58. Stickgold R, Whidbee D, Schirmer B, et al: Visual discrimination task improvement: a multi-step process occurring during sleep. J Cogn Neurosci 12(2):246–254, 2000.

59. Steiger A: Neurochemical regulation of sleep. J Psychiatr Res 2006; in press ("Epub ahead of print"). Available online at www.sciencedirect.com.

60. Van Cauter E: Endocrine physiology. In Kryger MH, Roth T, Dement WC (eds): *Principles and Practice of Sleep Medicine*, 4th ed. Philadelphia, Elsevier Saunders, 2005, pp 266–282.

61. Verrier RL, Harper RM, Hobson JA: Cardiovascular physiology: central and autonomic regulation. In Kryger MH, Roth T, Dement WC (eds): *Principles and Practice of Sleep Medicine*, 4th ed. Philadelphia, Saunders, 2005, pp 192–202.

62. Volgin DV, Mackiewicz M, Kubin L: Alpha (1B) receptors are the main postsynaptic mediators of adrenergic excitation in brainstem motoneruons, a single-cell RT-PCR study. J Chem Neuroanat 22(3):147–166, 2001.

63. Walker M, Brakefield I, Morgan A, et al: Practice with sleep makes perfect: sleep-dependent motor skill learning. Neuron 35(1):205–211, 2002.

64. Weil JV: Respiratory physiology: sleep at high altitudes. In Kryger MH, Roth T, Dement WC (eds): *Principles and Practice of Sleep Medicine*, 4th ed. Philadelphia, Elsevier Saunders, 2005, pp 245–255.

65. White DP, Weil JV, Zwillick JW: Metabolic rate and breathing during sleep. J Appl Physiol 59(2):384–391, 1985.

66. Wiegand L, Zwillich CW, White DP: Collapsibility of the human upper airway during normal sleep. J Appl Physiol 66(4):1800–1808, 1989.

67. Yoon IY, Kripke DF, Elliott JA, et al: Age-related changes of circadian rhythms and sleep-wake cycles. Am Geriatr Soc 51(8):1085–1091, 2003.

68. Young JK, Wu M, Manaye KF, et al: Orexin stimulates breathing via medullary and spinal pathways. J Appl Physiol 98:1387–1395, 2005.

Mechanisms of Sleep Neuroscience

CHRISTOPHER M. SINTON

Questions

1. Circadian and homeostatic processes that govern sleep propensity are integrated in a simple additive two-process model. Process S is dependent on prior wakefulness, and process C is a single period oscillator dependent on circadian time. A patient presents with an unusual syndrome: process S is normal but process C has a 12-hour, instead of the normal 24-hour, cyclicity. Assuming no interaction between the two processes, which of the following symptoms would have been reported to suggest this diagnosis as a possibility?
   A. Difficulty staying awake in the evening
   B. Difficulty waking up in the morning
   C. Abnormally sleepy during the day
   D. All of the above
   E. Either A or C

2. Adenosine is an extracellular factor that inhibits neural activity throughout the brain by an action at specific receptors. But experiments have shown that adenosine may act as a mediator of sleepiness in which of the following areas?
   A. The ventrolateral preoptic area of the hypothalamus
   B. The suprachiasmatic nucleus (SCN)
   C. The basal forebrain
   D. The lateral geniculate nucleus

3. Neurons in the hypothalamic ventrolateral preoptic area (VLPO) are an important group of cells involved in sleep-wake neurophysiology. VLPO cells send projections throughout the neuraxis, but which of the following statements is true about VLPO projections?
   A. They inhibit cells in the hypothalamic paraventricular nucleus.
   B. They inhibit cells in the laterodorsal tegmental nucleus.
   C. They excite cells in the thalamic reticular nucleus.
   D. They excite cells in the locus coeruleus.
   E. They inhibit cells in the nucleus pontis oralis.

4. High-frequency electrical stimulation of the nucleus basalis of Meynert in the basal forebrain has been found to induce wakefulness. Which of the following neural pathways is the principal substrate for this effect?
   A. Glutamatergic innervation of the reticular activating system
   B. Indirect stimulation of fibers of passage that comprise the dorsal pathway of the ascending reticular activating system
   C. Cholinergic innervation of the intralaminar thalamic nucleus
   D. Cholinergic innervation of the cortex

5. A preparation named the *cerveau isole* is made by transecting the brainstem just above the junction of the pons and midbrain. It transects all afferent cranial nerves except I and II. Which of the following changes would you expect to see while examining the EEG of this preparation?
   A. Continuous high-amplitude δ (1–4 Hz) waves characteristic of stage 3–4 slow wave sleep (SWS)
   B. A brief, strong visual stimulation induces prolonged EEG arousal that outlasts the stimulus
   C. The cyclical alternating patterns of activation and synchronization characteristic of rapid eye movement (REM) and non-REM (NREM) sleep
   D. Spindles and continuous low-amplitude waves characteristic of stage 2 non-REM sleep

6. The ascending pathways of the pontine reticular formation are critical for central arousal and wakefulness. Which of the following is a component of these pathways?
   A. A ventral cholinergic projection to the subthalamus
   B. A dorsal glutamatergic projection to the midline thalamus
   C. A ventral noradrenergic projection to the posterior hypothalamus
   D. All of the above

7. Cataplexy is important for the diagnosis of narco-lepsy. Which of the following are possible explanations for the occurrence of cataplexy?
   A. Insurmountable sleepiness
   B. The intrusion of the signs of REM sleep into wakefulness
   C. A unique state reflecting the occurrence of δ (1–4 Hz) waves during wakefulness
   D. All of the above

8. The generation of δ (1–4 Hz) waves, a characteristic observation from EEG records during SWS, is dependent primarily on:
   A. Depolarization of cortical pyramidal cells by basal forebrain cholinergic projections
   B. Synchronization of oscillations through the septohippocampal system
   C. Intrinsic membrane properties of thalamic GABAergic interneurons
   D. GABAergic innervation from thalamic reticular to thalamic relay cells

9. REM sleep can be induced by localized microinjection of carbachol into which of the following brain areas?
   A. Pontine reticular formation
   B. Ventral tegmental area
   C. Ventrolateral preoptic area
   D. Posterior lateral hypothalamic region

10. Act 4 of *Macbeth* begins with a famous scene that includes a recitation of the ingredients for a witch's brew as they are added one by one to the cauldron. One ingredient that Shakespeare left out was belladonna (containing atropine), believed to be an important component of the brew because of the hallucinations it can produce. Which of the following is the best description of how ingestion of nontoxic amounts of belladonna might induce hallucinations?
    A. A dissociated state resembling hypnosis
    B. REM sleep induction and intense vivid dreaming remembered on awakening
    C. A drug-induced, cataplectic-like state with hypnopompic hallucinations
    D. Intense arousal and anxiety

11. When the anatomy of the orexin (hypocretin) projections was described, and before the relationship between orexin and narcolepsy was discovered, it was evident that the neuropeptide might be important in the regulation of sleepwakefulness. Which of the following projection areas of the orexinergic neurons was important in reaching that conclusion?

A. The pedunculopontine tegmental region
B. The suprachiasmatic nucleus
C. The thalamic lateral geniculate nucleus
D. The arcuate nucleus

12. After the discovery of the relationship between orexin (hypocretin) and narcolepsy, investigations continued concerning the normal function of orexin. Which of the following is a putative function of orexin in the normal animal?
    A. Postprandial sleepiness
    B. The circadian wakefulness signal
    C. Increase in the duration of REM sleep bouts
    D. Reduction in metabolism when food sources are restricted
    E. All of the above

13. When compared with wakefulness, sleep is accompanied by a fall in body temperature. Which of the following is the cause of this drop in temperature?
    A. Reduction in metabolic rate
    B. Enhanced heat loss to the environment
    C. Reduced thermoregulatory response in REM sleep
    D. Downregulation of hypothalamic thermosensitivity
    E. All of the above

14. The suprachiasmatic nucleus (SCN) is critical for the circadian organization of behavior, including the sleep-wake cycle, and photic information is important in setting the circadian cycle. Neuronal projections from which of the following areas of the brain reach the SCN with this information?
    A. The intergeniculate leaflet of the thalamus
    B. The pineal gland
    C. The median raphe nucleus
    D. The dorsomedial hypothalamus

15. A 25-year-old healthy male subject in a research protocol has been in England for several months and flies from London to Chicago. Two days later he undergoes a sleep evaluation together with an endocrine analysis. By this time his sleep-wake schedule is reasonably well adapted to the new clock time, but which of the following results would you expect from the endocrine analysis?
    A. A growth hormone (GH) peak soon after sleep onset and a cortisol peak just before awakening
    B. Coincident GH and cortisol peaks soon after sleep onset
    C. Coincident GH and cortisol peaks just prior to awakening
    D. A GH peak during the afternoon and a cortisol peak soon after sleep onset

16. Fatal familial insomnia is a rare prion disorder marked by gliosis and cell loss primarily in the dorsomedial thalamic nucleus. The neuropathology of this condition has affected our understanding of the neuroanatomy of sleep processes because:

A. The ventral ascending cholinergic activating system terminates in the dorsomedial thalamus.

B. Thalamic nucleus reticularis neurons project to the dorsomedial thalamic nucleus.

C. The basal forebrain cholinergic system innervates the same cortical areas that receive projections from the dorsomedial thalamus.

D. Orexin (hypocretin) projections from the lateral hypothalamus terminate in the dorsomedial thalamus.

17. Which of the following effects on sleep architecture are observed following typical therapeutic doses of the benzodiazepine hypnotics (e.g., triazolam, flurazepam, or temazepam)?

A. An increase in EEG spectral power in the beta (14–30 Hz) frequency range

B. A decrease in stage 1 and 2 NREM sleep

C. An increase in SWS

D. All of the above

18. Antihistamines that act at the H_1 receptor and cross the blood-brain barrier (e.g., diphenhydramine) cause drowsiness and promote sleep. These compounds have this effect by postsynaptic antagonism of a neuronal system with cell bodies in which of the following areas?

A. The raphe dorsalis nucleus

B. The lateral hypothalamus

C. The tuberomammillary nucleus

D. The thalamic reticularis nucleus

19. Drugs that enhance dopaminergic (DA) transmission increase wakefulness and arousal. Which of the following is a likely explanation for this effect on wakefulness?

A. The discharge rate of DA cells in the substantia nigra varies across the sleep-wakefulness cycle.

B. The discharge rate of DA cells in the periaqueductal gray varies across the sleep-wakefulness cycle.

C. The discharge rate of DA cells in the arcuate and periventricular hypothalamic nuclei varies across the sleep-wakefulness cycle.

D. All of the above

20. The cyclical occurrence of sleep spindles (waxing and waning 7–14 Hz bursts on the electroencephalogram [EEG]) is one of the defining features of

stage 2 sleep as sleep begins and before it deepens into stage 3. Which of the following neurophysiological events are correlated with the occurrence of spindles on the EEG?

A. Cyclical depolarization of cells in the thalamic nucleus reticularis

B. Cyclical hyperpolarization of cells in the thalamic nucleus reticularis

C. Cyclical depolarization of thalamocortical projection cells

D. The thalamocortical projection cells discharge at a high frequency, which is cyclically modulated at the spindle frequency

21. Narcolepsy is a disabling sleep disorder that is typically characterized by excessive daytime sleepiness and cataplexy. The clinical picture of narcolepsy, however, can be complicated by which of the following additional symptoms?

A. Nocturnal insomnia

B. Semiautomatic behavior during a conversation

C. Visual hallucinations on awakening

D. Weight gain

E. All of the above

22. The pro-inflammatory cytokine, tumor necrosis factor-α (TNF-α), is produced in the brain and its level varies with the sleep-wake cycle. Its level is also increased by sleep deprivation. Knowing this and the interrelated pathways of cytokine production and regulation, which consequence would you expect when levels of the following are increased in brain?

A. Cyclooxygenase (COX)-2 inhibitors will decrease sleep.

B. Prostaglandin (PG) D_2 will decrease sleep.

C. The transcription factor, nuclear factor-κB (NF-κB) will decrease sleep.

D. All of the above

23. A cat is subjected to localized bilateral lesions of areas just medial to the locus subcoeruleus region in the pontine reticular formation. While exhibiting the polygraphic characteristics of sleep, the cat begins to move. This is a model of which of the following human sleep disorders?

A. Restless legs syndrome

B. REM sleep behavior disorder

C. Somnambulism

D. Periodic limb movement disorder

E. Rhythmic movement disorder

24. A 4-year-old child is brought to the sleep clinic because his parents are concerned by regular nocturnal awakenings with screaming and hypertonia.

After completion of a polysomnographic evaluation, your diagnosis is one of night terrors because:

A. These episodes are observed during REM sleep.

B. After being reassured on awakening, the child has a lucid memory of the cause of the event.

C. The child shows little autonomic activation and no polypnea or mydriasis.

D. The episodes are observed at the beginning of the night during stage 4 SWS.

25. Various groups of central monoaminergic neurons are known to change their discharge firing rate with the different states of sleep and wakefulness. Which of the following statements describes these changes?

A. Dorsal raphe serotoninergic cells increase their discharge rate in REM sleep, but locus coeruleus noradrenergic cells decrease their firing rate during this state.

B. Dorsal raphe serotoninergic, as well as substantia nigra dopaminergic cells, decrease their discharge rate in SWS.

C. Dorsal raphe serotoninergic, as well as locus coeruleus noradrenergic cells, decrease their discharge rate in SWS.

D. Tuberomammillary nucleus histaminergic cells, as well as substantia nigra dopaminergic cells, decrease their discharge rate in REM sleep.

26. Familial advanced sleep phase syndrome is a recently described autosomal dominant disorder of the circadian clock gene *per2*. These patients exhibit:

A. A normal duration of sleep but the sleep cycle occurs at different times each day, drifting by 1 to 2 hours each day

B. A normal duration of sleep but the sleep cycle occurs at the same, abnormal time each day

C. A sleep cycle that occurs at a normal time but is abnormally short in duration

D. Fragmentation of the typical 90-minute sleep-wake cycle, with some cycles as short as 30 minutes

27. The secretion of melatonin, a pineal hormone, is high during the dark phase. Which of the following statements also describes melatonin secretion?

A. Melatonin secretion is at a maximum during SWS but falls during REM sleep.

B. Melatonin secretion is less during nights that follow intense physical activity, an effect that is likely to cause delayed sleep onset after exercise.

C. Melatonin secretion inhibits dopaminergic cells.

D. Even in a regulated environment, melatonin secretion varies in an individual from one day to the next.

28. An EEG record of a complete night of sleep in a young adult is examined and the following waves are found to occur. Which of them would be considered abnormal and require further evaluation?

A. Bilateral negative synchronous sharp waves, occurring alone or at irregular intervals during light sleep

B. The biphasic or triphasic wave that is characteristic of the K-complex occurring in stage 3

C. Spindles, a burst of activity in the 11–15 Hz range lasting for a few seconds, occurring in stage 4

D. Alpha waves at a frequency slightly less than seen in wakefulness occurring in REM sleep

E. None of these characteristics is abnormal.

29. An important characteristic of the change from wakefulness to sleep at the cellular level is the change in the discharge pattern of the thalamocortical relay cells. Which of the following statements is the best summary of this change in discharge pattern?

A. A rapid discharge rate (>40 Hz) changes to a slow discharge rate (<10 Hz).

B. A burst discharge is replaced by tonic firing of single spikes.

C. Tonic firing of single spikes is replaced by a burst discharge.

D. The cells are not spontaneously active but then begin to fire very slowly (<4 Hz).

30. Intracellular recording of the thalamocortical relay cells has identified the currents through specific ion channels that are responsible for the change in the discharge pattern of these cells (cf. question 29) occurring between wakefulness and sleep. Which of the following is responsible for this change?

A. A calcium current that is activated when the cell is hyperpolarized

B. A voltage-dependent potassium current

C. A delayed-rectifier sodium current

D. All of the above

31. A group of effector neurons in the pontine reticular formation is responsible for the eye movement saccades that are one of the cardinal signs of REM sleep. These rapid eye movement effector neurons are *depolarized by*:

A. A cholinergic projection from the laterodorsal pontine tegmentum acting at muscarinic receptors

B. A serotoninergic projection from the dorsal raphe acting at $5HT_{1A}$ receptors

C. A noradrenergic projection from the locus coeruleus acting at α_2 receptors

D. A serotoninergic projection from the median raphe acting at $5HT_2$ receptors

E. A cholinergic projection from the nucleus basalis acting at nicotinic receptors

32. The ascending cholinergic projection systems are important for cortical arousal and the production of wakefulness and REM sleep. The cholinergic cell bodies are localized within two brain regions, one in the laterodorsal pontine tegmentum (LDT) and the other in the nucleus basalis of Meynert of the basal forebrain (BF). Which of the following statements describes their discharge patterns?

A. A subpopulation of LDT cholinergic cells discharges only in REM sleep.

B. A subpopulation of LDT cholinergic cells discharges only in wakefulness.

C. BF cholinergic cells reduce their discharge rate during REM sleep.

D. A subpopulation of BF cholinergic cells discharges only in REM sleep.

33. Ponto-geniculo-occipital (PGO) waves are an important component of REM sleep and are linked to the appearance of the eye movement saccades that also occur during this state. PGO waves can be recorded in the pons, the lateral geniculate nucleus (LGN) of the thalamus, and the occipital cortex. Which of the following statements is correct?

A. PGO waves follow the onset of muscle atonia and EEG activation in REM sleep.

B. Clustered low-amplitude PGO waves change to high-amplitude isolated waves as REM sleep continues.

C. Local injection of nicotinic ACh antagonists (e.g., hexamethonium) into the LGN suppresses PGO waves.

D. Local injection of muscarinic ACh antagonists (e.g., scopolamine) into the LGN suppresses PGO waves.

34. High plasma prolactin is associated with which of the following changes to sleep architecture in humans and animals?

A. An increase in δ waves in SWS

B. A decrease in spindle incidence

C. An increase in REM sleep

D. A decrease in total sleep time

E. An increase in sleep efficiency

35. Depression can be alleviated by sleep deprivation as well as by several different classes of antidepressant medications. Downregulation of which of the following receptors is a possible mechanism in common to these different treatments?

A. Dopaminergic D_1 receptor

B. Serotoninergic $5HT_2$ receptor

C. Noradrenergic β receptor

D. Serotoninergic $5HT_{1A}$ receptor

E. Orexinergic ORX_1 receptor

36. Noradrenergic projections from the locus coeruleus are fundamental for the control of sleep and wakefulness because:

A. Lesions of the noradrenergic system lead to a profound decrement in arousal.

B. Orexinergic processes depolarize the noradrenergic cells during REM sleep.

C. Noradrenergic innervation of cells in the LDT plays a role in REM sleep generation.

D. Noradrenergic innervation of thalamic relay cells maintains them in a hyperpolarized state during wakefulness.

37. Serotoninergic projections from the raphe dorsalis are important for the regulation of sleep and wakefulness because:

A. Serotoninergic innervation depolarizes neurons in the relay nuclei of the thalamus.

B. Serotonin autoreceptor antagonists, such as pindalol, increase REM sleep.

C. Electrical stimulation of the raphe dorsalis region is followed by drowsiness and sleep.

D. Serotoninergic cell discharge rate is coupled to the light-dark cycle.

38. During a research protocol, d-amphetamine is given to volunteers for a 2-day period of enforced wakefulness and compared with placebo treatment under the same protocol. Compared with placebo, which of the following best describes the effect of the drug treatment on *subsequent* sleep and wakefulness?

A. REM sleep recovery is partial and delayed.

B. There is no recovery of SWS.

C. The total sleep time lost during the procedure is recovered.

D. There is a REM sleep and SWS rebound that overcompensates for the loss of sleep.

39. The alerting properties of caffeine are now known to result primarily from its effect as an adenosine receptor antagonist in the brain;

however, caffeine has several other mechanisms of action. Considering only those mechanisms that would be effective at the concentrations in brain that could be achieved by reasonable consumption of caffeine-containing beverages and over-the-counter compounds containing caffeine, which of the following mechanisms will also contribute to the *central* effects of caffeine?
A. Antagonist at the GABA benzodiazepine receptor
B. Inhibition of cyclic nucleotide phosphodiesterase
C. Changes in intracellular calcium concentrations with effects on calcium channels
D. None of these mechanisms

40. Encephalitis lethargica was characterized by intense and continuous somnolence. Following the encephalitis lethargica pandemic, von Economo published in 1930 a seminal study based on autopsy results. He reported that the prolonged sleepiness in this condition was correlated with pathology in:
A. The posterior hypothalamus
B. A region of the hypothalamus close to the optic chiasm
C. The mediodorsal thalamus
D. The locus coeruleus
E. The dentate gyrus

41. Which of the following is co-localized in orexin-containing (hypocretin-containing) neurons?
A. Nitric oxide synthase
B. Melanin-concentrating hormone
C. Histadine carboxylase
D. Neuropeptide Y
E. Dynorphin

42. Orexinergic (hypocretinergic) projections to which of the following areas is believed to be critical for the influence of the neuropeptide on the stabilization of transitions between wakefulness and sleep?
A. Tuberomammillary nucleus
B. Ventral bed nucleus of stria terminalis
C. Lateral lemniscus
D. Paraventricular thalamus

43. A 60-year-old female patient is evaluated at the sleep clinic. She presents with kicking or jerking movements of the legs that worsen in the evening and particularly affect the early sleep period. The movements occur daily and are severe. Which of the following treatments would be expected to alleviate this condition?
A. Risperidole
B. Paxil

C. Imipramine
D. Diphenhydramine
E. None of the above

44. Post-traumatic stress disorder (PTSD) and depression are frequently associated with similar abnormalities in sleep architecture, including increased phasic events of REM sleep and increased total REM sleep time. Which of the following neurochemical changes might be associated with both of these disorders and affect sleep architecture?
A. Increased cholinergic activity and decreased noradrenergic activity
B. Increased orexinergic (hypocretinergic) activity and decreased noradrenergic activity
C. Decreased noradrenergic activity and increased serotoninergic activity
D. Decreased cholinergic activity and increased orexinergic activity

45. Alcohol can be used as a self-medicating aid to induce sleep. Taken at bedtime, however, alcohol affects sleep architecture by:
A. Increasing REM sleep
B. Increasing total sleep time
C. Increasing SWS
D. Decreasing sleep fragmentation

46. As an important sign of REM sleep, many studies have elucidated the mechanisms by which muscle atonia is produced during this state. For example, electrical stimulation of the medulla will elicit atonia, but which of the following statements is also true?
A. Glutamatergic stimulation of the nucleus magnocellularis in the medulla produces atonia.
B. Nicotinic cholinergic stimulation of the nucleus magnocellularis in the medulla produces atonia.
C. The final common descending pathway from the medulla for the production of atonia depends on GABAergic postsynaptic inhibition of motoneurons.
D. Medullary stimulation produces atonia in a preparation transected at the pontomedullary junction.
E. Changes in blood pressure have no effect on atonia produced by electrical stimulation of the medulla.

47. Pentobarbital has been previously used as a hypnotic and still finds application as a sedative. At the brain concentrations achieved for the hypnotic action, which of the following is a known mechanism of action?
A. Increasing the frequency of the GABA-dependent opening of the GABA chloride channel

B. Increasing the GABA-dependent opening time of the GABA chloride channel

C. Displacing endogenous ligands from the GABA-benzodiazepine receptor complex

D. Inhibiting the voltage-dependent sodium channel

E. Increasing the calcium-dependent release of GABA and glycine

48. Many of the neurophysiological changes that occur during sleep and wakefulness are dependent on GABA, the principal inhibitory neurotransmitter in brain. The regulation of the synthesis of GABA from glutamate is complex. For example, the enzyme, glutamate decarboxylase (GAD), exists in different isoforms. All of the following statements are true, *except*:

A. Aspartate is also a substrate for GAD.

B. The isoforms of GAD have different intracellular distributions.

C. All isoforms of GAD are regulated by the same cofactor, pyridoxal-P.

D. Unlike many enzymes, GAD is not regulated by phosphorylation.

49. The use of PET scanning with ^{15}O-labeled water to measure regional cerebral blood flow (rCBF) has identified certain areas of the brain that are specifically more or less active during the different states of sleep. Which of the following statements is true?

A. During SWS, rCBF increases in the thalamus.

B. During REM sleep, rCBF increases in the prefrontal cortex.

C. During REM sleep, rCBF decreases in the amygdala.

D. During SWS, rCBF decreases in the basal forebrain.

50. Use of the forced desynchrony protocol has enabled researchers to differentiate the circadian and homeostatic processes that govern sleep at different phases of the circadian cycle. These studies have shown that the elderly exhibit earlier waking and reduced sleep consolidation because of:

A. A reduction in the period of the circadian oscillator

B. A reduction in the amplitude of the circadian rhythm of melatonin release

C. A reduction in the homeostatic pressure for sleep

D. An increase in the amplitude of the circadian component of temperature rhythm

Answers

1. E. Difficulty staying awake in the evening or abnormally sleepy during the day

The normal 24-hour cycle in process C is such the drive for wakefulness reaches a maximum in the evening just before the sleep phase, and, conversely, the drive for sleep is at a maximum in the early morning hours just before the time of normal awakening. In this way, sleep can be consolidated into a single period during the night because process C essentially acts to antagonize the accumulation/dissipation of process S during the day/night (Figure 13-1). Here we are presented with a patient with a 12-hour cycle in process C, but the phase relationship between the circadian and homeostatic processes is unknown. Thus C could vary such that the maximum wakefulness signal will still be in the evening, in which case its minimum will be at about noon (i.e., answer C), or conversely with a maximum wakefulness signal around noon, the minimum will be in the evening (i.e., answer A). The maximum drive for wakefulness of process C could also lie between these time points (i.e., answer A). There is no effect on morning sleepiness (answer B), because process C is at a minimum drive for wakefulness at that time, so this patient would be normal in this regard.

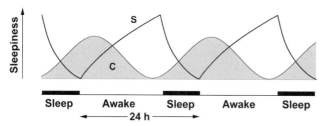

FIGURE 13-1 ■ Schematic representation of the contribution to sleepiness from a circadian factor C, and a homeostatic factor S. Each 24-hr period is designated by an awake phase followed by a sleep phase, and the repetitive nature of each process is shown by concatenating three sleep phases and the intervening two awake phases. S, which can be considered an "hourglass" factor, increases gradually as waking continues and then dissipates during sleep. C, a "clock-like" process, varies continuously over the nychthemeron and is shown here as a simple single-period oscillator that reaches a minimum at the end of the wake period and a maximum at the end of the sleep period. This representation is based on exemplar data from adolescent subjects when they were scored on the multiple sleep latency test (MSLT) at different times (cf. page 370, Sinton and McCarley [*Neuropsychiatry*, 2nd ed. 2003, pp 358–394] for a summary of these data from Carskadon). In the elderly population, process C is shifted to an earlier phase, and process S is reduced in amplitude, and these changes contribute to the poor sleep in this population.

2. C. The basal forebrain

Both sleep-active and wake-active neurons are found in the basal forebrain, and the balance between the activity in these neuronal groups is critical for determining the wakefulness-sleep transition. Adenosine, although a ubiquitous extracellular factor, has been found to accumulate selectively in the basal forebrain during wakefulness, and furthermore, to inhibit wake-active neurons in this region. By acting in this way, adenosine will shift the balance toward sleepiness. Adenosine is therefore a good candidate for the substrate of the homeostatic accumulation of sleepiness with continued wakefulness. Adenosine will also probably function in the same way in other regions of the brain that contain cells that are specifically wake-active, but such cells are not found in the other areas provided as alternate answers.

3. B. They inhibit cells in the laterodorsal tegmental nucleus.

Neurons in the VLPO are selectively active during sleep and contain the inhibitory neurotransmitters, GABA and galanin. These neurons have been shown to project to the wakefulness-promoting neurons of the pontine and forebrain nuclei important in EEG arousal, including the cholinergic cell group of the laterodorsal tegmental nucleus. As activity of the VLPO cells increase, in coordination with the BF sleep-active cells, the transition from wakefulness to sleep occurs. VLPO cells are not excitatory, and they do not send projections to the other brain regions that are provided as alternate answers.

4. D. Cholinergic innervation of the cortex

The two principal cholinergic components of the ascending arousal system project from the laterodorsal tegmental region in the pons, and the basal forebrain, specifically the nucleus basalis of Meynert (NBM). Electrical stimulation of either region produces immediate cortical arousal and wakefulness. Some effect of stimulation in the NBM might be mediated through fibers of passage, as such an effect can never be totally eliminated in a stimulation experiment; but the dorsal pathway, as specified in answer B, terminates in the thalamus and does not innervate the BF area. Conversely, the BF does not directly innervate the intralaminar thalamic nucleus. All descending influences from this area are sleep-inducing.

5. D. Spindles and continuous low-amplitude waves characteristic of stage 2 NREM sleep

The *cerveau isolé* preparation and the results obtained were critical for the initial studies that led eventually to the concept of the ascending reticular activating system (ARAS). See Figure 13-2 for the

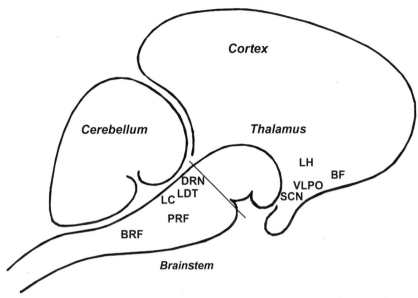

FIGURE 13-2 ■ Schematic representation of a sagittal section from a mammalian brain showing the transection for the *cerveau isole* preparation, which demonstrates continuous light sleep. Nuclei and regions that are important for the control of sleeping and waking are also annotated: BRF, bulbar reticular formation, containing the magnocellular field; PRF, pontine reticular formation, containing cell groups, known as *effector* neurons, that are critical for the cardinal signs of REM sleep such as muscle atonia; LDT, laterodorsal tegmental nucleus/pedunculopontine tegmental nucleus, which is the principal brainstem site containing cholinergic cells, important for REM sleep and wakefulness; LC, locus coeruleus, containing most of the central noradrenergic cells; DRN, dorsal raphe nucleus, containing a major cluster of serotoninergic cells that are important for vigilance state control; SCN, hypothalamic suprachiasmatic nucleus, the principal center for the endogenous circadian oscillator; VLPO, ventrolateral preoptic nucleus, containing the sleep-active GABAergic cells; BF, basal forebrain, a region that contains cortically projecting cholinergic cells that are important for arousal; LH, lateral hypothalamus, which uniquely contains the orexinergic cell body field.

location of the transection in this preparation, which shows a permanently "sleeping" EEG, with continuous spindling-like stage 2 sleep with low-amplitude waves; any high-amplitude δ waves develop for only brief periods. Because almost no sensory input can reach the portion of the brain above the transection, most behavioral measures were not possible, although the EEG (and pupillary reflex) resembled those of the normal, lightly sleeping animal. Attempts to arouse this preparation with strong visual stimulation were unsuccessful, and the weak EEG pattern of arousal that resulted never outlasted the stimulus. Also the REM generator mechanisms are in the pons, so we would not expect to see any signs of REM sleep in this preparation. At the time of Bremer's study (Comptes Rendus des Seances de la Societe de Biologie 118:1235, 1935), the conclusion was that this brain is sleeping because there is no sensory stimulation to arouse it, but the subsequent classic studies of Moruzzi and Magoun (Electroencephalog Cl Neurophys 1:455, 1949) showed that the ARAS is required for normal arousal.

6. D. All of these projections

In addition to the cholinergic components of the ascending arousal system (cf. question 4), a ventral

noradrenergic projection from the locus coeruleus sends projections throughout the neuraxis, including the posterior hypothalamus. Also critically involved in the processes of arousal and wakefulness is the dorsal projection of the ascending arousal system that originates in the medulla and contains glutamate as the neurotransmitter. These neurons send widespread projections to the thalamus and cortex.

7. B. The intrusion of the signs of REM sleep into wakefulness

Because consciousness is maintained in cataplexy and because wakefulness frequently returns at the end of a cataplectic episode in the narcoleptic patient, cataplexy has been considered a separate, unique state. Furthermore, there is evidence from animal studies that brain sites and mechanisms for triggering cataplexy in narcoleptic canines are distinct from those that trigger REM sleep. The state of cataplexy, however, combines wakefulness with characteristics of REM sleep, in particular, muscle atonia. Thus cataplexy could be the partial intrusion of REM sleep signs into wakefulness, or it could be an intermediate state between wakefulness and REM sleep. Cataplexy is not the result of insurmountable sleepiness, which is a separable symptom of narcolepsy. Although narcoleptic patients exhibit slow δ waves during wakefulness, this also is a correlate of insurmountable sleepiness. Also see Figures 13-3 and 13-4 for more details of the pathophysiology.

8. D. GABAergic innervation from thalamic reticular to thalamic relay cells

Thalamocortical cells have intrinsic membrane properties that allow them to oscillate at δ frequencies once they are hyperpolarized by more than 10 mV. This oscillation, however, does not become widespread, nor does it recruit large populations of thalamocortical cells in synchrony or drive the cortical mantle at the same frequency, without additional network connectivity. This connectivity requires a feedback loop from the thalamocortical cells to the cortical cells, which in turn project to the thalamic reticular nucleus. The thalamic reticular cells thus provide a critical stage in this network by transferring impulses back to the thalamic relay neurons to complete the loop. In fact, corticothalamic volleys reinforce and synchronize the δ oscillation throughout the thalamocortical network as a result of the innervation through the reticular nucleus. Local interneurons provide some interconnectivity, but it is insufficient for the synchronous cortical δ oscillations that characterize the EEG.

9. A. Pontine reticular formation

A cholinoceptive area localized to the medial pontine reticular formation (see Figure 13-2) is very sensitive to muscarinic agonists, and localized injection of these agents in this area creates a state that closely mimics REM sleep. Injections slightly removed from the target area do not have this effect. Projections from the laterodorsal tegmentum (LDT) cholinergic region innervate this area, and LDT cholinergic cells begin to discharge before the onset of REM sleep and remain active throughout this phase of sleep, thereby providing the cholinergic drive that is being modeled by the carbachol injection.

10. A. A dissociated state resembling hypnosis

Atropine induces a state of cortical slow waves during behavioral wakefulness by inhibiting the cholinergic arousal centers of the pons and BF. This state is similar to that induced by hypnosis and is also seen in the dissociated states or automated behaviors of hypersomnolence, particularly narcolepsy. Hallucinations, dissociation, and automatic behavior are corollaries of this state. Belladonna is believed to be a likely cause for at least some of the psychotropic effects that resulted from the ingestion of the "witch's brew." Atropine suppresses REM sleep, and it has a somnolent rather than an arousing effect.

11. A. The pedunculopontine tegmental region

When first described, the anatomy of the orexin projection system was remarkable because of the innervation of many of the areas that were known to be critical for sleep-wakefulness regulation. These included the pedunculopontine tegmental region, which, together with the adjacent laterodorsal pontine tegmentum, is the source of the cholinergic arousal system that drives cortical activation during wakefulness and REM sleep. Orexinergic fibers were not found in the suprachiasmatic nucleus or the thalamic lateral geniculate nucleus, and the arcuate nucleus is implicated in feeding behavior, another function of orexin. Also see Figure 13-4.

12. B. The circadian wakefulness signal

The intrusion of REM sleep into wakefulness and the inability to maintain wakefulness summarize the primary symptoms of narcolepsy. Thus the absence of orexin will cause these effects (Figure 13-4). In the normal animal, orexin is wake-inducing and induces arousal when administered centrally. In fact, an important role for the neuropeptide, and clearly related to this induction of arousal, is likely to be in setting the balance between behavioral activation and sleepiness when food sources are scarce. Another arousal-related function, however, has been noted from animal studies. There is evidence that orexin may be linked with the circadian wakefulness signal (i.e., the additional circadian wakefulness drive that builds during the wake period to counteract the effect of homeostatic sleepiness). Also see Figure 13-1. Orexin does not cause reduced arousal or sleepiness (i.e., these effects would be contrary to the action of orexin), nor does orexin increase the duration of REM sleep bouts. Orexin controls the gate for the intrusion of REM sleep into wakefulness, as seen in narcolepsy, but its absence makes little difference to the mean duration of REM sleep episodes. In fact, narcoleptic animal models lacking orexin tend to have slightly increased REM sleep bout duration.

13. E. All the responses are true.

The transition to a lower temperature set point during sleep is accompanied by all the changes that are listed here. The thermoregulatory response during REM sleep is reduced even further. The potential energy savings that result from these changes has been used as evidence that energy conservation might be a possible function of sleep.

14. A. The intergeniculate leaflet of the thalamus

The primary source of photic information to the SCN is from the retinohypothalamic tract (RHT). The RHT also sends projections to the thalamic

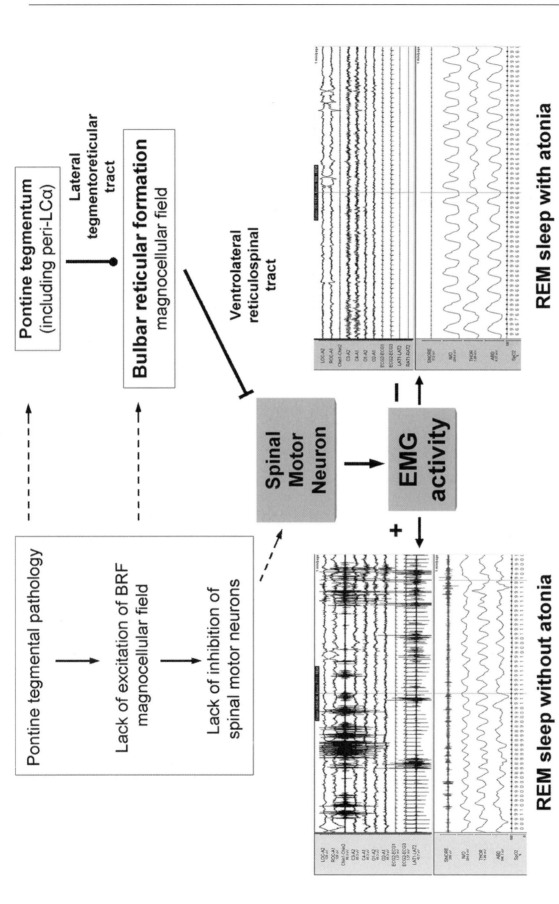

FIGURE 13-3 ■ Mechanisms of muscle atonia during REM sleep. Cells within localized areas of the PRF (i.e., pontine tegmentum), including a group that lies dorsal and medial to the LC, the peri-LCα, send excitatory projections via the lateral tegmental tract to the magnocellular (also known as the gigantocellular) field in the BRF. The latter cells send glycinergic inhibitory axons, via the ventrolateral reticulospinal tract, to synapse on the motor neurons of the ventral horn of the spinal cord. During REM sleep, cholinergically mediated depolarization of cells in the nucleus magnocellularis and thus hyperpolarization of spinal motor neurons. The result is REM sleep with atonia. One of the mechanisms of REM sleep behavior disorder (RBD) is thus pathology in the PRF. This is modeled by animals with lesions in the region of the peri-LCα. In RBD patients, depolarization of cells in the BRF magnocellularis field does not occur during REM sleep, and hence the descending hyperpolarization of the ventral horn spinal motor neurons is also absent. The result, as shown in the polygraphic tracing, is muscle activity during REM sleep in these patients. The filled circle represents excitatory synapses, and T-bar represents inhibitory synapses. (Adapted from Avidan AY: Sleep disorders in the older patient. Prim Care 32:563–586, 2005.)

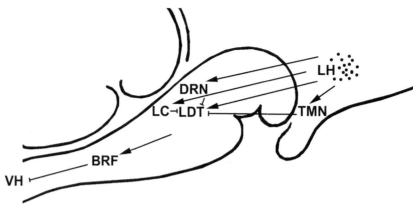

FIGURE 13-4 ■ Schematic of some of the more important neuronal projections involved in the symptoms of narcolepsy, caused by pathology of the orexin cells (dots) that are located around the lateral hypothalamus (LH). Orexin cells send excitatory projections, *inter alia*, to the tuberomammillary nucleus (TMN), the locus coeruleus (LC), the dorsal raphe nucleus (DRN) and the cholinergic cells of the laterodorsal pontine tegmentum/pedunculopontine tegmental nucleus (LDT). Inhibitory inputs from the LC, DRN and TMN project to the "REM-on" cells of the LDT, thus maintaining these cells in a quiescent state during normal wakefulness. The lack of orexinergic influence in narcolepsy thus has two principal effects. One results from the absence of a depolarizing input onto important ascending activating systems, causes reduced arousal and sleepiness. The second principal effect is by reducing excitatory drive onto cell groups that normally inhibit the pontine cholinergic LDT "REM-on" cells alters the balance of activity of these cells, allowing them to become active during wakefulness. One of the results of this activity is an excitatory drive onto cells of the magnocellularis nucleus in the basal reticular formation (BRF), which in turn send an inhibitory, hyperpolarizing input to spinal motor neurons in the ventral horn (VH). This induces muscle atonia during wakefulness (i.e., cataplexy). Arrowheads represent excitatory synapses, and T-bars represent inhibitory synapses.

intergeniculate leaflet, which in turn also projects to the SCN. Note that the pineal does not send neuronal projections to the SCN, and the feedback from the pineal to the SCN is therefore hormonal via the release of melatonin.

15. B. Coincident GH and cortisol peaks soon after sleep onset:

In young healthy subjects, the sleep cycle will adjust relatively quickly to the circadian disturbances induced by jet lag. GH is closely coupled to the sleep-wake cycle and also adjusts quickly, so the GH peak will occur at the normal time in the subject in this study (i.e., soon after sleep onset). Cortisol rhythms, however, take much longer to adapt, typically about 2 weeks to be completely adjusted. Dissociation between sleep and cortisol rhythms may contribute to jet lag. In this case, therefore, after only 2 days, the cortisol peak will remain at the same circadian time as it occurred in London, which would have been about 6 hours after sleep onset, toward the end of the sleep phase. But in Chicago, with a 6-hour time difference, the cortisol peak will now occur 6 hours earlier with respect to local time (i.e., coincident with the GH peak and soon after sleep onset).

16. B. Thalamic nucleus reticularis neurons project to the dorsomedial thalamic nucleus.

The dorsomedial thalamus exhibits severe gliosis in fatal familial insomnia (FFI). The onset of sleep requires the gradual hyperpolarization of thalamic reticularis cells and then the transfer of burst discharges through the network of oscillatory loops between the cortex and the thalamus (cf. questions 8 and 20). The dorsomedial thalamic nucleus receives projections from the reticularis nucleus and also sends projections to cortical areas, specifically the prefrontal cortex. Hence the dorsomedial thalamus plays a role in the thalamocortical network that initiates and sustains sleep, and the symptoms of FFI reveal that this is a vital role. The dorsal (not the ventral) cholinergic innervation of cells in this nucleus would also decrease with the onset of sleep, and so enable the burst mode of firing that aids synchrony as network oscillations begin. The network, however, is more fundamental to this process, especially at sleep onset.

17. A. An increase in EEG spectral power in the beta (14–30 Hz) frequencies

Pharmaco-EEG studies of the benzodiazepine hypnotics have consistently shown an increase in power in the beta (14–30 Hz) frequency band. This may be the result of changes in the oscillatory frequency of the thalamocortical network loops as GABA chloride channel effects change membrane properties and cell coupling. The normal sleep changes seen after benzodiazepines include an increase in stage 1 to 2 NREM and a decrease in SWS.

18. C. The tuberomammillary nucleus

Histamine is produced by neurons of the tubero-mammillary nucleus (TMN) in the posterior hypothalamus. Histamine is one of the components of the arousal system, and TMN histaminergic cells send widespread excitatory projections throughout the neuraxis, including an innervation to the sleep-promoting cells of the ventrolateral preoptic nucleus. Histamine cells also show the state-related changes in discharge rate that is characteristic of other monoaminergic cell groups and begin to slow their discharge rate with sleep onset.

19. B. The discharge rate of dopaminergic cells in the periaqueductal gray varies across the sleep-wakefulness cycle.

Dopamine cell bodies in the brain are found clustered in several distinct nuclei in different brain areas. Neurons in each of these clusters have different projection systems. Of interest, only dopamine cells of the periventricular system, with cell bodies in the central gray (which surrounds the cerebral aqueduct at the level of the rostral midbrain [i.e., just rostral to the transection marked on Figure 13-2]) appear to show the state-related change in discharge rate that is characteristic of other monoaminergic cell groups. Significantly, these dopaminergic cells project to the principal components of the sleep-wakefulness system, including the mediodorsal thalamus, basal forebrain ventrolateral preoptic nucleus, the lateral hypothalamic orexin cell group, laterodorsal tegmental nucleus, and locus ceruleus (see Figure 13-2). This pattern of projections to areas that are implicated in arousal, in conjunction with the wake-active nature of this group of cells, indicate a role in sleep-wakefulness control and/or arousal.

20. A. Cyclical depolarization of cells in the thalamic nucleus reticularis

Like δ waves, spindle waves are generated by network oscillations in thalamic nucleus reticularis cells, thalamocortical cells, and cortical pyramidal cells. They are the first sign of sleep from this network as depolarizing influences on the thalamic cells begin to decrease at the onset of sleep and the membrane potential starts to shift to a hyperpolarized level. Intracellular recordings have shown that nucleus reticularis cells exhibit rhythmic bursting on a depolarizing envelope during spindles. These bursts, at the spindle frequency, in turn send a strong and cyclical hyperpolarizing influence to the thalamocortical cells, which also show burst firing but on a hyperpolarizing envelope. The spindle frequency is reinforced and network oscillations are set up as the bursts are transferred to the cortical pyramidal cells. The inherent properties of the nucleus reticularis cells are such that they spindle even when deafferented, although it is the transfer properties of the

network that is required for the synchronized spindling at a cortical level. Note therefore that the thalamocortical cells fire in bursts at spindle frequencies, and these bursts wax and wane as the spindles appear and disappear. They do not discharge at higher frequencies, thus precluding answer D.

21. E. All of these additional symptoms are observed in narcolepsy.

All these symptoms are explicable in terms of the functional effects of the loss of orexinergic innervation. In particular the effect of orexin on state boundary control between the different vigilant states is apparent: slow δ waves appearing on the EEG during behavioral wakefulness (B), wakefulness intruding into sleep (A), and the signs of REM sleep intruding into wakefulness (C). The orexinergic influence on feeding behavior (D) is also evident in these patients.

22. B. Cyclooxygenase (COX)-2 inhibitors will decrease sleep.

TNF-α activates the transcription nuclear factor NF-κB, which is enhanced in brain during sleep deprivation (i.e., in a concatenated response with TNF-α to sleep deprivation). Inhibition of NF-κB is therefore associated with decreased sleep. COX is the rate-limiting enzyme that catalyzes the synthesis of the prostanoids, including prostaglandin (PG) D_2, and NF-κB promotes transcription of the COX-2 gene (the COX variant that exists in brain). Therefore a COX-2 inhibitor will decrease sleep, and PG D_2 will enhance sleep. There is thus a logical progression among the steps in this cytokine cascade, and each component has an effect on sleep that would be predicted from the others. Preclinical studies have confirmed these results. (Yoshida et al, Am J Physiol Regul Integr Comp Physiol 285:R99, 2003).

23. B. REM sleep behavior disorder

Bilateral lesions in the cat of an area medial to the locus subcoeruleus region in the dorsal pontine reticular formation produces a preparation that shows all the characteristic signs of REM sleep except muscle atonia (i.e., the cat demonstrates cortical arousal, PGO waves, and eye movements). This is equivalent to REM sleep behavior disorder (RBD) in the human. RBD is a parasomnia associated with dream mentation during REM sleep in the presence of skeletal muscle tone (i.e., without the normal atonia of REM sleep). The disorder is strongly associated with synucleopathies such as Parkinson's disease and diffuse Lewy body dementia. It can be distinguished clinically from other movements that occur during sleep, listed here as alternative responses, as these do not occur during REM sleep; however, palatal myoclonus is another movement disorder that can occur in this state. Figure 13-3 illustrates the underlying neuropathology of RBD based on the animal models of REM sleep without atonia.

24. D. The episodes are observed at the beginning of the night during stage 4 slow wave sleep (SWS).

Arousal disorders (somnambulism, confusional arousals, and night terrors) form a symptomatic cluster that shows several similarities. In particular, they occur toward the beginning of the night during stage 4 SWS at a time when a REM sleep period would be expected. This suggests that the appearance of these disorders is linked with a deficit in the mechanism that ensures the transition from SWS into REM sleep. They occur primarily in younger children, but significantly, there is a familial pattern of incidence, implying genetic linkage. Night terrors are marked by intense anxiety with autonomic arousal. Furthermore, the child shows no lucidity after the event and no recollection.

25. C. Dorsal raphe serotoninergic, as well as locus coeruleus noradrenergic cells, decrease their discharge rate in SWS.

The discharge rates of monoaminergic cells, including the noradrenergic cells of the locus coeruleus, the serotoninergic cells of the dorsal raphe, the histaminergic cells of the tuberomammillary nucleus, and the dopaminergic cells of the periaqueductal gray (cf. question 19) change in the following way during the different vigilance states: The discharge rate begins to decrease during stage 2 NREM sleep, decreases further during SWS, and almost completely ceases firing during REM sleep. Dopaminergic cells of the substantia nigra and ventral tegmentum are an exception. The discharge rates of these cells are not correlated with vigilance state.

26. B. A normal duration of sleep but the sleep cycle occurs at the same, abnormal time each day

Advanced sleep phase syndrome (ASPS) is characterized by a normal duration of sleep but the major sleep period is out of phase with that of normal subjects; specifically the sleep cycle occurs several hours earlier. The finding that in one family this disorder could be linked to the circadian clock gene *per2* was important because it was the first demonstration of the genetic regulation of the circadian system in humans. This result will thus likely have implications for a better understanding of the underlying pathophysiology of ASPS and other circadian rhythm disorders.

27. C. Melatonin secretion inhibits dopaminergic cells.

Inhibition of dopamine release by melatonin has been demonstrated in several specific brain areas, including the hypothalamus, hippocampus, medulla, and retina. One important interaction, for example, is in the retina where melatonin is synthesized and where dopaminergic amacrine cells possess presynaptic melatonin receptors. Melatonin inhibits dopamine release from these cells. Interindividual variation in melatonin secretion is very high, but within individuals it is remarkably constant. Stress affects melatonin secretion, but in humans, physical exercise has been shown either to have no effect on melatonin secretion or to increase it. The variation in plasma melatonin follows a 24-hour rhythm, which is coupled to the light-dark cycle, and sleep has no effect on its release.

28. E. None of these characteristics is abnormal.

Although spike and sharp waves are frequently abnormal, all the listed waves can occur on an EEG record of a normal healthy young adult. Vertex sharp transients (A), for example, can occur spontaneously, or in response to alerting stimuli, in stage 1 or 2; K-complexes (B), although characteristic of stage 2, occur frequently in stage 3 and, with slow waves, in stage 4. Spindles (C) also occur in stage 4; this is important because our understanding of the neurophysiological mechanisms of spindle and delta wave generation shows that they are mutually exclusive (cf. questions 8 and 20). Thus these instances of spindles during stage 4 must reflect brief changes in the level of arousal. Alpha waves (D), typically at a frequency that is 1–2 Hz less than that in wakefulness, can be observed during REM sleep. The importance of the generation of the specific frequencies of alpha waves by the thalamocortical network is unknown.

29. C. Tonic firing of single spikes is replaced by a burst discharge.

30. A. A calcium current that is activated when the cell is hyperpolarized

Both questions 29 and 30 refer to the beginning of sleep and the correlated events that occur in the thalamus, a region that is critical for orchestrating the changes in brain state between wakefulness and sleep. The beginning of sleep is associated with a significant change in the discharge pattern of thalamocortical cells, as the depolarizing inputs to these cells during wakefulness gradually reduce and the cells become hyperpolarized. As sleep deepens, the EEG pattern demonstrating the waxing and waning pattern of spindle oscillations (cf. question 20) is replaced by thalamocortical oscillations of slower frequencies, particularly the δ frequencies (1–4 Hz). At a cellular level, the tonic regular firing of single spikes of the thalamic relay cells during wakefulness is replaced by the rhythmic and periodic burst discharges of slow wave sleep (i.e., response C, question 29). The latter induce the widespread synchronized network oscillations that are seen on the EEG as δ waves. The critical ionic channel for the burst discharge as the cell becomes hyperpolarized is the low-threshold calcium channel. This is activated when the membrane potential drops below approximately $-65 \, mV$ and is thus responsible for the change in discharge pattern of the thalamocortical cells as sleep replaces wakefulness (i.e., response A, question 30). The calcium current that results from activation of this channel then depolarizes the cell back above the spike threshold, and a burst of fast-action potentials results from the interplay of a voltage-dependent sodium channel and a delayed-rectifier potassium current.

31. A. A cholinergic projection from the laterodorsal pontine tegmentum acting at muscarinic receptors

The effector neurons that are responsible for the cardinal signs of REM sleep are located in the median pontine reticular formation (PRF) (Figure 13-2). One group of neurons, for example, is responsible for eye movement saccades, and these neurons are depolarized as REM sleep begins. Cholinergic agonists such as carbachol, when locally administered in this region, mimic the neuronal depolarization seen during REM sleep and in fact produce a state that is essentially the same as REM sleep. Anatomical tracing has shown that the cholinergic projection to the PRF originates in the laterodorsal pontine tegmentum. The alternative responses provided are either inhibitory or do not project to the median PRF. Hence they are not responsible for the depolarization of effector neurons in the PRF observed during REM sleep.

32. A. A subpopulation of laterodorsal pontine tegmentum (LDT) cholinergic cells discharges only in REM sleep.

The critical cholinergic projection that drives the depolarization of pontine reticular formation neurons during REM sleep originates in the LDT. This projection is composed of a subgroup of cells that are active only during REM sleep (cf. question 31). Other cholinergic cells in this region discharge both during wakefulness and REM sleep. Cholinergic cells in the BF have not been found to discharge specifically during REM sleep.

33. C. Local injection of nicotinic ACh antagonists (e.g., hexamethonium) into the lateral geniculate nucleus (LGN) suppresses ponto-geniculo-occipital (PGO) waves.

Studies of the thalamic transfer of PGO waves have shown that they depend on nicotinic excitation of LGN relay cells by an ascending cholinergic projection from the pons. Muscarinic antagonists have no effect on PGO wave transfer in the thalamus. PGO waves are also one of the first signs of the onset of REM sleep and appear before muscle atonia and EEG activation. They also begin as high-amplitude isolated waves and become clustered and lower in amplitude as REM sleep continues.

34. C. An increase in REM sleep

In humans, plasma levels of prolactin are related to REM sleep and are highest in the early morning hours. Considerable evidence is also available from preclinical studies to show that intracerebral or systemic injection of prolactin increases REM sleep but has no effect on NREM sleep or other measures of sleep architecture. For a review, see Roky et al (Sleep 18:536, 1995).

35. D. Serotoninergic $5HT_{1A}$ receptor

A putative relationship between depression and decreased efficacy of the serotonin system and increased efficacy of cholinergic neurotransmission has a long history. The sleep changes, especially the REM sleep differences, seen in some depressed patients have been linked to impaired serotoninergic neurotransmission. Selective serotonin reuptake inhibitors and the monoamine oxidase inhibitors enhance serotonin. Sleep deprivation has been shown to stimulate the serotonin system, thus providing a possible common mechanistic link between this technique and medications for their antidepressant effects. The $5HT_{1A}$ receptor, unlike the $5HT_2$ receptor, is a presynaptic autoreceptor, so that its downregulation is associated with enhanced serotoninergic neurotransmission.

36. C. Noradrenergic innervation of cells in the laterodorsal tegmental nucleus (LDT) plays a role in REM sleep generation.

Like other monoaminergic cell groups, noradrenergic cells in the locus coeruleus are "REM-off" (i.e., they are hyperpolarized and cease firing during REM sleep). The inhibitory influence of these cells on the LDT cholinergic "REM-on" cells is therefore removed during REM sleep (Figure 13-4). This is of primary importance for the initiation of the REM sleep state; for example, the subsequent cholinergic depolarizing influence from the LDT on the various groups of REM sleep effector neurons in the median PRF is necessary for the appearance of REM sleep signs. Lesions of the noradrenergic cells of the locus coeruleus have no influence on arousal or cortical activation because of the redundancy of the ascending arousal systems. Noradrenaline, like other components of the arousal system, maintains thalamic relay cells in a depolarized state during wakefulness.

37. A. Serotoninergic innervation depolarizes neurons in the relay nuclei of the thalamus.

Serotonin, like other components of the ascending arousal system, maintains thalamic relay neurons in a depolarized state during wakefulness. As serotonin release diminishes during NREM sleep, the relay cells gradually hyperpolarize, thereby allowing the change into the burst discharge mode that is characteristic of NREM sleep. Pindolol, a $5HT_{1A}$ receptor antagonist, produces a dose-dependent decrease in REM sleep, probably because serotonin release is increased by this compound. The discharge rate of serotonin cells is related to vigilance state; for example serotonin cells are "REM-off," but their rate is not affected by the light-dark cycle. Electrical stimulation of the nucleus raphe dorsalis (DRN, see Figure 13-2) is followed by arousal and alertness, as would be expected of a component of the ascending arousal system.

38. A. REM sleep recovery is partial and delayed.

During recovery sleep after amphetamine, SWS is almost completely recovered—a response similar to that seen after combined placebo treatment and enforced wakefulness. However, total sleep time is not recovered after amphetamine, and notably, the REM sleep lost is only minimally recovered and after a 24-hour delay. These results affect our understanding of the REM sleep homeostat and how it can be separated from the sleep homeostat, or process S, that is typically measured as SWS and power in the EEG δ frequency band.

39. D. None of these mechanisms

Methylxanthines were known to inhibit cyclic nucleotide phosphodiesterases and to mobilize intracellular calcium before their action as adenosine antagonists was recognized. Both the phosphodiesterase and calcium effects, however, occur at concentrations much higher than those that are achieved in brain by ingestion of even very high doses of caffeine. Similarly, although caffeine can act as an antagonist at the benzodiazepine receptor, the required concentrations are about 5 to 10 times greater than those that act as adenosine antagonists. Thus it is unlikely that normal consumption of caffeine would result in an action at the benzodiazepine receptor in humans. A review of the effects and mechanisms of caffeine as a central nervous system stimulant is provided by Nehlig et al (Brain Res Rev 17:139, 1992).

40. A. Posterior hypothalamus

Following the recent discovery of the orexin (hypocretin) system, the posterior hypothalamus is now known to encompass the region (the LH, see Figure 13-4) that contains the orexin cell bodies. These results thus confirm von Economo's prediction (J Nerv Ment Diseases 71:249, 1930) that this region would contain neurons that promote wakefulness. More recent data have also demonstrated the importance of the hypothalamic region near the optic chiasm as the localization of sleep-promoting neurons. Lesions to this area, the BF, and preoptic area, caused prolonged insomnia. The mediodorsal thalamus was not found to be affected in encephalitis lethargica but is now known to be the region most affected in fatal familial insomnia (cf. question 16).

41. E. Dynorphin

To date, only dynorphin has been found to be co-localized in orexin (hypocretin) neurons. The presence of dynorphin in this cell population may affect the phenotype of narcolepsy.

42. A. Tuberomammillary nucleus

An important function of orexin (hypocretin) appears to be the stabilization of vigilance state transitions, and a model has been proposed for vigilance state stability to provide a mechanistic explanation for organized transitions between states (Saper et al., Trends Neurosci 24:726, 2001). This model is based on reciprocal innervation between sleep-promoting neurons of the hypothalamic ventrolateral preoptic nucleus and aminergic wake-promoting neurons of the principal arousal nuclei, including the tuberomammillary nucleus. Mutual inhibition between these two groups would form a bistable ("flip-flop") switch, which could maintain state stability despite slowly accumulating circadian or homeostatic pressures to the contrary. At a certain point, a threshold is reached and the switch suddenly flips to the opposite pole. As an additional factor, the excitatory influence of orexin on wake-promoting neurons predominates during the active phase, thus maintaining this side of the circuit, and stabilizing arousal. Also see Figure 13-4.

43. E. None of the above

This patient would be diagnosed with restless legs syndrome (RLS), and all of the listed medications aggravate RLS. The underlying pathology of RLS remains unknown, although the response of these patients to compounds that affect central dopaminergic neurotransmission has been used as evidence that dopamine may be involved. As dopaminergic antagonists, antipsychotics such as risperidole worsen RLS, whereas dopamimetics, including dopamine agonists and L-dopa, almost always alleviate the condition. In fact, the symptoms of RLS are typically responsive to dopamine agents and, combined with the circadian effect of lowered dopamine levels at night, have led to the hypothesis of a dopaminergic dysfunction in RLS; however, no data are yet available to support the hypothesis convincingly. The other listed compounds also aggravate the condition but have not led to hypotheses concerning the underlying pathology, primarily because, for these agents, there is no evidence that the opposite treatment will alleviate RLS.

44. A. Increased cholinergic activity and decreased noradrenergic activity

Preclinical and clinical studies have consistently demonstrated that the changes in sleep architecture most typically associated with both depression and PTSD can be modeled by increasing central cholinergic activity and/or decreasing central noradrenergic activity. In particular, these changes to sleep include the effects on REM sleep, for which the relevant brainstem mechanisms are now relatively well understood (i.e., cholinergic REM-on cells are inhibited by the noradrenergic and serotoninergic REM-off cells) (see Figure 13-4). Therefore in terms of both effective treatments and underlying sleep architecture differences, increased cholinergic activity combined with decreased noradrenergic and serotoninergic activity is a likely neurochemical imbalance in depression and PTSD. To date, there is no evidence of differences in orexinergic activity in these disorders. Note also question 35.

45. C. Increasing slow wave sleep (SWS)

Alcohol increases SWS in normal healthy adults but decreases REM sleep time and total sleep time. Alcohol also disturbs sleep continuity by increasing the number of nocturnal awakenings.

46. A. Glutamatergic stimulation of the nucleus magnocellularis in the medulla produces atonia.

The atonia mechanism is complex, and it is feasible that more than one anatomically separate system is involved. The medial medullary muscle inhibitory area, for example, where electric stimulation produces atonia, can be divided into two areas. One of these zones, the nucleus magnocellularis, is sensitive to glutamate but not to cholinergic stimulation. See Figure 13-3 for the pathways involved in this system. The other area, located more caudally, is sensitive to muscarinic agonists. Atonia depends on descending glycinergic inhibitory neurons via the reticulospinal tract that innervate spinal motor neurons: inhibitory postsynaptic potentials (IPSPs) can be recorded in the

motor neurons during REM sleep, and the IPSPs can be blocked by strychnine, a glycine antagonist. Note that structures above the pontomedullary junction are required for the production of atonia because a preparation transected at this level does not show atonia when the medullary inhibitory area is stimulated. Atonia is also very sensitive to blood pressure, and a fall in blood pressure as little as 10 mm Hg can prevent the induction of atonia.

47. B. Increasing the GABA-dependent opening time of the GABA chloride channel

Barbiturates facilitate GABA-ergic neurotransmission by promoting the GABA-induced chloride current. They achieve this effect by prolonging the periods during which the burst of channel openings can occur, rather than by increasing the frequency of the burst of channel openings (the mechanism by which benzodiazepines enhance GABAergic neurotransmission). Pentobarbital is also a weak enhancer of binding of GABA and benzodiazepines at the GABA-benzodiazepine receptor complex, and at very high doses it can inhibit voltage-dependent Na^+ channels. Also at high doses, pentobarbital reduces the Ca^{2+}–dependent release of neurotransmitters. These latter effects occur, however, at doses that are higher than those that achieve anesthesia, and GABAergic mechanisms are also unlikely to explain the anesthetic action of the barbiturates.

48. D. Unlike many enzymes, glutamate decarboxylase (GAD) is not regulated by phosphorylation.

GAD can be regulated by phosphorylation, resulting in an increase or decrease in activity, depending on whether the enzyme is membrane bound or soluble. Of interest, a large proportion of GAD in brain is inactive, as it is unbound to the cofactor, pyridoxal-P. Although both of the isoforms of GAD are regulated by pyridoxal-P, they have different intracellular distributions. Aspartate is also a substrate for the enzyme. This question highlights the complexities of the synthesis of GABA, and in particular the regulation of GAD, although the functional importance of these complexities remains to be elucidated. GABAergic neurons, however, are implicated in many of the neurophysiological changes associated with sleep and wakefulness, GABA levels change in specific brain areas during sleep, and most of the currently available hypnotics act at the GABA-chloride ionophore. Thus advances in the knowledge of GABA synthesis not only are likely to translate into improved understanding of the mechanisms of sleep-wakefulness but also allow development of more specific hypnotics.

TABLE 13-1 ■ Summary of Some of the Significant Regional Changes That Occur in rCBF During Sleep in Comparison with Wakefulness

	Stage 3–4 NREM Sleep (SWS)	REM sleep
Pons/mesencephalon	↓	↑
Thalamus	↓	–
Caudate/striatum	↓/↓	↑/–
Basal forebrain/hypothalamus	↓	↑
Orbitofrontal cortex/PFC	↓	↓
Anterior cingulate cortex	↓	↑
Posterior cingulate cortex	–	↓
Precuneus	↓	↓
Medial temporal cortex	–	–
Superior/inferior temporal gyrus	–	↑
Amygdala	–	↑
Cerebellar vermis	–	↑
Parietal/occipital cortex	–	↓/↑

This table summarizes the results from several studies* that have measured a relative increase (↑), decrease (↓), or no change (–) in rCBF in regions of the human brain during sleep in comparison with preceding wakefulness. PFC, Prefrontal cortex.
*Maquet P, et al. J Neurosci 17:2807, 1997; Braun AR, et al. Brain 120(Pt7):1173, 1997; Maquet P, et al. Nature 383:163, 1996; Born AP, et al. Neuroimmage 17:1325, 2002; Dang–Vu TT, et al. Neuroimage 28:14, 2005; Kajimura N, et al. J Neurosci 19:10065, 1999.

49. D. During slow wave sleep (SWS), regional cerebral blood flow (rCBF) decreases in the basal forebrain.

During SWS, global CBF is known to decrease. However, particularly notable decreases in rCBF have been observed, *inter alia*, in the BF and the thalamus. A different pattern of rCBF is seen during REM sleep, including a decrease in the prefrontal cortex and an increase in the amygdaloid complex. Table 13-1 summarizes these and other significant changes in rCBF that have been determined during sleep.

50. C. A reduction in the homeostatic pressure for sleep

Aging in the human is associated with changes in the timing and duration of the sleep cycle. Sleep fragmentation and early morning awakening are particularly troublesome for older adults. The circadian pacemaker had been considered primary to these sleep differences, and a reduction in the period of the circadian oscillator was a possible explanation for their occurrence. When younger and older subjects were compared in a forced desynchrony protocol, however, the period of the circadian oscillator in older adults did not change, but the oscillator was entrained to an earlier time. Of importance, this study also revealed a reduced homeostatic drive for sleep in older subjects, combined with a putative reduction in the amplitude of the circadian wakefulness signal in the early morning (see Figure 13-1). Melatonin rhythm was found to be unaffected by age, but a reduced amplitude of the circadian component of the temperature rhythm was noted in older subjects.

REFERENCES

1. Aldrich MS: Narcolepsy. Neurology 42:34–43, 1992.

2. Avidan AY: Sleep disorders in the older patient. Prim Care 32:563–586, 2005.

3. Bach V, Telliez F, Libert JP: The interaction between sleep and thermoregulation in adults and neonates. Sleep Med Rev 6:481–492, 2002.

4. Bao J, Cheung WY, Wu JY: Brain L-glutamate decarboxylase. Inhibition by phosphorylation and activation by dephosphorylation. J Biol Chem 270:6464–6467, 1995.

5. Basheer R, Porkka-Heiskanen T, Strecker RE, et al: Adenosine as a biological signal mediating sleepiness following prolonged wakefulness. Biol Signals Recept 9:319–327, 2000.

6. Beuckmann CT, Sinton CM, Williams SC, et al: Expression of a poly-glutamine-ataxin-3 transgene in orexin neurons induces narcolepsy-cataplexy in the rat. J Neurosci 24:4469–4477, 2004.

7. Born AP, Law I, Lund TE, et al: Cortical deactivation induced by visual stimulation in human slow-wave sleep. Neuroimage 17:1325–1335, 2002.

8. Braun AR, Balkin TJ, Wesenten NJ, et al: Regional cerebral blood flow throughout the sleep-wake cycle. An H2(15)O PET study. Brain 120(Pt 7):1173–1197, 1997.

9. Bremer F: Cerveau isole et physiologie du sommeil. Comptes Rendus des Seances de la Societe de Biologie 118:1235–1241, 1935.

10. Buguet A, Montmayeur A, Pigeau R, Naitoh P: Modafinil, d-amphetamine and placebo during 64 hours of sustained mental work. II. Effects on two nights of recovery sleep. J Sleep Res 4:229–241, 1995.

11. Chase MH, Soja PJ, Morales FR: Evidence that glycine mediates the postsynaptic potentials that inhibit lumbar motoneurons during the atonia of active sleep. J Neurosci 9:743–751, 1989.

12. Chemelli RM, Willie JT, Sinton CM, et al: Narcolepsy in orexin knockout mice: molecular genetics of sleep regulation. Cell 98:437–451, 1999.

13. Chou TC, Lee CE, Lu J, et al: Orexin (hypocretin) neurons contain dynorphin. J Neurosci 21:RC168, 2001.

14. Cornwall J, Phillipson OT: Afferent projections to the dorsal thalamus of the rat as shown by retrograde lectin transport. II. The midline nuclei. Brain Res Bull 21:147–161, 1988.

15. Dang-Vu TT, Desseilles M, Laureys S, et al: Cerebral correlates of delta waves during non-REM sleep revisited. Neuroimage 28:14–21, 2005.

16. Dijk DJ, Czeisler CA: Paradoxical timing of the circadian rhythm of sleep propensity serves to consolidate sleep and wakefulness in humans. Neurosci Lett 166:63–68, 1994.

17. Dijk DJ, Duffy JF, Riel E, et al: Aging and the circadian and homeostatic regulation of human sleep during forced desynchrony of rest, melatonin and temperature rhythms. J Physiol 516(Pt 2):611–627, 1999.

18. el Mansari M, Sakai K, Jouvet M: Unitary characteristics of presumptive cholinergic tegmental neurons during the sleep-waking cycle in freely moving cats. Exp Brain Res 76:519–529, 1989.

19. Esclapez M, Tillakaratne NJ, Kaufman DL, et al: Comparative localization of two forms of glutamic acid decarboxylase and their mRNAs in rat brain supports the concept of functional differences between the forms. J Neurosci 14:1834–1855, 1994.

20. Guilleminault C, Gelb M: Clinical aspects and features of cataplexy. Adv Neurol 67:65–77, 1995.

21. Hishikawa Y, Shimizu T: Physiology of REM sleep, cataplexy, and sleep paralysis. Adv Neurol 67:245–271, 1995.

22. Hu B, Bouhassira D, Steriade M, Deschenes M: The blockage of ponto-geniculo-occipital waves in the cat lateral geniculate nucleus by nicotinic antagonists. Brain Res 473:394–397, 1988.

23. Jacobs BL, Trimbach C, Eubanks EE, Trulson M: Hippocampal mediation of raphe lesion- and PCPA-induced hyperactivity in the rat. Brain Res 94:253–261, 1975.

24. Janowsky DS, el-Yousef MK, Davis JM, Sekerke HJ: A cholinergic-adrenergic hypothesis of mania and depression. Lancet 2:632–635, 1972.

25. John J, Wu MF, Boehmer LN, Siegel JM: Cataplexy-active neurons in the hypothalamus: implications for the role of histamine in sleep and waking behavior. Neuron 42:619–634, 2004.

26. Jones BE: Activity, modulation and role of basal forebrain cholinergic neurons innervating the cerebral cortex. Prog Brain Res 145:157–169, 2004.

27. Jones BE: The organization of central cholinergic systems and their functional importance in sleep-waking states. Prog Brain Res 98:61–71, 1993.

28. Kajimura N, Uchiyama M, Takayama Y, et al: Activity of midbrain reticular formation and neocortex during the progression of human non-rapid eye movement sleep. J Neurosci 19:10065–10073, 1999.

29. Kales A, Soldatos CR, Bixler EO, et al: Hereditary factors in sleepwalking and night terrors. Br J Psychiatry 137:111–118, 1980.

30. Kokkotou E, Jeon JY, Wang X, et al: Mice with MCH ablation resist diet-induced obesity through strain-specific mechanisms. Am J Physiol (Regul Integr Comp Physiol) 289:R117–R124, 2005.

31. Kupfer DJ, Ehlers CL: Two roads to rapid eye movement latency. Arch Gen Psychiatry 46:945–948, 1989.

32. Lai YY, Siegel JM, Wilson WJ: Effect of blood pressure on medial medulla-induced muscle atonia. Am J Physiol 252:H1249–H1257, 1987.

33. Lai YY, Siegel JM: Medullary regions mediating atonia. J Neurosci 8:4790–4796, 1988.

34. Lu J, Jhou TC, Saper CB: Identification of wake-active dopaminergic neurons in the ventral periaqueductal gray matter. J Neurosci 26:193–202, 2006.

35. Majumdar S, Mallick BN: Increased levels of tyrosine hydroxylase and glutamic acid decarboxylase in locus coeruleus neurons after rapid eye movement sleep deprivation in rats. Neurosci Lett 338:193–196, 2003.

36. Maquet P, Degueldre C, Delfiore G, et al: Functional neuroanatomy of human slow wave sleep. J Neurosci 17:2807–2812, 1997.

37. Maquet P, Peters J, Aerts J, et al: Functional neuroanatomy of human rapid-eye-movement sleep and dreaming. Nature 383:163–166, 1996.

38. Martin DL, Martin SB, Wu SJ, Espina N: Regulatory properties of brain glutamate decarboxylase (GAD): the apoenzyme of GAD is present principally as the smaller of two molecular forms of GAD in brain. J Neurosci 11:2725–2731, 1991.

39. Maudhuit C, Jolas T, Chastanet M, et al: Reduced inhibitory potency of serotonin reuptake blockers on central serotoninergic neurons in rats selectively deprived of rapid eye movement sleep. Biol Psychiatry 40:1000–1007, 1996.

40. McCarley RW, Greene RW, Rainnie D, Portas CM: Brainstem modulation and REM sleep. Semin Neurosc 7:341–354, 1995.

41. Mitani A, Ito K, Hallanger AE, et al: Cholinergic projections from the laterodorsal and pedunculopontine tegmental nuclei to the pontine gigantocellular tegmental field in the cat. Brain Res 451:397–402, 1988.

42. Moruzzi G, Magoun HW: Brain stem reticular formation and activation of the EEG. Electroencephalog Clin Neurophysiol 1:455–473, 1949.

43. Nehlig A, Daval JL, Debry G: Caffeine and the central nervous system: mechanisms of action, biochemical, metabolic and psychostimulant effects. Brain Res Rev 17:139–170, 1992.

44. Nishino S, Riehl J, Hong J, et al: Is narcolepsy a REM sleep disorder? Analysis of sleep abnormalities in narcoleptic Dobermans. Neurosci Res 38:437–446, 2000.

45. Peyron C, Tighe DK, van den Pol AN, et al: Neurons containing hypocretin (orexin) project to multiple neuronal systems. J Neurosci 18:9996–10015, 1998.

46. Porkka-Heiskanen T, Strecker RE, McCarley RW: Brain site-specificity of extracellular adenosine concentration changes during sleep deprivation and spontaneous sleep: an in vivo microdialysis study. Neuroscience 99:507–517, 2000.

47. Prinz PN, Roehrs TA, Vitaliano PP, et al: Effect of alcohol on sleep and nighttime plasma growth hormone and cortisol concentrations. J Clin Endocrinol Metab 51:759–764, 1980.

48. Roky R, Obal F Jr, Valatx JL, et al: Prolactin and rapid eye movement sleep regulation. Sleep 18:536–542, 1995.

49. Saper CB, Chou TC, Scammell TE: The sleep switch: hypothalamic control of sleep and wakefulness. Trends Neurosci 24:726–731, 2001.

50. Sastre JP, Jouvet M: Oneiric behavior in cats. Physiol Behav 22:979–989, 1979.

51. Schenck CH, Bundlie SR, Ettinger MG, Mahowald MW: Chronic behavioral disorders of human REM sleep: a new category of parasomnia. Sleep 9:293–308, 1986.

52. Seifritz E, Stahl SM, Gillin JC: Human sleep EEG following the 5-HT1A antagonist pindolol: possible disinhibition of raphe neuron activity. Brain Res 759:84–91, 1997.

53. Sherin JE, Elmquist JK, Torrealba F, Saper CB: Innervation of histaminergic tuberomammillary neurons by GABAergic and galaninergic neurons in the ventrolateral preoptic nucleus of the rat. J Neurosci 18:4705–4721, 1998.

54. Sherin JE, Shiromani PJ, McCarley RW, Saper CB: Activation of ventrolateral preoptic neurons during sleep. Science 271:216–219, 1996.

55. Sinton CM, McCarley RW: Neurophysiological mechanisms of sleep and wakefulness: a question of balance. Semin Neurol 24:211–223, 2004.

56. Sinton CM, McCarley RW: Neurophysiology and neuropsychiatry of sleep and sleep disorders. In Schiffer RB, Rao SM, Fogel BS (eds): *Neuropsychiatry*, 2nd ed. Philadelphia: Lippincott, Williams & Wilkins, 2003, pp 358–394.

57. Snyder SH, Brown B, Kuhar MJ: The subsynaptosomal localization of histamine, histidine decarboxylase and histamine methyltransferase in rat hypothalamus. J Neurochem 23:37–45, 1974.

58. Steiger A: Sleep and the hypothalamo-pituitary-adrenocortical system. Sleep Med Rev 6:125–138, 2002.

59. Steriade M, McCormick DA, Sejnowski TJ: Thalamocortical oscillations in the sleeping and aroused brain. Science 262:679–685, 1993.

60. Strecker RE, Morairty S, Thakkar MM, et al: Adenosinergic modulation of basal forebrain and preoptic/anterior hypothalamic neuronal activity in the control of behavioral state. Behav Brain Res 115:183–204, 2000.

61. Szymusiak R: Magnocellular nuclei of the basal forebrain: substrates of sleep and arousal regulation. Sleep 18:478–500, 1995.

62. Toh KL, Jones CR, He Y, et al: An hPer2 phosphorylation site mutation in familial advanced sleep phase syndrome. Science 291:1040–1043, 2001.

63. Trulson ME, Jacobs BL: Raphe unit activity in freely moving cats: lack of diurnal variation. Neurosci Lett 36:285–290, 1983.

64. Twyman RE, Rogers CJ, Macdonald RL: Differential regulation of gamma-aminobutyric acid receptor channels by diazepam and phenobarbital. Ann Neurol 25:213–220, 1989.

65. Vanni-Mercier G, Sakai K, Jouvet M: Specific neurons for wakefulness in the posterior hypothalamus in the cat. C R Acad Sci III 298:195–200, 1984.

66. von Economo C: Sleep as a problem of localization. J Nerv Ment Dis 71:249–259, 1930.

67. Willie JT, Chemelli RM, Sinton CM, Yanagisawa M: To eat or to sleep? Orexin in the regulation of feeding and wakefulness. Annu Rev Neurosci 24:429–458, 2001.

68. Yoshida H, Kubota T, Krueger JM: A cyclooxygenase-2 inhibitor attenuates spontaneous and TNF-alpha-induced non-rapid eye movement sleep in rabbits. Am J Physiol Regul Integr Comp Physiol 285:R99–R109, 2003.

69. Zeitzer JM, Buckmaster CL, Parker KJ, et al: Circadian and homeostatic regulation of hypocretin in a primate model: implications for the consolidation of wakefulness. J Neurosci 23:3555–3560, 2003.

70. Zisapel N: Melatonin-dopamine interactions: from basic neurochemistry to a clinical setting. Cell Mol Neurobiol 21:605–616, 2001.

Cardiopulmonary Disorders

VAHID MOHSENIN ■ VLAD DIMITRIU

Questions

1. The non-rapid eye movement (NREM) sleep and particularly slow-wave stages of sleep are associated with one of the following cardiovascular changes:
   A. Increase in heart rate
   B. Increase in cardiac output
   C. Decrease in vascular resistance
   D. Increase in blood pressure

2. Regarding obstructive apneic events, one of the following changes occur:
   A. Surges in sympathetic nervous system activity at the beginning of an apnea
   B. Vasodilation of peripheral vasculature
   C. Systemic blood pressure is usually lowest during the early to middle portion of most apneic episodes.
   D. Increased cardiac output

3. During obstructive sleep apnea the intrathoracic pressure can be as low as –80 cm H_2O. Which of the following changes in the cardiovascular system is expected as a result?
   A. Decreased venous return
   B. Rightward shift of the interventricular septum
   C. Increased left ventricular compliance
   D. Increased left ventricular afterload

4. Patients with obstructive sleep apnea (OSA) are at risk for developing persistent systemic hypertension. Which one of the following systems is the primary cause of hypertension in obstructive sleep apnea?
   A. Endothelin
   B. Renin-angiotensin system
   C. Chemoreceptor stimulation
   D. Decreased nitric oxide production

5. Left ventricular hypertrophy is seen more commonly in normotensive patients with OSA than in control subjects. The mechanism (s) underlying this includes:
   A. Myocardial ischemia
   B. Nocturnal surges in blood pressure during apneic episodes
   C. Cardiac myocyte injury or necrosis owing to increased catecholamine levels
   D. All of the above

6. Patients with congestive heart failure are at higher risk for central apneas. The mechanisms underlying central apnea and Cheyne-Stokes respiration in this setting include:
   A. Hyperventilation
   B. Short circulation time
   C. Blunted chemoreception
   D. Brainstem stroke

7. In healthy persons, activation of baroreflex results in attenuation of which of the following responses to peripheral chemoreflex excitation?
   A. Ventilatory
   B. Sympathetic
   C. Bradycardic
   D. All of the above

8. Which one of the following is observed during normoxic daytime wakefulness in patients with obstructive sleep apnea?
   A. Fast heart rate
   B. Blunted heart rate variability
   C. Increased blood pressure variability
   D. All of the above

9. A 60-year-old man was recently discharged from the hospital after a transient ischemic attack. There was no evidence for hypertension, atrial fibrillation, lipid disorders, or diabetes mellitus. He lives alone. Occasionally, he falls asleep in the chair in the afternoon, but otherwise is able to function well at work. He works within the security department at a small town hospital. He smokes 10 cigarettes a day and is overweight. Which one of the following is the best course of action?

A. Order polysomnography to rule out sleep apnea.

B. In the absence of known risk factors, the chance of having a stroke is low, and the patient should be given assurance and be counseled for smoking cessation.

C. Order smoking cessation counseling and daily aspirin.

D. Order nocturnal oximetry to further evaluate the ischemic attack.

10. Sleep breathing disorders are associated with an increased incidence of cardiovascular events. Among the mechanisms implicated, altered coagulation seems to play an important role. Sleep apnea is associated with which one of the following humoral changes?
    A. Decreased C-reactive protein
    B. Increased platelet aggregation
    C. Decreased plasma fibrinogen levels
    D. Increased high-density lipoprotein

11. Regarding the cerebral circulation and the influence of obstructive apnea episodes, which statement is correct?
    A. The cerebral blood flow velocity remains unaffected during apneic episodes.
    B. The cerebral autoregulation is abnormal during wakefulness in OSA patients.
    C. Hypocapnia causes cerebral vasodilation.
    D. Hypoxia causes cerebral vasodilation.

12. A 35-year-old obese man, otherwise healthy, is undergoing diagnostic polysomnography for suspected sleep apnea. The polysomnography technologists notify you about a 4-second sinus pause in REM sleep with no associated apnea. Which one of the following statements is correct?
    A. Wake the patient up and take further history.
    B. Initiate continuous positive airway pressure (CPAP).
    C. Reassure the technologist and continue monitoring.
    D. Send the patient to the emergency department.

13. A 65-year-old man with a history of coronary artery disease but no known cardiac arrhythmias is noted to have a 7-beat run of ventricular tachycardia (VT) while asleep during polysomnography. Which of these statements is *incorrect*?
    A. In the absence of known history of ventricular arrhythmias, VT with symptoms will require an emergency evaluation to rule out cardiac ischemia.

B. Ventricular tachycardia of this kind during sleep is common and does not warrant interruption of polysomnography.

C. If the patient is known for VT and is asymptomatic, no further action is necessary.

D. Sleep-related VT is indicative of cardiac ischemia and increased sympathetic tone.

14. One of the following statements is true:
    A. Five percent of patients undergoing elective cardioversion for atrial fibrillation have significant sleep-disordered breathing.
    B. Patients with sleep-disordered breathing are more likely to remain in sinus rhythm after cardioversion if the sleep-disordered breathing is treated with CPAP.
    C. Cardiac pacing ameliorates the sleep-disordered breathing.
    D. Slow wave sleep is typically a time of fast atrioventricular node conduction, shortened cardiac refractory cycles, and tachyarrhythmias.

15. Risk factors for central sleep apnea in patients with congestive heart failure include all of the following *except*:
    A. Male gender
    B. Hypercapnia
    C. Atrial fibrillation
    D. Age over 60

16. The following statement is true about pulmonary hypertension (PH) in OSA:
    A. The prevalence of PH is high in OSA.
    B. The pulmonary artery pressures tend to be in the range of 40–50 mm Hg.
    C. Daytime hypocapnia is associated with higher prevalence of PH.
    D. CPAP lowers the pulmonary artery pressure.

17. CPAP treatment of patients with sleep apnea and known coronary artery disease results in all of the following *except*:
    A. Reduced risk of acute coronary syndrome
    B. Decreased hospitalization for heart failure
    C. No effect on cardiovascular death
    D. Decreased coronary revascularization

18. A 61-year-old man is referred to the sleep clinic by his cardiologist for evaluation of sleep apnea. He has a history of hypertension, atrial fibrillation, and congestive heart failure. He reports not feeling well-rested when he wakes up in the morning and being hypersomnolent throughout the rest of the day. He is retired from an accountant job and is not very active, spending most of his time in front of the

TV, napping once or twice a day. He lives alone. He has a 60 pack-year smoking history but quit smoking 10 years ago. His medications include long-acting metoprolol, enalapril, a diuretic, and coumadin. His last left ventricular ejection fraction was 30%. Your physical examination reveals an average-built man, with a short neck and Mallampati class II orophaynx. The auscultation of his chest reveals no rales or crackles. On heart examination, he has an irregularly irregular rate and a grade III systolic murmur at the apex. His Epworth score is 12. A sleep study is ordered, and a representative fragment is shown in Figure 14-1. His apnea hypopnea index is 45. Which statement is true regarding the patient's condition?

A. This condition is present in about 10% of patients with heart failure.

B. Oxygen supplementation can worsen his condition.

C. The apnea-hypopnea index can improve with theophylline.

D. His 2-year mortality is about 10%.

19. A 35-year-old woman is referred for a sleep evaluation by her primary care physician. She is obese and a heavy smoker. She reports feeling very tired when she wakes up in the morning and has a difficult time staying awake at work. She snores loudly, and her husband notices apneas lasting close to 1 minute. She can trace these symptoms as far back as college, but everything has worsened since she gave birth 1 year ago. Her mother had similar symptoms but was never diagnosed with sleep apnea and died at age 55 with massive intracranial bleeding. This patient's Epworth score is 12. You suspect OSA. A polysomnogram is ordered and you explain the procedure and potential therapies. The patient asks whether sleep apnea and hypertension are related. Which one of the following statements is true?

A. There is no relationship between hypertension and OSA.

B. CPAP use decreases the nighttime blood pressure and increases the daytime blood pressure.

C. CPAP use decreases both the nighttime and the daytime blood pressure.

D. CPAP use increases both the nighttime and the daytime blood pressure.

E. The relationship between CPAP use and blood pressure has never been studied.

20. A 75-year-old man is diagnosed with obstructive sleep apnea by polysomnography. His apnea-hypopnea index is 80/h. He undergoes a CPAP titration study, and it is determined that his respiratory events are significantly reduced by applying a CPAP of 12 cm H_2O. Regarding his risk of sudden death from cardiac causes, which one of the following statements is true?

A. The risk is higher in the evening hours (6–10 PM).

B. The risk is higher in the morning hours (6 AM–12 PM).

C. The risk is higher during sleeping hours (10 PM–6 AM).

D. The risk is the same throughout the 24-hour cycle.

21. Numerous studies have shown a strong association between sleep-disordered breathing and the development of stroke. Which one of the following mechanisms has been found to contribute to the increased risk of stroke in subjects with OSA?

A. Hypocoagulability

B. Paradoxical embolism

C. Use of dental appliances

D. Increased cerebral blood flow

E. Supplemental oxygen

22. A 60-year-old man is referred to the sleep center for evaluation. He is complaining of hypersomnolence, poor performance at work owing to inability to concentrate, and fatigue. He has a medical history of hypertension, hyperlipidemia, diabetes, and depression. He is an ex-smoker and an ex-alcoholic. He is employed as a respiratory therapist at a nearby hospital. He takes captopril, hydrochlorothiazide, atorvastatin, and rosiglitazone. He is obese and snores loudly. His neck circumference is 18 inches. When asked about additional medical history, he remembers that 6 months ago he had numbness in his right arm for about 3 hours, which subsided spontaneously and never recurred. His neurological examination is normal. You decide to start him on aspirin and notify his primary care physician. His sleep study shows an obstructive apnea-hypopnea index of 40, with an arousal index of 55. You tell the patient that:

A. OSA is an independent risk factor for stroke.

B. OSA is seen mostly secondary to stroke.

C. OSA is not a risk factor for stroke, but central sleep apnea is.

D. There is a strong association between the stroke location and the apnea type.

E. OSA is present in 10% of patients with stroke.

23. A 75-year-old man returns to your clinic 2 months after being started on CPAP. He was diagnosed

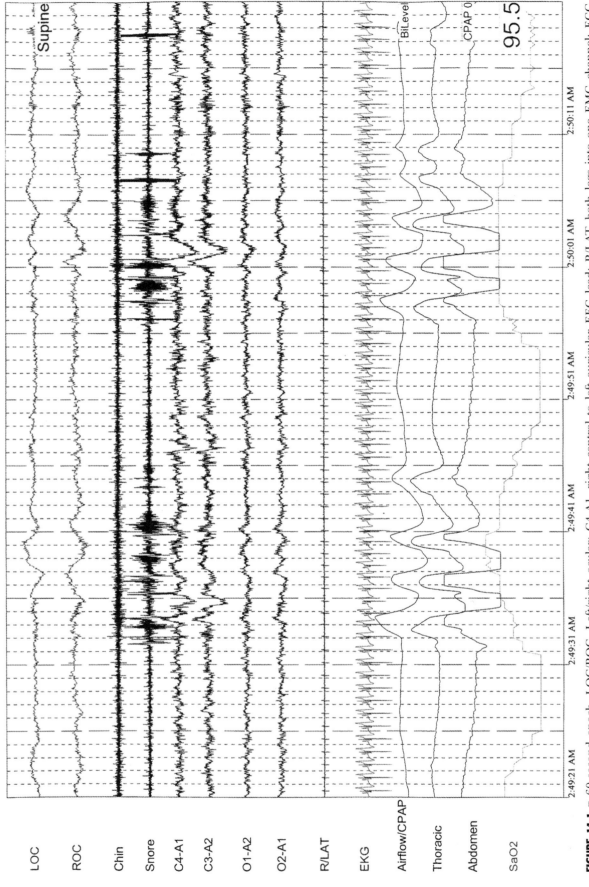

FIGURE 14-1 ■ 60-second epoch. LOC/ROC, Left/right ocular; C4-A1, right central to left auricular EEG lead; R/LAT, both legs into one EMG channel; ECG, electrocardiogram; "Airflow/continuous positive airway pressure (CPAP)" is only an airflow channel with no CPAP on this patient.

with OSA by polysomnography, which revealed 45 apneas and hypopneas per hour with concomitant desaturations, as low as 85%. He has a history of coronary artery disease and, despite medical treatment, was still having nocturnal angina before being placed on CPAP. Today he reports he has not had chest pain in the past 2 months, feels more energetic, and wants to know more about the effects of sleep apnea and CPAP treatment on coronary artery disease. You tell him that:

A. He is probably just sleeping better; the CPAP has no effect on nocturnal angina.

B. OSA always causes nocturnal ischemia, even in people with no coronary artery disease.

C. When present, nocturnal angina is accompanied by elevation in cardiac troponin.

D. Nocturnal angina is not related to the severity of OSA.

E. CPAP reduces the duration of ST-segment depression.

24. A 59-year-old man is seen in the sleep clinic. He is complaining of not getting a restful night's sleep, being hypersomnolent during the day, and not being able to concentrate on his work. He has snored loudly all his adult life, to the point that he is disturbing his wife's sleep. He did not have any traffic accidents but stated that he no longer drives long distances because he is afraid he might fall asleep. He has a medical history of allergic rhinitis for which he takes loratadine over the counter. His Epworth sleepiness score is 13. He does not smoke and drinks only occasionally. He has a body mass index (BMI) of 30 kg/m^2. The physical examination is positive for swollen nasal turbinates, a low soft palate, tachycardia, and fungal nail infection. You schedule him for a sleep study. His apnea hypopnea index is 8, and his oxygen saturation drops below 90%. Short episodes of bradycardia were noted in relationship with apneas. The technologist reports that he slept on his side 90% of the time. Which of the following statements is true regarding this patient's findings?

A. The presence of bradycardia warrants a full cardiac workup.

B. Expedite arrangements for a cardiac pacemaker.

C. Nocturnal desaturations cause bradycardia and tachycardia.

D. Apnea can trigger the diving reflex and result in significant tachycardia.

25. After reviewing the polysomnogram of one of your patients, you diagnose her with OSA. Her apnea-hypopnea index is 30. She also has multiple comorbidities: hypertension, diabetes, obesity, and atrial fibrillation. She underwent cardioversion 3 months ago after transesophageal echocardiography, but now the atrial fibrillation is present on the electrocardiogram (ECG) channel of the polysomnograph. Which one of the following factors was most probably decisive in the recurrence of her arrhythmia?

A. Diabetes mellitus

B. Obesity

C. Systemic hypertension

D. Obstructive sleep apnea

E. Her gender

Answers

1. C. Decrease in vascular resistance

Multiple physiologic changes accompany the transition between wakefulness and NREM sleep. In general, respiration in the deeper stages of NREM sleep comes mainly under metabolic control. Changes in the cardiovascular autonomic control parallel those of respiratory system. The decrease in sympathetic discharge is reflected in the notable decrease in heart rate, blood pressure, stroke volume, cardiac output, and systemic vascular resistance. As a consequence, myocardial oxygen consumption is reduced. The connections between the respiratory-related neurons and the central cardiovascular sympathetic neurons, both located in the brainstem, can explain the parallel decline in central respiratory and sympathetic neuronal outflow.

2. C. Systemic blood pressure is usually lowest during the early to middle portion of most apneic episodes.

Apneic events result in brief surges in sympathetic nervous system activity, vasoconstriction, and transient hypertension. Systemic blood pressure is usually lowest during the early to middle portion of most apneic episodes. A gradual increase in pressure is then observed, and a sudden elevation occurs after termination of the apnea event. During apneic episodes 35–40 seconds long, cardiac output decreases by approximately one third. After termination of the apnea, cardiac output increases by 10–15% above baseline. The combination of increasing systemic pressure and decreasing cardiac output indicates that systemic vascular resistance increases during the apnea. Systemic vasoconstriction is believed to be mediated by alpha sympathetic neural activity because patients with Shy-Drager syndrome, who are sympathetically denervated, have minimal changes in heart rate or systemic pressures in response to apnea.

3. D. Increased left ventricular afterload

During obstructive apneic episodes, exaggerated inspiratory efforts against an occluded upper airway can drop the intrathoracic pressure to as low as –80 cm H_2O. The pressure gradient that drives the venous return to the right heart increases, and more blood is filling the right ventricle. The increased venous return causes a leftward shift of the interventricular septum (ventricular interdependence), thereby reducing left ventricular compliance and decreasing left ventricular end-diastolic volume.

The exaggerated negative intrathoracic pressure also increases the gradient between intracardiac and extracardiac pressures (i.e., transmural pressure), thus increasing the left ventricular afterload. The combination of decreased left ventricular end-diastolic volume and increased left ventricular afterload results in decreased stroke volume and cardiac output. As a result of these hemodynamic changes and the surges in catecholamine levels, systemic blood pressure increases cyclically during sleep. The blood pressure falls during the apneic episode mainly as a result of an acute drop in stroke volume, as explained previously. Toward the end of the apneic episode, however, there is an increase in the sympathetic outflow in response to apnea-related hypoxia. This will induce a surge in both blood pressure and heart rate in the postapneic ventilatory phase.

4. C. Chemoreceptor stimulation

The mechanism for persistent hypertension is systemic vasoconstriction, mediated by chemoreceptor activation and alpha sympathetic neural activity. Patients with Shy-Drager syndrome who are sympathetically denervated have minimal changes in heart rate or systemic pressures in response to apnea. Humans and rats with carotid body surgery or denervation, respectively, do not develop hypertension with apnea or hypoxia. Hypoxia appears to be the main factor for the development of hypertension through sympathetic nervous system activation associated with alterations in chemoreflex sensitivity and baroreceptor set point.

Multiple other factors have been implicated in the development of OSA-induced hypertension, but so far no causal relationship has been clearly established. Endothelin-1 is a potent vasoconstrictor produced in the endothelial cells that has been found to have an essential role in the development of pulmonary hypertension; however, no significant increase in endothelin has been demonstrated in patients with OSA. Recent reports indicate that inhibition of renin-angiotensin system may actually improve sleep apnea and that nitric oxide is increased in subjects with OSA, possibly in connection with upper airway inflammation.

5. D. All of the above

Hypertension is the single most important predisposing factor for the development of left ventricular hypertrophy and systolic and diastolic left ventricular failure; however, normotensive patients with OSA have a higher incidence of left ventricular hypertrophy than control subjects without OSA. There are consequences of nocturnal changes in physiology in OSA that trigger structural alterations in the left ventricle. Increases in ventricular transmural pressure, hypoxemia, and repeated surges in sympathetic neural activity are all induced by the exaggerated negative intrathoracic pressure during apneic episodes. Swings in cardiac output combined with intermittent hypoxia induce elaboration of free radicals and ischemia-reperfusion injury to the vascular walls. Studies have shown that compliance with CPAP treatment for at least 6 months in subjects with OSA (both with and without hypertension) results in reduction of left ventricular mass.

6. A. Hyperventilation

Cheyne-Stokes respiration (CSR) associated with central sleep apnea is present in 30–40% of patients with congestive heart failure. There is now significant evidence that the mechanisms underlying this complex phenomenon involve the respiratory, cardiovascular, and nervous systems. First, the $PaCO_2$ is lower and closer to the apnea threshold in subjects with CSR. Hyperventilation, which is common is CSR, can easily decrease the $PaCO_2$ below this threshold. The causes of hyperventilation in CSR are not fully understood, but stimulation of pulmonary vagal irritant receptors by increased left ventricular volumes and pressures, as well as hypoxia, have been suggested. Second, there is increased central and peripheral chemoreceptor sensitivity to CO_2 and O_2, which can stimulate hyperventilation as well. Finally, the concept of delayed circulatory time in congestive heart failure and its capacity of inducing Cheyne-Stokes breathing were demonstrated by Guyton in a classic experiment. Stroke is associated with transitory increase in central sleep apnea associated with Cheyne-Stokes breathing, but not with development of heart failure. Also, the location of stroke within the central nervous system is not related to the development of periodic breathing. In conclusion, CSR appears to be the result of instability of the central control of respiration. This pattern of periodic breathing is thought to result from increased loop gain in the ventilatory control system owing to overcompensation in response to hyperventilation that occurs in congestive heart failure. The hyperventilation and periodic breathing may be the result of stimulation of pulmonary vagal-irritant receptors by pulmonary congestion.

7. D. All of the above

Chemoreflexes mediate the ventilatory response to hypercapnia and hypoxemia. Peripheral chemoreceptors primarily respond to blood oxygen tension, whereas brainstem central chemoreceptors are most sensitive to carbon dioxide and acid-base balance. Neural reflexes initiated at the chemoreceptor level modulate both the inspiratory and upper airway muscles to coordinate the inspiratory effort with upper airway tone. In healthy persons, activation of the baroreflexes attenuates ventilatory, sympathetic, and bradycardic responses to peripheral chemoreceptor excitation. Compared with healthy subjects, patients with OSA have heightened peripheral chemoreflex sensitivity, resulting in an increased ventilatory response and sympathetic activity to hypoxemia. Hypoxemia also increases cardiac vagal activity, which can manifest as severe bradyarrhythmias during apneic events.

8. D. All of the above

Patients with sleep apnea have been found by numerous studies to be at increased risk of developing cardiovascular diseases. Cardiovascular variability is part of the normal physiology and is considered to be the natural response of the autonomic nervous system to different situations encountered in everyday life. Altered cardiovascular variability in itself is a prognostic indicator for cardiovascular events. Narkiewicz and collaborators have shown that patients with OSA have a faster heart rate and increased sympathetic burst frequency. In addition, the heart rate variability is decreased and blood pressure variability is markedly increased in these patients. The magnitude of these alterations seems to be related to the severity of the sleep disorder, as patients with moderate OSA had significantly decreased heart rate variability compared with the mild disease group. In the author's opinion, repetitive sympathetic activation and blood pressure surges that occur in response to apneic episodes during sleep cause an impairment of baroreflex and other cardiovascular reflex functions that carry over even into daytime wakefulness.

9. A. Order polysomnography to rule out sleep apnea.

Patients with transient ischemic attack or stroke have a high prevalence (>50%) for OSA. Sleep apnea has been shown to increase the risk of stroke independent of known risk factors. These patients should be screened for underlying sleep apnea with polysomnography. Smoking cessation and aspirin use are important measures in the long-term stroke prevention program, but at this point obtaining a sleep study is paramount for our patient. Nocturnal trend oximetry cannot replace polysomnography for many reasons, especially as the absence of hypoxia does not rule out a sleep breathing disorder.

10. B. Increased platelet aggregation

Patients with OSA have increased morning levels of fibrinogen and higher plasma viscosity, and their magnitude correlates with OSA severity. Of interest, these changes were found to be independent of the other cardiovascular risk factors. This suggests that increased coagulability may be an intrinsic part of the OSA pathophysiology. During the obstructive apnea events, throughout the night there are repetitive surges in plasma catecholamines. The elevated catecholamine levels increase platelet aggregability. Other factors involved in coagulation that are higher in patients with OSA than in control subjects include XIIa, VIIa, thrombin-antithrombin, and soluble P-selectin. Sleep apnea was found to be an independent predictor of C-reactive protein elevation, and it correlates negatively with high-density lipoprotein cholesterol serum levels.

In conclusion, the procoagulation pathways are enhanced in patients with OSA, including increased platelet activation and aggregation. Treatment with CPAP partially mitigates these changes.

11. B. The cerebral autoregulation is abnormal during wakefulness in patients with OSA.

There is major fluctuation in cerebral blood flow (CBF) velocity during apnea. During the early part of an OSA event, the CBF decreases and then markedly increases with increasing arterial carbon dioxide tension and after termination of apnea, subjecting the brain to ischemia and vascular wall strain. Simultaneous monitoring of intracranial pressure, intra-arterial blood pressure, and central venous pressure in patients with OSA disorder while awake and during sleep-induced apnea demonstrated a marked increase in intracranial pressure and a decrease in cerebral perfusion pressure during obstructive apneas. Hypercapnia (not hypocapnia) is normally a powerful stimulus for vasodilation. Abnormalities of cerebral vascular response to hypercapnia that persist during wakefulness have been found in patients with sleep apnea, suggesting impaired cerebral autoregulation. During wakefulness the normal cerebral response to hypoxia is vasodilation and increased cerebral blood flow. Meadows et al showed that in sleep this reactivity is lost, and decreasing oxygen tension of the blood perfusing the brain triggers vasoconstriction and reduction in cerebral blood flow.

12. C. Reassure the technologist, and continue monitoring.

REM sleep–related sinus arrest is a cardiac rhythm disorder that affects otherwise healthy young adults of either gender and is characterized by sinus arrest during REM sleep, usually in clusters, with asystoles lasting up to 9 seconds. Daytime ECG, including Holter monitoring, is usually normal, and angiography, when performed, is unremarkable. Treatment is usually not indicated; however, the situation is different for patients with sleep apnea. Using an insertable loop recording device and about 2 months of recording in 23 sleep apnea patients who were free of other cardiac disease, Simantirakis and colleagues found that 46% of sleep apnea patients had rhythm disturbances, which mostly occurred at night. Five of these patients (22%) had multiple severe bradycardic events and frequent

sinus pauses or complete heart block, including one who had a 12-second episode of ventricular asystole. The frequency and severity of these events correlated with BMI, the degree of oxygen desaturation, and the apnea-hypopnea index recorded during polysomnography. These findings support another previously reported study that patients with heart block during sleep were more obese and had more severe sleep-disordered breathing. Perhaps most important, when these same patients were treated with CPAP, the rate of arrhythmias fell markedly and they were virtually eliminated after 4 months of CPAP treatment.

13. B. Ventricular tachycardia of this kind during sleep is common and does not warrant interruption of polysomnography.

Ventricular tachycardia occurs in 2% of the patients with sleep apnea. These patients generally have more severe oxygen desaturations. Ventricular ectopy peaks between 6:00 and 11:00 A.M. (as does all cause mortality). The peak prevalence of ventricular tachycardia and fibrillation appears to be at the time of wakening, both for those with cardiac disease and for normal individuals. Beta blockade eliminates this circadian variation in ventricular arrhythmias, suggesting that it is sympathetically mediated.

14. B. Patients with sleep-disordered breathing are more likely to remain in sinus rhythm after cardioversion if the sleep-disordered breathing is treated with CPAP.

Despite initial reports of beneficial effects of overdrive pacing in patients with sleep-disordered breathing, several subsequent studies did not confirm this effect. Simantirakis and collaborators found that overdrive pacing of the heart rate with an implantable pacemaker produced no differences in the apnea-hypopnea index, arousal index, desaturation index, mean or lowest arterial oxyhemoglobin saturation, total sleep time, or partial pressure of arterial carbon dioxide.

The prevalence of OSA in patients with atrial fibrillation was around 50% in a prospective study by Gami et al of patients undergoing electrocardioversion for atrial fibrillation. Maintaining a sinus rhythm after cardioversion in people with concomitant OSA has been found to be mainly dependent on correcting the elevated apnea-hypopnea index with CPAP. Generally, the deeper stages of sleep are a time of cardiovascular quiescence. The parasympathetic nervous system activity increases and that of the sympathetic system decreases, and consequently the atrioventricular node conduction slows down, refractory time lengthens, and there is a propensity towards bradycardia rather than tachycardia.

15. B. Hypercapnia

In patients with congestive heart failure, about 30–40% have CSR and central sleep apnea. It appears that congestive heart failure causes central sleep apnea by increased oscillation of $PaCO_2$ above and below the apneic threshold. These patients tend to have hypocapnia rather than hypercapnia. Having a $PaCO_2$ just above the threshold makes these patients much more sensitive to hyperventilation. Because of concomitant long circulatory time to the central chemoreceptors, the apnea-hyperpnea cycles are long and the response is delayed, resulting in the characteristic pattern. Raising $PaCO_2$ away from the apnea threshold ameliorates the CSR.

The prevalence of the syndrome is increased in men and increases with age together with the prevalence of heart failure. Dysrhythmia further alters the ejection fraction and prolongs the circulatory time. Cardiac resynchronization therapy (using atrial-synchronized biventricular pacing to coordinate right and left ventricular contraction) significantly improves the ejection fraction and reduces central sleep apnea.

16. D. CPAP lowers the pulmonary artery pressure.

The prevalence of pulmonary hypertension (PH) in sleep apnea is relatively low, most studies reporting values around 20%. Although OSA can cause elevation of the pulmonary arterial pressures, the pressure is generally lower than in primary pulmonary hypertension. The average pressure in the pulmonary artery is 25–30 mm Hg, and OSA rarely causes cor pulmonale by itself. Findings of pulmonary arterial pressures above this level should be investigated beyond the diagnosis of OSA. Patients with OSA in conjunction with PH tend to have left-sided heart disease, parenchymal lung disease, more obesity, and greater nocturnal oxygen desaturation. A consistent finding in the literature is that oxygen desaturation predicts the risk of PH better than does the apnea-hypopnea index. Hypercapnia (not hypocapnia) is associated with higher prevalence of PH. Pulmonary arterial pressure is reduced with CPAP therapy, with greater reductions observed in subjects with pulmonary hypertension.

17. C. No effect on cardiovascular death

The association between OSA and coronary artery disease (CAD) is now supported by a body of evidence. Even more important, studies have shown that irrespective of other confounding factors, the presence of OSA is a risk factor for the development of cardiac ischemia. Multiple mechanisms have been implicated in this association: hypoxia, repetitive sympathetic discharges induced by the apneic episodes, abnormal platelet and coagulation function, and various humoral alterations. Because the presence of CAD significantly increases the morbidity and mortality of the individuals affected, the ability of altering each of its risk factors is of paramount importance. The effect of CPAP on cardiac complications in people with known CAD has been addressed by two prospective studies. Both have shown decreased fatal and nonfatal myocardial infarction in patients with OSP treated with CPAP compared with the untreated group. The incidence of coronary revascularization was also reduced in subjects effectively treated.

18. C. The apnea-hypopnea index can improve with theophylline.

The epoch shown illustrates a central apnea event with Cheyne-Stokes respirations.

Left ventricular dysfunction resulting in heart failure is frequently associated with sleep disorders. In contrast with the general population, in which OSA is the most common sleep disturbance, in patients with heart failure, central sleep apnea has a higher prevalence. In a prospective study of 81 patients with heart failure, 40% had central sleep apnea versus 11% with OSA. Symptoms such as hypersomnolence, fatigue, nocturia, or nocturnal dyspnea can be due to either heart failure or its treatment; therefore sleep apnea may not be readily suggested by history. Furthermore, because snoring and obesity may be absent in subjects with heart failure and central sleep apnea, the clinical diagnosis is often difficult. The mortality of patients with low ejection fraction is related to their apnea-hypopnea index (AHI), as shown by Lanfranchi, et al. They demonstrated that the AHI was the most powerful independent predictor of survival, with a 2-year mortality rate of 50% in patients with an AHI >30, versus 26.2% in patients with an AHI <30. The therapy of central sleep apnea associated with heart failure usually starts with optimizing the cardiopulmonary function (beta-blockers, angiotensin converting enzyme inhibitors or angiotensin II receptor blockers, diuretics). For patients that still have a significant number of apneic events, positive pressure devices (CPAP, BiPAP) and nocturnal oxygen have been shown to improve the AHI. Supplemental oxygen decreases the ventilatory response to CO_2, resulting in an increase in $PaCO_2$ above the apneic threshold that subsequently decreases central apneas. Theophylline, a respiratory stimulant, was proven to be beneficial in treating central sleep apnea. In a study by Javaheri et al (N Engl J Med 335:562, 1996), a 5-day course of theophylline reduced the AHI by 50% and central sleep apnea index from 26/hr to 6/hr. The use of theophylline has to be weighed against its narrow therapeutic range and the need for frequent monitoring because of potential arrhythmic complications.

19. C. CPAP decreases both the nighttime and the daytime blood pressures.

There is solid evidence that OSA and hypertension are related in a cause-and-effect manner. In a prospective epidemiological study, (Peppard PE et al: N Engl J Med 342:1378–1384, 2000), an increased apnea-hypopnea index at baseline predicts the risk of hypertension in the years to come in a dose-response relationship. The odds ratio for developing hypertension was 1.42 for subjects with an AHI within normal limits (0–4.9). The same odds ratio increased to 2.03 for an AHI of 5–14.9, and furthermore to 2.89 for an AHI greater than 15.

The sympathetic surge related to the apneic episodes not only increases the blood pressure during the night, but is carried over during the daytime, occasionally being diagnosed as idiopathic hypertension. There is a high incidence of undiagnosed OSA in patients with hypertension refractory to treatment. Randomized studies of CPAP versus sham in normotensives and mild hypertensives showed that CPAP consistently lowered the blood pressure during both nighttime and daytime.

20. C. The risk is higher during sleeping hours (10 P.M.–6 A.M.).

This issue was addressed in a study by Gami et al, which reviewed polysomnograms and death certificates of 112 Minnesota residents who died suddenly from cardiac causes.

In contrast with the general population, people with sleep apnea died more frequently during sleeping hours (10 P.M.–6 A.M.). The severity of sleep apnea also correlated directly with the risk of nocturnal death from cardiac causes. In people with an AHI of 40, the relative risk for sudden cardiac death was 40% higher than in those with lower AHI (5–39). The sympathetic drive and frequency of cardiac arrhythmias are diminished during normal sleep; however, quite the opposite is true for subjects with sleep apnea. The repetitive apneic episodes can trigger sympathetic surges that increase the blood pressure, promote platelet aggregation, and induce hypoxemia. All these factors favor cardiac ischemia and ventricular arrhythmias. Fatal rhythm disturbances occur during sleep in people with obstructive apnea, and applying effective therapy can diminish their occurrence.

21. B. Paradoxical embolism

The relationship between various cardiovascular risk factors and OSA was the object of both cross-sectional and cohort studies. Shahar et al (AJRCCM 163:19, 2001) have shown an association between OSA and the risk for hypertension, stroke, congestive heart failure, and coronary artery disease in a large, cross-sectional study. More recently Yaggi and collaborators (N Engl J Med 353:2034, 2005) have demonstrated that OSA significantly increases the risk of stroke independently of other risk factors. The pathophysiological mechanisms through which OSA influences the risk of stroke are complex. Cerebral blood flow velocity decreases after apnea termination concomitant with changes in arterial pressure. Low cerebral blood flow, low arterial pressure, and hypoxemia after apnea termination may predispose to nocturnal cerebral ischemia. Hypercoagulability (not hypocoagulability) has been implicated also in increasing the risk of stroke in subjects with OSA. Increased platelet activation and aggregation occur during sleep in patients with OSA, and this effect is greatly reduced by CPAP use. The incidence of patent foramen ovale was found to be increased in both OSA and stroke patients. A causal relationship between the right-to-left shunt and obstructive apneas has been described by Beelke et al (Sleep 25:856, 2002). Supplemental oxygen and dental appliance usage has not been associated with increased incidence of cerebrovascular accidents.

22. A. OSA is an independent risk factor for stroke.

The most compelling evidence regarding the effect of OSA on the risk of stroke come from a recent large observational cohort study by Yaggi et al (N Engl J Med 353:2034, 2005). Subjects underwent polysomnography, and subsequent events (strokes and deaths) were verified. The authors found that OSA is associated with an increased incidence of stroke independent of other cardiovascular or cerebrovascular risk factors. The study also showed that the risk of stroke or death increased further with the severity of sleep apnea, as measured by the AHI.

Stroke is the third leading cause of death and produces the most cases of long-term disability. Among subjects who suffered a stroke, the prevalence of sleep apnea is 43–91%, with the vast majority having the obstructive type. The fact that the OSA precedes stroke in most patients is supported by the findings that: (1) there is no difference in the frequency and severity of OSA between the patients with stroke versus those with transient ischemic attack (TIA), and (2) the frequency of obstructive apneas do not decline in time after a stroke. In contrast, the central type of apneas tend to disappear with time, probably related to decreasing local inflammation. These data suggest that acute stroke predisposes to development of central sleep apnea, and that OSA most likely was already present at the time of stroke. There was no association found between stroke location and apnea type.

23. E. CPAP reduces the duration of ST-segment elevation.

Analyzing the cohort of the Sleep Heart Health Study, Shahar et al (AJRCCM 163:19, 2001) found that OSA is an independent risk factor for CAD, with an odds ratio of 1.27 for an AHI >11. This confirmed previous observations by Hung et al (Lancet 8710:261, 1990) that an AHI >5.3 is an independent risk factor for myocardial ischemia. OSA induces several physiologic effects that could predispose to myocardial ischemia during sleep. Experimentally, in animals with induced coronary disease, obstructive apnea can lead to myocardial ischemia, even in the absence of hypoxia. In the absence of coronary stenosis, however, myocardial ischemia was not observed. Results of studies in patients with OSA but without CAD have not been consistent. Although most of them did not find signs of nocturnal ischemia, one study described ST-segment depressions at night in 30% of patients. Application of CPAP in these patients significantly reduced the duration of ST-segment elevation. The ST changes are thought to be caused by the increased myocardial oxygen demand during the postapneic surges in blood pressure and heart rate, at a time when the oxyhemoglobin saturation is at its lowest point. Measurements of cardiac markers during sleep in patients who have both CAD and OSA have not shown elevations of troponin T, even with repeated measurements.

24. D. Nocturnal desaturations cause bradycardia and tachycardia.

Hypoxia has different influences on the heart rate according to the presence or absence of airflow and the balance between its sympathetic and parasympathetic effects.

During apnea, with no airflow, hypoxic stimulation of the carotid body stimulates the vagus nerve endings and causes bradycardia. Once the apnea is terminated, in the presence of the airflow, the stretching of the lungs inhibits vagal outflow to the heart, sympathetic discharge is unopposed, and reflexive tachycardia can result. Bradycardia responds in time to therapy with CPAP, and its frequency and severity correlate well with the AHI and magnitude of the desaturations. In some individuals, hypoxia increases sympathetic output to vascular beds through peripheral chemoreceptors, whereas activation of cardiac vagal activity results in bradycardia. The net result is peripheral vasoconstriction plus bradycardia, a phenomenon called the *diving reflex*. This mechanism maintains homeostasis during prolonged periods of apnea and may be activated in some patients with OSA, causing severe bradycardia during apneic events.

25. D. Obstructive sleep apnea (OSA)

Atrial fibrillation (AF) is common in people with OSA. One study estimated that OSA is present in approximately 50% of patients with AF. The prevalence of OSA in AF is higher than in any other cardiovascular disease without associated atrial fibrillation. These findings support the concept that it is not only the associated conditions of OSA (most important, hypertension) that may lead to AF, but there may be a unique interaction between the pathophysiology of OSA and AF. In patients with OSA, intermittent hypoxemia, hypercapnia, chemoreceptor excitation, markedly increased sympathetic drive, and severe pressor surges can all occur nightly for years if untreated and may initiate or predispose to AF. In a prospective study of 118 patients with OSA, Kanagala et al (Circulation 107:2589, 2003) showed that patients with untreated OSA have a higher recurrence of AF after cardioversion than patients without a polysomnographic diagnosis of sleep apnea. This high rate of recurrence is not secondary to differences in age, sex, antiarrhythmic therapy, BMI, functional status, ECG measures, or coexisting diabetes or hypertension. Therapy with CPAP at an appropriate level improves significantly the chances of remaining in sinus rhythm after conversion.

REFERENCES

1. Andreas S, Schulz R, Werner G, et al: Prevalence of obstructive sleep apnoea in patients with coronary disease. Coron Artery Dis 7:541–545, 1996.

2. Atwood Jr, Charles W: Pulmonary artery hypertension and sleep-disordered breathing. Chest 126:72S, 2004.

3. Bassetti C, Aldrich MS: Sleep apnea in acute cerebrovascular diseases: final report on 128 patients. Sleep 22:217–223, 1999.

4. Beelke M, Angeli S, Del Sette M: Obstructive sleep apnea can be provocative for right-to-left shunting through a patent foramen ovale. Sleep 25:856–862, 2002.

5. Bokinsky G, Miller M, Ault K, et al: Spontaneous platelet activation and aggregation during obstructive sleep apnea and its response to therapy with nasal continuous positive airway pressure. A preliminary investigation. Chest 108(3):625–630, 1995.

6. Borgel J, Sanner BM, Bittlinsky A, et al: Obstructive sleep apnoea and its therapy influence high-density lipoprotein cholesterol serum levels. Eur Respir J 27(1):121–127, 2006.

7. Brown HW, Plum F: The neurological basis of Cheyne-Stokes respiration. Am J Med 30:849–861, 1961.

8. Caples M, Gami A, Somers VK: Ann Intern Med 142:187–197, 2005.

9. Chaouat A, Weitzenblum E, Krieger J, et al: Pulmonary hemodynamics in obstructive sleep apnea syndrome. Results in 220 consecutive patients. Chest 109:380–386, 1996.

10. Cicolin A, Mangiardi L, Mutani R, et al: Angiotensin-converting enzyme inhibitors and obstructive sleep apnea. Mayo Clin Proc 81(1):53–55, 2006.

11. Cloward and Tom: Left ventricular hypertrophy is a common echocardiographic abnormality in severe obstructive sleep apnea and reverses with nasal continuous positive airway pressure. Chest 124(2):594, 2003.

12. Daly MDB, Scott MJ: The cardiovascular responses to stimulation of the carotid chemoreceptors in the dog. J Physiol 165:179–197, 1963.

13. Davies RJO, Crosby J, Prothero A, et al: Ambulatory blood pressure and left ventricular hypertrophy in subjects with untreated obstructive sleep apnoea and snoring compared with matched control subjects and their response to treatment. Clin Res 86:417–424, 1994.

14. Franklin KA: Cerebral haemodynamics in obstructive sleep apnoea and Cheyne-Stokes respiration. Sleep Med Rev 6(6):429–441, 2002.

15. Gami AS, Howard DE, Olson EJ, Somers VK: Day-night pattern of sudden death in obstructive sleep apnea. N Engl J Med 352(12):1206–1214, 2005 Mar 24.

16. Gami AS, Pressman G, Caples SM, et al: Association of atrial fibrillation and obstructive sleep apnea. Circulation 110:364–367, 2004.

17. Gami AS, Svatikova A, Wolk R, et al: Cardiac troponin T in obstructive sleep apnea. Chest 125:2097–2100, 2004.

18. Grimpen F, Kanne P, Schulz E, et al: Endothelin-1 plasma levels are not elevated in patients with obstructive sleep apnoea. Eur Respir J 15:320–325, 2000.

19. Guilleminault CS, Motta J, Mihm F, et al: Obstructive sleep apnea and cardiac index. Chest 89:331–334, 1986.

20. Guyton AC: Basic oscillating mechanism of Cheyne-Stokes breathing. Am J Physiol 187:395–398, 1956.

21. Hla KM, Young TB, Bidwell T, et al: Sleep apnea and hypertension. A population based study. Ann Intern Med 120:382–388, 1994.

22. Hung J, Whitford EG, Parsons RW, Hillman DR: Association of sleep apnoea with myocardial infarction in men. Lancet 336(8710):261–264, 1990.

23. Javaheri S, Parker TJ, Wexler L, et al: Effect of theophylline on sleep-disordered breathing in heart failure. N Engl J Med 335:562–567, 1996.

24. Javaheri S, Parker TJ, Liming JD, et al: Sleep apnea in 81 ambulatory male patients with stable heart failure: types and their prevalences, consequences, and presentations. Circulation 97:2154–2159, 1998.

25. Jennum P, Borgesen SE: Intracranial pressure and obstructive sleep apnea. Chest 95:279–283, 1989.

26. Kanagala R, Murali NS, Friedman PA, et al: Obstructive sleep apnea and the recurrence of atrial fibrillation. Circulation 107:2589–2594, 2003.

27. Khoo MC, Kronauer RE, Strohl KP, Slutsky AS: Factors inducing periodic breathing in humans: a general model. J Appl Physiol 53:644–659, 1982.

28. Khatri IM, Freis ED: Hemodynamic changes during sleep. J Appl Physiol 22:867–873, 1967.

29. Laks L, Lehrhaft B, Grustein RR, et al: Pulmonary artery pressure response to hypoxia in sleep apnea. Am J Respir Crit Care Med 155:193–198, 1997.

30. Lanfranchi P, Braghirol A, Bosimini E, et al: Prognostic value of nocturnal Cheyne-Stokes respiration in congestive hear failure. Circulation 99:1435–1440, 1999.

31. Leung RS, Bradley TD: Sleep apnea and cardiovascular disease. Am J Respir Crit Care Med 164:2147–2165, 2001.

32. Lindberg E, Janson C, Gislason T, et al: Sleep apnea and hypertension: a 10 year follow-up. Eur Respir J 11:884–889, 1998.

33. Lindberg E, Janson C, Svardsudd K, et al: Increased mortality among sleepy snorers: a prospective population based study. Thorax 53:631–637, 1998.

34. Marin JM, Carrizo SJ, Vincente E, et al: Long-term cardiovascular outcomes in men with obstructive sleep apnoea-hypopnea with or without treatment with continuous positive airway pressure: an observational study. Lancet 365:1046–1053, 2005.

35. Meadows GE, O'Driscoll DM, Simonds AK, et al: Cerebral blood flow response to isocapnic hypoxia during slow-wave sleep and wakefulness. J Appl Physiol 97:1343–1348, 2004.

36. Miller JC, Horvath SM: Cardiac output during human sleep. Aviat Space Environ Med 47:1046–1051, 1976.

37. Milleron O, Pilliere R, Foucher A, et al: Benefits of obstructive sleep apnoea treatment in coronary artery disease: a long-term follow-up study. Eur Heart J 25(9):728–734, 2004.

38. Mooe T, Rabben T, Wiklund U, et al: Sleep-disordered breathing in men with coronary artery disease. Chest 109:659–663, 1996.

39. Mooe T, Rabben T, Wiklund U, et al: Sleep-disordered breathing in women, occurrence and association with coronary disease. Am J Med 101:251–256, 1996.

40. Motta J, Guilleminault CS, Schroeder JS, et al: Tracheostomy and hemodynamic changes in sleep-induced apnea. Ann Intern Med 89:454–458, 1978.

41. Narkiewicz K, Montano N, Cogliati C, et al: Altered cardiovascular variability in obstructive sleep apnea. Circulation 98:1071–1077, 1998.

42. Peled N, Abinader EG, Pillar G, et al: Nocturnal ischemic events in patients with obstructive sleep apnea syndrome and ischemic heart disease: effects of continuous positive air pressure treatment. J Am Coll Cardiol 34:1744–1749, 1999.

43. Parra O, Arboix A, Bechich S, et al: Time course of sleep-related breathing disorders in first-ever stroke or transient ischemic attack. Am J Respir Crit Care Med 161:375–380, 2000.

44. Peppard PE, Young T, Palta M, et al: Prospective study of the association between sleep-disordered breathing and hypertension. N Engl J Med 342:1378–1384, 2000.

45. Pepperell JCT, Ramdassingh-Dow S, Crosthwaite N, et al: Ambulatory blood pressure after therapeutic and subtherapeutic nasal continuous positive airway pressure for obstructive sleep apnoea: a randomized parallel trial. Lancet 359:204–210, 2002.

46. Sajkov D, Cowie RJ, Thornton AT: Pulmonary hypertension and hypoxemia in obstructive sleep apnea syndrome. Am J Respir Crit Care Med 149:193–198, 1994.

47. Sajkov D, Wang T, Saunders NA, et al: Continuous positive airway pressure treatment improves pulmonary hemodynamics in patients with obstructive sleep apnea. Am J Respir Crit Care Med 165:152–158, 2002.

48. Schafer H, Koehler U, Ploch T, et al: Sleep-related myocardial ischemia, and sleep structure in patients with obstructive sleep apnea, and coronary artery disease. Chest 111:387–393, 1997.

49. Scharf SM, Graver LM, Balaban K: Cardiovascular effects in periodic occlusions of the upper airways in dogs. Am Rev Respir Dis 146:321–329, 1992.

50. Schroeder JS, Motta J, Guilleminault CS: Hemodynamic studies in sleep apnea. In Guilleminault C, Dement WC (eds): *Sleep Apnea Syndrome.* New York, Alan R Liss, 1978, pp 177–196.

51. Shahar E, Whitney CW, Redline S, et al: Sleep-disordered breathing and cardiovascular disease: cross-sectional results of the Sleep Heart Health Study. Am J Respir Crit Care Med 163:19–25, 2001.

52. Shepard JW: Cardiopulmonary consequences of obstructive sleep apnea. Mayo Clin Proc 65:1250–1259, 1990.

53. Simantirakis EN, Schiza SI, Chrysostomakis SI, et al: Atrial overdrive pacing for the obstructive sleep apnea-hypopnea syndrome. N Engl J Med 353(24):2568–2577, 2005.

54. Simatirakis EN, Schiza SI, Marketou ME, et al: Severe bradyarrhythmias in patients with sleep apnoea: the effect of continuous positive airway pressure treatment: a long-term evaluation using an insertable loop recorder. Eur Heart J 25(12):1070–1076, 2004.

55. Sin DD, Fitzgerald F, Parker JD, et al: Risk factors for central and obstructive sleep apnea in 450 men and women with congestive heart failure. Am J Respir Crit Care Med 160:1101–1106, 1999.

56. Sinha AM, Skobel EC, Breithardt OA, et al: Cardiac resynchronization therapy improves central sleep apnea and Cheyne-Stokes respiration in patients with chronic heart failure. J Am Coll Cardiol 44:68–71, 2004.

57. Smith M, Neidermaier O, Hardy S, et al: Role of hypoxemia in sleep apnea-induced sympathoexcitation. J Autonomic Nervous System 56:184–190, 1996.

58. Somers VK, Mark AL, Zavala DC, et al: Contrasting effect of hypoxia and hypercapnia on ventilation and sympathetic activity in humans. J Appl Physiol 67:2101–2106, 1989.

59. Steiner and Stephan, et al: Altered blood rheology in obstructive sleep apnea as a mediator of cardiovascular risk. Cardiology 104(2):92–96, 2005.

60. Tilkain AG, Guilleminault CS, Schroeder JS, et al: Hemodynamics in sleep induced apnea. Studies during wakefulnesss and sleep. Ann Intern Med 85:714–719, 1976.

61. Yaggi HK, Concato J, Kernan WN, et al: Obstructive sleep apnea as a risk factor for stroke and death. N Engl J Med 353:2034–2041, 2005.

62. Yaggi HK, Mohsenin V: Obstructive sleep apnoea and stroke. Lancet Neurol 3:333–342, 2004.

63. Young T, Finn L, Hla KM, et al: Snoring as part of a dose-response relationship between sleep-disordered breathing and blood pressure. Sleep 19:S202–S205, 1996.

Neurological Sleep Disorders

MASSIMILIANO M. SICCOLI ■ CLAUDIO L. BASSETTI

Questions

Stroke

Patient 1: Questions 1 and 2 refer to patient 1.
52-year-old man with acute ischemic stroke and frequent apneas during night sleep.

Case:

A 52-year-old man with known arterial hypertension and coronary heart disease reported a sudden weakness of the left arm and the left-sided face muscles, speech disturbances, and gait unsteadiness. He came to the emergency department 24 hours (h) after onset of symptoms.

In the clinical examination, a slight left-sided hemiparesis of the face, arm, and leg and a left hemisensory loss were found. The National Institutes of Health (NIH) stroke scale was 5. A computed tomography (CT) scan of the head showed a right-sided ischemic infarction in the territory of the middle cerebral artery with involvement of the insula (Figure 15-1A). Blood pressure was 175/110 mm Hg, heart rate 88/min. Respiration during the day was unremarkable, but frequent apneas as well as irregular breathing were observed during sleep. Transesophageal echocardiography revealed plaques of 4. degree in the aortic arch and an aneurysm of the left ventricle (residual, after myocardial infarction) as possible embolic sources, but no patent foramen ovale.

Sleep studies:

Respirography performed the first night after stroke onset (Figure 15-1B):

Frequent apneas and hypopneas (apnea-hypopnea index [AHI] 50/h), almost exclusively of central type, with frequent oxygen desaturations (oxygen-desaturation index [ODI] 49/h, minimal O_2 saturation 85%). Central periodic breathing in sleep was documented during about 50% of the recording time.

A polysomnography performed 3 months after acute stroke showed normal findings; the AHI was 1/h.

1. Which of the following sentences about sleep apnea in acute stroke is correct?

A. Sleep apnea is much more frequent in cerebral hemorrhage than in ischemic stroke.

B. Cheyne-Stokes respiration and central periodic breathing are found only in patients with bilateral strokes, brainstem stroke, heart failure, or profound disturbances of consciousness.

C. Sleep apnea does not usually spontaneously improve after stroke.

D. Sleep apnea is common in acute ischemic stroke (50–70% of patients).

E. Heart insufficiency is rarely present in patients with central breathing disorders.

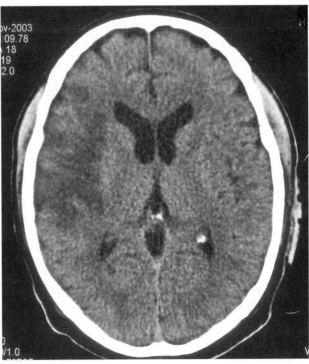

FIGURE 15-1A ■ Brain CT scan (2 days after stroke onset), showing a right-sided ischemic infarction in the territory of the middle cerebral artery. (Courtesy of the Institute of Neuroradiology, University Hospital of Zurich, Zurich, Switzerland.)

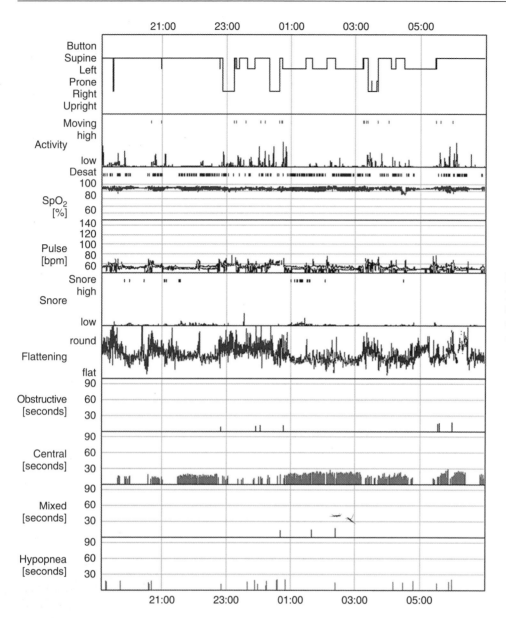

FIGURE 15-1B ■ Respirography performed in the first night after ischemic stroke, showing a severe central sleep apnea (AHI 50/h).

2. Should treatment of sleep apnea in an acute stroke setting be considered? Which sentence about continuous positive airway pressure (CPAP) treatment in acute stroke reflects the data currently existing in the literature?

A. CPAP treatment in the acute phase should be considered in all patients with obstructive and central sleep apnea.

B. CPAP treatment in acute stroke can be started in about 50% of patients with sleep-disordered breathing, but it can be maintained chronically in only a minority of patients.

C. CPAP treatment after acute stroke reduces stroke outcome and mortality.

D. CPAP treatment in patients with central sleep apnea improves sleep apnea severity, cardiac function, and survival.

Patient 2: Questions 3 and 4 refer to patient 2.

72-year-old woman with disturbed night sleep and recurrent nightmares after ischemic stroke.

Case:

A 72-year-old woman was referred to the emergency department because of acute neurological symptoms of slurred speech and impaired consciousness. In the morning she experienced a few hours of a transient sensation of pain in the right eye with moving shapes on the right side of the visual field. In the evening, during a telephone call, slurred speech suddenly appeared, followed within a few minutes by an impairment of consciousness. During the transport to the hospital the patient became comatose. In the emergency room, no spontaneous movements and no reaction to acoustic and painful stimuli were noted. Glasgow coma scale was 5. A skew deviation (left eye higher than right) with reduced reaction of the pupil to light, as well as a bilateral Babinski sign, were observed. Within the following 5 hours, the neurological deficits dramatically recovered, and a slight skew deviation, a gait ataxia, and a slight impairment of frontal cognitive functions remained as residual symptoms. Furthermore, the patient was not able to remember what happened shortly before and during the first hours after hospitalization. Magnetic resonance imaging (MRI) revealed a T2-hyperintensity in the left and a small one in the right thalamus, suggestive of an acute ischemic lesion (Figure 15-2A). The etiology of the stroke remained unclear despite extensive examinations.

During the first 2 days after stroke, she experienced recurring unpleasant dreams: she saw a big, awkward-looking hand with rough skin ("elephant skin") floating before her face. She saw then an embossed red point rising from the back of this hand that became larger.

The third day after the stroke, these dreams disappeared, and the patient did not report any dreams during the next week. After the first week, she noticed an increasing fatigue with excessive sleep needs, but without daytime sleepiness (Epworth sleepiness scale = 4). She denied sleep paralysis, cataplectic phenomena, snoring, restless legs symptoms, and hallucinations.

In a control examination 4 months after the stroke, she still complained about fatigue and excessive sleep needs, but to a lesser extent than during the acute phase. This improvement was also documented actigraphically.

Sleep studies:

First actigraphy, performed 1 week after stroke (Figure 15-2B):

Quite stable rest/activity pattern with constant bedtimes; increased amount of time "asleep" (rest and sleep)/24 h (55%, 11h07′) with reduced activity in the early afternoon; rest during the day 2h43′; normal rest/sleep efficiency (85%) and night phase fragmentation (index 27).

Polysomnography, performed 3 weeks after stroke:

Normal sleep latency (24′); markedly reduced sleep efficiency (44%) with 56% of time awake; distribution of sleep stages: NREM1 6%, NREM2 18%, NREM3 + NREM4 15%, reduced REM sleep (6%); profound reduction of the spindle activity; AHI 2/h, mean oxygen saturation 95%; preserved rapid eye movement (REM) sleep atonia; no periodic limb movements in sleep.

Second actigraphy, performed 4 months after stroke (Figure 15-2C):

Quite stable rest/activity pattern with constant bedtimes; increased amount of time "asleep"/24 h (44%, 10h47′) with reduced activity in the early afternoon; rest during the day 1h49′; normal rest/sleep efficiency (82%) and night phase fragmentation (index 25).

3. Which of the following sentences about hypersomnia after stroke is correct?

    A. The majority of stroke hypersomnias arises from a disruption of the ascending reticular activating system (ARAS) and corresponds to decreased arousal.

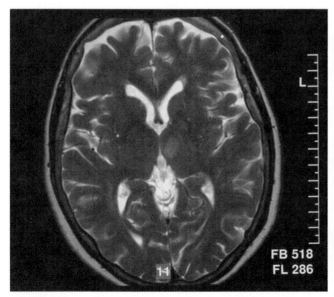 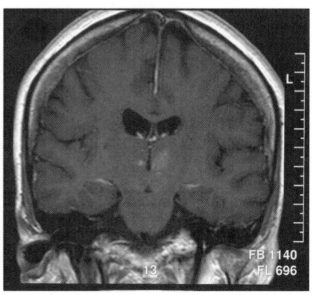

FIGURE 15-2A ■ Brain magnetic resonance image examination (T2-weighted, T1-weighted after contrast medium) performed 5 days after stroke onset, showing a bilateral thalamic stroke. (Courtesy of the Institute of Neuroradiology, University Hospital of Zurich, Zurich, Switzerland.)

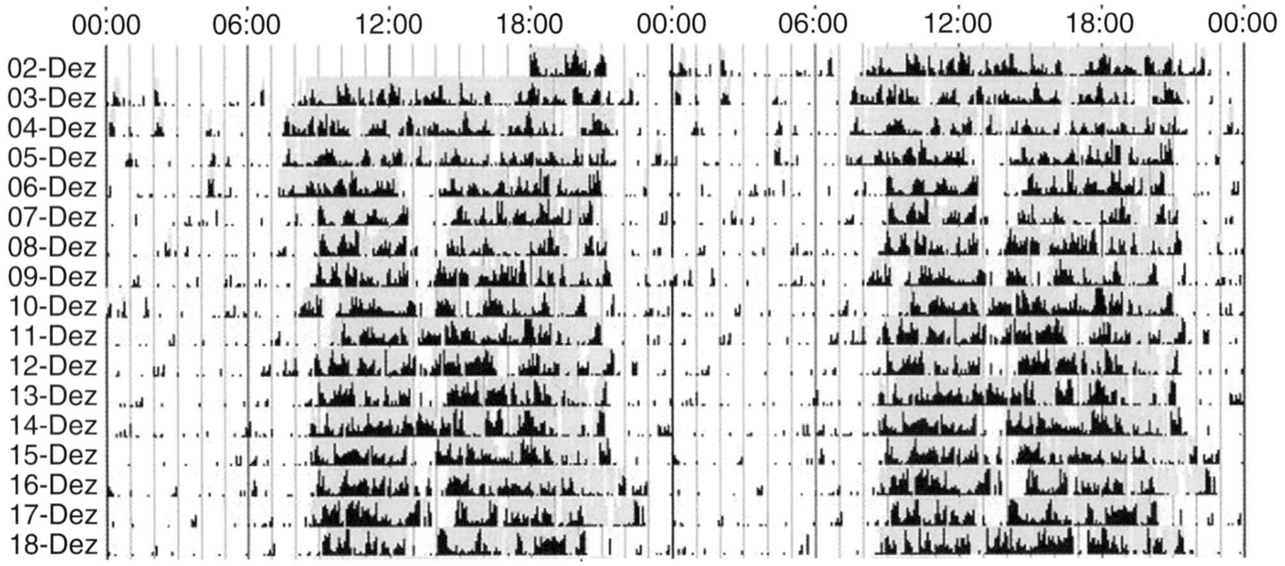

FIGURE 15-2B ■ Actigraphy performed one week after ischemic stroke, showing an increased amount of time "asleep"/24 h (11h07′).

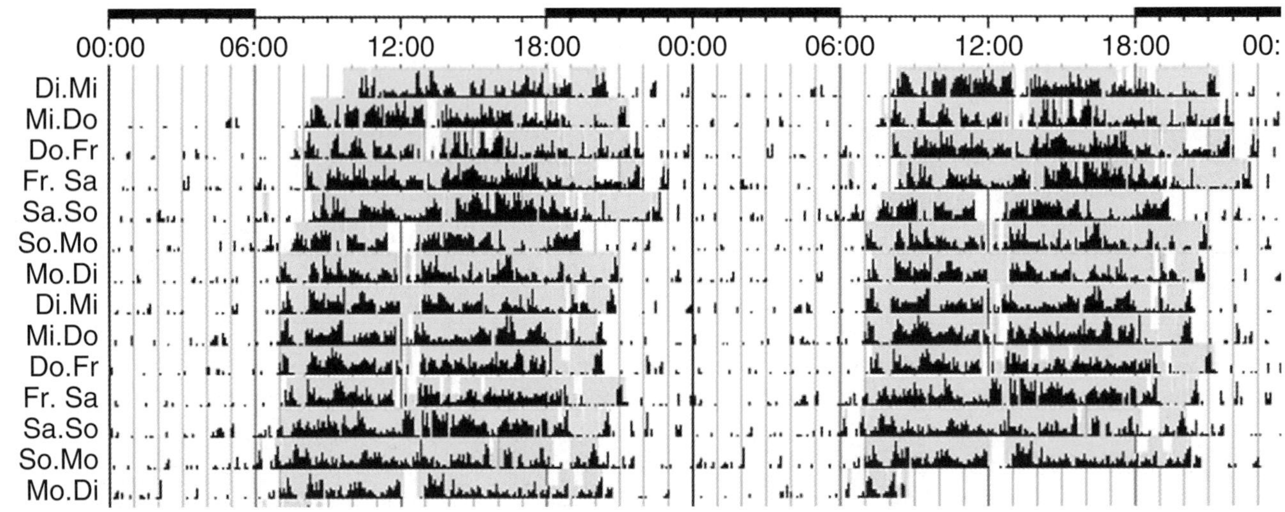

FIGURE 15-2C ■ Actigraphy performed 4 months after ischemic stroke, showing a slight improvement of the previous findings.

B. Small ischemic lesions are not associated with hypersomnia.
C. Hypersomnia is found only in patients with thalamic, hypothalamic, or mesencephalic strokes.
D. NREM sleep is usually increased in patients with thalamic strokes and hypersomnia.

4. Which of the following stroke topographies may be associated with a new-onset REM sleep behavior disorder after stroke?
A. Paramedian thalamus
B. Tegmentum pontis

C. Parietal lobe
D. Occipital lobe
E. Hypothalamus

Extrapyramidal diseases

Patient 3: Questions 5 and 6 refer to patient 3.
69-year-old man with asymmetric parkinsonism, increasing gait unsteadiness, and disturbed night sleep.
Case:
A 69-year-old man with parkinsonism was referred to our neurological ward. The first symptoms appeared 5 years previously, consisting in slowness/rigidity of movements and unsteadiness in walking

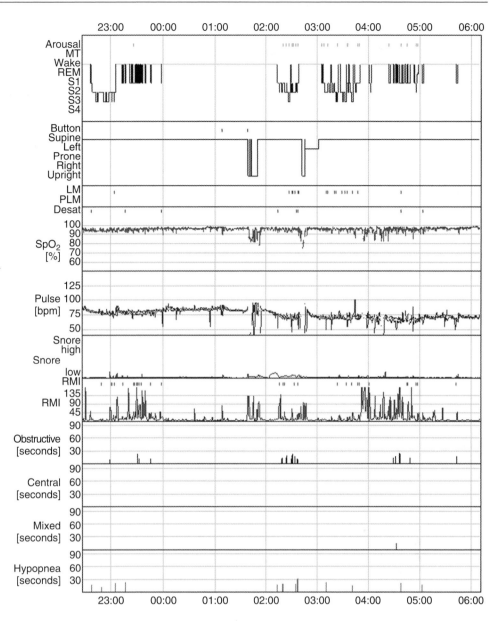

FIGURE 15-3 ■ Hypnogram of patient 3, showing a marked insomnia with arousals (no reason indicated) and only mild obstructive sleep apnea (AHI 17/h).

with repeated falls. Two years later, a right-sided tremor, increased salivation, speech disturbances, and some degree of memory impairment (mini mental test 28/30 points) appeared. Treatment with L-dopa, ropinirole, and donepezil was gradually established, with a partial improvement of the symptoms but appearance of transient confusion and hallucinations ("angels with trumpet") during the night. Considering clinical findings and evolution, an idiopathic etiology of parkinsonism was assumed.

The patient reported frequent awakenings during the night associated with difficulty in turning when lying in bed, as well as slight excessive daytime sleepiness (Epworth sleepiness scale = 9) with increased sleep needs (frequent naps) during the day. He denied snoring, restless legs symptoms, sleep paralysis, sleep walking, sleep talking or screaming, and cataplexy.

Sleep studies:

Polysomnography (Figure 15-3):

Normal sleep latency (14′); markedly reduced sleep efficiency (28%) with 72% of time awake; almost no REM sleep (0.3%); AHI 17/h (mainly of obstructive type), no oxygen desaturations <90%; preserved REM sleep atonia; no periodic limb movements in sleep.

Multiple sleep latency test (MSLT):

Normal mean sleep (non-REM [NREM]1) latency (12.4′); no sleep onset REM periods.

5. Which of the following factors can lead to sleep fragmentation and disruption in patients with Parkinson's disease?
   A. Parkinsonian tremor and inability to turn in and get off of bed
   B. Nycturia

C. Restless legs and leg cramps
D. Depression
E. All of the above

6. Which of the following groups of drugs are considered to be first-choice medication in the treatment of insomnia in patients with Parkinson's disease?
A. Benzodiazepines and hypnotics
B. Tricyclic antidepressants
C. Anticholinergic drugs
D. Atypical antipsychotics (clozapine, quetiapine)
E. L-dopa and dopaminergic drugs

Patient 4: Questions 7 and 8 refer to patient 4.
61-year-old man with idiopathic Parkinson's disease and excessive daytime sleepiness.

Case:

A 61-year-old patient with known idiopathic Parkinson's disease, treated for 3 years with L-dopa, ropinirole, and amitriptyline was referred to our outpatient department because of very disturbing excessive daytime sleepiness (Epworth sleepiness scale = 20). Subjective estimation of night sleep was maintained, and the quality of sleep was reported to be satisfactory. He denied insomnia, snoring, restless legs symptoms, hallucinations, and nightmares, as well as pain, off-motor phenomena, and dyskinesias during the night. During the day he felt permanently tired and sleepy, and daytime naps were frequently reported. Amitriptyline was tentatively withdrawn for 1 week, but night sleep worsened and daytime sleepiness did not improve.

Sleep studies:

Polysomnography (Figure 15-4):

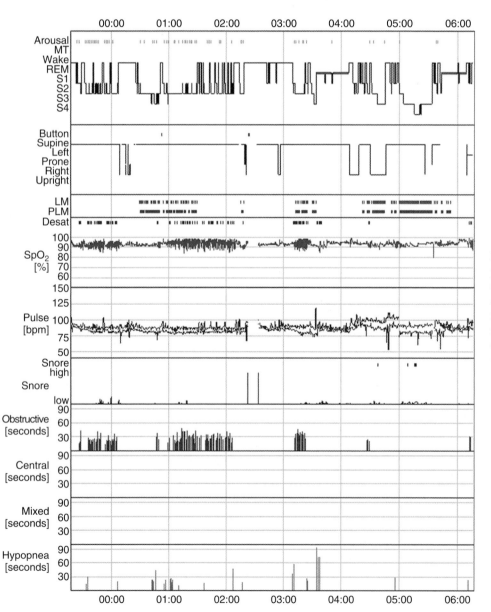

FIGURE 15-4 ■ Hypnogram of patient 4, showing a marked amount of periodic (PLM) and nonperiodic (LM) limb movements in sleep (PLMS index 81/h). In addition moderate obstructive sleep apnea (AHI 28/h).

Normal sleep latency (12′); reduced sleep efficiency (70%) with 30% of time awake; prolonged REM-sleep latency (246′); distribution of sleep stages: NREM1 12%, NREM2 33%, NREM3 + NREM4 11%, REM sleep 14%; AHI 28/h (only of obstructive type, obstructive apnea index 23/h, ODI 26/h, time with oxygen saturation <90% [CT90%] 16′); preserved REM sleep atonia; very high number of periodic and nonperiodic limb movements in sleep (PLMS index 81/h), partly associated with arousals (arousal index 33/h).

MSLT:

Moderately reduced mean sleep (NREM1) latency (5′); no sleep-onset REM periods (SOREMPs)

Maintenance of wakefulness test (MWT):

Slightly reduced mean sleep (NREM1) latency (15″); no SOREMPS.

7. Which of the following etiologies should be considered in the differential diagnosis of excessive daytime sleepiness in patients with parkinsonian syndromes?
   A. Sleep-disordered breathing
   B. Restless legs symptoms and periodic limb movements in sleep
   C. L-dopa and dopaminergic agents
   D. All of the above
   E. NREM-sleep parasomnia

8. Which of the following treatment options can be considered in this patient?
   A. Reduce ropinirole or levodopa.
   B. Continuous positive airway pressure treatment.
   C. Add modafinil in the morning.
   D. Replace the antidepressant.
   E. All the mentioned options can be considered.

Patient 5: Questions 9, 10, and 11 refer to patient 5.
61-year-old woman with gait unsteadiness, double vision, and screaming/talking during sleep.

Case:

A 61-year-old woman noticed a slowly progressive double vision looking to the left side, then in all directions. At the same time, a gait unsteadiness and a slowness of the movement on the right side of the body with repeated falls appeared. A right-sided tremor and a feeling of stiffness in the neck and of discomfort in the right leg, as well as autonomic disturbances (excessive sweating, orthostatic hypotension, frequent and imperative micturition), were also progressively noticed. The neurological examination revealed an asymmetrical parkinsonism (right more than left) with a vertical gaze-evoked nystagmus. A brain MRI scan was unremarkable. The suspicion of a multiple-system atrophy of type P was raised. Her husband reported also episodes with talking and screaming

during sleep occurring almost every night for a few years, as well as frequent nightmares; however, no overt acting out of the dreams was observed. She denied excessive daytime sleepiness (Epworth sleepiness scale = 4), snoring, restless legs symptoms, hallucinations, sleep paralysis, cataplexy, and sleep walking. Sleep medication and alcohol consumption were denied.

Sleep studies:

Hypnogram (Figure 15-5):

Slightly prolonged sleep latency (32′); reduced sleep efficiency (83%) with 17% of time awake; normal REM-sleep latency (291′); distribution of sleep stages: NREM1 11%, NREM2 47%, NREM3 + NREM4 10%, REM sleep 15%; AHI 0/h, ODI 0/h; very high amount of periodic leg movements in sleep (PLMS index 113/h); pathological electroencephalogram (EEG) findings in sleep (slow background activity, reduced spindle activity) with excessive sleep fragmentation and reduced sleep efficiency; only partially preserved atonia with persistent PLMS during REM sleep; in the video registration, no abnormal movements in sleep, no inspiratory stridor.

MSLT:

Normal NREM1 mean sleep latency (20′); no SOREMPs.

9. Which diagnostic suspicion can be raised based on clinical picture and sleep examination?
   A. NREM-sleep parasomnia
   B. REM-sleep behavior disorder
   C. Restless legs syndrome
   D. Sleep-disordered breathing
   E. Nocturnal seizures (of frontal type)

10. Which conditions are typically associated with REM-sleep behavior disorder?
    A. Parkinson's disease
    B. Lewy body dementia
    C. Progressive supranuclear palsy
    D. Multiple system atrophy
    E. A, B, and D

11. Which treatment should be considered in this patient?
    A. L-dopa
    B. Dopaminergic agents
    C. Anticholinergic drugs
    D. Clonazepam
    E. Tricyclic antidepressants

Dementia

Patient 6: Questions 12 and 13 refer to patient 6.
59-year-old man with progressive mental deterioration and insomnia.

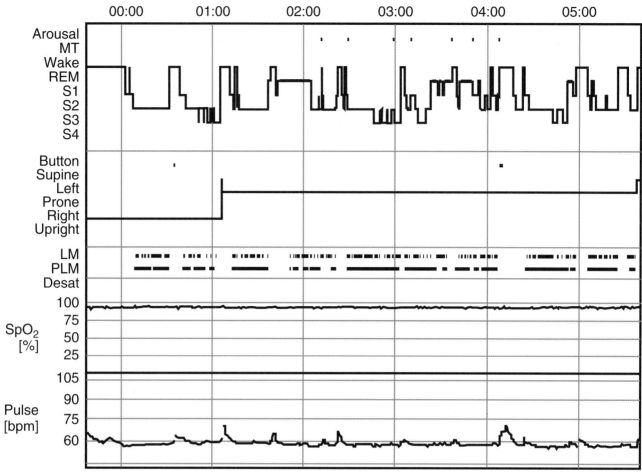

FIGURE 15-5 ■ Hypnogram of patient 5, showing a marked amount of periodic (PLM) and nonperiodic (LM) limb movements in sleep (PLMS index 113/h).

Case:

A 59-year-old man presented to our outpatient department because of a progressive deterioration of mental functions. The first symptoms were observed about 1 year previously, when he noticed difficulty remembering names of well-known persons, appointments, or dates. Performing the usual daily activities became then more and more difficult, and spatial orientation (e.g., driving) also became affected. Behavioral abnormalities with personality changes (loss of personal interests, impaired emotional swinging, and loss of distance in social contacts) were progressively observed. The patient also noticed difficulties in initiating and maintaining sleep, as well as fatigue and excessive daytime sleepiness (Epworth sleepiness scale = 15) with frequent naps during the day. In the last weeks before examination, gait unsteadiness with repeated falls and speech disorders were also reported.

The neuropsychological (impaired flexibility, conceptual thinking, impulse control, short-term memory, and inadequate social behavior) and the neurological (positive palmomental reflexes, paratonia of the limbs) findings suggested the clinical diagnosis of a frontotemporal dementia. Family history, however, was negative for dementia and other neurological disorders. MRI examination of the brain and EEG were unremarkable. Cerebrospinal fluid (CSF) examination revealed normal findings except for the presence of 14-3-3 protein.

Sleep studies:

First polysomnography (Figure 15-6A):

Prolonged sleep latency (74′) with one SOREMP markedly reduced sleep efficiency (39%) with 70% of time awake; altered sleep patterns with NREM1 16%, reduced NREM2 (6%), NREM3 + NREM4 4%, 12% "high-density" REM sleep; no sleep-disordered breathing (AHI 1/h); excessive phasic activity of the tibial muscle in REM sleep without videographic abnormalities, Broughton myoclonus in NREM sleep.

MSLT:

In three of four tests the patient did not fall asleep; in 1 test, NREM sleep latency 10′; no SOREMPs.

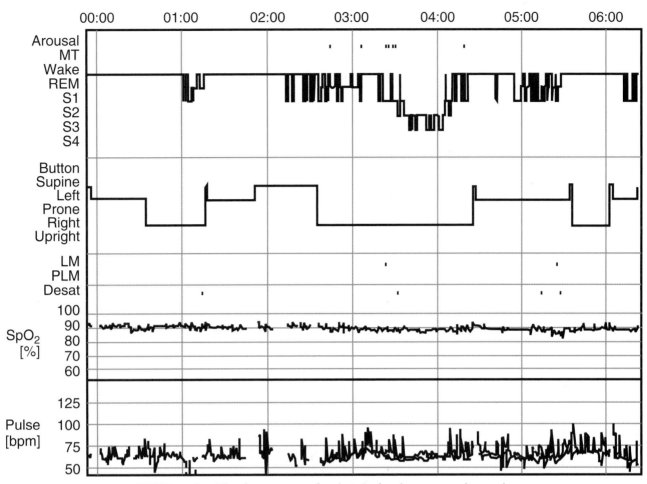

FIGURE 15-6A ■ First hypnogram of patient 6, showing a severe insomnia.

Second polysomnography, performed after 2 months (Figure 15-6B):

Prolonged sleep latency (135′) with one SOREMP, markedly reduced sleep efficiency (27%) with 73% of time awake; altered sleep patterns with NREM1 9%, reduced NREM2 (4%), NREM3 + NREM4 1.5%, 13% REM; in deep sleep stages, atypical "high frequent" beta-spindles were registered, K-complexes were present, and morphological unremarkable; REM atonia was preserved; no videographic abnormalities in NREM and REM sleep were observed.

12. Which further diagnostic procedure would you perform as the next step for this patient?
    A. Genetic analysis
    B. Maintenance of wakefulness test
    C. Video-EEG
    D. Actigraphy (Figure 15-6C)

13. Which factors may contribute to insomnia in patients with dementia?
    A. Lack of light exposure with repeated naps during the day
    B. Lack of physical activity during the day
    C. Nocturnal pain
    D. Inadequate medication
    E. All of the above

Patient 7: Question 14 refers to patient 7.

70-year-old man with mental deterioration and excessive sleep needs during the day.

Case:

A 70-year-old man was referred to our outpatient department because of increasing difficulty remembering names of persons and objects, beginning 4 years ago. He also noticed difficulties finding his way home or orientating himself in a nonfamiliar environment. His social life became more and more impaired, with increasing isolation. Changes in personality and behavior were also noticed, with irritability and fluctuations between excessive sadness and gladness. Furthermore, he complained about episodes occurring many times every day, characterized by dizziness followed by a compelling need to lie down and sleep for 30–60 minutes. No changes in blood pressure or heart rate were observed during these episodes. These

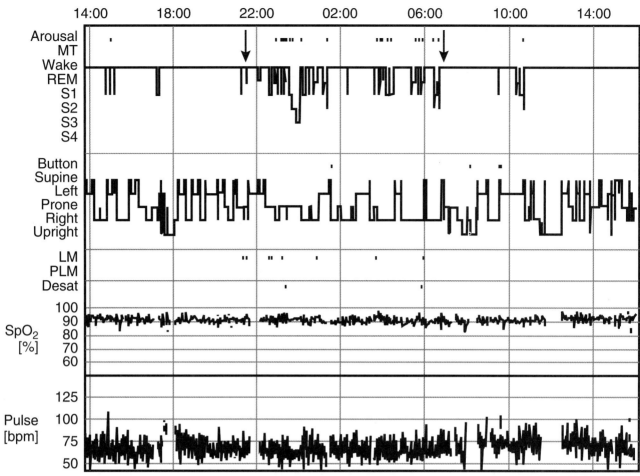

FIGURE 15-6B ■ Second hypnogram of patient 6 (2 months after the first), showing a worsening of insomnia. Arrows, administration of 1 tablet zopiclone 10 mg.

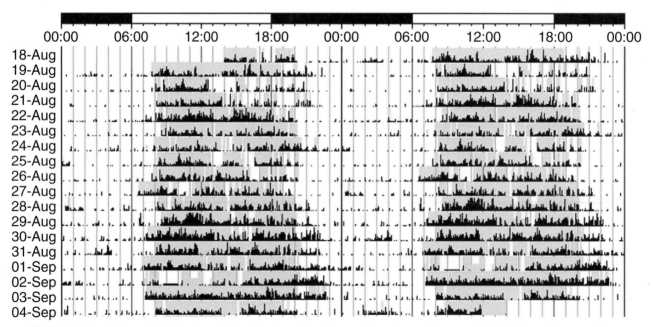

FIGURE 15-6C ■ Actigraphy of patient 6, showing irregular sleep-wake cycles and increased night sleep fragmentation.

phenomena are accompanied by a permanent feeling of fatigue and of increased sleep needs during the day. His wife observed repeated episodes with movements of the limbs and speaking during sleep. He denied snoring, hallucinations, restless legs symptoms, cataplexy, or sleep paralysis. Epworth sleepiness scale was 12.

Sleep studies:

Polysomnography (Figure 15-7A):

Normal sleep latency (10′) and sleep efficiency (90%) with 10% of time awake; reduced REM-sleep latency (41′); distribution of sleep stages: NREM1 7%, NREM2 57%, NREM3 + NREM4 12%, REM-sleep 10%; slight snoring, many apneic events almost exclusively of central type (AHI 59/h, OAI 0/h, CAI 53/h, ODI 49/h, CT90% 6′), associated with arousals (arousal index 22/h); slightly increased phasic activity of the limbs during REM sleep; no periodic limb movements in sleep (PLMS index 6/h).

MSLT:

Moderately reduced sleep (NREM1) latency (6); no SOREMPs.

Actigraphy (Figure 15-7B):

Stable rest/activity pattern with constant bedtimes; increased amount of time "asleep"/24 hours (50%, 9h25′) with reduced activity in the afternoon; normal rest/sleep efficiency (89%) and night phase fragmentation (index 31).

14. Which one of the following conditions is usually associated with severe excessive daytime sleepiness and excessive sleep needs?
    A. Chronic sleep deprivation
    B. Narcolepsy
    C. Sleep-disordered breathing
    D. REM-sleep behavior disorder
    E. Restless legs syndrome

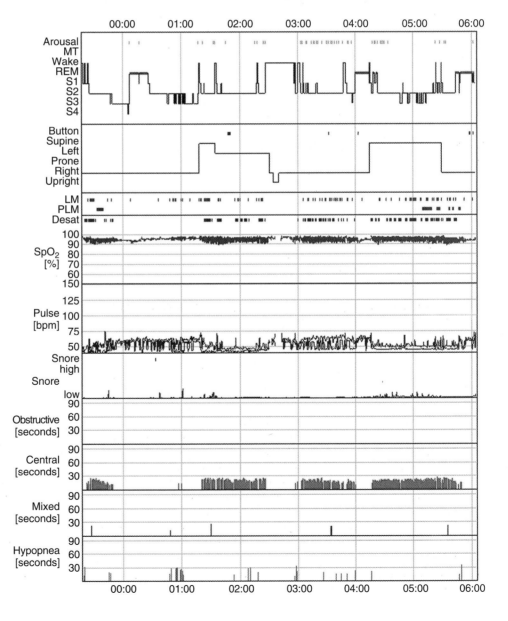

FIGURE 15-7A ■ Hypnogram of patient 7, showing a severe, mainly central sleep apnea (AHI 59/h).

Head trauma

Patient 8: questions 15 and 16 refer to patient 8

35-year-old man with excessive sleep needs after a bike accident.

Case:

A 35-year-old man was referred to our outpatient department because of excessive sleep needs. These symptoms appeared after a bike accident 1 year previously, which was associated with transient loss of consciousness and persisting retrograde and anterograde amnesia, but without further major neurological complications. Before the accident, medical history and sleep habits were unremarkable. Since the accident, he noticed a dramatic change of sleep habits: he fell asleep at 11 P.M. and awakened between 6:30 and 8:00 A.M. One time per week he slept until noon because he did not hear the alarm clock. If he did lie down in the afternoon, he fell asleep for 2–6 hours, sometimes sleeping until the next day. He denied excessive daytime sleepiness (Epworth sleepiness scale = 2), snoring, restless legs symptoms, sleep paralysis, hallucinations, and cataplexy. He also noticed some degree of difficulty in activation and concentration. He was no longer working since the accident. The neurological examination, as well as an MRI examination of the brain, were unremarkable.

Sleep studies:

Actigraphy, performed 1 year after head trauma (Figure 15-8):

Unstable rest/activity pattern with variable bedtimes and rest times (7–13.5 h, median 8.5 h). Increased amount of time "asleep"/24 hours (47%). Within 2 weeks, progressive delay of the sleep and awake time.

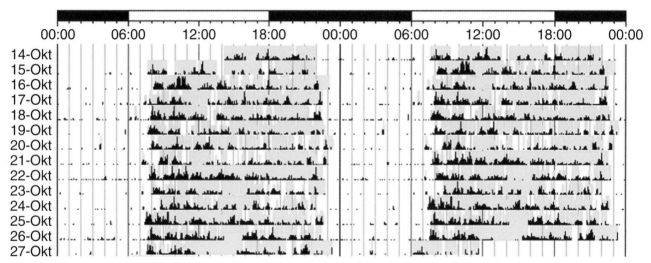

FIGURE 15-7B ■ Actigraphy of patient 7, showing increased rest/sleep needs and a slight night phase fragmentation.

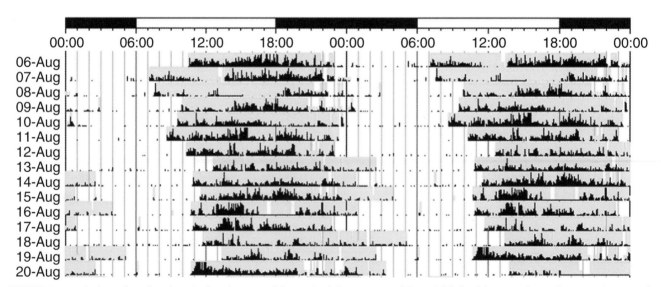

FIGURE 15-8 ■ Actigraphy of patient 8, showing unstable rest/activity pattern with variable bedtimes and rest times, an increased amount of time "asleep"/24 hours, increased rest/sleep needs, and progressive delay of the sleep and awakening time.

Polysomnography:

Short latency to NREM2 (13′) and to REM sleep (47′); normal sleep pattern; no sleep-disordered breathing (AHI 0/h); preserved REM atonia; normal videographic examination.

Hypocretin in the CSF: 456 pg/mL (within normal range).

15. Which of the following diagnoses should be considered according to medical history and sleep examinations?
   A. Chronic sleep deprivation
   B. Chronobiological disturbance
   C. Post-traumatic hypersomnia
   D. Idiopathic hypersomnia
   E. Combination of B and C

16. Which treatment would you consider in this patient?
   A. Methylphenidate
   B. Fluoxetine
   C. Modafinil
   D. Melatonin (in the evening)
   E. All of the above

Multiple sclerosis

Patient 9: Questions 17 and 18 refer to patient 9.
50-year-old woman with discomfort and burning sensation of the legs and feet and disturbed night sleep.
Case:

A 50-year-old woman was referred to our outpatient department because of a permanent discomfort of a burning and heat sensation in her feet and ankles for a few years. These complaints were not only more pronounced in the evening and during the night and were associated with repeated awakenings and disturbed night sleep, but were also constantly present during the day. While standing up and walking around she experienced a partial release of the discomfort. Many times per week she reported shock-like sensations in the feet, legs, and hips, which were sometimes triggered by movements and often associated with back pain. The clinical examination showed an afferent disorder of the right pupil, left foot extensor palsy, a reduction of the vibration sense in hands and feet, and an impaired stereognosis of the hands. The MRI examination of the brain revealed multiple T2-hyperintense periventricular lesions without enhancement. MRI of the cervical spine showed an intramedullary T2-hyperintensity at the level of the fourth cervical bone. Oligoclonal bands in CSF were positive. Visual evoked potentials were abnormal on the right side, showing a prolonged P100 latency. The diagnosis of multiple sclerosis was raised.

Sleep studies:
Polysomnography (Figure 15-9):

Normal sleep latency (13′); reduced sleep efficiency (69%) with 31% of time awake; slightly increased REM-sleep latency (100′); distribution of sleep stages: NREM1 7%, NREM2 51%, NREM3 + NREM4 5%, REM sleep 5%; AHI 0/h; preserved REM sleep atonia; slightly increased number of periodic limb movements in sleep (PLSM index 19/h), often without arousals (arousal index 6/h).

17. How common are difficulties initiating or maintaining sleep in patients with multiple sclerosis?
   A. Less than 10%
   B. 10–30%
   C. 30–50%
   D. More than 50%

18. Which of the following sentences about restless legs syndrome (RLS) in patients with multiple sclerosis (MS) is correct?
   A. RLS is the most common cause of insomnia in patients with MS.
   B. There is no association between severity of periodic limb movements in sleep (PLMS) and topography of the MS lesions.
   C. Incidence and prevalence of RLS and PLMS are higher in patients with MS than in the general population.
   D. Patients with MS usually do not respond to dopaminergic treatment for RLS.

Patient 10: Question 19 refers to patient 10.
65-year-old man with primary progressive multiple sclerosis and habitual nocturnal snoring.
Case:

A 65-year-old man with clinically definite primary progressive multiple sclerosis was referred to our inpatient ward because of a rapid progression of the neurological deficits and of functional disability. The clinical examination revealed severe paraparesis, cerebellar ataxia, reduction of proprioception and vibration sense of the limbs, and mild-moderate cognitive impairment. MRI examination of the brain revealed multiple, in parts confluent supratentorial and infratentorial T2-hyperintensities, mostly without gadolinium enhancement. MRI of the spine showed multiple T2-hyperintensities at level C4, Th7–Th9, and Th8–Th9. A treatment with mitoxantrone was started.

He also reported about habitual nocturnal snoring. His wife noticed many episodes with breathing pauses of which the patient was not aware. Excessive daytime sleepiness was denied (Epworth sleepiness scale = 1).

Sleep studies:
Respirography (Figure 15-10):

High amount of obstructive, mixed, and central sleep apneas (AHI 40/h), mainly in supine position, associated with pronounced oxygen desaturations

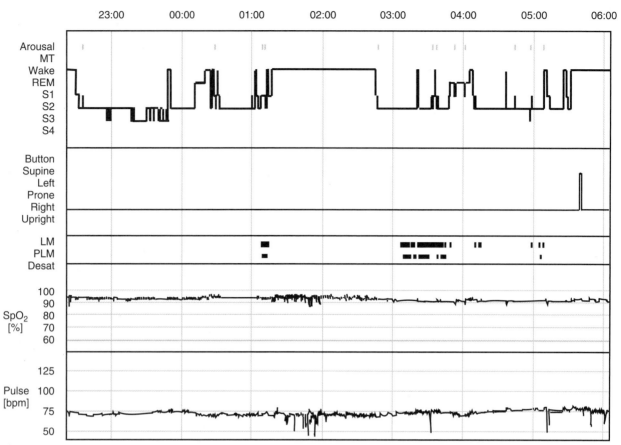

FIGURE 15-9 ■ Hypnogram of patient 9, showing insomnia with a slightly increased number of periodic limb movements (PLM) in sleep (PLMS index 19/h), often associated with arousals (arousal index 6/h).

(mean oxygen desaturations 90%, minimal oxygen desaturations 66%, ODI 35/h).

19. In which situation would you recommend CPAP for sleep apnea in this patient with advanced primary progressive multiple sclerosis?
   A. If snoring is very disturbing
   B. If the disability is progressing
   C. If a nocturnal dyspnea appears
   D. If the patient develops excessive daytime sleepiness or disabling fatigue
   E. None of the above

Encephalitis

Patient 11: Question 20 refers to patient 11.

70-year-old woman with rapidly progressive memory disturbance, increased sleep needs, and daytime sleepiness.

Case:

A 70-year-old woman was referred to our emergency unit because of a confusional state. Four months before referral, she had a short-lasting feeling of "alienation" in her own apartment. After 3 weeks she got lost trying to find her good friend's house. Two months before referral, she went on a journey. Thereafter, she was not able to remember the details of the trip, as well as the faces and names of the fellow passengers. A few days after her return, memory disturbances worsened, and she developed nausea and vomiting. A pronounced fatigue appeared, together with increased sleep needs (15–20 h/day) and excessive daytime sleepiness. Clinical examination revealed a striking deficit of anterograde recent memory with preserved attention (forward digit span 5/5). The mini mental examination was 27/30. MRI examination showed extensive T2-hyperintensities in both mesiotemporal regions, with involvement of the hippocampus, parahippocampal gyrus, and uncus (Figure 15-11A). CSF examination revealed a mononuclear pleocytosis (15 cells/μL) with slight protein elevation (0.63 g/L). Serological examination in serum and CSF was strongly positive for herpes simplex virus (HSV) type 1. The diagnosis of a herpetic encephalitis was raised. The patient denied snoring, nocturnal dyspnea, hallucinations, sleep paralysis, and cataplectic phenomena. Epworth sleepiness scale was 12.

Sleep studies:

First actigraphy (Figure 15-11B), *performed in the first week after hospitalization:*

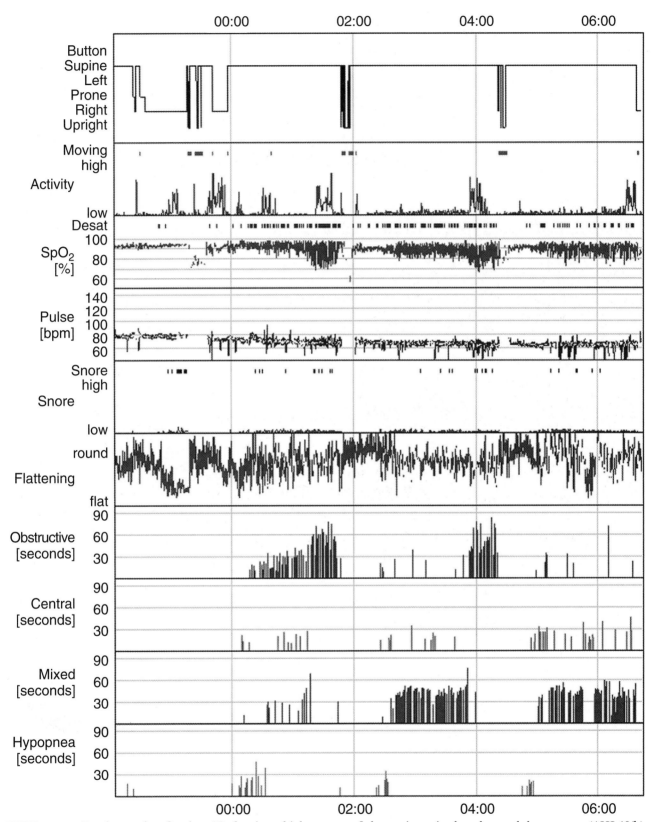

FIGURE 15-10 ■ Respirography of patient 10, showing a high amount of obstructive, mixed, and central sleep apneas (AHI 40/h), mainly in supine position, associated with severe oxygen desaturations (minimal oxygen saturation of 66%).

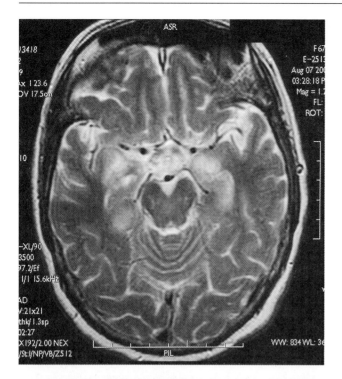

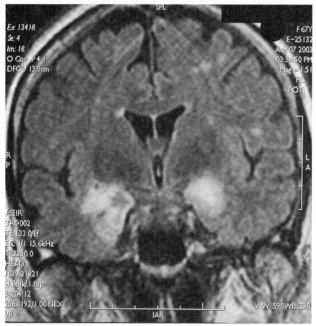

FIGURE 15-11A ■ Brain MRI examination (T2-weighted and FLAIR) performed on admission, 4 months after beginning of symptoms, showing T2-hyperintensities in both mesiotemporal regions, with involvement of the hippocampus, parahippocampal gyrus, and uncus. (Courtesy of the Institute of Neuroradiology, University Hospital, Zurich, Switzerland.)

Unstable rest/activity pattern with variable bedtimes and rest times. Increased amount of time "asleep"/24 h (49%) with repeated phases characterized by reduced activity during the day ("naps").

Second actigraphy, after 2 months (Figure 15-11C):

Unstable rest/activity pattern with variable bedtimes and rest times. Increased amount of time "asleep"/24 h (51%) with repeated phases characterized by reduced activity during the day. Compared with the previous examination, the findings are unchanged.

Third actigraphy, performed after 1 year (Figure 15-11D): Rather stable rest/activity pattern with regular bedtimes and rest times. Increased amount of time "asleep"/24 h (58%) with repeated phases characterized by reduced activity during the day (rest time during the day 5.5 h). Compared with the previous examination, there is overall worsening of the actigraphic findings.

20. Which of the following conditions may be associated with acute or subacute viral encephalopathy?
   A. Hypersomnia and excessive daytime sleepiness
   B. Transient sleep apnea
   C. Fatigue
   D. Fever and myalgias
   E. All of the above

Epilepsy

Patient 12: Question 21 refers to patient 12.
35-year-old man with refractory epilepsy and excessive daytime sleepiness.
Case:
A 35-year-old man with mental retardation was referred to our outpatient department because of refractory epilepsy with diurnal and nocturnal seizures. At the age of 7 years the patient was diagnosed with a hamartoma of the tuber cinereum. Radiation therapy and radical extirpation of the hamartoma were performed. The patient had experienced refractory generalized tonic-clonic and partial (gelastic) epileptic seizures occurring mostly on awakening, and only occasionally at night, since early childhood. The medical attendant and his parents also reported markedly increased sleep needs and excessive daytime sleepiness (Epworth sleepiness scale = 19) with repeated episodes of falling asleep during the day, as well as habitual snoring. He is on treatment with lamotrigine, clobazam, quetiapine, and thyroxine.

In the clinical examination, a pronounced obesity (109 kg; 161 cm; body –43.6 kg/m^2 mass index) was noted. Blood pressure was 120/80 mm Hg, pulse was 110/min. Neck circumference was 45 cm, a moderate narrowing of the oropharyngeal opening (Mallampati classification grade II) was found, and the palatine tonsils were moderately enlarged.
Sleep studies:
Respirography
Frequent obstructive sleep apneas, AHI 106/h; oxygen saturation <90% during ≥45% of recording time, in 16% of recording time <80%.

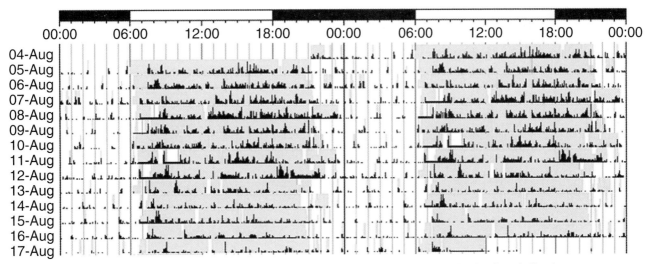

FIGURE 15-11B ■ First actigraphy of patient 11, performed in the first week after hospitalization.

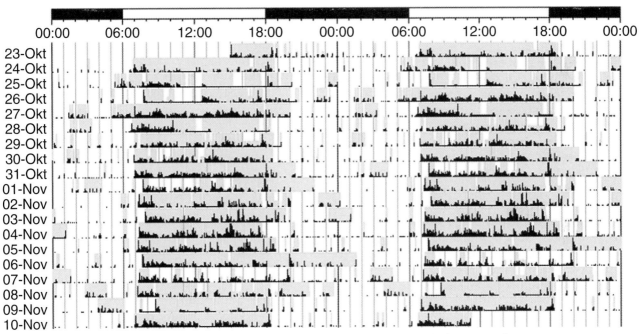

FIGURE 15-11C ■ Second actigraphy of patient 11, performed after 2 months.

21. Which statement about epilepsy and sleep apnea is correct according to the current literature data?
    A. Sleep apnea is much more frequently found in patients with epilepsy than in controls.
    B. Excessive daytime sleepiness is rare in patients with sleep apnea epilepsy.
    C. The appearance of sleep apnea symptoms in patients with epilepsy is associated with an increase in seizure frequency.
    D. Treatment with CPAP in patients with sleep apnea and epilepsy did not lead to a reduction of seizure frequency in treated patients.

Spinal cord diseases

Patient 13: Questions 22, 23, and 24 refer to patient 13. 70-year-old man with slowly progressive gait difficulties and jerks of the legs during sleep.

Case:

A 70-year-old man was referred to our outpatient clinics complaining about a slowly progressive feeling

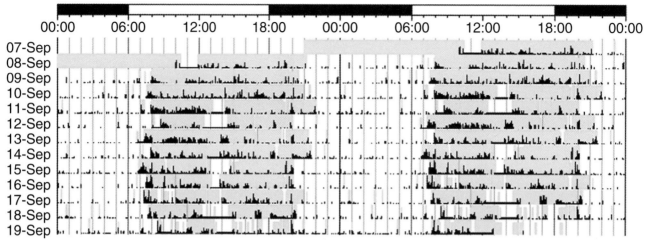

FIGURE 15-11D ■ Third actigraphy of patient 11, performed after 1 year.

of stiffness and traction in his legs that had been present for about 20 years. He noticed also increasing gait difficulties for 2 years with pain and cramps in the legs, leading to the permanent use of a walking stick during the past year. The pain and cramps were mainly present in the evening and night after going to bed and were accompanied by short jerks of the legs. Trying to alleviate the symptoms, the patient pressed and squeezed his legs, then stood up and walked around the bed. The use of clonazepam allowed him to reduce these complaints. The family history was unremarkable. The clinical examination showed a spastic paraparesis with increased tendon reflexes, Babinski signs bilaterally, and bilateral reduction of vibration sense. The examination of the cranial nerves and of the upper limbs was normal. MRI examination of the brain and spinal cord, CSF examination, and an extensive blood examination were unremarkable. The diagnosis of a sporadic spastic paraplegia was made. He denied habitual snoring, sleep paralysis, cataplectic phenomena, or excessive daytime sleepiness (Epworth sleepiness scale = 5).

Sleep studies:

Polysomnography (Figure 15-12):

Markedly prolonged sleep latency (121′), sleep episode started only after 10 mg zolpidem, normal REM-latency (81′); high sleep efficiency (98%); distribution of sleep stages: NREM1 9%, NREM2 53%, NREM3 + NREM4 14%, REM sleep 22%; AHI 0/h; preserved REM sleep atonia; markedly increased number of periodic limb movements while awake and during sleep (PLSM index 263/h), beginning in the distal muscles (M. tibialis anterior), then spreading to the proximal muscles (thigh, glutei, hips) but not, however, to the trunk or upper limbs, 3–7 seconds duration, occurring in intervals of 9–13 seconds, mainly not associated with arousals (arousal index 6/h);

the PLMS movements look Babinski-like, with dystonic and jerklike appearance.

22. Which of the following sentences about periodic limb movements in sleep (PLMS) is correct?
    A. PLMS are mostly (>95%) present in patients with clinically definite restless legs syndrome.
    B. PLMS also occur in a wide range of neurological and sleep disorders, including neurodegenerative diseases, spinal cord lesions, stroke, narcolepsy, REM-sleep behavior disorder, and obstructive sleep apnea.
    C. PLMS are absent in healthy subjects.
    D. PLMS are usually more pronounced in young than in older individuals.
    E. There is a good correlation between severity of PLMS and excessive daytime sleepiness in restless legs patients.

23. Which of the following diseases is usually *not* associated with secondary restless legs syndrome?
    A. Pregnancy
    B. Addison's disease
    C. Rheumatoid arthritis
    D. Charcot-Marie-Tooth disease type 2
    E. Spinocerebellar ataxia type 3

24. Which group of drugs may worsen restless legs syndrome and/or PLMS?
    A. Dopaminergic agents
    B. Opioids
    C. Anticonvulsants
    D. Antidepressants
    E. Benzodiazepines

Polyneuropathy/polyradiculopathy

Patient 14: Question 25 refers to patient 14.

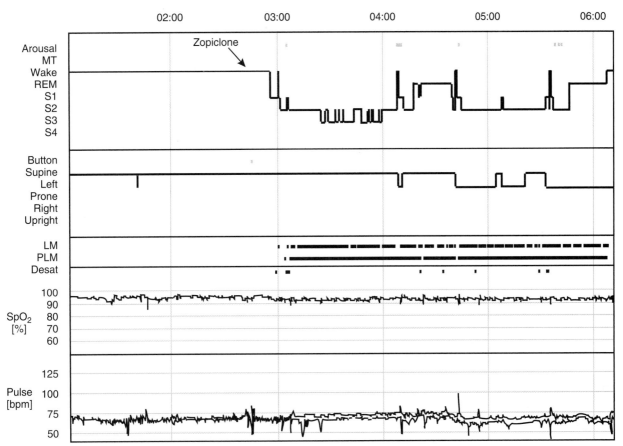

FIGURE 15-12 ■ Hypnogram of patient 12, showing a markedly increased number of periodic limb movements during sleep (PLMS index 263/h).

74-year-old man with acute tetraparesis and nocturnal apneas.

Case:

A 74-year-old man went to his physician because of strong pain in the right shoulder. After receiving an injection the pain partially subsided. After a few days, numbness in both hands/fingers and feet appeared. Within the next 3 to 4 days the numbness arose to the elbows and knees, and a weakness in both legs occurred, such that walking was possible only with two canes. His medical history was unremarkable, except for an allergy to penicillin. He particularly denied any history of infections or vaccinations in the past weeks, as well as blurred or double vision, hearing disturbances or vertigo, speech, swallowing, or micturition disturbances.

The clinical examination revealed a slight bilateral peripheral facial palsy, as well as sensory and motor (M4/M4+) deficits of the limbs and a generalized areflexia. CSF examination showed a slight increased protein (0.85 g/L). Glucose concentration and cell count were unremarkable. Electrodiagnostic examination showed a demyelinating neuropathy.

The diagnosis of an autoimmune acute inflammatory demyelinating polyneuropathy was raised, and a treatment with intravenous immunoglobulins was started.

Shortly after the patient was hospitalized, frequent episodes of breathing pauses (duration up to 45 seconds) were observed during the day and at night.

Sleep studies:

Respirography (Figure 15-13):

Oxygen saturation 96%; AHI 14/h, obstructive apnea index (AI) 1/h, central AI 6/h, mixed AI 8/h; duration of apneas up to 76 seconds; oxygen saturation <90% during 31 minutes (6%) of recording time.

25. Which of the following mechanisms may lead to a respiratory dysfunction in patients with acute polyradiculoneuritis?
    A. Diaphragmatic weakness
    B. Alveolar hypoventilation
    C. Obstructive apneas
    D. Microatelectasis with ventilation-perfusion mismatch
    E. All of the above

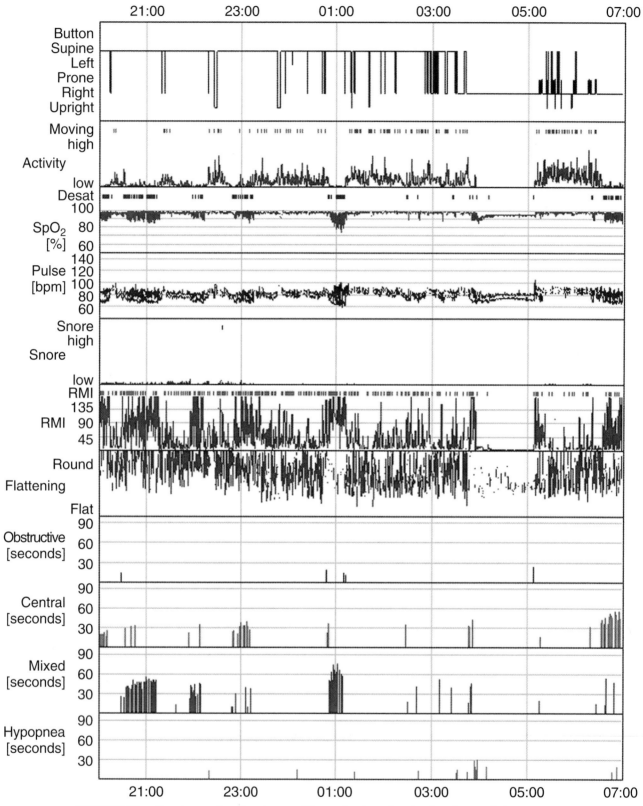

FIGURE 15-13 ■ Respirography, showing a mild, predominantly mixed and central sleep apnea.

Answers

1. D. Sleep apnea is common in acute ischemic stroke (50–70% of patients).

Sleep apnea (SA), defined as apnea-hypopnea index (AHI) ≥ 10, affects 9% of females and 24% of males aged 30 to 60 years and in 2% of women and 4% of men and is combined with excessive daytime sleepiness. In the last 15 years, sleep apnea has been recognized as an independent risk factor for cardiovascular morbidity and mortality and stroke. Compared with the general population, SA is very common (50–70%) in patients with transitory ischemic attack and acute stroke, and may affect the duration of hospitalization, stroke outcome, and mortality. No clear association between stroke type, topography, etiology, and severity of sleep apnea has been reported thus far. Furthermore, SA was shown to spontaneously improve after acute stroke, and an AHI ≥ 10 is still found in about 50% of patients.

Central sleep apnea (CSA) and central periodic breathing in sleep (CPBS) are common phenomena in acute stroke and are found in 10–30% of patients. Ischemic lesions affecting the medullary respiratory neurons or the cortical, corticobulbar, or corticospinal structures involved in breathing control, especially if bilateral and extensive, can be traditionally associated with CSA or Cheyne-Stokes respiration in wakefulness or during sleep. Conversely, CSA or Cheyne-Stokes respiration presenting exclusively during sleep can also be observed in patients with unilateral lesions of variable topography and without a disturbed level of consciousness or clinically overt heart failure. In subjects and patients without stroke, the presence of left ventricular systolic dysfunction has been shown to be a frequent predisposing factor to CPBS.

2. B. Continuous positive airway pressure (CPAP) treatment in acute stroke can be started in about 50% of patients with sleep-disordered breathing but can be maintained chronically in a minority of patients.

Few data exist about CPAP treatment during the acute stroke phase in patients with sleep apnea. Bassetti et al studied 152 patients with acute ischemic stroke and started a CPAP treatment acutely in patients with AHI ≥ 15 or AHI ≥ 10 and excessive daytime sleepiness. Initial AHI was shown to decreased in the subacute phase. CPAP was started in about 50% of SA patients and continued chronically in 15%. SA was associated with higher mortality after stroke (follow-up 60 $\pm$ 16 months); However, there were no differences between the patients receiving CPAP treatment and those receiving no treatment. Therefore CPAP treatment in the acute stroke setting remains a controversial issue, and further studies are needed to better define its potential benefits on stroke outcome and mortality.

CPAP treatment for central SA in patients with cardiac failure has been investigated in an extensive trial (CANPAP) by Bradley et al to assess the effect on survival rate in patients without heart transplantation. CPAP attenuated CSA, improved nocturnal oxygenation, increased the ejection fraction, lowered norepinephrine levels, and increased the distance walked in 6 minutes, but it did not affect survival. Results of this study suggest that CPAP does not improve mortality in patients who have CSA and heart failure.

3. A. The majority of stroke hypersomnias are due to a disruption of the ascending reticular activating system (ARAS) in terms of decreased arousal.

Hypersomnia, defined as excessive sleep needs and/or increased sleep propensity with excessive daytime sleepiness, is found in up to 40% of patients after ischemic stroke. The most likely underlying mechanism is a dysfunction of the ARAS in terms of a de-arousal. Bilateral ischemic stroke localized in the thalamus, subthalamic area, tegmental midbrain, and upper pons are traditionally associated with this type of hypersomnia. Smaller unilateral lesions in the mentioned areas, as well as cortical or deep hemispheric lesions with different topography, may also lead to the same condition, although they are usually less pronounced and/or transient. Occasionally, hypersomnia with clearly documented increased sleep needs has been described in patients with thalamic, hypothalamic, mesencephalic, and pontine strokes, sometimes with a narcolepsy-like phenotype. A reduced NREM and REM sleep is found in polysomnography.

4. B. Tegmentum pontis

Generalized atonia during REM sleep results from an active inhibition of motor activity by centers of the locus coeruleus region located in the tegmentum pontis on spinal motor neurons through the reticularis magnocellularis nucleus. Lesions in the area of the tegmentum pontis may therefore lead to REM sleep behavior disorder because of a loss of physiologic REM atonia. Other dreamlike or hallucinatory visual phenomena can be observed in patients with mesencephalic (peduncular hallucinosis), thalamic, or hemispheric strokes. Alteration of dreams with increased dreaming, recurrent nightmares, syndrome of dream-reality confusion, or decrease/cessation of dreams was reported in strokes of variable topography, including thalamic, frontal, temporal, parietal, or occipital lesions.

5. E. All of the above

Parkinson's disease is a common neurodegenerative disease, and sleep disorders are frequently associated with this condition. The most common complaints observed in these patients are excessive daytime sleepiness, insomnia, and parasomnia. Insomnia, defined as a perception of insufficient or poor-quality sleep, can become manifest as difficulty in initiating sleep (sleep, onset insomnia), difficulty in maintaining sleep (sleep maintenance insomnia), or early morning awakening.

There are multiple potential mechanisms leading to insomnia in patients with Parkinson's disease. Complaints related to impaired mobility and pain (e.g., rigidity with impairment in turning and getting off the bed, tremor, dystonic movements, painful cramps) are important factors. Associated sleep disorders (restless legs, periodic limb movements in sleep, REM sleep behavior disorder, obstructive and central sleep-disordered breathing, hallucinations, vivid dreams, and nightmares are frequently found), as well as a disease-related alteration of sleep patterns, may contribute to insomnia. Medical problems such as excessive nocturia, breathlessness, and excessive sweating should also be considered. Furthermore, cognitive impairment and associated psychiatric disorders (anxiety, depression) lead to agitation, nocturnal restlessness, confusion and frequent awakenings and wanderings (the so-called "sundowning" syndrome). Finally, various drugs, such as levodopa, dopaminergic agents, anticholinergics, and antidepressants, may detrimentally affect sleep quality in patients with Parkinson's disease.

6. D. Atypical antipsychotics (clozapine, quetiapine)

The treatment of insomnia in Parkinson's disease is a difficult issue. Benzodiazepines and hypnotics can lead to paradoxical reactions and habituation. Its use in the treatment of insomnia therefore should be evaluated carefully. These drugs, however, can be considered in young patients with Parkinson's disease. Conversely, these medications can be useful in treatment of anxiety, affective, or psychotic disorders in Parkinson's disease, and clonazepam is the medication of choice for the treatment of REM sleep behavior disorder, which is often associated with Parkinson's disease. Anticholinergic drugs are primarily used for the treatment of tremor in Parkinson's disease and may worsen cognitive functions and disrupt sleep. Many tricyclic antidepressants also have anticholinergic effect and are for the same reasons not recommended for the treatment of insomnia in patients with Parkinson's disease. Levodopa and dopaminergic agents were shown to promote arousals and to reduce slow wave and REM sleep and to be associated with excessive daytime sleepiness in patients with Parkinson's disease. These drugs are not used to treat insomnia unless the insomnia is due to uncontrolled nocturnal motor disturbances including PLMS in Parkinson's disease. Atypical antipsychotics, such as clozapine and quetiapine, improve behavior during night in patients with Parkinson's disease and are recommended in the treatment of insomnia in Parkinson's disease.

7. D. All of the above

Approaching a patient with excessive daytime sleepiness (EDS), a wide range of medical (heart, lung, kidney, liver, rheumatological, or endocrinological diseases), neurological, and psychiatric disorders, as well as side effects of medication, must be considered as possible underlying causes. In terms of sleep disorders leading to EDS, chronic sleep insufficiency, sleep-disordered breathing, restless legs syndrome/periodic limb movements in sleep, and narcolepsy must be considered in the differential diagnosis as main groups of diseases associated with this condition.

In patients with Parkinson's disease, EDS is more frequently found (15–50%) than in the general population, and the multiple causes of EDS often coexist in the same patient. Also, sleep disruption resulting from impaired mobility, pain, medical problems, cognitive impairment, associated psychiatric disorders, and altered biologic rhythms with nocturnal agitation and confusion have to be considered. REM-sleep behavior disorder should be taken into account as a further factor disrupting night sleep, which can rarely lead to pronounced daytime sleepiness.

Respiratory dysfunction in sleep is more common in patients with Parkinson's disease than in control subjects. Impairment of breathing control and of respiratory muscle function, as well as laryngeal spasms resulting from hypokinesia/akinesia and rigidity, are possible underlying mechanisms. Obstructive, central, and mixed apneas can be found in Parkinson's disease; their prevalence is poorly known.

Restless legs syndrome and periodic leg movements in sleep occur in Parkinson's disease more frequently than in the control population and are more often associated with off phases in patients with motor fluctuations.

In the past years, EDS and sleep attacks, as well as sleep attacks without EDS, have been reported in association with levodopa or dopaminergic medication.

8. E. All of the above

Because multiple factors may potentially contribute to EDS in this patient, all the options are valid and should be considered. Because the apneas are exclusively obstructive in this patient, CPAP treatment should be discussed. A certain degree of cooperation and of motor skills is necessary to consider this option. Amitriptyline can promote daytime sleepiness and worsen periodic limb movements in sleep and should be possibly replaced. Serotonin reuptake inhibitors and modafinil have been reported to be effective in the treatment of EDS in Parkinson's disease and should be considered as main treatment options. Finally, a reduction of ropinirole or levodopa should be considered.

9. B. REM-sleep behavior disorder

The medical history with episodes of talking and screaming during sleep occurring almost every night, because a few years in a patient with a clinical suspicion of multisystemic atrophy of type P strongly suggests a REM behavior disorder (RBD). The diagnostic hypothesis was supported by the presence of only partially preserved atonia with persistent periodic limb movements during sleep (PLMS) during REM sleep, although other motor phenomena could not be registered in the polysomnogram. The medical history and the polysomnographic findings did not show any evidence of a NREM-parasomnia or a sleep-disordered breathing.

Central, obstructive, or mixed apneas are a common finding in patients with multisystemic atrophy, as well as respiratory dysrhythmias with nocturnal (mostly inspiratory) stridor as highly characteristic findings.

Despite the patient not noticing any restless legs symptoms, we found a very high amount of periodic and non- PLMS. PLMS and limb movements in general have been reported to be a common finding in patients with multiple system atrophy.

Nocturnal seizures of frontal type must always be considered in the differential diagnosis of recurrent nocturnal motor phenomena. Medical history, as well as videographic and EEG findings, usually allows distinguishing this entity from RBD or NREM parasomnias.

10. E. A, B, and D (A. Parkinson's disease; B. Lewy-body dementia; D. multiple system atrophy).

REM sleep behavior disorder (RBD) is reported to have a prevalence of 0.5% in the general population. In extrapyramidal diseases, RBD is highly prevalent and reported in up to 50–70% of patients. In this group, RBD has been shown to be mostly associated with synucleinopathies such as Parkinson's disease, Lewy body disease, and multisystemic atrophy. RBD can often be the first sign of disease and may precede the extrapyramidal symptoms and signs by more than 10 years. This reflects the results of previous studies,

suggesting that brainstem structures are among the first affected in most of the extrapyramidal diseases. In contrast, RBDs are rarely only reported in tauopathies, such as progressive supranuclear palsy and corticobasal degeneration, although recent reports suggest higher prevalence of RBD and REM sleep without atonia in this disease group.

11. D. Clonazepam

The treatment of choice in patients with REM sleep behavior disorder is clonazepam. Clonazepam is effective in up to 90% of patients, and response to treatment is also high in terms of duration. Tolerance or abuse has been reported to be rare, even in patients treated for many years. The initial recommended dose is 0.5 mg at bedtime; the dose may be increased up to 1.0 mg. Most patients respond to treatment within a few days, and withdrawal of treatment is usually associated with a rebound. The mechanism of action of clonazepam is unknown, although stimulation of gamma-aminobutyric acidergic inhibition is presumed.

Melatonin, levodopa or pramipexole, carabamazepine, gabapentin, monoamine oxidase inhibitors, donepezil, and clonidine have also reported to be effective in single patients.

12. D. Actigraphy

Wrist actigraphy is a movement detector (accelerometer) recording of the activity of the arm/hand during the sleep and wake phase and represents a simple, cost-effective examination allowing the clinician to obtain information about sleep and behavior of the patient in his/her natural environment over a period of 24 hours during 2 weeks. The raw movement data are then processed by computer algorithms to obtain information about total sleep time, percentage of time spent asleep, total wake time, percentage of time spent awake, number of awakenings, time between awakenings, and sleep onset latency. The first model was developed in the 1970s by Kupfer and colleagues. This method was shown to have high reliability (80–90%) compared with polysomnography in the distinction of wake from sleep. Many studies have shown the validity of this method for evaluation of insomnia, circadian rhythm disorders, excessive sleepiness, and periodic limb movements during sleep, and for the study of sleep/wake rhythms in special populations such as children or patients with dementia.

Actigraphy (see Figure 15-6C) allowed our patient to better assess sleep/wake rhythms and to optimize treatment.

13. E. All of the above (lack of light exposure with repeated naps during the day; lack of physical

activity during the day; nocturnal pain; inadequate medication)

As with patients with Parkinson's disease, many factors may contribute to the development of insomnia in patients with neurodegenerative dementia. Basically, factors leading to insomnia in patients with dementia can be divided in (1) anatomical-functional (disease-related) and (2) environmental. Disruption of sleep-wake patterns with increased extent and frequency of wakefulness during the night and sleep/rest during the day (so-called "sundowning" phenomenon) can occur early in the course of the disease. Polysomnographically, an increase of stage 1 sleep and a reduced percentage of slow-wave sleep are common findings, whereas REM-sleep is usually not affected in early stages of the disease. In later stages, REM sleep may also become affected and usually reduced. An alteration of the neuronal network regulating sleep-wake rhythms was suggested as a possible underlying mechanism. Environmental factors, such as keeping patients in quiet and dark rooms during the day, repeated daytime naps, and lack of physical activity during the day, as well as other medical factors (e.g., pain, nycturia, anxiety, and inadequate medications), play also an important role in entertaining and aggravating insomnia in patients with dementia.

14. B. Narcolepsy

While investigating a patient with excessive daytime sleepiness (EDS), a wide differential diagnosis including medical, psychiatric, and neurological disorders, as well as side effects of medication, has to be taken into account. As already mentioned, chronic sleep insufficiency, sleep-disordered breathing, restless legs syndrome/PLMS, and narcolepsy are among the most important groups of sleep disorders leading to EDS. Whereas chronic sleep deprivation, sleep-disordered breathing, restless legs syndrome, and REM-sleep behavior disorder may be associated with various degrees of EDS, a certain number of patients in these groups of disorder does not complain about EDS. In contrast, pronounced EDS is a typical complaint in patients with narcolepsy, and Epworth sleepiness scales >14 are frequently found, with mean values of typically 17–20 minutes. MSLT typically shows a mean sleep latency <5 minutes in most (about 90%) patients with narcolepsy with cataplexy, with two or more sleep-onset REM periods (SOREMPs) and a mean latency to NREM of 2–3 minutes. Maintenance of wakefulness test typically shows a sleep latency <12 minutes (mean 5–7) and the presence of one or more SOREMPs.

15. E. Combination of B and C (B. delayed sleep phase syndrome; C. post-traumatic hypersomnia)

In this patient, excessive sleep needs newly appeared after a bike accident without other neurological sequelae. Based on the medical records and on the MRI examination, the patient had probably a mild traumatic brain injury. Sleep fragmentation and a decrease in sleep quality is a common finding that has been reported after mild traumatic brain injury.

Post-traumatic hypersomnia has been described in patients with severe brain injury involving components of the arousal system at a different level, but also in patients with mild head trauma not associated with loss of consciousness or with detectable cerebral lesions. Excessive sleep needs, excessive daytime sleepiness, disturbed and not restorative sleep, difficulties performing habitual tasks, inability to maintain work, headache (of tension type or migraine-like), poor concentration, deterioration in the quality of life, and depressive disorders are common complaints in this setting. Recently, decreased hypocretin-1 levels have been documented in patients with acute traumatic brain injury, reflecting a possible hypothalamic dysfunction as an underlying mechanism. In our patient, excessive sleep needs were not associated with excessive daytime sleepiness, and hypocretin-1 levels in CSF (determined, however, 1 year after accident) were within normal range. Also, we found in the actigraphy (see Figure 15-8) a shift of the sleep onset time suggesting a disturbance of the internal clock. Circadian rhythm disorders have been described following traumatic brain injury, mainly in patients with severe or extensive cerebral lesions. In our patient, brain trauma was mild, and other factors such as alteration of day structure may play a role contributing to the manifestation of delayed sleep phase after brain injury.

16. E. All the mentioned treatment options can theoretically be considered (methylphenidate; fluoxetine; modafinil; melatonin in the evening).

Regarding the treatment of this condition, all mentioned medications can be considered. Methylphenidate and modafinil have been reported to be effective in the treatment of hypersomnia after traumatic brain injury. Fluoxetine may also be considered, especially if depressed mood or apathy are present. Administration of exogenous melatonin at 10 P.M. combined with morning bright light (chronotherapy) has shown to be effective in treatment of chronobiological disturbance and might be considered in this patient.

17. C. 30–50%

Compared with the general population, sleep-related complains are frequently found in patients with multiple sclerosis (MS). In one study performed by Tachibana et al, 11 of 28 patients with MS (40%) had difficulties initiating or maintaining sleep. In a larger study published by Alarcia et al, 36 of 100 patients (36%) reported sleep disorders in any form. An association between sleep disorders and disease activity and severity, respectively, has been reported. As in our patients, the most frequently reported causes for insomnia in MS are restless legs syndrome (RLS) and PLMS pain related to spinal cord lesions, spasticity and muscle spasms, nycturia, psychiatric disorders including depression, and effect of medication (especially steroids). Polysomnographic studies show a significantly reduced sleep efficiency and increased arousals during sleep.

18. C. Incidence and prevalence of restless legs syndrome (RLS) and periodic limb movements during sleep (PLMS) are higher in patients with MS than in the general population.

Although an accurate estimation of the frequency of RLS in patients with MS is not available, prevalence is reported to be higher than in the general population. In a polysomnographic study, Ferini-Strambi et al reported an incidence of PLMS of 36%, higher than in the general population. Moreover, MRI suggested an association between lesions in the infratentorial region and PLMS in the same study. However, RLS and PLMS are probably not the most frequent cause of insomnia in patients with MS, as nocturia or urinary incontinence, pain, and depression are much more frequently found than the first condition. The treatment of choice includes dopaminergic agents and anticonvulsants.

19. D. If the patient develops excessive daytime sleepiness or disabling fatigue

Obstructive sleep apnea, central sleep apnea, paroxysmal hyperventilation, hypoventilation, respiratory muscle weakness, and respiratory arrest have been previously reported in patients with MS, particularly in association with brainstem inflammatory lesions affecting respiratory control. Nevertheless, the incidence of obstructive sleep apnea in patients with MS does not seem to be higher than in the general population.

In our patient, initiation and CPAP treatment at home may be linked with practical difficulties owing to the severe motor disability and the cognitive impairment. Because of this reason, CPAP would be considered in cases of severe excessive daytime sleepiness or disabling fatigue, after having excluded other possible concomitant factors leading to the same symptoms. Nocturnal dyspnea in patients with MS is usually due to different causes but rarely to sleep apnea alone. Potential underlying etiologies (e.g., respiratory muscle weakness, cardiac diseases,

anxiety) must be investigated before considering CPAP treatment. Considering the clinical situation and the fact that the patient does not complain about any symptoms, we did not recommend CPAP treatment in this case.

20. E. All of the above (hypersomnia and excessive daytime sleepiness; transient sleep apnea; fatigue; fever and myalgias)

This patient complains about excessive sleep needs (hypersomnia) and excessive daytime sleepiness, which appeared in the course of acute herpetic encephalitis and still persisted relatively unchanged 1 year after infection. This condition has rarely been reported in the literature.

Acute or subacute viral infections (typically mononucleosis, pneumonia), as well as viral encephalitis, are reported to be associated with chronic fatigue, excessive daytime sleepiness, and hypersomnia. Fever, myalgias, headache, cognitive disorders, focal neurological symptoms and signs, poor mood, and anxiety were observed as accompanying symptoms. Severe hypersomnia was the main feature of the encephalitis lethargica occurring in the 1920s. Transient obstructive sleep apnea and episodes of tachybradycardia with asystole have been described in association with viral encephalopathy.

21. C. The appearance of sleep apnea symptoms in patients with epilepsy is associated with an increase in seizure frequency.

Despite a striking association between epilepsy and sleep, few publications exist at the present time about the relationships between epilepsy and sleep apnea (SA), as well as its extent, nature, and clinical relevance. This issue was addressed by Hollinger et al, who studied characteristics of epilepsy, sleep history, presence of excessive daytime sleepiness, and polysomnographic findings in 29 patients with epilepsy and obstructive SA. 52% of the patients had excessive daytime sleepiness. In 21 of 29 patients, the appearance of SA symptoms coincided with a clear increase in seizure frequency or with the first appearance of status epilepticus. Treatment with CPAP was continued for a longer time in 12 patients and was associated with a significant reduction of both excessive daytime sleepiness (Epworth sleepiness scale) and seizure frequency in 4 patients. In another study performed by Khatami et al, with 100 consecutive patients with epilepsy and 90 control subjects, frequency of sleep apnea was not significantly higher in patients with epilepsy compared with controls, and a history of habitual snoring predicted the presence of excessive daytime sleepiness. These data corroborate the importance of considering and investigating obstructive sleep apnea in patients with epilepsy, especially in the presence of poor seizure control or by reappearance of seizures after a seizure-free interval.

22. B. Periodic limb movements during sleep (PLMS) also occur in a wide range of neurological and sleep disorders, including neurodegenerative diseases, spinal cord lesions, stroke, narcolepsy, REM-sleep behavior disorder, and obstructive sleep apnea.

PLMS are a supportive criterion for the diagnosis of restless legs syndrome (RLS) in addition to the presence of a response to dopaminergic treatment and to a positive family history for RLS. They are defined as a sequence of at least four muscle contractions usually localized in the feet, ankles, or legs lasting 0.5–5 seconds, recurring at intervals of 5–90 seconds, and being at least 25% of the amplitude of the voluntary leg movements the patient is asked to do for calibration before the start of a sleep study. PLMS are found in about 80% of patients with a clinically defined RLS. PLMS are not specific for the RLS condition and can be found in other disorders including neurodegenerative diseases, spinal cord lesions, stroke, narcolepsy, REM-sleep behavior disorder, obstructive sleep apnea, insomnia, hypersomnia, and medication with antidepressant or neuroleptic drugs, as well as in asymptomatic individuals. The amount of PLMS tends to increase with age, and its frequency is higher in older individuals, with more than 50% of individuals having PLMS. Furthermore, correlation between PLMS and severity of RLS symptoms or excessive daytime sleepiness is weak.

23. B. Addison's disease

Among the potential causes of secondary RLS, iron deficiency, end-stage renal disease, and pregnancy are common and clearly established. In patients with iron deficiency, including anemia and blood donation, RLS and PLMS are frequently found. Serum and CSF levels of ferritin were shown to be lower, and CSF transferrin levels were higher in patients than in control subjects, and a defect of iron metabolism and iron regulatory proteins is postulated. In patients with end-stage renal disease requiring hemodialysis, the prevalence of RLS is reported to be 30–60%; of PLMS, about 70%; and RLS and PLMS are associated with higher morbidity and mortality. In pregnancy, RLS was documented in about 23% of women. RLS has been reported also in association with peripheral polyneuropathy, especially small fibers polyneuropathy, Charcot-Marie-Tooth disease type 2, and cryoglobulinemic neuropathy.

Spinocerebellar ataxia type 3, rheumatoid arthritis, low back pain, myelopathy, radiculopathy, stenosis of the spinal canal, and fibromyalgia have been reported to be associated with RLS.

24. D. Antidepressants

Dopaminergic agents, such as pramipexole, ropinirole, pergolide, and cabergoline, are at the present time first-choice medications in the treatment of RLS. Because the occurrence of valvular heart disease with pergolide treatment has recently been reported, benefits and potential risks to treatment should be evaluated individually. Second-choice drugs are opioids, anticonvulsants, and benzodiazepines. Tricyclic antidepressants and serotonine/noradrenaline reuptake inhibitors are reported to worsen RLS and PLMS. Their use may be considered in patients with RLS and concomitant depression.

25. E. All of the above (diaphragmatic weakness; alveolar hypoventilation; obstructive apneas; microatelectasis with ventilation-perfusion mismatch)

Respiratory failure is a common and a substantial complication in patients with acute polyradiculoneuritis (Guillain-Barré syndrome [GBS]) and should be identified early to prevent major problems. Early manifestations of impending respiratory failure detectable at bedside are as reported by Rabinstein et al: the inability to pronounce long sentences without taking a breath (the so-called staccato speech), activation of accessory muscles during inspiration, tachypnea, paradoxical breathing, and symptoms/signs of hyperactivity of the sympathetic nervous system (tachycardia, profuse sweating). Rapid disease progression, bilateral facial weakness, signs of bulbar dysfunction, signs of autonomic failure, as well as a reduction of vital capacity of more than 30% or below 20 mL/kg, predict progression of respiratory failure.

Various and distinct mechanisms may contribute to the occurrence of respiratory dysfunction and insufficiency in GBS. Weakness of diaphragm and other respiratory muscles, alveolar hypoventilation, and microatelectasis with secondary ventilation-perfusion mismatch, as well as decreased tonus of oropharyngeal muscles together with muscle weakness, were all described as possible underlying mechanisms that can lead to episodes of obstructive apnea. The occurrence of central apneas in our patient remains unexplained. A latent cardiac abnormality in this case should be considered as a possible explanation for this phenomenon.

REFERENCES

Stroke

1. Bassetti C, Aldrich MS, Chervin RD, Quint D: Sleep apnea in patients with transient ischemic attack and stroke: a prospective study of 59 patients. Neurology 47:1167–1173, 1996.
2. Bassetti C, Aldrich MS, Quint D: Sleep-disordered breathing in patients with acute supra- and infratentorial strokes. A prospective study of 39 patients. Stroke 28:1765–1772, 1997.
3. Bassetti C, Aldrich MS: Sleep apnea in acute cerebrovascular diseases: final report on 128 patients. Sleep 22:217–223, 1999.
4. Bassetti C, Mathis J, Gugger M, et al: Hypersomnia following paramedian thalamic stroke: a report of 12 patients. Ann Neurol 39:471–480, 1996.
5. Bassetti CL, Milanova M, Gugger M: Sleep disordered breathing and acute stroke: diagnosis, risk factors, treatment, evolution and outcome. Stroke 37(4):967–972, 2006.
6. Bassetti C, Valko P: Poststroke hypersomnia. Sleep Med Clin 1:139–155, 2006.
7. Bischof M, Bassetti CL: Total dream loss: a distinct neuropsychological dysfunction after bilateral PCA stroke. Ann Neurol 56:583–586, 2004.
8. Bradley TD, Logan AG, Kimoff RJ, et al: Continuous positive airway pressure for central sleep apnea and heart failure. N Engl J Med 353:2025–2033, 2005.
9. Castaigne P, Escourolle R: [Topographical study of anatomical lesions in hypersomnias.]. Rev Neurol (Paris) 116:547–584, 1967.
10. Dyken ME, Somers VK, Yamada T, et al: Investigating the relationship between stroke and obstructive sleep apnea. Stroke 27:401–407, 1996.
11. Geller TJ, Bellur SN: Peduncular hallucinosis: magnetic resonance imaging confirmation of mesencephalic infarction during life. Ann Neurol 21:602–604, 1987.
12. Harbison J, Ford GA, James OFW, Gibson GJ: Sleep-disordered breathing following acute stroke. QJM 95:741–747, 2002.
13. Hui DSC, Choy DKL, Wong LKS, et al: Prevalence of sleep-disordered breathing and continuous positive airway pressure compliance: results in Chinese patients with first-ever ischemic stroke. Chest 122:852–860, 2002.
14. Hung J, Whitford EG, Parsons RW, Hillman DR: Association of sleep apnoea with myocardial infarction in men. Lancet 336:261–264, 1990.
15. Iranzo A, Santamaria J, Berenguer J, et al: Prevalence and clinical importance of sleep apnea in the first night after cerebral infarction. Neurology 58:911–916, 2002.
16. Javaheri S, Parker TJ, Wexler L, et al: Occult sleep-disordered breathing in stable congestive heart failure. Ann Intern Med 122:487–492, 1995.
17. Kimura K, Tachibana N, Kohyama J, et al: A discrete pontine ischemic lesion could cause REM sleep behavior disorder. Neurology 55:894–895, 2000.
18. Kumral E, Ozturk O: Delusional state following acute stroke. Neurology 62:110–113, 2004.
19. Lee MC, Klassen AC, Resch JA: Respiratory pattern disturbances in ischemic cerebral vascular disease. Stroke 5:612–616, 1974.
20. Leung RST, Bradley DT: Sleep apnea and cardiovascular disease. Am J Respir Crit Care Med 164:2147–2165, 2001.
21. Mahowald MW, Schenk CH: REM sleep parasomnias. In Kryger MH, Roth T, Dement WC (eds): *Principles and Practice of Sleep Medicine*, 4th ed. Philadelphia, Elsevier, 2005.
22. Nachtmann A, Siebler M, Rose G, et al: Cheyne-Stokes respiration in ischemic stroke. Neurology 45:820–821, 1995.
23. Nieto FJ, Young TB, Lind BK, et al: Association of sleep-disordered breathing, sleep apnea, and hypertension in a large community-based study. Sleep Heart Health Study. JAMA 283:1829–1836, 2000.
24. Parra O, Arboix A, Bechich S, et al: Time course of sleep-related breathing disorders in first-ever stroke or transient ischemic attack. Am J Respir Crit Care Med 161:375–380, 2000.
25. Parra O, Arboix A, Montserrat JM, et al: Sleep-related breathing disorders: impact on mortality of cerebrovascular disease. Eur Respir J 24:267–272, 2004.
26. Partinen M, Jamieson A, Guilleminault C: Long-term outcome for obstructive sleep apnea syndrome patients. Mortality. Chest 94:1200–1204, 1988.
27. Passouant P, Cadilhac J, Baldy-Moulinier M: [Physiopathology of hypersomnias]. Rev Neurol (Paris) 116:585–629, 1967.
28. Scammell TE, Nishino S, Mignot E, Saper CB: Narcolepsy and low CSF orexin (hypocretin) concentration after a diencephalic stroke. Neurology 56:1751–1753, 2001.
29. Sin DD, Fitzgerald F, Parker JD, et al: Risk factors for central and obstructive sleep apnea in 450 men and women with congestive heart failure. Am J Respir Crit Care Med 160:1101–1106, 1999.
30. Turkington PM, Allgar V, Bamford J, et al: Effect of upper airway obstruction in acute stroke on functional outcome at 6 months. Thorax 59:367–371, 2004.
31. Turkington PM, Bamford J, Wanklyn P, Elliott MW: Prevalence and predictors of upper airway obstruction in the first 24 hours after acute stroke. Stroke 33:2037–2042, 2002.
32. Vock J, Achermann P, Bischof M, et al: Evolution of sleep and sleep EEG after hemispheric stroke. J Sleep Res 11:331–338, 2002.
33. Wessendorf TE, Teschler H, Wang YM, et al: Sleep-disordered breathing among patients with first-ever stroke. J Neurol 247:41–47, 2000.
34. Yaggi HK, Concato J, Kernan WN, et al: Obstructive sleep apnea as a risk factor for stroke and death. N Engl J Med 353:2034–2041, 2005.
35. Young T, Palta M, Dempsey J, et al: The occurrence of sleep-disordered breathing among middle-aged adults. N Engl J Med 328:1230–1235, 1993.
36. Young T, Peppard P, Palta M, et al: Population-based study of sleep-disordered breathing as a risk factor for hypertension. Arch Intern Med 157:1746–1752, 1997.

Extrapyramidal Diseases

37. Adler CH, Caviness JN, Hentz JG, et al: Randomized trial of modafinil for treating subjective daytime sleepiness in patients with Parkinson's disease. Mov Disord 18:287–293, 2003.

38. Adler CH: Nonmotor complications in Parkinson's disease. Mov Disord 20(Suppl 11):S23–S29, 2005.

39. Arnulf I, Konofal E, Merino-Andreu M, et al: Parkinson's disease and sleepiness: an integral part of PD. Neurology 58:1019–1024, 2002.

40. Arnulf I, Merino-Andreu M, Bloch F, et al: REM sleep behavior disorder and REM sleep without atonia in patients with progressive supranuclear palsy. Sleep 28:349–354, 2005.

41. Bamford CR: Carbamazepine in REM sleep behavior disorder. Sleep 16:33, 1993.

42. Bannister R, Gibson W, Michaels L, Oppenheimer DR: Laryngeal abductor paralysis in multiple system atrophy. A report on three necropsied cases, with observations on the laryngeal muscles and the nuclei ambigui. Brain 104:351–368, 1981.

43. Bhatt MH, Podder N, Chokroverty S: Sleep and neurodegenerative disease. Semin Neurol 25(1):39–51, 2005.

44. Boeve BF, Silber MH, Ferman TJ, et al: Association of REM sleep behavior disorder and neurodegenerative disease may reflect an underlying synucleinopathy. Mov Disord 16:622–630, 2001.

45. Boeve BF, Silber MH, Ferman TJ: Melatonin for treatment of REM sleep behavior disorder in neurologic disorders: results in 14 patients. Sleep Med 4:281–284, 2003.

46. Boeve BF, Silber MH, Parisi JE, et al: Synucleinopathy pathology and REM sleep behavior disorder plus dementia or parkinsonism. Neurology 61:40–45, 2003.

47. Braak H, Braak E: Pathoanatomy of Parkinson's disease. J Neurol 247(Suppl 2):II3–II10, 2000.

48. Braak H, Rub U, Sandmann-Keil D, et al: Parkinson's disease: affection of brain stem nuclei controlling premotor and motor neurons of the somatomotor system. Acta Neuropathol (Berl) 99:489–495, 2000.

49. Brotini S, Gigli GL: Epidemiology and clinical features of sleep disorders in extrapyramidal disease. Sleep Medicine 5:169–179, 2004.

50. Chadwick D, Hallett M, Harris R, et al: Clinical, biochemical, and physiological features distinguishing myoclonus responsive to 5–hydroxytryptophan, tryptophan with a monoamine oxidase inhibitor, and clonazepam. Brain 100:455–487, 1977.

51. Chokroverty S: Sleep and degenerative neurologic disorders. Neurol Clin 14:807–826, 1996.

52. Comella CL, Nardine TM, Diederich NJ, Stebbins GT: Sleep-related violence, injury, and REM sleep behavior disorder in Parkinson's disease. Neurology 51:526–529, 1998.

53. Cummings JL: Depression and Parkinson's disease: a review. Am J Psychiatry 149:443–454, 1992.

54. Factor SA, McAlarney T, Sanchez-Ramos JR, Weiner WJ: Sleep disorders and sleep effect in Parkinson's disease. Mov Disord 5:280–285, 1990.

55. Fantini ML, Gagnon JF, Filipini D, Montplaisir J: The effects of pramipexole in REM sleep behavior disorder. Neurology 61:1418–1420, 2003.

56. Ferini-Strambi L, Zucconi M: REM sleep behavior disorder. Clin Neurophysiol 111(Suppl 2):S136–S140, 2000.

57. Fernandez HH: Quetiapine for l-dopa-induced psychosis in PD. Neurology 55:899, 2000.

58. Frucht S, Rogers JD, Greene PE, et al: Falling asleep at the wheel: motor vehicle mishaps in persons taking pramipexole and ropinirole. Neurology 52:1908–1910, 1999.

59. Frucht SJ, Greene PE, Fahn S: Sleep episodes in Parkinson's disease: a wake-up call. Mov Disord 15:601–603, 2000.

60. Ghorayeb I, Yekhlef F, Chrysostome V, et al: Sleep disorders and their determinants in multiple system atrophy. J Neurol Neurosurg Psychiatry 72:798–800, 2002.

61. Green RA, Gillin JC, Wyatt RJ: The inhibitory effect of intraventricular administration of serotonin on spontaneous motor activity of rats. Psychopharmacology (Berl) 51:81–84, 1976.

62. Hogl B, Saletu M, Brandauer E, et al: Modafinil for the treatment of daytime sleepiness in Parkinson's disease: a double-blind, randomized, crossover, placebo-controlled polygraphic trial. Sleep 25:905–909, 2002.

63. Hollister AS, Breese GR, Kuhn CM, et al: An inhibitory role for brain serotonin-containing systems in the locomotor effects of d-amphetamine. J Pharmacol Exp Ther 198:12–22, 1976.

64. Kumar S, Bhatia M, Behari M: Sleep disorders in Parkinson's disease. Mov Disord 17:775–781, 2002.

65. Kunz D, Bes F: Exogenous melatonin in periodic limb movement disorder: an open clinical trial and a hypothesis. Sleep 24:183–187, 2001.

66. Larsen JP, Tandberg E: Sleep disorders in patients with Parkinson's disease: epidemiology and management. CNS Drugs 15:267–275, 2001.

67. Lesser RP, Fahn S, Snider SR, et al: Analysis of the clinical problems in parkinsonism and the complications of long-term levodopa therapy. Neurology 29:1253–1260, 1979.

68. Mahowald MW, Bornemann MC, Schenck CH: Parasomnias. Semin Neurol 24(3):283–292, 2004.

69. Menza MA, Rosen RC: Sleep in Parkinson's disease. The role of depression and anxiety. Psychosomatics 36:262–266, 1995.

70. Montplaisir J, Petit D, Decary A, et al: Sleep and quantitative EEG in patients with progressive supranuclear palsy. Neurology 49:999–1003, 1997.

71. Ohayon MM, Caulet M, Priest RG: Violent behavior during sleep. J Clin Psychiatry 58:369–376, 1997; quiz 377.

72. Ondo WG, Dat Vuong K, Khan H, et al: Daytime sleepiness and other sleep disorders in Parkinson's disease. Neurology 57:1392–1396, 2001.

73. Partinen M: Sleep disorder related to Parkinson's disease. J Neurol 244:S3–S6, 1997.

74. Paus S, Brecht HM, Koster J, et al: Sleep attacks, daytime sleepiness, and dopamine agonists in Parkinson's disease. Mov Disord 18:659–667, 2003.

75. Plazzi G, Corsini R, Provini F, et al: REM sleep behavior disorders in multiple system atrophy. Neurology 48:1094–1097, 1997.

76. Ringman JM, Simmons JH: Treatment of REM sleep behavior disorder with donepezil: a report of three cases. Neurology 55:870–871, 2000.

77. Sitaram N, Moore AM, Gillin JC: Experimental acceleration and slowing of REM sleep ultradian rhythm by cholinergic agonist and antagonist. Nature 274:490–492, 1978.

78. Starkstein SE, Preziosi TJ, Robinson RG: Sleep disorders, pain, and depression in Parkinson's disease. Eur Neurol 31:352–355, 1991.

79. Stiasny-Kolster K, Doerr Y, Moller JC, et al: Combination of 'idiopathic' REM sleep behaviour disorder and olfactory dysfunction as possible indicator for alpha-synucleinopathy demonstrated by dopamine transporter FP-CIT-SPECT. Brain 128:126–137, 2005.

80. Sweet RD, McDowell FH: Five years' treatment of Parkinson's disease with levodopa. Therapeutic results and survival of 100 patients. Ann Intern Med 83:456–463, 1975.

81. Takeuchi N, Uchimura N, Hashizume Y, et al: Melatonin therapy for REM sleep behavior disorder. Psychiatry Clin Neurosci 55:267–269, 2001.

82. Tan A, Salgado M, Fahn S: Rapid eye movement sleep behavior disorder preceding Parkinson's disease with therapeutic response to levodopa. Mov Disord 11:214–216, 1996.

83. Vetrugno R, Provini F, Cortelli P, et al: Sleep disorders in multiple system atrophy: a correlative video-polysomnographic study. Sleep Med 5:21–30, 2004.

84. Zucconi M, Ferini-Strambi L: NREM parasomnias: arousal disorders and differentiation from nocturnal frontal lobe epilepsy. Clin Neurophysiol 111(Suppl 2): S129–S135, 2000.

Dementia

85. Aldrich MS, Chervin RD, Malow BA: Value of the multiple sleep latency test (MSLT) for the diagnosis of narcolepsy. Sleep 20:620–629, 1997.

86. Ancoli-Israel S, Cole R, Alessi C, et al: The role of actigraphy in the study of sleep and circadian rhythms. Sleep 26:342–392, 2003.

87. Ancoli-Israel S, Martin JL, Kripke DF, et al: Effect of light treatment on sleep and circadian rhythms in demented nursing home patients. J Am Geriatr Soc 50:282–289, 2002.

88. Baumann CR, Dauvilliers Y, Mignot E, Bassetti CL: Normal CSF hypocretin-1 (orexin A) levels in dementia with Lewy bodies associated with excessive daytime sleepiness. Eur Neurol 52(2):73–76, 2004.

89. Bhatt MH, Podder N, Chokroverty S: Sleep and neurodegenerative disease. Semin Neurol 25(1):39–51, 2005.

90. Carskadon MA, Acebo C, Richardson GS, et al: An approach to studying circadian rhythms of adolescent humans. J Biol Rhythms 12:278–289, 1997.

91. Cole RJ, Kripke DF, Gruen W, et al: Automatic sleep/wake identification from wrist activity. Sleep 15:461–469, 1992.

92. Furuta H, Kaneda R, Kosaka K, et al: Epworth Sleepiness Scale and sleep studies in patients with obstructive sleep apnea syndrome. Psychiatry Clin Neurosci 53:301–302, 1999.

93. Gigli GL, Adorati M, Dolso P, et al: Restless legs syndrome in end-stage renal disease. Sleep Med 5:309–315, 2004.

94. Guilleminault C, Partinen M, Quera-Salva MA, et al: Determinants of daytime sleepiness in obstructive sleep apnea. Chest 94:32–37, 1988.

95. Haba-Rubio J, Janssens JP, Rochat T, Sforza E: Rapid eye movement-related disordered breathing: clinical and polysomnographic features. Chest 128:3350–3357, 2005.

96. Harper DG, Stopa EG, McKee AC, et al: Differential circadian rhythm disturbances in men with Alzheimer disease and frontotemporal degeneration. Arch Gen Psychiatry 58:353–360, 2001.

97. Johns MW: Sensitivity and specificity of the multiple sleep latency test (MSLT), the maintenance of wakefulness test and the Epworth Sleepiness Scale: failure of the MSLT as a gold standard. J Sleep Res 9:5–11, 2000.

98. Kupfer DJ, Weiss BL, Foster G, et al: Psychomotor activity in affective states. Arch Gen Psychiatry 30:765–768, 1974.

99. Lavie P, Tzischinsky O, Epstein R, Zomer J: Sleep-wake cycle in shift workers on a "clockwise" and "counterclockwise" rotation system. Isr J Med Sci 28:636–644, 1992.

100. Lopes LA, Lins Cde M, Adeodato VG, et al: Restless legs syndrome and quality of sleep in type 2 diabetes. Diabetes Care 28:2633–2636, 2005.

101. Martin J, Marler M, Shochat T, Ancoli-Israel S: Circadian rhythms of agitation in institutionalized patients with Alzheimer's disease. Chronobiol Int 17:405–418, 2000.

102. McPartland RJ, Foster FG, Kupfer DJ, Weiss BL: Activity sensors for use in psychiatric evaluation. IEEE Trans Biomed Eng 23:175–178, 1976.

103. Mitler MM, Walsleben J, Sangal RB, Hirshkowitz M: Sleep latency on the maintenance of wakefulness test (MWT) for 530 patients with narcolepsy while free of psychoactive drugs. Electroencephalogr Clin Neurophysiol 107:33–38, 1998.

104. Moe KE, Vitiello MV, Larsen LH, Prinz PN: Symposium: Cognitive processes and sleep disturbances: sleep/wake patterns in Alzheimer's disease: relationships with cognition and function. J Sleep Res 4:15–20, 1995.

105. Motohashi Y, Maeda A, Wakamatsu H, et al: Circadian rhythm abnormalities of wrist activity of institutionalized dependent elderly persons with dementia. J Gerontol A Biol Sci Med Sci 55:M740–M743, 2000.

106. Petit D, Montplaisir J, Boeve BF: Alzheimer's disease and other dementias. In Kryger MH, Roth T, Dement WC (eds): *Principles and Practice of Sleep Medicine*, 4th ed. Philadelphia, Elsevier, 2005.

107. Prinz PN, Vitaliano PP, Vitiello MV, et al: Sleep, EEG and mental function changes in senile dementia of the Alzheimer's type. Neurobiol Aging 3:361–370, 1982.

108. Reynolds CF III, Kupfer DJ, Taska LS, et al: EEG sleep in elderly depressed, demented, and healthy subjects. Biol Psychiatry 20:431–442, 1985.

109. Sforza E, Johannes M, Claudio B: The PAM-RL ambulatory device for detection of periodic leg movements: a validation study. Sleep Med 6:407–413, 2005.

110. Sforza E, Zamagni M, Petiav C, Krieger J: Actigraphy and leg movements during sleep: a validation study. J Clin Neurophysiol 16:154–160, 1999.

111. Skomro RP, Ludwig S, Salamon E, Kryger MH: Sleep complaints and restless legs syndrome in adult type 2 diabetics. Sleep Med 2:417–422, 2001.

112. Sturzenegger C, Bassetti CL: The clinical spectrum of narcolepsy with cataplexy: a reappraisal. J Sleep Res 13:395–406, 2004.

Head Trauma

113. Alster J, Pratt H, Feinsod M: Density spectral array, evoked potentials, and temperature rhythms in the evaluation and prognosis of the comatose patient. Brain Inj 7:191–208, 1993.

114. Baumann CR, Bassetti CL: Hypocretins (orexins) and sleep-wake disorders. Lancet Neurol 4:673–682, 2005.

115. Baumann CR, Stocker R, Imhof HG, et al: Hypocretin-1 (orexin A) deficiency in acute traumatic brain injury. Neurology 65:147–149, 2005.

116. Billiard M, Negre C, Besset A, et al: [Sleep organization by subjects in chronical post-traumatic inconscience (author's transl)]. Rev Electroencephalogr Neurophysiol Clin 9:171–178, 1979.

117. Challman TD, Lipsky JJ: Methylphenidate: its pharmacology and uses. Mayo Clin Proc 75:711–721, 2000.

118. Dahlitz M, Alvarez B, Vignau J, et al: Delayed sleep phase syndrome response to melatonin. Lancet 337:1121–1124, 1991.

119. Francisco GE, Ivanhoe CB: Successful treatment of post-traumatic narcolepsy with methylphenidate: a case report. Am J Phys Med Rehabil 75:63–65, 1996.

120. Guilleminault C, Faull KF, Miles L, van den Hoed J: Posttraumatic excessive daytime sleepiness: a review of 20 patients. Neurology 33:1584–1589, 1983.

121. Levin HS, Mattis S, Ruff RM, et al: Neurobehavioral outcome following minor head injury: a three-center study. J Neurosurg 66:234–243, 1987.

122. Mundey K, Benloucif S, Harsanyi K, et al: Phase-dependent treatment of delayed sleep phase syndrome with melatonin. Sleep 28:1271–1278, 2005.

123. Song C, Phillips AG, Leonard BE, Horrobin DF: Ethyl-eicosapentaenoic acid ingestion prevents corticosterone-mediated memory impairment induced by central administration of interleukin-1beta in rats. Mol Psychiatry 9:630–638, 2004.

124. Teitelman E: Off-label uses of modafinil. Am J Psychiatry 158:1341, 2001.

Multiple Sclerosis

125. Alarcia R, Ara JR, Martin J, et al: [Sleep disorders in multiple sclerosis]. Neurologia 19:704–709, 2004.

126. Amarenco G, Kerdraon J, Denys P: [Bladder and sphincter disorders in multiple sclerosis. Clinical, urodynamic and neurophysiological study of 225 cases]. Rev Neurol (Paris) 151:722–730, 1995.

127. Auer RN, Rowlands CG, Perry SF, Remmers JE: Multiple sclerosis with medullary plaques and fatal sleep apnea (Ondine's curse). Clin Neuropathol 15:101–105, 1996.

128. Ferini-Strambi L, Filippi M, Martinelli V, et al: Nocturnal sleep study in multiple sclerosis: correlations with clinical and brain magnetic resonance imaging findings. J Neurol Sci 125:194–197, 1994.

129. Fleming WE, Pollak CP: Sleep disorders in multiple sclerosis. Semin Neurol 25:64–68, 2005.

130. Howard RS, Wiles CM, Hirsch NP, et al: Respiratory involvement in multiple sclerosis. Brain 115(Pt 2):479–494, 1992.

131. Montplaisir J, Boucher S, Poirier G, et al: Clinical, polysomnographic, and genetic characteristics of restless legs syndrome: a study of 133 patients diagnosed with new standard criteria. Mov Disord 12:61–65, 1997.

132. Rae-Grant AD, Eckert NJ, Bartz S, Reed JF: Sensory symptoms of multiple sclerosis: a hidden reservoir of morbidity. Mult Scler 5:179–183, 1999.

133. Sadovnick AD, Remick RA, Allen J, et al: Depression and multiple sclerosis. Neurology 46:628–632, 1996.

134. Tachibana N, Howard RS, Hirsch NP, et al: Sleep problems in multiple sclerosis. Eur Neurol 34:320–323, 1994.

See also reference 42 above.

Encephalitis

135. Culebras A: Other neurological disorders. In Kryger MH, Roth T, Dement WC (eds): *Principles and Practice of Sleep Medicine*, 4th ed. Philadelphia, Elsevier, 2005.

136. Dyken ME, Yamada T, Berger HA: Transient obstructive sleep apnea and asystole in association with presumed viral encephalopathy. Neurology 60:1692–1694, 2003.

137. Guilleminault C, Mondini S: Mononucleosis and chronic daytime sleepiness. A long-term follow-up study. Arch Intern Med 146:1333–1335, 1986.

138. Howard RS, Lees AJ: Encephalitis lethargica. A report of four recent cases. Brain 110(Pt 1):19–33, 1987.

139. Merriam AE: Kleine-Levin syndrome following acute viral encephalitis. Biol Psychiatry 21:1301–1304, 1986.

Epilepsy

140. Devinsky O, Ehrenberg B, Barthlen GM, et al: Epilepsy and sleep apnea syndrome. Neurology 44:2060–2064, 1994.

141. Hollinger P, Khatami R, Gugger M, et al: Epilepsy and obstructive sleep apnea. Eur Neurol 55:74–79, 2006.

142. Khatami R, Zutter D, Siegel A, et al: Sleep-wake habits and disorders in a series of 100 adult epilepsy patients: a prospective study. Seizure 15:299–306, 2006.

143. Malow BA, Levy K, Maturen K, Bowes R: Obstructive sleep apnea is common in medically refractory epilepsy patients. Neurology 55:1002–1007, 2000.

144. Manni R, Terzaghi M, Arbasino C, et al: Obstructive sleep apnea in a clinical series of adult epilepsy patients: frequency and features of the comorbidity. Epilepsia 44:836–840, 2003.

Spinal Cord Diseases

145. Agargun MY, Kara H, Ozbek H, et al: Restless legs syndrome induced by mirtazapine. J Clin Psychiatry 63:1179, 2002.

146. Allen RP, Picchietti D, Hening WA, et al: Restless legs syndrome: diagnostic criteria, special considerations, and epidemiology. A report from the restless legs syndrome diagnosis and epidemiology workshop at the National Institutes of Health. Sleep Med 4:101–119, 2003.

147. Bastuji H, Garcia-Larrea L: Sleep/wake abnormalities in patients with periodic leg movements during sleep: factor analysis on data from 24-h ambulatory polygraphy. J Sleep Res 8:217–223, 1999.

148. Connor JR, Wang XS, Patton SM, et al: Decreased transferrin receptor expression by neuromelanin cells in restless legs syndrome. Neurology 62:1563–1567, 2004.

149. Earley CJ, Connor JR, Beard JL, et al: Abnormalities in CSF concentrations of ferritin and transferrin in restless legs syndrome. Neurology 54:1698–1700, 2000.

150. Haba-Rubio J, Staner L, Krieger J, Macher JP: What is the clinical significance of periodic limb movements during sleep? Neurophysiol Clin 34:293–300, 2004.

151. Hogl B, Poewe W: Restless legs syndrome. Curr Opin Neurol 18:405–410, 2005.

152. Hui DS, Wong TY, Ko FW, et al: Prevalence of sleep disturbances in Chinese patients with end-stage renal failure on continuous ambulatory peritoneal dialysis. Am J Kidney Dis 36:783–788, 2000.

153. Lesage S, Hening WA: The restless legs syndrome and periodic limb movement disorder: a review of management. Semin Neurol 24:249–259, 2004.

154. Mizuno S, Mihara T, Miyaoka T, et al: CSF iron, ferritin and transferrin levels in restless legs syndrome. J Sleep Res 14:43–47, 2005.

155. Montplaisir J, Allen RP, Walters AS, et al: Restless legs syndrome and periodic limb movements during sleep. In Kryger MH, Roth T, Dement WC (eds): *Principles and Practice of Sleep Medicine*, 4th ed. Philadelphia, Saunders, 2005, pp 839–852.

156. Nicolas A, Lesperance P, Montplaisir J: Is excessive daytime sleepiness with periodic leg movements during sleep a specific diagnostic category? Eur Neurol 40:22–26, 1998.

157. Polydefkis M, Allen RP, Hauer P, et al: Subclinical sensory neuropathy in late-onset restless legs syndrome. Neurology 55:1115–1121, 2000.

158. Rascol O, Pathak A, Bagheri H, Montastruc JL: Dopaminagonists and fibrotic valvular heart disease: further considerations. Mov Disord 19:1524–1525, 2004.

159. Rascol O, Pathak A, Bagheri H, Montastruc JL: New concerns about old drugs: valvular heart disease on ergot derivative dopamine agonists as an exemplary situation of pharmacovigilance. Mov Disord 19:611–613, 2004.

160. Rijsman RM, de Weerd AW, Stam CJ, et al: Periodic limb movement disorder and restless legs syndrome in dialysis patients. Nephrology (Carlton) 9:353–361, 2004.

161. Sanz-Fuentenebro FJ, Huidobro A, Tejadas-Rivas A: Restless legs syndrome and paroxetine. Acta Psychiatr Scand 94:482–484, 1996.

162. Suzuki K, Ohida T, Sone T, et al: The prevalence of restless legs syndrome among pregnant women in Japan and the relationship between restless legs syndrome and sleep problems. Sleep 26:673–677, 2003.

163. Trenkwalder C, Paulus W, Walters AS: The restless legs syndrome. Lancet Neurol 4:465–475, 2005.

164. Walters AS: Toward a better definition of the restless legs syndrome. The International Restless Legs Syndrome Study Group. Mov Disord 10:634–642, 1995.

165. Wilson S, Argyropoulos S: Antidepressants and sleep: a qualitative review of the literature. Drugs 65:927–947, 2005.

Polyneuropathy/Radiculopathy

166. Chokroverty S: Sleep-disordered breathing in neuromuscular disorders: a condition in search of recognition. Muscle Nerve 24:451–455, 2001.

167. Lawn ND, Fletcher DD, Henderson RD, et al: Anticipating mechanical ventilation in Guillain-Barré syndrome. Arch Neurol 58:893–898, 2001.

168. Rabinstein AA, Wijdicks EF: Warning signs of imminent respiratory failure in neurological patients. Semin Neurol 23:97–104, 2003.

169. Ropper AH, Kehne SM: Guillain-Barré syndrome: management of respiratory failure. Neurology 35:1662–1665, 1985.

170. Ferini-Strambi L, Filippi M, Martinelli V, et al: Nocturnal sleep study in multiple sclerosis: correlations with clinical and brain magnetic resonance imaging findings. J Neurol Sci 125(2):194–197, 1994.

171. Rae-Grant AD, Eckert NJ, Bartz S, et al: Sensory symptoms of multiple sclerosis: a hidden reservoir of morbidity. Mult Scler 5(3):179–183, 1999.

Sleep-Wake Disorders

BARUCH EL-AD

Questions

Questions 1–3: A 23-year-old student complains about insomnia and excessive daytime sleepiness that interfere with his daytime activities. The symptoms had begun when he was about 17 years old. He would go to bed at about 11 P.M. and lie awake for about 2 hours until he fell asleep. In the morning he had to wake up at about 7:30 A.M. to be on time for school; he frequently slept in until 9 A.M. and was often late for his classes. After graduation he took a night job as a bartender, three times per week, working from 8 P.M. until 3 A.M. He found out that "wearing himself out" this way assisted him in falling asleep easier. Today, as a student, he avoids taking morning courses for fear of not showing up for them. He is physically healthy. He consulted a psychologist for his sleep problems, was diagnosed with mild anxiety, and was advised to try relaxation techniques before sleep. This treatment did not help. The patient is unwilling to take any pills or medications.

1. Which of the following is the most likely diagnosis?
   A. Adjustment insomnia
   B. Delayed sleep phase disorder (DSPD)
   C. Insomnia associated with mental disorder
   D. Long sleeper
   E. Shift work disorder

2. Employment of which of the following aids to confirm the clinical diagnosis is most appropriate?
   A. History alone
   B. Multiple sleep latency test (MSLT)
   C. Polysomnography
   D. Sleep log and actigraphy
   E. Psychiatric assessment

3. Which of the following is your single best advice to this specific patient?
   A. Avoid shift work.
   B. Continue psychological therapy.
   C. Avoid stimulating activities in the evening.
   D. Curtail your time in bed.
   E. Be exposed to bright light on awakening.

Questions 4–5: A 68-year-old patient complains about difficulties staying awake for her favorite evening TV show, which is broadcast at 9 P.M. During the last few years she has become increasingly sleepy from 7 P.M. onward. She usually goes to bed at about 10 P.M. and wakes up at 4 A.M. The patient's husband describes embarrassing situations in which she dozes off during evening social events. The patient tried to engage in stimulating evening activities to delay going to bed early but would still get up at 5 A.M. and have difficulties reinitiating her sleep. She sought psychiatric help for frustration and depression resulting from her propensity to feel sleepy during the early evening and reduced social activity. She was also concerned that her symptoms represented an early sign of dementia, as her father, who died of dementia, had the same sleep pattern before developing cognitive decline. The patient occasionally snores, but otherwise her airway and neurological examinations are normal.

4. What is the most likely diagnosis?
   A. Early morning awakening as part of major depression
   B. Advanced sleep phase disorder
   C. Changes in sleep pattern owing to normal aging
   D. Sleep apnea with ensuing sleepiness in passive circumstances
   E. Irregular sleep-wake rhythm

5. Which of the following treatments has the greatest chance of improving this patient's sleep problem?
   A. Antidepressants
   B. Bright light therapy
   C. Melatonin
   D. Hypnotics
   E. Stimulants

Questions 6–8: A 35-year-old female patient complains of chronic insomnia. She works as a freelance columnist for an Internet magazine. She is usually unable to fall asleep at night, so she works until she feels tired, which can happen at any time during day or night. She sleeps for a few hours in a row, then wakes up and stays awake until she feels sleepy again. Her sleep during the day consists of two to three sleep sessions of 2–3 hours each. The patient is otherwise physically healthy, is single, and leads a secluded life with few social contacts. The main conduit of interpersonal interaction is through the Internet. She suspects that her present sleep schedule may prevent her from leading a more active social life, but she is unable to change her schedule independently. She is therefore presenting for consultation.

6. Which of the following is the most plausible diagnosis in this case?
   A. Inadequate sleep hygiene
   B. Irregular sleep-wake rhythm
   C. Insomnia resulting from mental disorder
   D. Shift work disorder
   E. Psychophysiological insomnia

7. Which of the following investigations should be carried out first to diagnose the condition?
   A. Psychiatric assessment
   B. Polysomnography
   C. Actigraphy and sleep log
   D. 24-hour fractional salivary melatonin excretion measurement
   E. Brain imaging

8. The initial management of this patient would consist of which of the following measures?
   A. Antidepressants
   B. Hypnotics
   C. Improvement of sleep hygiene and melatonin
   D. Psychotherapy

Questions 9–10: A 49-year-old male patient seeks advice for insomnia that started 2 days ago. On the day the insomnia began, he arrived from Santiago, Chile (altitude 600 meters, local time Greenwich Mean Time [GMT] − 4:00), to New York City (altitude 1 meter, local time GMT − 5:00) after an 11-hour night flight with a 2-hour layover. The purpose of his visit is an important presentation to be given in 3 days. The patient is afraid his insomnia will interfere with the presentation. He has never suffered from insomnia before, except during jet lag.

9. Which of the following diagnoses is the most probable in this case?
   A. Adjustment insomnia
   B. Altitude insomnia
   C. Jet lag
   D. Insomnia resulting from mental disorder

10. Which of the following treatments best suits this patient needs?

A. Hypnotic
B. Melatonin
C. Reassurance
D. Sedative antidepressant

Questions 11–13: A 67-year-old blind patient seeks help for her chronic sleep problem. Her right eye was enucleated in childhood after an accident. She suffered from longstanding glaucoma in her left eye, which eventually rendered her totally blind 7 years ago. She suffers from periodic nocturnal insomnia accompanied by excessive daytime sleepiness. Alternatively, she may have a few weeks of nearly normal night sleep. The sleep disturbance has been present for about 4 years. The patient is hypertensive and diabetic and is treated with enalapril and metformin.

11. What is the most plausible explanation for the fact that this patient had retained a normal sleep pattern until 4 years ago, despite being blind?
   A. Because entrainment continues for several years after light cues disappear.
   B. Because she may have retained circadian photoreception independent of visual photoreception.
   C. Because she entrained to social environmental stimuli.
   D. Because her sleep disorder is unrelated to her blindness.

12. What will be the *initial* step in evaluating this patient's sleep disorder, if history seems insufficient?
   A. 2-night polysomnography
   B. Long-term actigraphy and sleep log
   C. 24-hour fractional salivary melatonin excretion measurement
   D. Electroretinography
   E. Polysomnography followed by MSLT

13. What will be the first-line treatment in this case?
   A. Hypnotics
   B. Melatonin
   C. Sedative antidepressants
   D. Cognitive-behavioral therapy
   E. Bright light therapy

14. A 65-year-old businessman travels from London, United Kingdom (local time GMT) to Sydney, Australia (local time GMT + 10:00) aboard an eastward flight and plans to stay for 1 month. Which statement best describes the expected adaptation of this individual to the new circadian timing?
   A. Full adaptation process is expected to last between 1 and 2 weeks.
   B. After eastward flights, adaptation process is usually orthodromic (advancing).

C. Adaptation is not assisted by melatonin after eastward flights.

D. Hypnotics used during the flight may prevent circadian adaptation.

15. A 74-year-old male patient is brought in by a family member. The patient was diagnosed with Alzheimer's disease 4 years previously. The family caregiver complains about the patient's disruptive sleep habits. He frequently dozes off during the daytime and is unwilling to go for a walk, saying that he is "too tired." However, he is frequently agitated and restless in the evening when put to bed. At nights, he frequently wanders about the house, turns on the lights, and interferes with others' sleep. The patient leads a sedentary life and has limited social interactions. His social contacts are limited to family members. The patient is treated for dementia with rivastigmine (centrally-acting cholinesterase inhibitor, Exelon) and memantine (N-methyl-D-aspartate antagonist, Namenda). His general practitioner prescribed eszopiclone for insomnia, which caused further agitation at night and sedation in the morning. A trial of quetiapine (atypical antipsychotic, Seroquel) reduced evening agitation but did not improve sleep. What is the potential *primary* pathophysiology of this patient's sleep disruption?
A. Insufficient social interaction
B. Medication side effects
C. Degeneration of the suprachiasmatic nuclei and their connections
D. Insufficient exposure to bright daylight
E. Inadequate sleep hygiene

16. A 21-year-old patient with delayed sleep phase disorder is treated daily with 5 mg immediate-release melatonin at 8 P.M. Before treatment, her usual bedtime and wake-up time were 3 A.M. and 11 A.M., respectively. With treatment, these times have advanced to 11 P.M. and 7 A.M., respectively. The patient becomes drowsy 1 hour after taking melatonin, and this interferes with her evening activities. What will be the initial advice to the patient?
A. Delay taking melatonin until 10 P.M.
B. Engage in physical activity when drowsy.
C. Reduce the dose of melatonin to 3 mg.
D. Try light therapy in the morning instead of melatonin.
E. Discontinue melatonin; take a hypnotic at bedtime.

17. A 30-year-old patient with shift work disorder works sedentary night shifts five times a week (11 P.M. to 7 A.M., Mondays through Fridays). His sleep schedule at home is 9 A.M. to 5 P.M. The patient keeps a similar sleep-wake schedule during days off work. He has significant difficulties with sleepiness at work and insomnia during his bedtime. What is the main reason for this patient's inability to impose the desired sleep-wake schedule on his intrinsic circadian rhythm so that the latter suits his work schedule?
A. Insufficient exposure to light at night
B. Insufficient exercise at night
C. Exposure to daylight during morning home commute
D. Age-dependent loss of adaptation of the circadian rhythm

18. A healthy 40-year-old shift worker was involved in a near-collision as a result of sleepiness while driving during his night shift at 4 A.M. He admitted feeling drowsy between 3 A.M. and 5 A.M. during most nights he worked in the last 3 years. He said he was reluctant to share this problem with his superiors for fear of losing his job. The patient asks for medical advice to improve his alertness at night. What will be your best evidence-based management of this patient?
A. Advise him to drink a lot of coffee at night.
B. Prescribe modafinil before the night shift.
C. Write a prescription for melatonin, 3 mg in the morning after the night shift.
D. Suggest that his workplace be well-lit.
E. Allow for a short break during work to exercise.

19. An 18-year-old student's habitual sleep and wake times are 11 P.M. and 7 A.M., respectively. During summer vacation he slept between 3 A.M. and 11 A.M., even when not "going out" with his friends. He spends hours on the Internet at night playing videogames. His parents are worried about his sleep time, particularly about adapting to the school schedule when classes resume. What would you advise?
A. Start the patient on melatonin, 3 mg at 8 P.M.
B. Educate the patient about sleep hygiene.
C. Get psychological evaluation.
D. Wait until the vacation ends; the previous sleep pattern may then reemerge.
E. Reassure the parents that this is a normal sleep pattern in teenagers.

20. A patient with the DSPD needs to wake up early for an important appointment. His usual

sleep-wake times are 3 A.M. and 11 A.M., respectively. He skips a night of sleep 2 nights before the appointment, stays awake until the following night, goes to bed at 10 P.M. the night before the appointment, and wakes up at 7 A.M. to make the appointment at 9 A.M. This patient is making use of which of the following mechanisms?
A. Increasing homeostatic sleep drive
B. Delaying the circadian rhythm further to suit changing needs
C. Switching to free-running type of circadian rhythm sleep disorder
D. Using the morning light to advance the circadian rhythm on the next night

21. A blind patient suffers from circadian rhythm sleep disorder, free-running type. The lack of output of which of the following structures of the visual pathway may be involved in the pathogenesis of this disorder?
A. Rod and cone photoreceptors
B. Retinal ganglion cells
C. Optic tract
D. Lateral geniculate bodies
E. Optic radiation

22. A 27-year-old woman complains of chronic problems with her sleep. A nearly 4-week actigraphy study was done of this patient, shown in Figure 16-1. Her corrected visual acuity is 20/30 on the right and no light perception on the left. The neurological examination and brain magnetic resonance imaging scan are normal. Which of the following investigations is most helpful in management of this patient?
A. Psychiatric assessment
B. 24-hour fractionated salivary melatonin excretion
C. Electroretinography
D. Visual-evoked potentials
E. Polysomnography

23. In a hypertensive patient with dementia and irregular sleep-wake rhythm, which of the following classes of antihypertensive medications (assumed to be of equal efficacy) is best avoided?
A. Angiotensin-converting enzyme inhibitors
B. Angiotensin II antagonists
C. Beta-blockers
D. Calcium channel blockers
E. Diuretics

24. A 17-year-old patient complained of falling asleep and getting up at later times than his daytime schedule demands. This pattern emerged after studying late for exams for a few weeks 1 month

ago. The patient seems to be unable to switch back to his previous sleep-wake schedule, despite trying hard to do so. You wish to correct the patient's schedule as soon as possible and prescribe classic chronotherapy. What would be your specific instructions for this patient?
A. Each day, delay going to sleep by 2–3 hours, until you reach the desired sleep time.
B. Each week, advance your wake time by 15 to 30 minutes, until you reach the desired sleep time.
C. Avoid sleeping on Friday night, and go to bed 90 minutes earlier than usual from Saturday night onward; repeat each week until you reach the desired sleep time.
D. Wake up at the desired time regardless of bedtime, until your sleep schedule becomes normal.

25. If the retinohypothalamic tract is completely destroyed, which of the following circadian rhythm sleep disorders will ensue?
A. Advanced sleep phase disorder
B. DSPD
C. Irregular sleep wake rhythm
D. Circadian rhythm sleep disorder, free-running type

Questions 26–27: A patient suffers from DSPD. It was determined that the onset of her dim-light endogenous melatonin secretion was at 9 P.M., 3 hours after the sunset, while the nadir of her core body temperature was at 8 A.M.

26. Bright light exposure at which of the following times is expected to produce the largest phase advance?
A. 9 P.M.
B. 1 A.M.
C. 5 A.M.
D. 9 A.M.
E. 1 P.M.

27. Melatonin administration at which of the following times is expected to produce the largest phase advance?
A. 8 P.M.
B. 12 A.M.
C. 4 A.M.
D. 8 A.M.
E. 12 P.M.

28. Generation of circadian rhythms is an intrinsic quality of most tissues. The synchronization of these multiple rhythms is probably achieved by which of the following mechanisms?

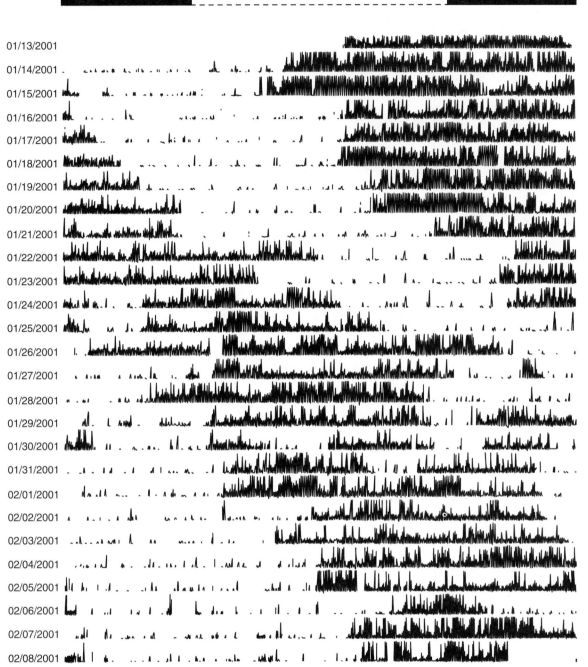

FIGURE 16-1 ■ An actigraph recording of a patient in question 22. This is a 27-day recording of the patient. Each row represents a 24-hour period between 12 A.M. on a given day and 12 A.M. on the following consecutive day. The hours are in the "military" 24-hour format (HH:MM). The dates in each row are in mm/dd/yyyy format. (Modified from Dagan Y: Circadian rhythm sleep disorders [CRSD]. Sleep Med Rev 6:45–55, 2002; with permission.)

A. Extraocular circadian phototransduction
B. Nonphotic entrainment of rhythms (behavior, feeding, etc.)
C. Neurohumoral influences orchestrated by the suprachiasmatic nuclei
D. Direct sleep-wake influences on tissue metabolism

Questions 29–31 are based on the followings case: The following actigraph recording (Figure 16-2) depicts the sleep pattern of a 27-year-old patient complaining of longstanding insomnia. The patient was instructed by the physician to go to bed only when sleepy and wake up without an alarm clock for the duration of the study. The device is worn on the right (dominant) wrist.

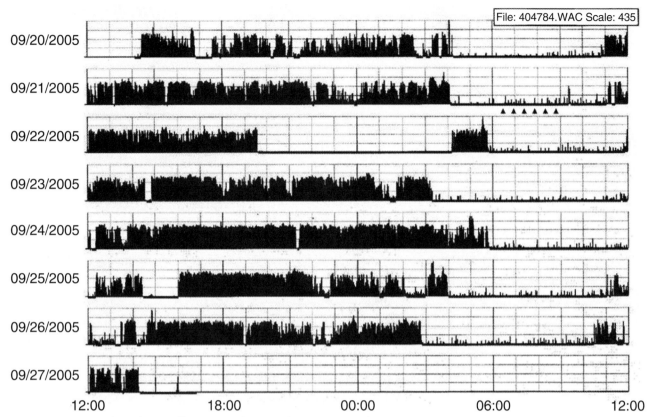

File: 404784.WAC Scale: 435

FIGURE 16-2 ■ An actigraph recording concerning questions 29–31. Each row represents a 24-hour period between 12 P.M. on a given day and 12 P.M. on the following consecutive day. The hours are in the "military" 24-hour format (HH:MM). The dates in each row are in mm/dd/yyyy format.

29. Judging by this recording alone, this patient suffers from which of the following conditions?
    A. Psychophysiological insomnia
    B. DSPD
    C. Circadian rhythm sleep disorder, free-running type
    D. Periodic limb movement disorder

30. What is happening on 09/22/2005 between 19:30 and 04:10 hours?
    A. The patient is asleep.
    B. The patient is not wearing the actigraph.
    C. There is a hardware malfunction.
    D. The patient is lying awake quietly.

31. What are the small vertical lines in the parts of the recording representing sleep times (e.g., on 09/21/2005 between 04:00 and 10:50 hours) (marked with small black triangles)?
    A. Awakenings
    B. Artifacts
    C. Normal movements in sleep
    D. Periodic limb movements in sleep

Questions 32–34 concern the actigraph recording shown in Figure 16-3, which was recorded in a 38-year-old male patient who complained of poor sleep and excessive daytime sleepiness. He reports awakenings from sleep, during which he is completely aware of himself. The patient was instructed by the physician to go to bed when sleepy and wake up without an alarm clock for the duration of the study. The device is worn on the right (dominant) wrist.

32. With which of the following circadian rhythm sleep disorders is his major sleep pattern compatible?
    A. Advanced sleep phase disorder
    B. DSPD
    C. Irregular sleep-wake rhythm
    D. Circadian rhythm sleep disorder, free-running type

33. Based on the visual inspection of the recording, from which of the following additional sleep disorders may this patient suffer?
    A. Psychophysiological insomnia
    B. Inadequate sleep hygiene

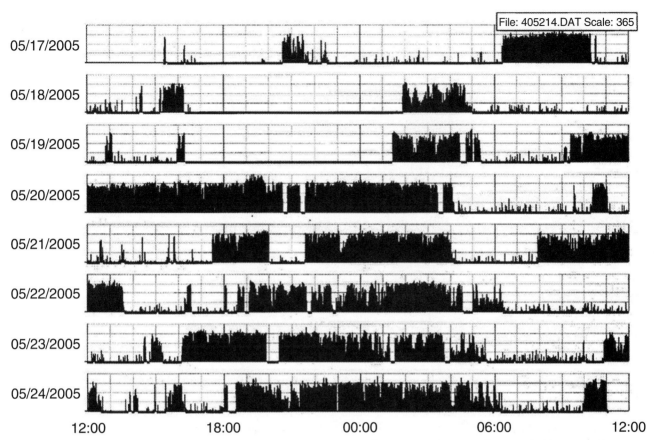

FIGURE 16-3 ■ An actigraph recording concerning questions 32–34. Each row represents a 24-hour period between 12 P.M. on a certain day and 12 P.M. on the consecutive day. The hours are in the "military" 24-hour format (HH:MM). The dates in each row are in mm/dd/yyyy format.

C. Periodic limb movement disorder
D. Sleepwalking

34. What is the patient doing between 22:30 and 06:30 on 05/17/2005?
A. Sleeping
B. Lying awake quietly
C. Lying awake and kicking his leg from time to time
D. Napping but waking up a lot

35. A normal individual in a time-isolation facility lives on a forced desynchrony protocol using a 28-hour schedule. For a period of 21 days, he lives there in dim light with a strictly imposed feeding and activity schedule. In these conditions, his intrinsic circadian period measured by the core body temperature curve is likely to be:
A. Slightly more than 28 hours
B. Slightly less than 28 hours

C. About 25 hours
D. Slightly more than 24 hours

36. The actigraph recording shown in Figure 16-4 was performed on a 72-year-old patient living at home with his wife. The patient complained about insomnia. His wife described the patient's nocturnal wanderings and occasional confusion at night. She also complained of his sleepiness during the day, sometimes to the point of sleeping throughout the daytime hours and being awake all night. This recording, considered together with the patient's history, is compatible with which of the following sleep disorders?
A. Circadian rhythm sleep disorder, free-running type
B. Inadequate sleep hygiene
C. Irregular sleep-wake rhythm
D. Psychophysiological insomnia

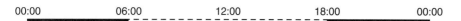

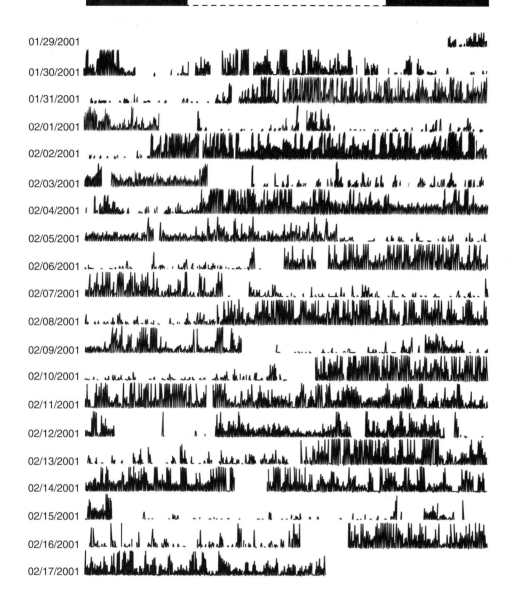

FIGURE 16-4 ■ An actigraph recording of a patient in question 36. This is a 20-day recording of the patient. Each row represents a 24-hour period between 12 A.M. on a given day and 12 A.M. on the following consecutive day. The hours are in the "military" 24-hour format (HH:MM). The dates in each row are in mm/dd/yyyy format. (Modified from Dagan Y: Circadian rhythm sleep disorders [CRSD]. Sleep Med Rev 6:45–55, 2002; with permission.)

Answers

1. B. Delayed sleep phase disorder (DSPD)

The history suggests chronic unremitting inability to comply with a socially sound schedule. The patient adjusts to his limitation by taking on night work, afternoon classes, etc. All these are highly characteristic of DSPD. Adjustment insomnia is unlikely because there was no identifiable trigger, and the sleep disorder lasts for too long a time. Anxiety may cause prolonged insomnia, but habitually late awakening is uncommon; therefore insomnia associated with mental disorder is an unlikely diagnosis. The patient is not a long sleeper judging by his habitual sleep hours. Although the patient works part-time night shifts, his sleep disorder started before he took this job. Shift work disorder is probably not a consideration here but is rather the patient's attempt at leading a normal life with his disorder.

2. D. Sleep log and actigraphy

Although diagnosis of DSPD may frequently be made by history alone, if an auxiliary investigation is desired, sleep log and actigraphy provide the most valuable information about the patient's sleep patterns. Polysomnography and MSLT only provide information about a single-day pattern of sleep and are useless for diagnosis of DSPD. Psychiatric assessment may be indicated in insomnia associated with a mental disorder, or in evaluating the secondary emotional influences of DSPD, but it has no role in establishing the diagnosis itself.

3. E. Be exposed to bright light on awakening.

Although all listed advices have merit in this case, none but bright light has any potential in treating the patient's condition. Therefore choice C, bright light therapy, is the single most important advice in this case. Melatonin may also be used, but according to the case history, the patient is "unwilling" to take any pills. Sometimes the best advice would be to adjust the daily activities to the sleep-wake schedule, rather than attempting to do the opposite.

4. B. Advanced sleep phase disorder

The patient suffers from a typical presentation of advanced sleep phase disorder, with sleep onset and final awakening that are much earlier than socially acceptable. Her sleep duration and quality are otherwise normal. Early morning awakening is a manifestation of major depression, but early bed time is not. The patient is indeed depressed, but the depression is part of an adjustment disorder and was not present before the sleep disturbance. The patient's sleep pattern changed in the same direction, but the change was of much larger magnitude than would be expected from changes owing to normal aging. Sleep apnea is probably not a consideration, given the patient's normal airways and rare snoring.

5. B. Light therapy

Light therapy in the early evening has the best potential in delaying the patient's sleep-wake rhythm. The other listed therapies may occasionally be tried in similar patients, primarily because they are frequently incorrectly diagnosed. Antidepressants are not indicated in this patient, except perhaps for treating adjustment disorder. Melatonin in the morning may have a potential theoretical merit, similar to its use in the evening for DSPD but it has not been investigated in this disorder because of its relative rarity. The use of hypnotics to prolong night sleep in the context of advanced sleep phase disorder may cause daytime drowsiness in the elderly, whereas a stimulant in the second half of the day may interfere with nocturnal sleep.

6. B. Irregular sleep-wake rhythm

The patient's sleep-wake pattern of several sleep periods during a 24-hour period at irregular periods and her complaints are compatible with this diagnosis. Her lifestyle of seclusion and work without actual human contact may be suggestive of schizoid personality disorder, which is common in cognitively intact individuals with irregular sleep-wake rhythms. Inadequate sleep hygiene is a major differential diagnosis in this case; however, the patient's lifestyle and preferences, and inability to change the pattern, suggest the irregular sleep-wake rhythm as the most correct diagnosis. Insomnia resulting from mental disorder is an incorrect diagnosis, as the patient does not suffer from a major mental disorder, and her complaints are more than insomnia. Although the patient works nights frequently, her sleep pattern is incompatible with shift work disorder. Patients with psychophysiological insomnia usually do not sleep during the day, and insomnia is their main complaint, unlike this patient.

7. C. Actigraphy and sleep log

The most important step in the diagnosis is to ascertain the patient's sleep pattern; this can be achieved by using a sleep log and actigraphy. Psychiatric assessment is important in subsequent evaluation, but probably not for an initial diagnosis. Polysomnography is not indicated as a first step, as it only depicts 1 night of sleep, not a chronic pattern, and does not have a role in the absence of other potential comorbidities (such as sleep apnea). Melatonin salivary excretion will not help because even if abnormalities are discovered, they will probably not aid in the diagnosis, which is a clinical one. Brain imaging may be necessary in circadian rhythm disturbances owing to a medical condition (e.g., various types of dementia), but not in this case, and not as a first priority.

8. C. Improvement of sleep hygiene and melatonin

This cognitively intact patient suffers from irregular sleep-wake rhythm. The therapy should aim at the circadian rhythm disturbance that underlies the explicit irregularity of sleep-wake rhythm. Improving sleep hygiene is always desirable, particularly in cognitively intact patients. This disorder was indeed first described in cognitively intact patients suffering from extreme inadequacy of sleep hygiene. Melatonin is sometimes effective in cognitively impaired patients suffering from a similar disorder (formally, circadian rhythm sleep disorder resulting from a medical condition), and it may also be tried here, but there is no specific data regarding the use of melatonin under the circumstances in this case history.

Psychotherapy and antidepressants may be occasionally used in these patients if there is a specific indication, such as depression or personality disorder, but they have no role in correcting the circadian sleep disorder itself. Hypnotics are frequently abused by these patients, and they should be used sparingly, if at all.

9. A. Adjustment insomnia

There is a well-defined future event (presentation), which may be the trigger of the patient's acute insomnia. Altitude insomnia is an acute insomnia that occurs on ascent to high altitude, not a descent to sea level, as in this case. Jet lag is an incorrect option, as there is only a 1-hour time difference between the origin and the destination locations. The patient's acute anxiety over his presentation is not a mental disorder; therefore the diagnosis of insomnia resulting from a mental disorder is not justified.

10. A. Hypnotic

A brief course of hypnotic medication suits best the patient's need to improve his sleep in anticipation of the presentation. Melatonin could have been used in jet lag, which is not the case in this patient. Reassurance of the benign nature of this patient's insomnia may be enough to alleviate the patient's fears, but it will probably not help to improve his sleep. Sedative antidepressants (e.g., mirtazapine or trazodone) may be used in chronic insomnia, particularly in patients with underlying anxiety or mood disorders, but in acute

insomnia they are probably not indicated. There may also be a significant daytime sedation in the beginning of therapy, which will be counterproductive in this case.

11. B. Because she may have retained circadian photoreception independent of visual photoreception.

This blind patient suffers from the circadian rhythm sleep disorder, free-running type. She was completely blind for 7 years, but has suffered from a typical sleep disturbance for only for 4 years. This may be interpreted that she has retained her circadian entrainment for 3 years after becoming completely blind. Circadian photoreception is independent of rod and cone visual photoreception and is mediated via specialized melanopsin-containing photosensitive retinal ganglion cells. Many blind individuals retain the capacity to entrain to light stimuli despite being completely blind with no light perception and negative electroretinography, which is a test to measure the electrical response of the retinal rods and cones to flashes of light. Obviously, enucleated eye cannot transduce light stimuli, but her remaining eye afflicted with severe glaucoma can; because the retinal ganglion cells are still viable, light-induced circadian entrainment may continue. On the other hand, when light cues are prevented from reaching the suprachiasmatic nuclei, photic entrainment ceases immediately and does not continue for years; therefore option A is incorrect. Entrainment to social stimuli is possible, and in the blind even more so than in sighted individuals; however, social entrainment is probably not a tremendously effective compensatory mechanism, as it does not correct sleep disturbances in the vast majority of blind patients. The blindness and the sleep disorder are interconnected in this patient, as the majority of blind patients suffer from a chronic circadian rhythm sleep disorder, and as this blind patient suffers from a typical circadian rhythm sleep disorder, free-running type.

12. B. Long-term actigraphy and sleep log

The classic pattern of the circadian rhythm sleep disorder, free-running type, is several weeks of almost normal sleep-wake rhythm alternating with longer periods of progressively misaligned rhythm. To diagnose the disorder, long-term monitoring of sleep-wake patterns is necessary. This monitoring can be performed only by long-term actigraphy and sleep logs (see Figure 16-1). Therefore 2-night polysomnography or polysomnography followed by MSLT are insufficient to demonstrate this long-term alternating pattern. Electroretinography will document the excitability of the retina but has no role in documenting the circadian rhythm disturbance. Abnormalities of melatonin rhythm during any 24-hour period will not document the dynamic nature of the disturbance.

13. B. Melatonin

Melatonin may entrain circadian rhythms in blind individuals and normalize their sleep patterns. Bright light therapy may be tried in certain individuals, with the hope that their circadian photoreceptor system is at least partially intact. This approach, however, does not work in many patients. Hypnotics and sedative antidepressants, although improving sleep, have no role in the long-term management of this disorder, as it is optimal timing of sleep that is the problem, not the sleep itself. Cognitive-behavioral therapy is appropriate for psychophysiological insomnia, not circadian rhythm sleep disorders.

14. A. Full adaptation process is expected to last between 1 and 2 weeks.

The circadian adaptation is a process that changes the circadian phase at a pace of roughly about 1 hour per day under favorable circumstances; therefore the full adaptation to a 10-hour shift is expected to normally take between 1 and 2 weeks. After a long transmeridian travel (8 hours shift or more), circadian adaptation is frequently antidromic (e.g., in this case, *delaying* the rhythm by 14 hours rather than advancing it by 10 hours). Both timed melatonin use and in-flight hypnotics may *assist* the circadian adaptation, if administered at correct times.

15. C. Degeneration of the suprachiasmatic nuclei and their connections

This patient suffers from irregular sleep-wake rhythm brought about by Alzheimer's disease (formally, circadian rhythm sleep disorder owing to a medical condition). The *primary* pathophysiology in this case is likely due to neurodegenerative changes in the structures responsible for circadian time keeping, the suprachiastmatic nuclei. Other options probably also contribute to the explicit disorder, as patients with dementia do indeed suffer from insufficient social interaction, medication side effects, insufficient exposure to bright daylight and inadequate sleep hygiene, but these are not the primary causes of this disorder.

16. C. Reduce the dose of melatonin to 3 mg.

Drowsiness is a dose-dependent side effect of melatonin. The drowsiness may occur about an hour after administration and last for an hour or two. The best solution to this problem is to reduce the dose of melatonin. Delaying administration of melatonin may reduce its efficacy. Physical activity in the evening a few hours before sleep may delay sleep onset owing to rising body temperature, thus offsetting the effect of melatonin. Light therapy in the morning is also effective in DSPD, but it is more cumbersome, and many patients find it difficult to wake up in time for the optimal effect of bright light therapy to take place. There is also no need to change the effective treatment in this case. Hypnotics at bedtime are a poor choice in DSPD, as they will probably be needed as a chronic therapy, with all the attending problems in chronic hypnotic treatment.

17. C. Exposure to daylight during morning home commute

This patient tries to entrain his endogenous circadian rhythm to his work schedule by keeping his sleep-wake rhythm the same during both on-work and off-work days. However, the timing of the circadian rhythm of the vast majority of shift workers remains anchored to the environmental light-dark cycle. In this patient, this is seen primarily because of his exposure to light during the morning commute home, which occurs at the circadian time that is optimal to keep the rhythm locked to the environmental cycle. Exercise and light exposure at night may help shift workers adapt to their work hours, but their influence is insufficient to negate the "anchoring" effect of the morning light. The circadian rhythm in this 30-year-old patient is supposed to be flexible enough to allow for circadian adaptation if the conditions are right, so option D is incorrect.

18. B. Take modafinil before the night shift.

Modafinil has been approved by the FDA to treat drowsiness associated with shift work, based on controlled studies (Walsh et al: Sleep 27:434, 2004). Options A, D, and E may also help to combat fatigue; however, the evidence about their efficacy is less conclusive. In the United States, melatonin is considered a "food additive" and no prescription is needed. Melatonin in the morning may help to delay the circadian rhythm timing, but other variables in the typical shift worker probably offset this effect (exposure to morning light during the home commute, sleeping nights rather than days/during days off-work, etc.).

19. B. Educate the patient about sleep hygiene.

It is frequently difficult to draw a line between the culturally and genetically determined sleep habits of teenagers and genuine DSPD. Many teenagers have no problem rotating back to a normal schedule after living by delayed schedule during vacations. It is the inability to do so that distinguishes DSPD. Because this is the patient's first vacation with a delayed schedule, the most appropriate next step is to educate the patient about sleep hygiene, in order to prevent inadvertent gliding into DSPD in a predisposed patient. Of course, waiting until the vacation ends to see whether he can resume a normal sleep-wake pattern is a logical continuation of this approach, but not the first thing to do. Starting the patient on melatonin is premature under the circumstances. Psychological evaluation is unwarranted; reassuring the parents that this is a normal pattern is wrong, as it is a common but abnormal sleep-wake pattern.

20. A. Increasing homeostatic sleep drive

Patients with DSPD may have a relatively weak homeostatic sleep drive, judging by their inability to fall asleep at conventional hours at night, even when they wake up early in the preceding morning (to attend school, work, etc.). In the complex interplay of the circadian and the homeostatic drives for sleep, the former determines the sleep onset in these patients in usual circumstances (Figure 16-5). Skipping a night's sleep 2 nights before his appointment increases the homeostatic sleep drive, such that the patient was able to fall asleep at 10 P.M. on the night preceding the appointment, which would otherwise be difficult. Waking up at 7 A.M. before the appointment translates to waking in the middle of his subjective night, but after 9 hours of sleep, he is able to do so relatively easily. Option B is incorrect because skipping a night's sleep does not delay the rhythm. Option C is also incorrect. Although patients with DSPD may switch to free-running type of circadian rhythm sleep disorder occasionally, it does not reflect what the patient did. Skipping the night's sleep may indeed expose the patient to morning light; however, even if there was a phase advance, its magnitude would be insufficient to suit the patient's needs.

21. B. Retinal ganglion cells

Blind patients suffer from circadian rhythm sleep disorder, free-running type, because of the lack of environmental light input to the suprachiasmatic nuclei. The origin of the environmental light input is in the photosensitive specialized retinal ganglion cells, rather than rod and cone photoreceptors. Options C–E include retrochiasmatic structures that have no role in the pathogenesis of circadian rhythm sleep disorders in the blind (Figure 16-6).

22. A. Psychiatric assessment

This is a sighted patient whose actigraph recording shows a daily delay of habitual sleep and wake times, which encompasses about 24 hours during this nearly 4-week recording. This pattern is compatible with the circadian rhythm sleep disorder, free-running type; she apparently has no brain pathology. There is a

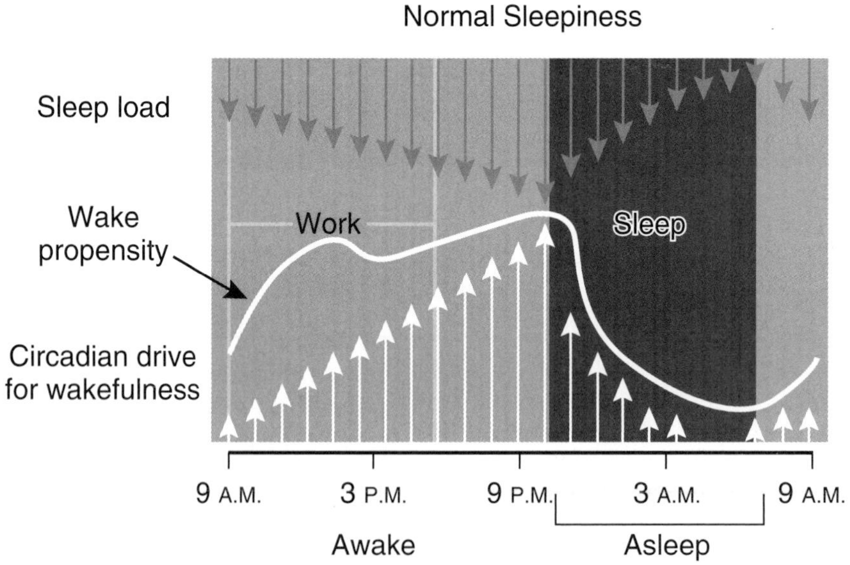

FIGURE 16-5 ■ The opponent process model of sleep regulation. In this schematic representation of the classic opponent process model of sleep regulation (Mistlberger: Brain Research Rev 49:429–454, 2005), the homeostatic sleep drive (sleep load) is represented by down arrows, while the circadian drive for wakefulness is represented by up arrows; the length of the arrows represents the intensity of the respective drives. The resulting wake propensity (the curved line between the arrowheads) is the final result of the complex interplay between the two drives. It can be readily seen that the habitual sleepiness times (early afternoon and night) are the reflection of the decreased wake propensity at these times. Increasing the sleep load (by a night of sleep deprivation, for example) may allow a person to fall asleep at a time when ordinarily the circadian drive for wakefulness would not allow it.

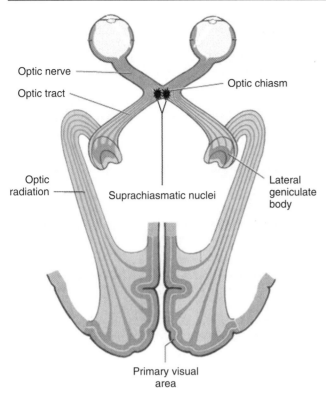

Optic nerve

Optic tract

Optic chiasm

Optic radiation

Suprachiasmatic nuclei

Lateral geniculate body

Primary visual area

FIGURE 16-6 ■ Schematic representation of the optic pathways. The suprachiasmatic nuclei (SCN) are slightly above the optic chiasm; in this bidimensional drawing, they are superimposed on the chiasm. It can be seen that the structures mentioned in the options C–E in question 21 are downstream from the SCN; therefore they have no role in the pathogenesis of the circadian rhythm sleep disorders.

high incidence of psychiatric and personality disorders in these rare patients; therefore a psychiatric evaluation is warranted. Because this patient is sighted, electroretinography and visual-evoked potentials are not helpful; apparently the patient does have light perception, so there is no issue of light impulse not reaching the suprachiasmatic nuclei. Twenty-four-hour fractionated salivary melatonin excretion provides only a picture of the circadian rhythm for the sampled period; it has no role in long-term assessment in this patient. Polysomnography will not further advance this patient's diagnosis and treatment unless there is clinical evidence for another sleep disorder in which polysomnography may be useful (e.g., obstructive sleep apnea syndrome or periodic limb movement disorder).

23. C. Beta-blockers

Patients with dementia and irregular sleep-wake rhythm presumably have a disorder of circadian rhythm secondary to degeneration of suprachiasmatic nuclei or their sources of input or destinations of output.

Endogenous melatonin secretion, which has an important role in the circadian regulation, is controlled by the suprachiasmatic nuclei via multineuronal sympathetic pathways (Figure16-7). Beta-blockers may further reduce the endogenous melatonin secretion by blocking this sympathetic pathway. In Smith-Magenis syndrome, a genetic disorder that manifests as dysmorphism, mental retardation, behavioral disturbances, and advanced sleep phase disorder, the latter is attributed to diurnal, rather than nocturnal, melatonin secretion. Morning use of beta-blockers effectively reduced daytime endogenous melatonin secretion, and evening use of exogenous melatonin significantly improved the sleep disturbance. Other antihypertensive medications listed have no effect on the melatonin secretion.

24. A. Each day, delay going to sleep by 2 to 3 hours, until you reach the desired sleep time.

The patient suffers from DSPD. Chronotherapy was originally described in these patients, the classic instructions being the one in option A. This method of chronotherapy allows reaching the desired bed and waking times within a few days. It uses the inherent tendency to phase delay in these patients and increases the homeostatic sleep drive by delaying sleep each day. On reaching the desired sleep time, however, one needs to adhere to a strict schedule, allowing for no exceptions, otherwise risking reemergence of the previous pattern. The method in option B uses mild sleep restriction in the morning to achieve increased homeostatic drive for sleep in the evening, thus allowing for earlier bedtime. This method takes longer than the one in option A and may be less effective. The method in option C was developed to allow for individuals unable to conduct the classic chronotherapy because of work or other obligations; it also takes longer than option A. Option D is not part of chronotherapy and is ineffective.

25. D. Circadian rhythm sleep disorder, free-running type

The retinohypothalamic tract is the main conduit of environmental light input to the suprachiasmatic nuclei (see Figure 16-7). If it was completely destroyed, no light information would reach the suprachiasmatic nuclei, thus making it unable to entrain the intrinsic circadian rhythm with the environmental light-dark cycle. A free-running rhythm would ensue, corresponding to option D. The circadian rhythm sleep disorders in options A–C ensue when the suprachiasmatic nuclei malfunction in various ways (out-of-phase in options A and B or "misfires" in option C) but still receives the environmental light input.

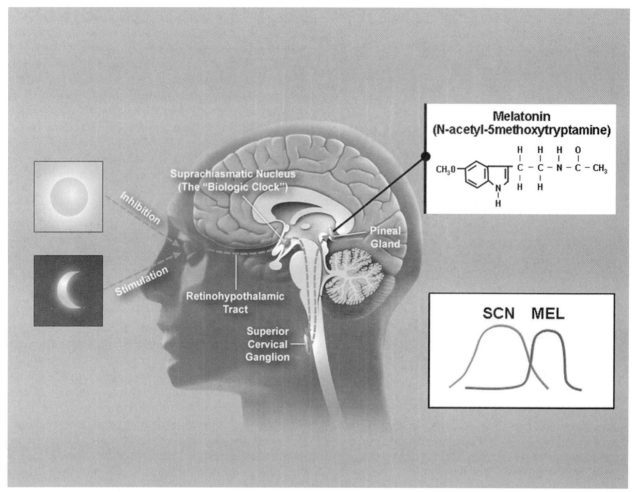

FIGURE 16-7 ■ The human circadian system outline. Melatonin (upper-right inset) is produced in the pineal gland. The production and secretion of melatonin are mediated largely by postganglionic retinal nerve fibers that pass through the retinohypothalamic tract to the suprachiasmatic nucleus, then to the superior cervical ganglion, and finally to the pineal gland. This neuronal system is activated by darkness and suppressed by light (left insets). The activation of α_1- and β_1-adrenergic receptors in the pineal gland raises cyclic AMP and calcium concentrations and activates arylalkylamine N-acetyltransferase, initiating the synthesis and release of melatonin. The daily rhythm of melatonin secretion is controlled by the endogenous master pacemaker located in the suprachiasmatic nuclei. The lower-right inset shows the temporal relationship between the activity of the suprachiasmatic nuclei and the secretion of melatonin within a period of 24 hours (not to scale). SCN, Suprachiasmatic nuclei; MEL, melatonin. (Adapted [2006], with permission, from Brzezinski A: Mechanisms of disease: melatonin in humans. New Engl J Med 336:186–195, 1997. Copyright 1997 Massachusetts Medical Society.)

26. D. 9 A.M.

Light stimulation just after the core body temperature nadir is expected to produce the largest phase advance. Therefore in this case, light exposure at 9 A.M. is supposed to be optimal in this regard. Exposure at 1 P.M. (option E) will produce a modest time advance, if at all. Exposure at times before 8 A.M. will produce phase delays, rather than advance (options A–C).

27. A. 8 P.M.

Exogenous melatonin administration at or just before the dim-light endogenous melatonin onset is expected to produce maximal phase advance. At other times, melatonin administration may have modest or no effect in phase advancing.

28. C. Neurohumoral influences orchestrated by the suprachiasmatic nuclei

Recent data suggest that circadian oscillation is an inherent property of many tissues. The synchronization of multiple tissue clocks needs a master unifying mechanism. At this point the only known master clock is in the suprachiasmatic nuclei, which exerts modulating influence through both neural influences on multiple brain areas and humoral mediators acting elsewhere. Extraocular circadian phototransduction in option A is a highly controversial concept, which postulates that extraocular sites (possibly the skin) provide light input to the circadian system. Even if this concept is correct, the phototransduction information must still reach the brain to exert its influence. It does not act directly on tissues; therefore it does not exert a direct synchronizing effect on the tissue clock. Regarding options B and D, there is no good evidence that, in humans, behavioral and feeding rhythms (e.g., recurring scheduled exercise or feeding) or sleep-wake rhythms act directly on entrainment of various tissue rhythms independently of the suprachiasmatic nuclei.

29. B. DSPD

This recording shows a consistently late sleep onset (between 3 A.M. and 6 A.M.) and sleep offset (between 11 A.M. and 1 P.M.), which is compatible with DSPD. The quality of sleep seems normal, and the sleep pattern seems consistent. These are incompatible with psychophysiological insomnia (characterized by disrupted sleep) or circadian rhythm sleep disorder, free-running type (characterized by progressively delayed sleep onset and offset). Movements during the sleep periods represent normal sleep movements and not periodic limb movement disorder for the following reasons: (1) the device is worn on the wrist, and it cannot reliably pick up the leg movements; and (2) periodic limb movements in sleep are not diagnosed by actigraphy, despite continuing effort to develop actigraphy-based devices that can do so reliably.

30. B. The patient is not wearing the actigraph.

The total absence of recorded movements during the period in question suggests that the device was still functioning but completely immobile. This can occur only if the patient is not wearing the device. Minor movements picked up by the device do occur during both sleep and quiet rest.

31. C. Normal movements in sleep

These lines represent normal adjustment movements in sleep picked up by the device. They correspond to minor movements that are too small in amplitude and frequency to qualify for full-scale awakenings. Wrist actigraphy does not usually pick up periodic limb movements in sleep.

32. B. DSPD

This patient falls asleep more or less consistently between 4 and 6 A.M. and wakes up in late afternoon, which suggests DSPD. In advanced sleep phase disorder (option A), early sleep onset and offset times are expected but are not seen here. In irregular sleep wake rhythm (option C) the sleep pattern is disorganized, but in this recording more or less regular major sleep periods are seen. For option D to be considered, progressively delayed sleep periods should be present (see Figure 16-1).

33. B. Inadequate sleep hygiene

Although the patient's sleep onset is more or less consistent, he wakes up at different times each day after varying periods of sleep. He may also doze off during the day, and his sleep quality is inadequate (e.g., on 05/24/2005 between 12:00 and 18:00 hours). Dozing off during the daytime impairs his night sleep, as can be seen further on during the same 24-hour period; he fell asleep only after 06:00, partly because of his daytime sleep. The patient is also not very compliant with instruction and does not wear the device on parts of 2 consecutive days (05/18/2005 and 05/19/2005 between about 16:30 to 02:00). The brief, intense-movement periods during sleep (e.g., 05/20/2005 between 10:30 and 11:00) most likely represent awakenings, rather then sleepwalking, as no history is given compatible with this diagnosis. Diagnosis of sleepwalking requires demonstration of ambulation during sleep *and* persistence of sleep or altered state of consciousness during the episode; in this case the patient gives the history of being fully conscious during awakenings. Also, actigraph cannot ascertain the state of consciousness; it only records movement, so an episode of intense movement amidst a sleep episode can represent awakening, sleepwalking, REM sleep behavior disorder, or a seizure, among other possibilities. The brief mild movements during sleep probably represent episodes of restless sleep rather than periodic limb movements, which cannot be picked up by wrist actigraphy.

34. A. Sleeping

This is a typical recording of quiet sleeping. Periods of wakefulness are characterized by continuous movements, represented by tall black lines; the taller the line, the more intense the movement pattern. Therefore periods of continuous wakefulness are represented in the recording by confluent black pattern (e.g., 05/20/2005 between 12:00 and 04:00, with three brief episodes of complete inactivity when the patient removed the device). Had the patient been lying awake, even quietly, his movement pattern would have been much more intense than in the segment in question, let alone if he had been kicking his leg. The minor movements during the period in question do not represent awakenings. The movements during awakenings are much more prominent, such as seen on 05/24/2005 between 12:00 and 18:00.

35. D. Slightly more than 24 hours

This question refers to the seminal publication by Czeisler et al (Science 284:2177, 1999) regarding the human circadian period. Under these conditions, the intrinsic human circadian period measured by core body temperature is about 24.2 hours. The human circadian pacemaker is unable to run with periodicity of 28 hours. The proposed cycle in the experiment is outside of "range of entrainment." The earlier estimate of the intrinsic human cycle of about 25 hours (Weitzman: Hum Neurobiol 1:173, 1982) was an error possibly brought about by an inadvertent exposure of subjects to ambient light in these conditions.

36. C. Irregular sleep-wake rhythm

The visual inspection of this recording shows a disorganized pattern of sleep and wake periods. There is no time during any 24-hour period at which the patient is consistently awake or asleep. This recording is incompatible with option D because patients with psychophysiological insomnia rarely sleep through the day, and their sleep, although disrupted, is mostly at night. The recording is also incompatible with option A because in patients with circadian rhythm sleep disorder, free-running type, a progressive delaying of sleep periods is expected to be demonstrated during a 20-day recording such as the one in consideration. The two plausible options judging only by the recording are an extreme example of inadequate sleep hygiene (option B) and irregular sleep-wake rhythm. If the history of confusion and nocturnal wanderings *(sundowning)* is considered, the irregular sleep-wake rhythm in a patient with dementia is the most probable diagnosis. Phenomenologically, this is irregular sleep-wake rhythm. This disorder should be categorized formally as circadian rhythm sleep disorder resulting from a medical condition.

REFERENCES

1. American Academy of Sleep Medicine: *The International Classification of Sleep Disorders: Diagnostic and Coding Manual*, 2nd ed. Westchester, IL, American Academy of Sleep Medicine, 2005, pp 117–136.

2. American Academy of Sleep Medicine: *International Classification of Sleep Disorders: Diagnostic and Coding Manual*, 2nd ed. Westchester, IL, American Academy of Sleep Medicine, 2005, pp 142–144.

3. Ancoli-Israel S, Cole R, Alessi C, et al: The role of actigraphy in the study of sleep and circadian rhythms. American Academy of Sleep Medicine Review Paper. Sleep 26(3):342–392, 2003.

4. Barger LK, Wright KP Jr, Hughes RJ, Czeisler CA: Daily exercise facilitates phase delays of circadian melatonin rhythm in very dim light. Am J Physiol Regul Integr Comp Physiol 286(6):R1077–R1084, 2004.

5. Berson DM, Dunn FA, Takao M: Phototransduction by retinal ganglion cells that set the circadian clock. Science 295:1070–1073, 2002.

6. Bliwise DL: Sleep in normal aging and dementia. Sleep 16:40–81, 1993.

7. Campbell SS, Murphy PJ: Extraocular circadian phototransduction in humans. Science 279:396–399, 1998.

8. Campbell SS, Murphy PJ, Suhner AG: Extraocular phototransduction and circadian timing systems in vertebrates. Chronobiol Int 18:137–172, 2001.

9. Cardinali DP, Brusco LI, Liberczuk C, et al: The use of melatonin in Alzheimer's disease. Neuroendocrinol Lett 23(Suppl 1):20–23, 2002.

10. Chesson AL Jr, Littner M, Davila D, et al: Practice parameters for the use of light therapy in the treatment of sleep disorders. Standards of Practice Committee. American Academy of Sleep Medicine. Sleep 22:641–660, 1999.

11. Cole RJ, Smith JS, Alcala YC, et al: Bright-light mask treatment of delayed sleep phase syndrome. J Biol Rhythms 17:89–101, 2002.

12. Czeisler CA, Buxton OM, Khalsa SBS: The human circadian timing system and sleep-wake regulation. In Kryger MH, Roth T, Dement WC (eds): *Principles and Practice of Sleep Medicine*, 4th ed. Philadelphia, Elsevier, 2005, pp 375–394.

13. Czeisler CA, Duffy JF, Shanahan TL, et al: Stability, precision, and near-24-hour period of the human circadian pacemaker. Science 284:2177–2181, 1999.

14. Czeisler CA, Richardson GS, Coleman RM, et al: Chronotherapy: resetting the circadian clock of patients with delayed sleep phase insomnia. Sleep 4:1–21, 35, 1981.

15. Czeisler CA, Shanahan TL, Klerman EB, et al: Suppression of melatonin secretion in some blind patients by exposure to bright light. N Engl J Med 332:6–11, 1995.

16. Deacon S, Arendt J: Adapting to phase shifts, I. An experimental model for jet lag and shift work. Physiol Behav 59:665–673, 1996.

17. Deacon S, Arendt R: Melatonin induced temperature suppression and its acute phase-shifting effects correlate in a dose-dependent manner in humans. Brain Res 688:77–85, 1995.

18. De Leersnyder H, Bresson JL, de Blois MC, et al: Beta 1-adrenergic antagonists and melatonin reset the clock and restore sleep in a circadian disorder, Smith-Magenis syndrome. J Med Genet 40:74–78, 2003.

19. Eastman CI, Stewart KT, Mahoney MP, et al: Dark goggles and bright light improve circadian rhythm adaptation to night-shift work. Sleep 17:535–543, 1994.

20. Gooley JJ, Saper CB: Anatomy of the mammalian circadian system. In Kryger MH, Roth T, Dement WC (eds): *Principles and Practice of Sleep Medicine*, 4th ed. Philadelphia, Elsevier, 2005, pp 335–350.

21. Hauri P: *The Sleep Disorders*, 1st ed. Scope Publication (Upjohn) 1977, p 10.

22. Hayakawa T, Uchiyama M, Kamei Y, et al: Clinical analyses of sighted patients with non-24-hour sleep-wake syndrome: a study of 57 consecutively diagnosed cases. Sleep 28:945–952, 2005.

23. Herxheimer A, Petrie KJ: Melatonin for the prevention and treatment of jet lag. Cochrane Database Syst Rev CD001520, 2002.

24. Hoelscher TJ, Bond T, Ware JC: Treatment of delayed sleep phase syndrome with sleep schedule manipulation. Sleep Res 21:211, 1992.

25. Khalsa SBS, Jewett ME, Cajochen C, et al: A phase response curve to single bright light pulses in human subjects. J Physiol 549:945–952, 2003.

26. Lewy AJ, Bauer VK, Ahmed S, et al: The human phase response curve (PRC) to melatonin is about 12 hours out of phase with the PRC to light. Chronobiol Int 15:71–83, 1998.

27. Liu RY, Zhou JN, Hoogendijk WJ, et al: Decreased vasopressin gene expression in the biological clock of Alzheimer disease patients with and without depression. J Neuropathol Exp Neurol 59:314–322, 2000.

28. Lowden A, Akerstedt T, Wibom R: Suppression of sleepiness and melatonin by bright light exposure during breaks in night work. J Sleep Res 13(1):37–43, 2004.

29. Mendelson WB: A review of the evidence for the efficacy and safety of trazodone in insomnia. J Clin Psychiatry 66:469–476, 2005.

30. Middletone B, Stone B, Arendt J: Complex effects of melatonin on human circadian rhythms in constant dim light. J Biol Rhytms 12:467–477, 1997.

31. Mistlberger RE: Circadian regulation of sleep in mammals: Role of the suprachiasmatic nucleus. Brain Research Rev 49:429–454, 2005.

32. Mistlberger RE, Skene DJ: Social influences on mammalian circadian rhythms: animal and human studies. Biol Rev Camb Philos Soc 79(3):533–556, 2004.

33. Moline ML, Pollak CP, Monk TH, et al: Age-related differences in recovery from simulated jet lag. Sleep 15:28–40, 1992.

34. Monk TH, Buysse DJ, Carrier J, et al: Inducing jet-lag in older people: directional asymmetry. J Sleep Res 9:101–116, 2000.

35. Morin CM: Cognitive-behavioral approaches to the treatment of insomnia. J Clin Psychiatry 65(Suppl 16):33–40, 2004.

36. Muehlbach MJ, Walsh JK: The effects of caffeine on simulated night-shift work and subsequent daytime sleep. Sleep 18:22–29, 1995.

37. O'Connor PJ, Youngstedt SD: Influence of exercise on human sleep. Exerc Sport Sci Rev 23:105–134, 1995.

38. Oren DA, Wehr TA: Hypernyctohemeral syndrome after chronotherapy for delayed sleep phase syndrome. N Engl J Med 327(24):1762, 1992.

39. Paul MA, Gray G, Sardana TM, et al: Melatonin and zopiclone as facilitators of early circadian sleep in operational air transport crews. Aviat Space Environ Med 75:439–443, 2004.

40. Sack RL, Brandes RW, Kendall AR, et al: Entrainment of free-running circadian rhythms by melatonin in blind people. N Engl J Med 343:1070–1077, 2000.

41. Schibler U, Sassone-Corsi P: A web of circadian pacemakers. Cell 111:919–922, 2002.

42. Sforza E, Johannes M, Claudio B: The PAM-RL ambulatory device for detection of periodic leg movements: a validation study. Sleep Med 6:407–413, 2005.

43. Stoschitzky K, Sakotnik A, Lercher P, et al: Influence of beta-blockers on melatonin release. Eur J Clin Pharmacol 55:111–115, 1999.

44. Terman M, Lewy AJ, Dijk DJ, et al: Light treatment for sleep disorders: consensus report. IV. Sleep phase and duration disturbances. J Biol Rhythms 10:135–147, 1995.

45. Uchiyama M, Okawa M, Shibui K, et al: Poor compensatory function for sleep loss as a pathogenetic factor in patients with delayed sleep phase syndrome. Sleep 23:553–558, 2000.

46. Walsh JK, Randazzo AC, Stone KL, Schweitzer PK: Modafinil improves alertness, vigilance, and executive function during simulated night shifts. Sleep 27(3):434–439, 2004.

47. Weitzman ED: Chronobiology of man, sleep, temperature and neuroendocrine rhythms. Hum Neurobiol 1:173–183, 1982.

48. Winokur A, Sateia MJ, Hayes JB, et al: Acute effects of mirtazapine on sleep continuity and sleep architecture in depressed patients: a pilot study. Biol Psychiatry 48:75–78, 2000.

Electroencephalography

CARL W. BAZIL ■ GREGORY L. SAHLEM ■ DEREK J. CHONG

Questions

1. Brain activity recorded with electroencephalography (EEG) is commonly obscured by the following factors:
   A. Electrical activity from scalp electromyography
   B. Skull
   C. Distance between the brain region of interest and the electrodes
   D. Fluid surrounding the brain
   E. All of the above

2. Electrical activity recorded at the scalp arises from:
   A. Muscles of the scalp
   B. Extracellular currents generated by the postsynaptic potentials of neurons
   C. Eye movements
   D. Electrode "pops"
   E. All of the above

3. According to the 10–20 system of electrode naming, odd-numbered electrodes indicate which location?
   A. Temporal lobe
   B. Frontal lobe
   C. Occipital lobe
   D. Left hemisphere
   E. Right hemisphere

4. Electrode C_z is located where, according to the 10–20 system of electrode placement?
   A. Central on the left
   B. Central on the midline
   C. Central on the right
   D. Parietally on the left
   E. Parietally on the right

5. Respiratory artifact seen on EEG may be attenuated by:
   A. Increasing the high-frequency filter
   B. Decreasing the high-frequency filter
   C. Increasing the low-frequency filter
   D. Decreasing the low-frequency filter
   E. Adjusting the nasal thermistor

6. The following EEG frequencies are typically seen in a normal awake adult:
   A. Alpha and theta
   B. Theta and delta
   C. Alpha and beta
   D. Alpha, beta, and delta
   E. Alpha, beta, delta, and theta

7. The posterior dominant ("alpha") rhythm may be absent in a normal awake adult owing to:
   A. Eye opening
   B. Concentration
   C. Hand movement
   D. Eye opening or concentration
   E. Eye opening or hand movement

8. By applying the notch filter, you achieve the following desirable and undesirable outcomes:
   A. Desirable: 60 Hz interference is decreased in the recording.
      Undesirable: Other signals close to this frequency are slightly attenuated and can be difficult to see.
   B. Desirable: 60 Hz interference is removed from the recording.
      Undesirable: There are no undesirable outcomes. The notch filter should always be left on.
   C. Desirable: All inconsequential information is removed (as in viewing only the useful notch).
      Undesirable: There are no undesirable outcomes. The notch filter should always be left on.
   D. Desirable: All inconsequential information is removed (as in viewing only the useful notch).
      Undesirable: It is possible to miss important information found outside of the notch range.

9. A patient is described as having a seizure. After viewing the video and EEG (six channel) polysomnography (PSG) recording, a classically appearing tonic-clonic seizure is observed; however, there is

no electrographic evidence of the event. Which is the most likely explanation?

A. The electrographic correlate of the seizure was obscured by artifact.

B. The patient became disconnected during the seizure.

C. Some generalized seizures do not have an EEG correlate.

D. High-amplitude EEG activity during seizures frequently blocks the recording.

10. You observe a high-amplitude wave that has a morphology consistent with a spike in one electrode pairing. The activity in all adjacent electrodes appears to be normal. What is the most likely conclusion?

A. You are observing a spike that suggests a risk of epilepsy.

B. You are observing electrode "pop." If it were an epileptic spike, there would be an electrical field, and similar activity would also be seen (at lower amplitude) in adjacent electrodes.

C. This is likely a vertex wave.

D. There is not enough information here to decide.

11. If the low-frequency filter is set on 1 Hz and the high-frequency filter is set on 70 Hz, how will the signal be altered?

A. All signals with frequencies below 1 Hz and above 70 Hz will be completely removed from the recording.

B. Those signals with frequencies below 1 Hz and above 70 Hz will be attenuated gradually, starting at the set number.

C. Those signals with frequencies below 1 Hz and above 70 Hz will be attenuated gradually, starting below/above the set number.

D. Those signals with frequencies of 1 Hz and 70 Hz will be removed from the recording. All other signals will remain unaltered.

12. When running an EEG/PSG concurrently, what type of adhesive is most effective for keeping electrodes in place?

A. Colodian

B. Conductive paste

C. Most electrodes are needle type and hold themselves in place.

D. A and B

13. K-complexes and sleep spindle activity are best viewed by using what electrodes?

A. Central electrodes

B. Occipital electrodes

C. Frontal electrodes.

D. Temporal electrodes

14. The observed amplitude of EEG activity is influenced by which of the following?

A. The interelectrode difference

B. The amount of brain involved in the discharge

C. The skin and skull thickness

D. All of the above

15. What is the standard paper speed for reading EEG?

A. 10 mm/sec

B. 10 sec/page

C. 30 mm/sec

D. B and C

16. A signal is considered to be in the alpha range if:

A. It has a frequency of 8–12 Hz.

B. It has an amplitude that is larger than beta but smaller than gamma.

C. It is sinusoidal in nature.

D. None of the above

17. When referring to the amplitude, frequency, and morphology of waveforms, how do the right and left hemispheres compare to one another in a normal patient?

A. They appear symmetrical.

B. The dominant hemisphere is always at least twice the amplitude of the nondominant hemisphere.

C. It has not been well established. Sometimes they are symmetrical, and at other times they are not.

D. The nondominant hemisphere is always at least twice the amplitude of the dominant hemisphere.

18. If mu rhythm is observed, what action should be taken?

A. The attending physician should be notified so that the patient is admitted for treatment.

B. This is a benign waveform.

C. The duration and amplitude should be noted and should be emphasized in the report.

D. The term *mu* is outdated. What was once referred to as *mu* is now referred to as *spiky alpha*.

19. Polymorphic focal slowing is typically indicative of which of the following?

A. A structural lesion in that area

B. It is a normal feature of sleep.

C. An ongoing seizure

D. A and C

E. None of the above

20. Nocturnal epileptiform activity is seen least in which state?
    A. Rapid eye movement (REM) sleep
    B. Wakefulness
    C. Slow wave sleep
    D. Light non-REM (NREM) sleep

21. In what channels are eye movements most often seen?
    A. Fp1, Fp2, F7, and F8
    B. C3 and C4
    C. O1 and O2
    D. Eye movements are usually observed equally in all EEG channels.

Questions 22 and 23 refer to Figure 17-1, which shows an EEG in typical PSG montage shown at the top, with a portion of the identical epoch in the longitudinal bipolar EEG montage below.

22. Differences between a typical PSG montage and a longitudinal bipolar EEG montage include:
    A. Waveform amplitudes in the PSG montage may appear larger because of the greater interelectrode differences.
    B. The PSG montage allows for more discrete localization of cerebral discharges because a larger area of the brain is covered.
    C. The "paper speed" for typical EEG reading is slower, thus increasing the amount of seconds of recording per page.
    D. Reducing the high-frequency filter to 30 Hz will have greater effects on the typical PSG

reading speed and cause frequencies of activity to decrease.

23. According to the EEG recording, which of the following is true about the patient?
    A. The patient is having a generalized seizure.
    B. There are abundant epileptiform discharges, but no evolution; therefore this is not a seizure.
    C. The patient is in stage 1 sleep.
    D. The patient is awake and alert.

Questions 24 and 25 refer to Figure 17-2, which shows an epoch in a typical PSG montage shown at the top, with the middle of the epoch shown in longitudinal bipolar montage below. A number of events are indicated.

24. The arrowhead is pointing to:
    A. Muscle artifact
    B. Focal beta activity starting in the right frontal region that is spreading in field, evolving in frequency and increasing in amplitude to meet criteria for a seizure
    C. Focal beta activity starting in the right anterior temporal region that is spreading in field, evolving in frequency and increasing in amplitude to meet criteria for a seizure
    D. Nystagmus

25. The large, dark arrows are pointing to:
    A. Focal spikes and spike-wave discharges
    B. Vertex waves
    C. "Pop" artifact
    D. None of the above

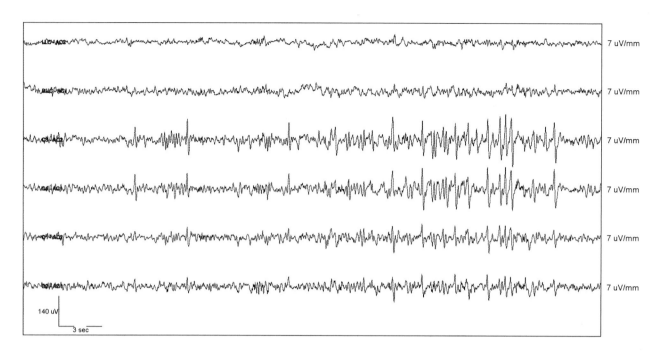

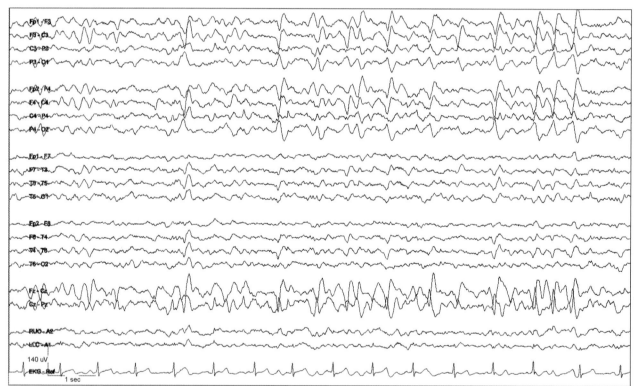

FIGURE 17-1 ■ An EEG in typical PSG montage is shown at the top, with a portion of the identical epoch in the longitudinal bipolar EEG montage below (for Questions 22 and 23).

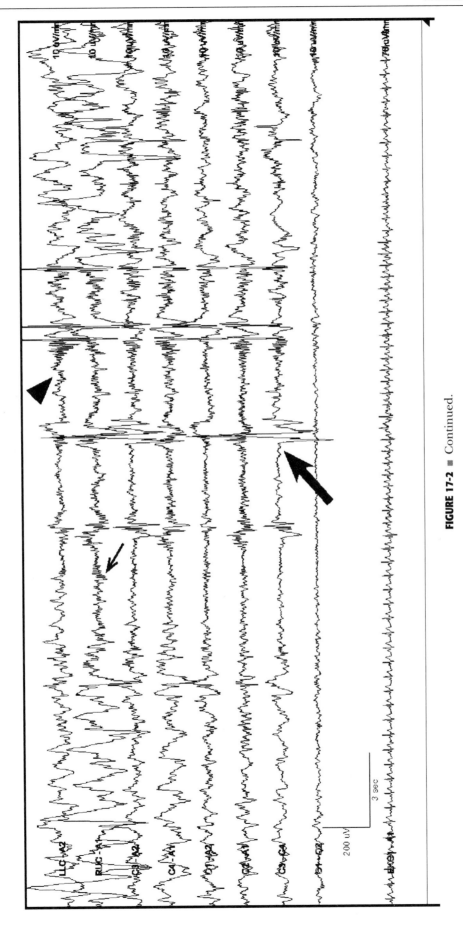

FIGURE 17-2 ■ Continued.

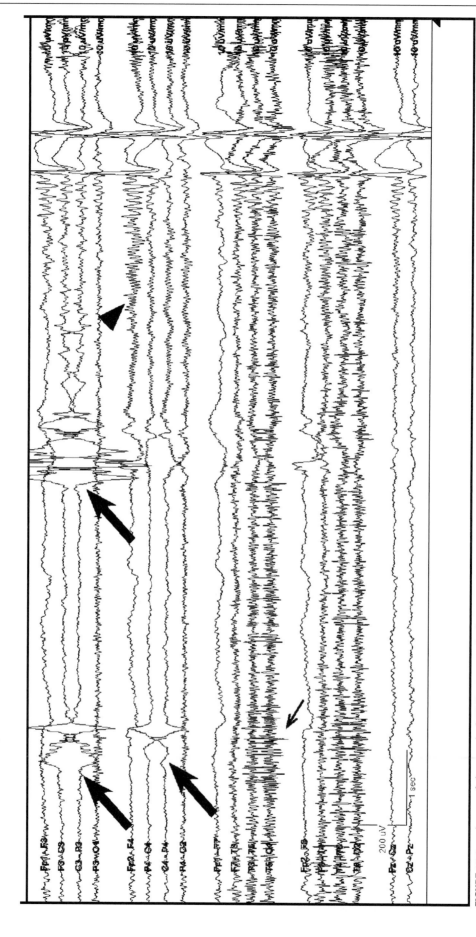

FIGURE 17-2 ■ An epoch in a typical PSG montage is shown at the top, with the middle of the epoch shown in longitudinal bipolar montage below. A number of events are indicated (for Questions 24 and 25).

Answers

1. E. All of the above

(Answers for questions 1 and 2 are combined.)

2. E. All of the above

The brain activity recorded by EEG is thought to arise from neuronal postsynaptic potentials, but there are many other potential sources of electrical activity recorded from the scalp. One common source is electromyography (EMG) from head muscles. Activity from temporalis and masseter muscles is most prominent in the temporal regions, and swallowing causes "glossokinetic" artifact arising from the tongue and muscles of the throat, which has a wide distribution. Eye movements also create electrical potentials (because of the electrical polarity of the cornea versus the retina), and small potentials can be seen from eye muscles (particularly the lateral rectus, typically causing a sharp potential in the temporal electrodes). The electrical activity generated by the heart is also seen on EEG; for this reason an electrocardiogram is usually recorded to distinguish this from brain. Electrical artifact localized to a single electrode is commonly called a "pop." In fact, any machinery or body organ that has electrical potential can appear on the EEG.

Conversely, any structure between the electrodes and the brain has the potential to attenuate brain electrical activity. Under normal conditions this occurs with scalp, skull, and cerebrospinal fluid. If there is an abnormal fluid collection (such as a subdural hematoma) or structure (as in a tumor or abscess), however, these can further attenuate brain activity.

3. D. Left hemisphere

(Answers for questions 3 and 4 are combined.)

4. B. Central in the midline

Electrodes for the measurement of EEG are named by a letter and (usually) a number. The letter indicates the brain region closest to the electrode (F, frontal; T, temporal; C, central; P, parietal; O, occipital). The numbers used are even on the right and odd on the left. Electrodes along the midline are labeled with a Z rather than a number. This system allows uniformity of electrode placement across a large variety of head sizes.

5. C. Increasing the low-frequency filter

Filters are used in EEG to reduce or eliminate unwanted signals while preserving the signals of interest (EEG activity). Breathing artifact is typically produced by movement of the electrodes during breathing. It is typically under 0.5 Hz (except in young infants);

therefore filtering frequencies below this frequency will attenuate the artifact. This is well below the range of most cerebral activity. An increase in the low-frequency filter is therefore indicated.

6. C. Alpha and beta

In a normal adult, faster-frequency activity predominates during wakefulness. There should be little or no theta (4–8 Hz) activity and no delta (1 < 4 Hz) activity. As drowsiness begins, theta activity will be seen and faster frequencies will decrease. No delta activity should be seen in a normal adult unless asleep.

7. D. Eye opening or concentration

The posterior dominant rhythm may be attenuated by either concentration or eye opening. It is best seen in a normal adult during a quiet, resting awake state with eyes closed. Decreased posterior dominant rhythm is one of the indicators of stage 1 sleep, where no more than 50% of the record can be occupied by this activity. Hand movement (or simply thinking about hand movement) attenuates mu activity, another normal rhythm that occurs during wakefulness.

8. A. Desirable: 60 Hz interference is decreased in the recording.

Undesirable: Other signals close to this frequency are slightly attenuated and can be difficult to see. The notch filter is designed to sharply attenuate power line interference, predominantly 60 Hz in North America. Although the notch filter is very effective in removing waveforms that have a frequency of 60 Hz, it also has the undesirable effect of altering the appearance of other waveforms. In particular, muscle activity can look like alpha frequency brain activity, and dislodged electrodes can appear to be recording properly.

9. A. The electrographic correlate of the seizure was obscured by artifact.

Muscle and movement artifact frequently obscures any electrographic correlate to a tonic-clonic seizure. In this case, a highly focal onset may have been seen with a complete EEG. Although some simple partial seizures have no EEG correlate, virtually all seizures with alteration of consciousness will show a change in brain activity provided the recording is not obscured. The activity during a seizure is not of sufficient amplitude in itself to obscure the recording; however, the gain may need to be decreased to view optimally.

10. B. You are observing electrode "pop." If it were an epileptic spike, there would be an electrical field and similar activity would also be seen (at lower amplitude) in adjacent electrodes.

Potentials that are isolated to a single electrode pairing are generally not cortical in nature. These are most commonly electrode artifact; this can be caused by interference with the connection between the electrode and the scalp and could indicate a poorly applied electrode. Any activity arising from the brain (including vertex waves) typically has a "field," meaning that it is also visible at lower amplitude in adjacent electrodes.

11. B. Those signals with frequencies below 1 Hz and above 70 Hz will be attenuated gradually, starting at the set number.

Filters act to gradually attenuate frequencies. Waveforms with frequencies at the filter setting are typically attenuated between 30% and 40% depending on the type of filter used. As the frequency diverges from the setting, attenuation is greater.

12. A. Colodian

Colodian is the most reliable method of holding a large number of electrodes in place for long periods of time (as in overnight). Although conductive paste can be used with careful wrapping, one or more electrodes are likely to become dislodged during the recording and result in the need to disturb the patient in order to reapply. Needle electrodes are rarely used because of the risk of infection transmission.

13. A. Central electrodes

The correct answer is A. Both K-complexes and sleep spindles have maximal amplitude at the vertex of the brain and therefore are best seen in channels using central leads. The alpha (posterior dominant) rhythm is important in distinguishing wakefulness and stage 1 sleep; it is best seen at the occipital electrodes (posteriorly). Frontal and temporal electrodes are less important in sleep staging and therefore are often not used in routine PSG.

14. D. All of the above

Each of the factors contribute to the recorded signal's amplitude. Larger interelectrode differences potentially magnify the difference in electrical potential measured on EEG. The amplitude of a given waveform on EEG is also related to the amount of brain tissue involved; a larger area (and therefore a larger number of neurons) will result in a higher amplitude, assuming the group of neurons is firing synchronously. Any substance between the structure producing the discharge (the brain) and the recording electrodes can attenuate the observed amplitude, including skin, skull, cerebrospinal fluid, and abnormal fluid collections such as a subdural hematoma.

15. D. B and C (B. 10 sec/page; C. 30 mm/sec)

If the paper is moving 30 mm every second, it will take 10 seconds to cover a page; this is standard for reading EEG. In most laboratories, however, "paper" is not used and the "page" consists of a single screen on the computer; 10 mm/sec is commonly used for reading PSG, resulting in 30 seconds per "page" (or screen).

16. A. It has a frequency of 8–12 Hz.

Waveform classifications are divided by frequency, not by amplitude. Although background waveforms are sinusoidal, this is not required. A waveform is said to be in the alpha range if the frequency is between 8 and 13 cycles per second. Beta frequency is faster than 13 Hz, theta is 4–8 Hz, and delta is slower than 4 Hz.

17. A. They appear symmetrical.

Although there may be some slight difference in amplitude, homologous regions should have similar amplitude, frequency, and morphology. Differences of more than 50% in the amplitude of a given frequency suggest an abnormality. The most common are fluid collection (such as a subdural hematoma), decreasing the amplitude on the affected side, or a skull defect, increasing the frequency. Both of these affect faster frequencies more than slower frequencies. Lesions of the brain, including tumors and strokes, will also affect amplitude and frequency of waveforms. Subcortical lesions typically cause increased slow activity on the affected side, whereas cortical abnormalities attenuate the amplitude of faster frequencies.

18. B. This is a benign waveform.

Mu is a normal waveform that is commonly seen in relaxed drowsy individuals. This can sometimes appear sharp and rhythmic and thus potentially confused with a seizure discharge. The best way to ensure that an observed rhythm is actually mu is by asking the individual to move one of his or her opposite sided limbs; this will attenuate mu (but not seizure activity).

19. A. A structural lesion in that area

Focal slow activity most likely results from a disruption in the normal thalamocortical projections in the involved region. Common etiologies include tumor, stroke, and abscess. Although structural lesions may increase the chance of seizure, focal slowing does not indicate ongoing seizure activity. Electrographically, a seizure is manifest by a rhythmic discharge that can be regional or generalized and represents large groups of neurons firing synchronously. Epileptic seizure activity is also stereotyped rather than polymorphic. Although slow activity is a manifestation of normal sleep, particularly stages 3 and 4, normal slow activity seen during sleep is diffuse rather than limited to a single region.

20. A. REM sleep

Seizure activity is most commonly seen during transitions between different stages of NREM sleep. There is rarely seizure activity found within REM sleep. Interictal epileptiform discharges are more commonly seen during NREM sleep but also are rare during REM. The reasons for this are unknown, although in theory the overall synchronization seen during NREM sleep makes it easier for seizures to begin and propagate.

21. A. Fp1, Fp2, F7, and F8

Each of these electrodes is close to the eye. Eye potentials are recordable owing to the cornea's relative electronegativity with respect to the retina. Centrally and occipitally placed electrodes are too far away from this potential difference to record it.

22. A. Waveform amplitudes in the PSG montage may appear larger because of the greater interelectrode differences.

The amplitude of brain activity (on PSG or EEG) is dependent on the amount of cortical activity, the distance from the cortex, the amount and properties of the material between the cortex and electrodes, and the difference in the voltage of the two channels being compared. The farther apart the electrodes, the more dissimilar the electrical activity in the underlying brain, which often translates to greater amplitudes. The fewer the electrodes, the wider the distances, increasing the amplitudes but decreasing the ability to localize the discharges. Paper speed refers to pre-digital recordings, where a slower paper speed under the pens would actually compress the study, allowing more seconds per page; by this measure the paper speed is slower for PSG than for standard EEG. Filter settings will change the appearance of the waveforms but not actually change their frequency; 12 Hz will remain 12 Hz.

23. C. The patient is in stage 1 sleep.

The tracing demonstrates classic vertex waves, with phase reversals seen maximally at the vertex. On the typical PSG recording (above), the very sharply contoured waves are best seen with the C3 and C4 electrodes referenced to the contralateral ears. Vertex and sleep activity in general is best seen on the EEG longitudinal bipolar (below) at central leads Fz-Cz, but also phase-reversing at C3-P3 and C4-P4. Repetitive vertex waves, as in this case, is a normal phenomenon in stage 1 sleep, particularly in the pediatric population, but can be mistakenly identified as epileptiform activity.

24. B. Focal beta activity starting in the right frontal region that is spreading in field, evolving in frequency and increasing in amplitude to meet criteria for a seizure

The arrowhead is at the midpoint of an evolving seizure. It is composed of an evolving, well-regulated beta frequency that meets all criteria for a seizure, initially focal and seen best at the right frontal region, with spread of the beta to the ipsilateral temporal region and contralateral hemisphere as the frequency slows before abruptly turning into a large-amplitude spike. This type of EEG pattern is characteristic of frontal lobe epilepsy with an underlying lesion or dysplastic region of cerebral cortex. Muscle artifact is typically not so uniform in frequency (unless a filter is applied) and should not evolve so clearly (see small arrows indicating temporalis muscle activation). On the PSG, the seizure could be overlooked as an arousal. In retrospect, the seizure appears maximal at the LLC-A2 channel, likely for two reasons: LLC is completely uninvolved, thus the difference between A2 (where the seizure evolves to late) and LLC is most pronounced, and the distance between the two electrodes is far. There is no coverage of the frontal lobes in a typical PSG, which argues for a full 10–20 EEG hookup if nocturnal epilepsy is in the differential diagnosis. Nystagmus is picked up best in the eye channels but should be seen as out-of-phase lateral eye movements. It can also be seen commonly at FP1, FP2, F7, and F8—all close to the eyes.

25. C. "Pop" artifact

The disturbance is due to poor electrode contact with the scalp, termed *electrode "pop" artifact*. The large-amplitude disturbances are seen best at C3 and somewhat at C4, but there is not a sensible field to the discharge to believe they are of cerebral origin. These particularly large-amplitude deflections did not cause a "ripple" effect; P3 and F3 should be involved secondarily with smaller amplitude deflections. This so-called field is seen with most discharges of cerebral origin, including both epileptiform discharges and sleep architecture. Also, although vertex waves are typically seen well at C3 and C4, in this recording they are conspicuously absent in the central channels, Fz or Cz. Both vertex waves and epileptiform discharges are also usually negative in polarity, but these deflections are not.

REFERENCES

1. Bazil CW, Malow BA: Sleep and epilepsy. In Guilleminault C (ed): *Clinical Neurophysiology of Sleep Disorders*, vol 6. New York, Elsevier, 2005, pp 281–291.

2. Bazil CW, Herman ST, Pedley TA: Focal electroencephalographic abnormalities. In Ebersole JS, Pedley TA (eds): *Current Practice of Clinical Electroencephalography*, 3rd ed. Philadelphia, Lippincott, Williams & Wilkins, 2003, pp 303–347.

3. Ebersole JS, Pedley TA (eds): *Current Practice of Clinical Electroencephalography*, 3rd ed. Philadelphia, Lippincott, Williams & Wilkins, 2003.

4. Fisch BJ: *Fisch and Spehlmann's EEG Primer*, 3rd ed. St Louis, Elsevier, 1999.

5. Kellaway P: Orderly approach to visual analysis: elements of the normal EEG and their characteristics in children and adults. In Ebersole JS, Pedley TA (eds): *Current Practice of Clinical Electroencephalography*, 3rd ed. Philadelphia, Lippincott, Williams & Wilkins, 2003, pp 100–159.

6. Olejniczak P: Neurophysiologic basis of EEG. J Clin Neurophysiol 23(3):186–189, 2006.

7. Pedley TA, Mendiratta A, Walczak TS: Seizures and epilepsy. In Ebersole JS, Pedley TA (eds): *Current Practice of Clinical Electroencephalography*, 3rd ed. Philadelphia, Lippincott, Williams & Wilkins, 2003, pp 506–587.

8. Rowan AJ, Tolunksy E: *Primer of EEG with a Mini-Atlas*. Philadelphia, Butterworth-Heinemann, 2003.

9. Tatum WO, Husain AM, Benbadis SR, Kaplan PW: Normal adult EEG and patterns of uncertain significance. J Clin Neurophysiol 23(3):194–207, 2006.

10. Westmoreland BF: Benign electroencephalographic variants and patterns of uncertain clinical significance. In Ebersole JS, Pedley TA (eds): *Current Practice of Clinical Electroencephalography*, 3rd ed. Philadelphia, Lippincott, Williams & Wilkins, 2003, pp 235–245.

Artifacts

JUDITH WIEBELHAUS ■ ALON Y. AVIDAN

Questions

1. A 26-year-old male with an apnea-hypopnea index (AHI) of 83 events per hour returns to the sleep laboratory for a continuous positive airway pressure (CPAP) titration. At the start of the recording, the technician notes artifact in the occipital leads. The technician replaces the electrodes even though the impedances on the leads were recorded as <5000 ohms. The technician elects to start the recording and later notes that the artifact is no longer in the occipital region but has now migrated to the C4 electrode. What is the artifact in Figures 18-1A and 18-1B and the most likely cause?
   A. Muscle artifact caused from the pressure of the patient lying on the electrodes
   B. 60 Hz artifact caused from a poorly prepped ground electrode
   C. 60 Hz artifact caused by environmental electrical interference
   D. Muscle artifact due to the patient's apprehension of wearing CPAP

2. A 58-year-old male presented for a diagnostic polysomnogram (PSG) for the evaluation of possible sleep apnea. The patient also complained of insomnia, which coincided with the death of a family member. What is the activity noted in the electroencephalographic (EEG) channels in Figures 18-2A and 18-2B?
   A. 60 HZ artifact
   B. Bruxism
   C. Muscle artifact in the A1 electrode
   D. Alpha intrusion

3. A 73-year-old male came to the sleep laboratory for a diagnostic PSG after an uvulopalatopharyngoplasty procedure. The patient was diagnosed with severe obstructive apnea 3 years ago. He was noncompliant to CPAP treatment. What best describes the cause of the artifact seen highlighted by the box in Figure 18-3?
   A. Movement artifact
   B. Respiratory artifact
   C. Muscle artifact
   D. Electrode "pop" artifact

4. Figure 18-4 is an example taken from a PSG of a 47-year-old female who presented with episodes of gasping arousals at night. The technician notes the activity indicated by the black arrows. What can be done to eliminate this activity?
   A. Replace the nasal cannula.
   B. It is a physiologic artifact, so it only needs to be monitored.
   C. Change the low pass filter.
   D. Engage the notch filter.

5. All of the following are true about the artifact noted in the C4-A1 electrode in Figure 18-5A, *except*:
   A. Respiratory artifact
   B. Electrode "popping" artifact
   C. Physiologic artifact
   D. Environmental artifact

6. A 43-year-old woman with a history of obstructive sleep apnea and coronary artery disease comes to the sleep laboratory for a follow-up evaluation using an oral appliance. While evaluating the electrocardiogram, the sleep fellow notes what appears to be an extra cardiac cycle. Please identify the cause of the activity indicated by the arrows in Figure 18-6.
   A. Electrode "pop"
   B. Pacemaker artifact
   C. Poor electrode application
   D. Bi-metallic artifact

7. On arrival to the sleep laboratory, a 27-year-old patient with a complaint of excessive daytime sleepiness indicates she is very anxious about her

Text continued on p. 341

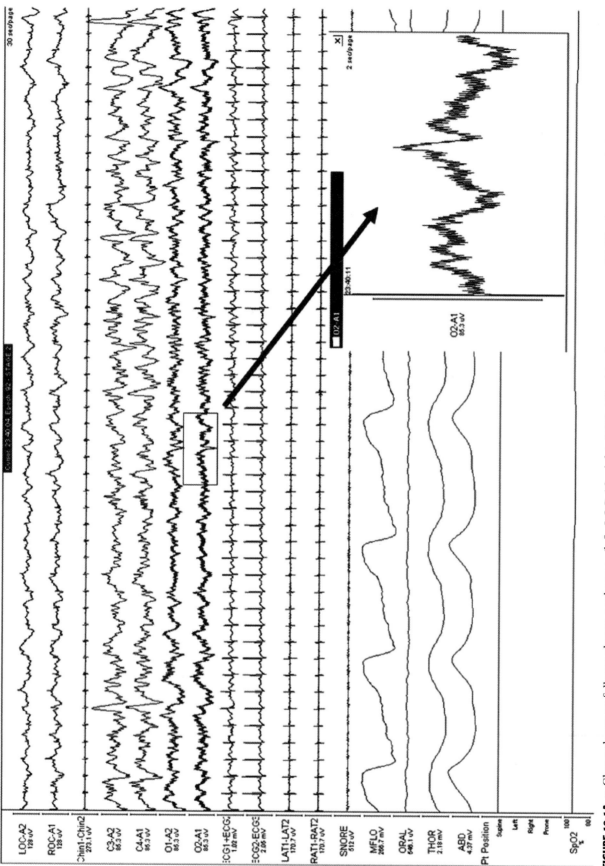

FIGURE 18-1A ■ Channels are as follows: electro-oculogram (left: LOC-A2, right: ROC-A1), chin electromyogram (EMG), electroencephalogram (left central, right central, left occipital, right occipital), two ECG channels, left and right limb EMG, snore channel, mask flow (MFLO), oral airflow, respiratory effort (thoracic, abdominal), position, and oxygen saturation (SpO2).

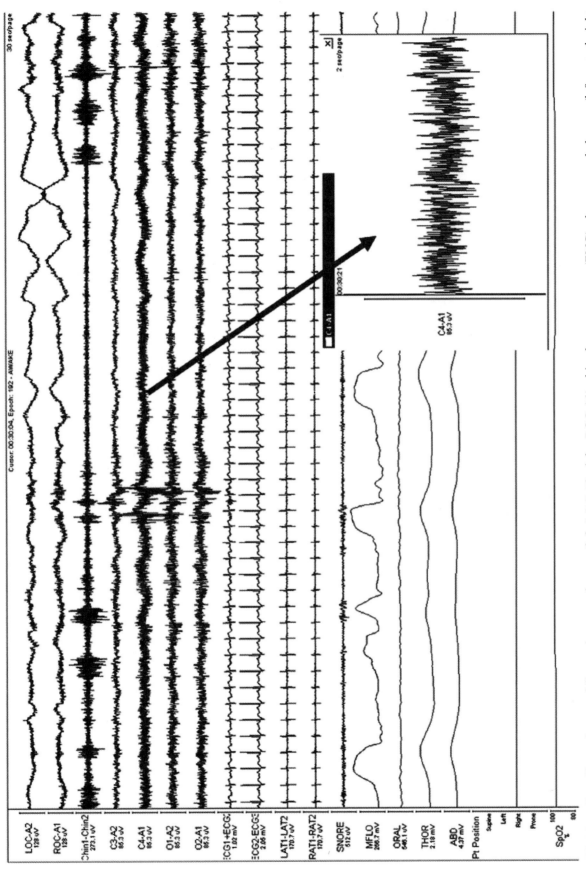

FIGURE 18-1B ■ Channels are as follows: electro-oculogram (left: LOC-A2, right: ROC-A1), chin electromyogram (EMG), electroencephalogram (left central, right central, left occipital, right occipital), two ECG channels, left and right limb EMG, snore channel, mask flow (MFLO), oral airflow, respiratory effort (thoracic, abdominal), position, and oxygen saturation (SpO₂).

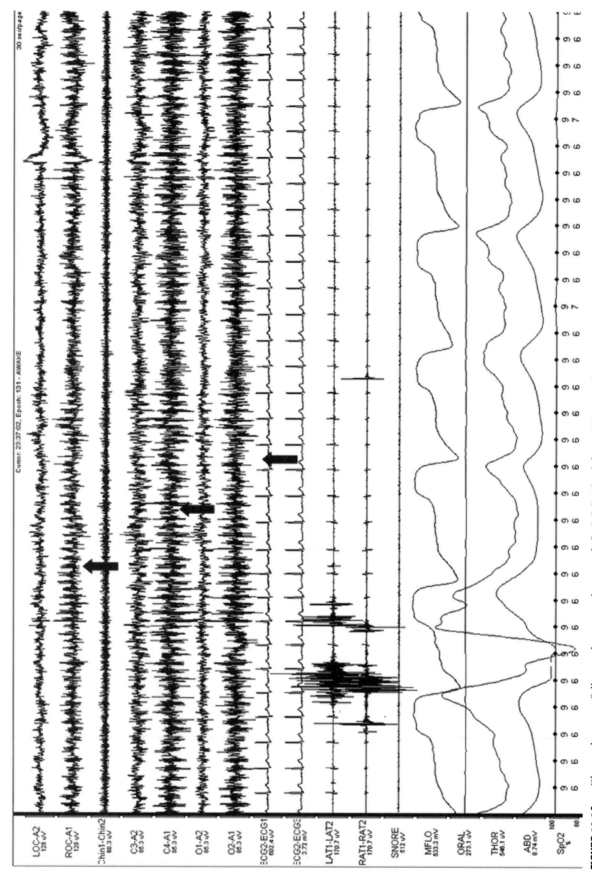

FIGURE 18-2A ■ Channels are as follows: electro-oculogram (left: LOC-A2, right: ROC-A1), chin electromyogram (EMG), electroencephalogram (left central, right central, right occipital, left occipital, right occipital), two ECG channels, left and right limb EMG, snore channel, mask flow (MFLO), oral airflow, respiratory effort (thoracic, abdominal), and oxygen saturation (SpO$_2$).

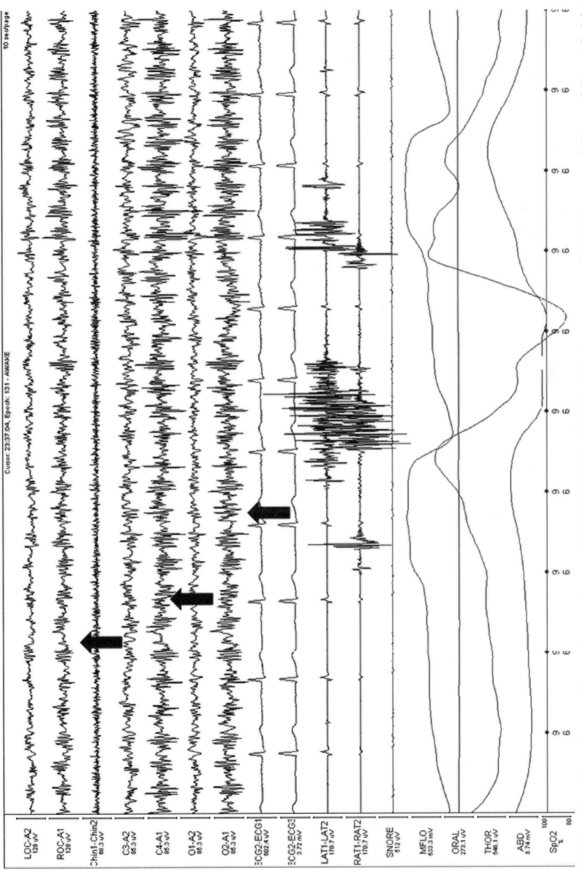

FIGURE 18-2B ■ Channels are as follows: electro-oculogram (left: LOC-A2, right: ROC-A1), chin electromyogram (EMG), electroencephalogram (left central, right central, left occipital, right occipital), two ECG channels, left and right limb EMG, snore channel, mask flow (MFLO), oral airflow, respiratory effort (thoracic, abdominal), and oxygen saturation (SpO₂).

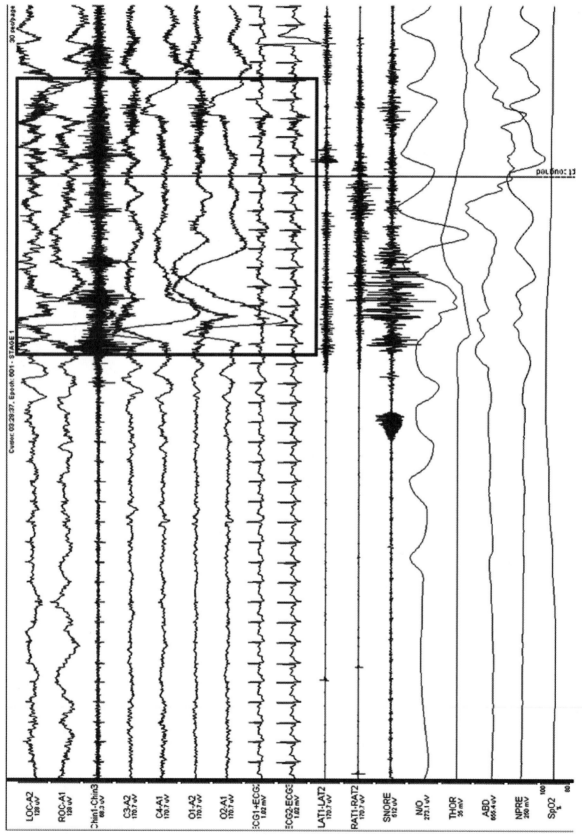

FIGURE 18-3 ▪ Channels are as follows: electro-oculogram (left: LOC-A2, right: ROC-A1), chin electromyogram (EMG), electroencephalogram (left central, right central, left occipital, right occipital), two ECG channels, left and right limb EMG, snore channel, nasal-oral airflow (N/O), respiratory effort (thoracic, abdominal), nasal pressure (NPRE), and oxygen saturation (SpO₂).

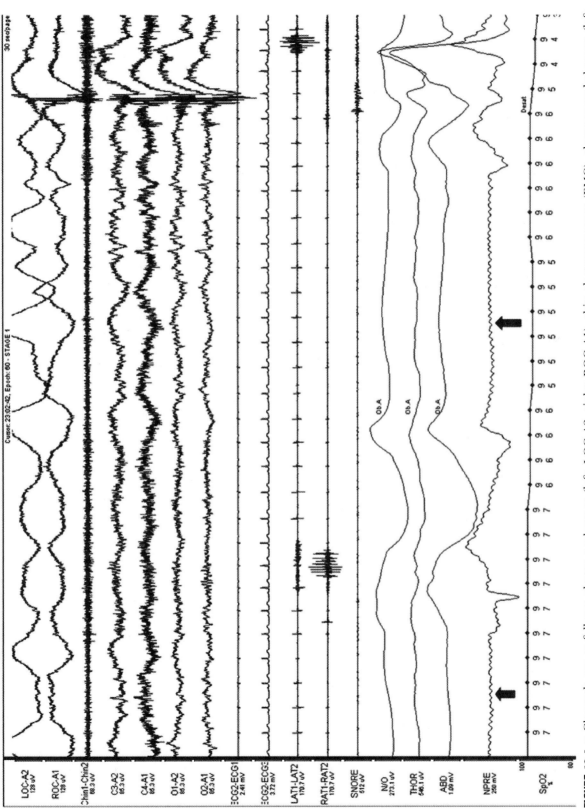

FIGURE 18-4 ■ Channels are as follows: electro-oculogram (left: LOC-A2, right: ROC-A1), chin electromyogram (EMG), electroencephalogram (left central, right central, left occipital, right occipital), two ECG channels, left and right limb EMG, snore channel, nasal-oral airflow (N/O), respiratory effort (thoracic, abdominal), nasal pressure (NPRE), and oxygen saturation (SpO₂).

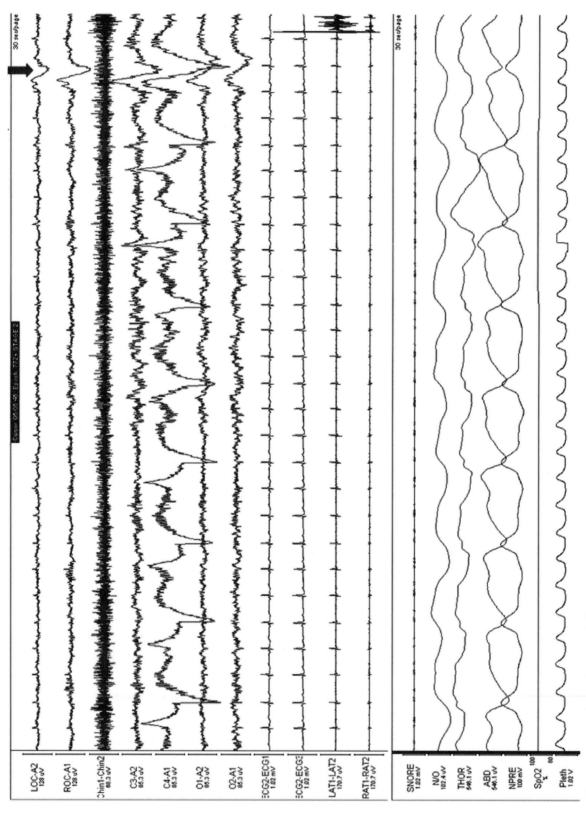

FIGURE 18-5A ■ Channels are as follows: electro-oculogram (left: LOC-A2, right: ROC-A1), chin electromyogram (EMG), electroencephalogram (left central, right central, left occipital, right occipital, two ECG channels, left and right limb EMG, snore channel, nasal-oral airflow (N/O), respiratory effort (thoracic, abdominal), nasal pressure (NPRE), oxygen saturation (SpO₂), and pleth waveform.

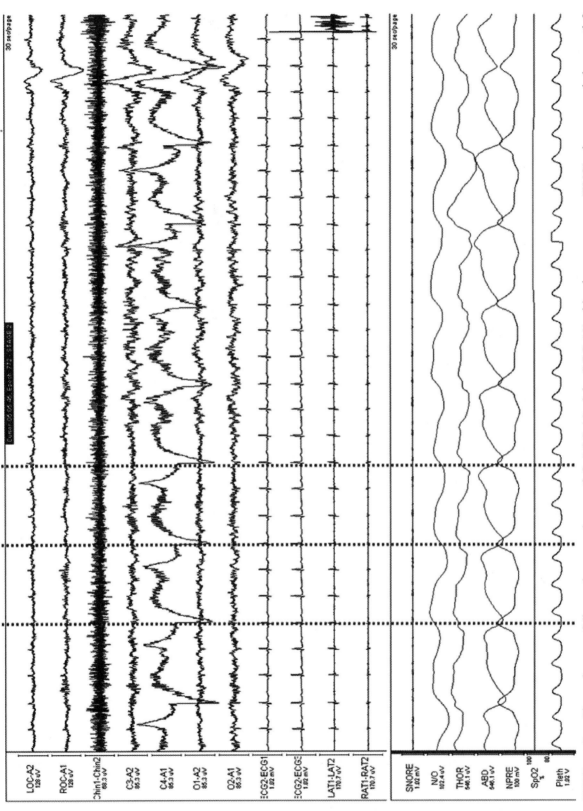

FIGURE 18-5B ■ Channels are as follows: electro-oculogram (left: LOC-A2, right: ROC-A1), chin electromyogram (EMG), electroencephalogram (left central, right central, left occipital, right occipital), two ECG channels, left and right limb EMG, snore channel, nasal-oral airflow (N/O), respiratory effort (thoracic, abdominal), nasal pressure (NPRE), oxygen saturation (SpO₂), and pleth waveform.

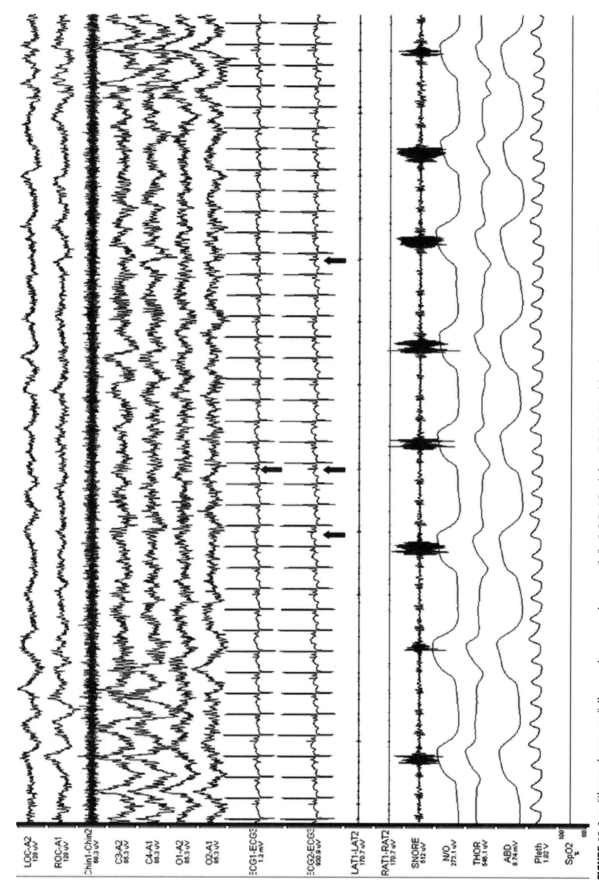

FIGURE 18-6 ■ Channels are as follows: electro-oculogram (left: LOC-A2, right: ROC-A1), chin electromyogram (EMG), electroencephalogram (left central, right central, left occipital, right occipital), two ECG channels, left and right limb EMG, snore channel, nasal-oral airflow (N/O), respiratory effort (thoracic, abdominal), oxygen saturation (SpO₂), and pleth waveform.

LOC-A2
128 uV

ROC-A1
128 uV

Chin1-Chin2
68.3 uV

C3-A2
85.3 uV

C4-A1
85.3 uV

O1-A2
85.3 uV

O2-A1
85.3 uV

ECG1-ECG
1.2 mV

ECG2-ECG
930.9 uV

LAT1-LAT2
170.7 uV

RAT1-RAT2
170.7 uV

SNORE
512 uV

N/O
273.1 uV

THOR
646.1 uV

ABD
8.74 mV

Pleth
1.02 V

SpO2
%

sleep study. In fact, her sleep latency was 2.6 hrs. What is the possible cause of the artifact indicated by arrows in Figure 18-7?
- A. Movement artifact from the patient getting settled
- B. Muscle artifact resulting from the patient's anxiety
- C. Chewing artifact from the patient's eating
- D. 60 Hz resulting from a bad ground lead

8. A 36-year-old male patient comes for an evaluation of loud snoring and witnessed apneas. The sleep technologists' summary of the night indicates they had to enter the patient's room several times to apply a cooling fan in an attempt to correct sweat artifact. The next day, the reviewing sleep fellow noted "an erratic nasal/oral signal." What is the most probable cause for the nasal/oral (N/O) signal disruption (underlined dotted line) in Figure 18-8?
- A. The thermocouple signal is not being displayed at the correct sensitivity.
- B. The thermocouple is not picking up necessary temperature changes.
- C. The thermocouple is displaying flow limitation resulting from snoring.
- D. The thermocouple is malfunctioning as a result of a loose connection.

9. A 55-year-old male patient with a history of restless legs syndrome presents for a diagnostic PSG because of concerns that he may also have sleep-disordered breathing. During the recording, the supervising technologist observes continuous high-amplitude deflections appearing in the chin electromyogram (EMG). What would be the next step in troubleshooting the origin of the signal (arrowheads) in Figure 18-9?
- A. Monitor and document the patient's activity until next arousal.
- B. Change the chin EMG configuration if additional input derivations are available.
- C. Apply additional EMG leads at the temporomandibular angle.
- D. Replace the chin EMG electrodes.

10. A 48-year-old female returns to the sleep laboratory for a CPAP titration. Her baseline PSG revealed obstructive sleep apnea with a respiratory disturbance index of 66.5 episodes per hour associated with oxygen desaturations down to the seventieth percentile. What is the artifact denoted by stars in Figure 18-10?
- A. Sweat artifact
- B. Respiratory artifact
- C. Ocular artifact
- D. Movement artifact

11. While reviewing the CPAP titration on a 30-year-old male patient with an unremarkable past medical history of obstructive sleep apnea, the sleep fellow notes a distinct difference in the amplitude of the central leads compared with the occipital leads. The fellow verifies that C3 and C4 leads are in the appropriate locations via video. What is the *least* likely explanation for the amplitude difference highlighted in the box shown in Figure 18-11?
- A. The leads associated with the software configuration for "averaging" are referenced incorrectly.
- B. A salt bridge has formed between C3, C4, and the reference lead.
- C. The ground lead is either faulty or detached from the patient's scalp.
- D. The sensitivity is decreased in the central leads.

12. An 18-year-old female comes to the sleep laboratory with the complaint of excessive daytime sleepiness and frequent nocturnal awakenings. What is the best explanation of the signal denoted by the arrows in Figure 18-12?
- A. A chemical reaction in the conductive gel of the electrode cup
- B. Movement of the electrode due to inhalation and exhalation
- C. A faulty electrode making intermittent contact with the scalp
- D. A correlating electrical potential change resulting from sucking

13. A 30-year-old male presents for a PSG to evaluate complaints of sleepiness and witnessed apnea. How would the artifact shown in Figure 18-13 (arrowheads) be corrected?
- A. "Jump" or average leads A1 and A2.
- B. Adjust the frequency filters.
- C. Reattach electrode at next arousal.
- D. Cool down the patient.

14. An 80-year-old male patient with complaints of frequent nocturnal awakenings presents for a sleep evaluation. An example from his PSG is displayed in Figure 18-14. What is the best description of the artifact illustrated between the two stars noted in the figure?
- A. Physiologic artifact
- B. Environmental artifact
- C. Instrumental artifact
- D. Noise artifact

15. A 40-year-old obese male returns to the sleep laboratory for a reevaluation of his CPAP. While reviewing the PSG, the sleep fellow notes the

Text continued on p. 350

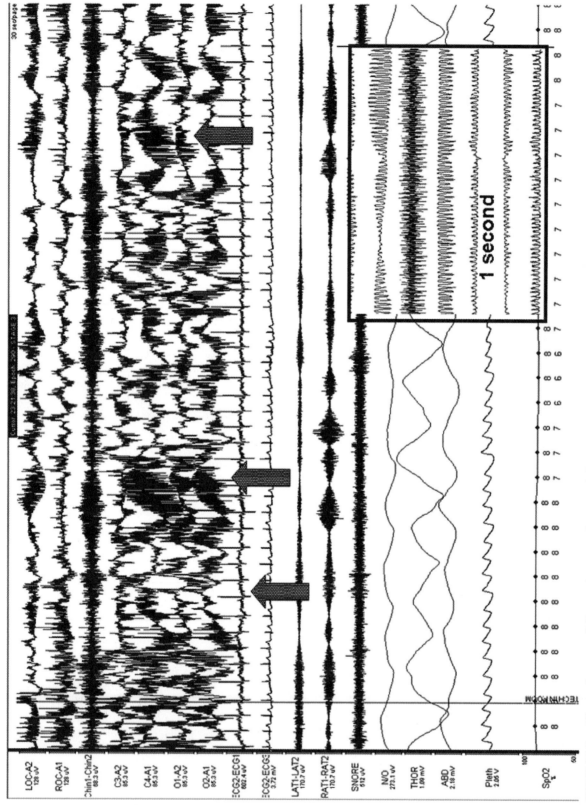

FIGURE 18-7 ■ Channels are as follows: electro-oculogram (left: LOC-A2, right: ROC-A1), chin electromyogram (EMG), electroencephalogram (left central, right central, left occipital, right occipital), two ECG channels, left and right limb EMG, snore channel, nasal-oral airflow (N/O), respiratory effort (thoracic, abdominal), oxygen saturation (SpO₂), and pleth waveform.

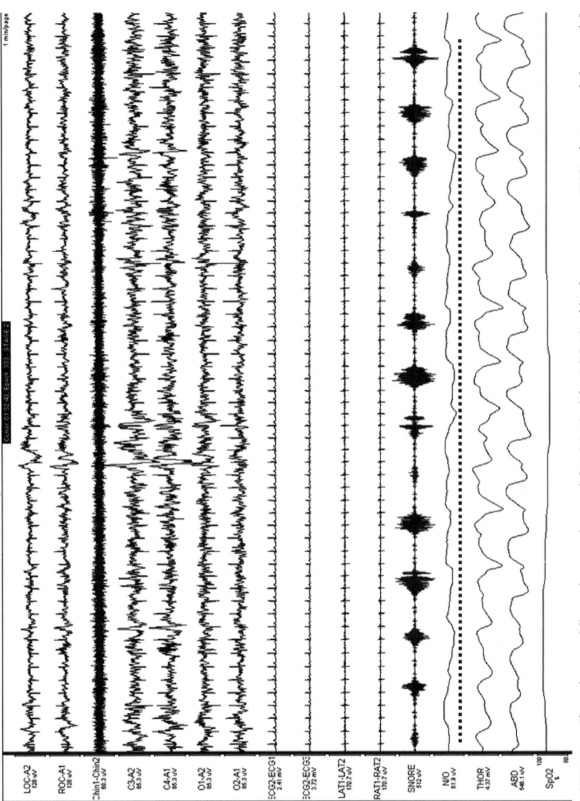

FIGURE 18-8 ■ Channels are as follows: electro-oculogram (left: LOC-A2, right: ROC-A1), chin electromyogram (EMG), electroencephalogram (left central, right central, left occipital, right occipital), two ECG channels, left and right limb EMG, snore channel, nasal-oral airflow (N/O), respiratory effort (thoracic, abdominal), and oxygen saturation (SpO₂).

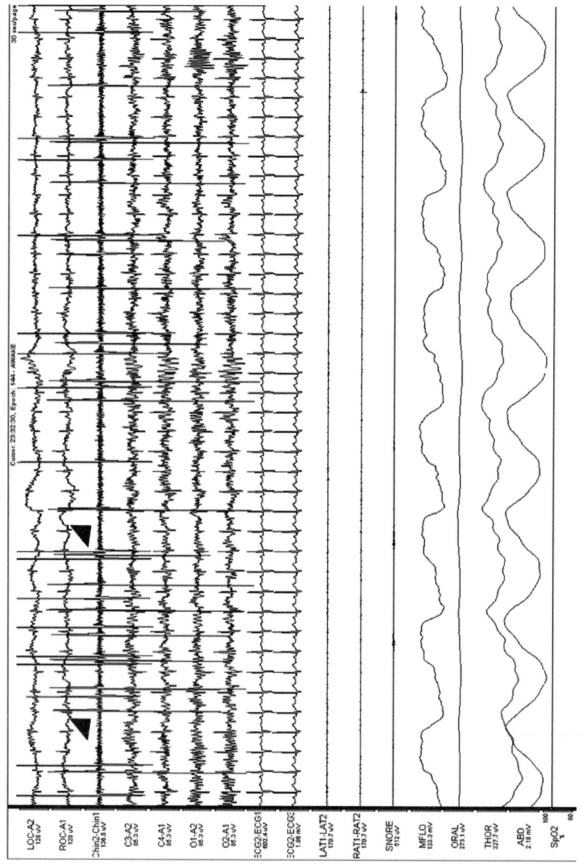

FIGURE 18-9 ■ Channels are as follows: electro-oculogram (left: LOC-A2, right: ROC-A1), chin electromyogram (EMG), electroencephalogram (left central, right central, left occipital, right occipital), two ECG channels, left and right limb EMG, snore channel, mask flow (MFLO), oral airflow, respiratory effort (thoracic, abdominal), and oxygen saturation (SpO2).

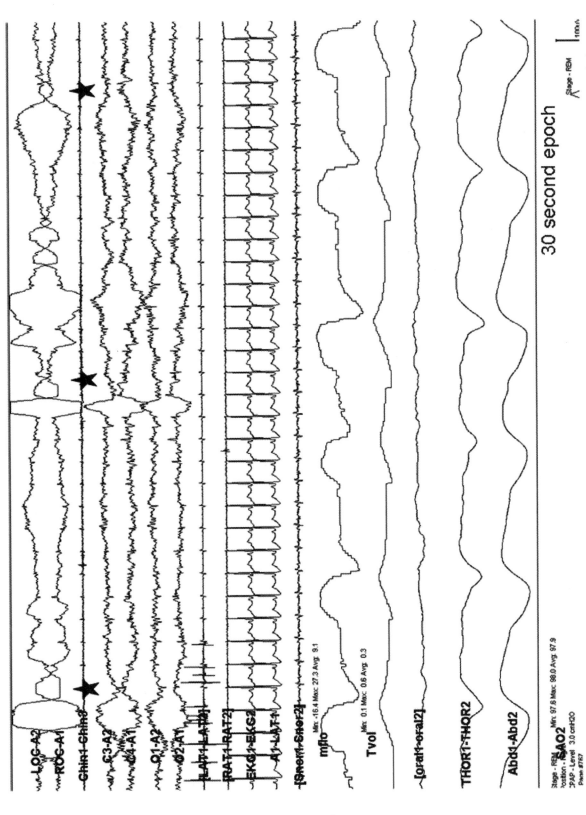

FIGURE 18-10 ■ Channels are as follows: electro-oculogram (left: LOC-A2, right: ROC-A1), chin electromyogram (EMG), electroencephalogram (left central, right central, left occipital, right occipital), two ECG channels, left and right limb EMG, snore channel, mask flow (MFLO), tidal volume (TVOL), oral airflow, respiratory effort (thoracic, abdominal), and oxygen saturation (SaO₂).

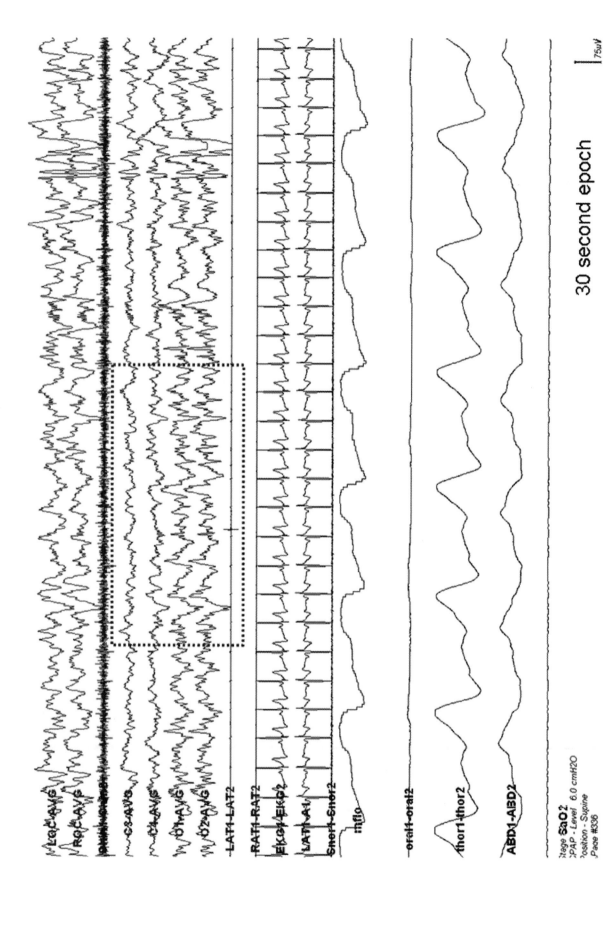

FIGURE 18-11 ■ Channels are as follows: electro-oculogram (left: LOC–A2, right: ROC–A1), chin electromyogram (EMG), electroencephalogram (left central, right central, left occipital, right occipital), two ECG channels, left and right limb EMG, snore channel, mask flow (MFLO), oral airflow, respiratory effort (thoracic, abdominal), and oxygen saturation (SaO₂).

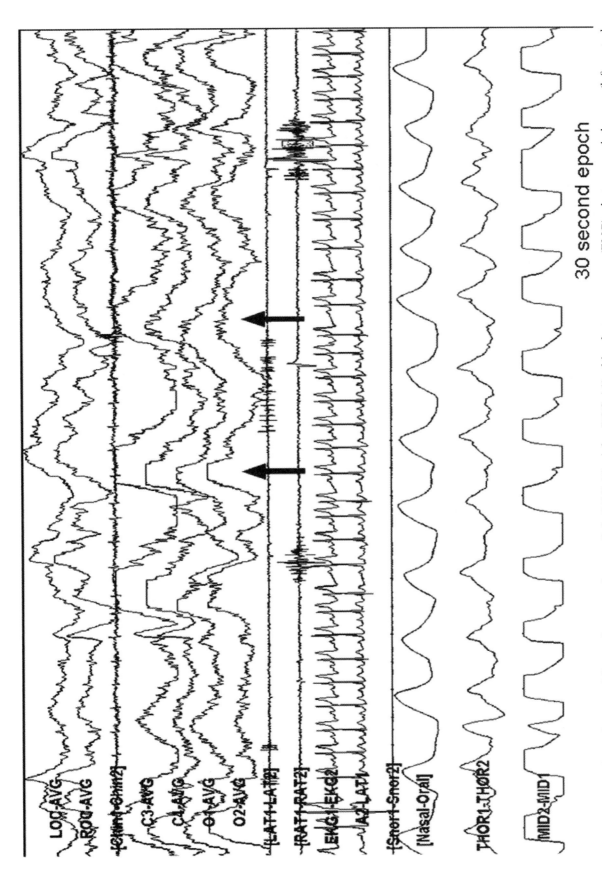

FIGURE 18-12 ■ Channels are as follows: electro-oculogram (left: LOC-A2, right: ROC-A1), chin electromyogram (EMG), electroencephalogram (left central, right central, left occipital, right occipital), two ECG channels, left and right limb EMG, snore channel, nasal-oral airflow, and respiratory effort (thoracic, abdominal).

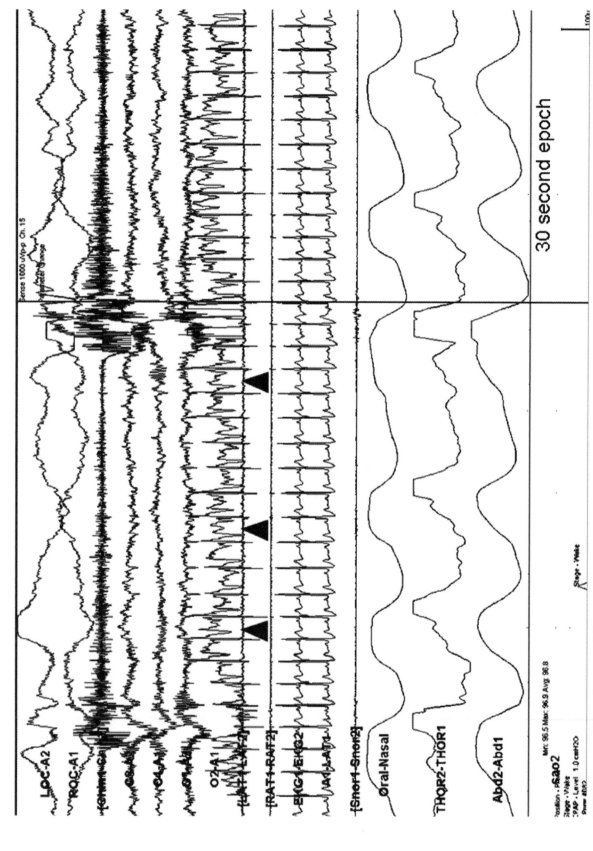

FIGURE 18-13 ■ Channels are as follows: electro-oculogram (left: LOC-A2, right: ROC-A1), chin electromyogram (EMG), electroencephalogram (left central, right central, left occipital, right occipital), two ECG channels, left and right limb EMG, snore channel, nasal-oral airflow, and respiratory effort (thoracic, abdominal).

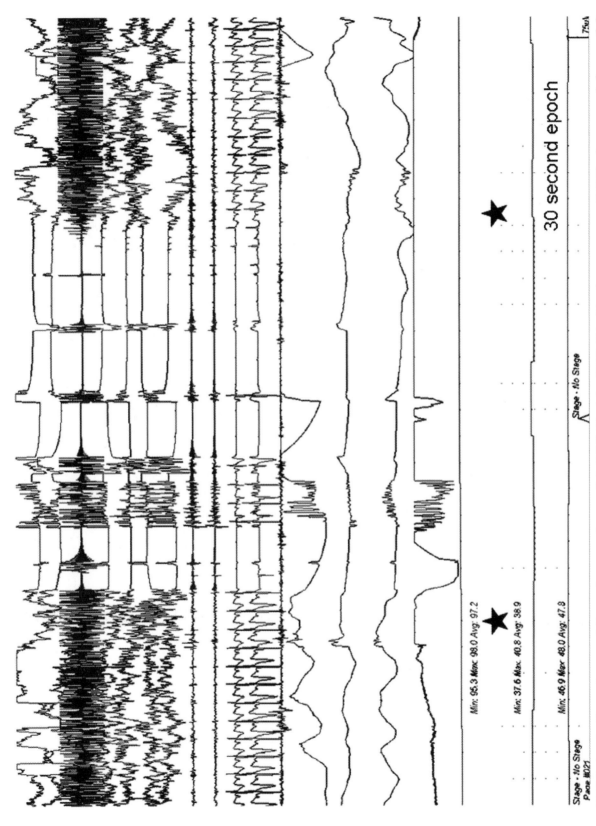

FIGURE 18-14 ■ Channels are as follows: electro-oculogram (left: LOC-A2, right: ROC-A1), chin electromyogram (EMG), electroencephalogram (left central, right central, left occipital, right occipital), two ECG channels, left and right limb EMG, snore channel, nasal-oral airflow, respiratory effort (thoracic, abdominal), esophageal monitoring, oxygen saturation, and end tidal.

phenomenon illustrated by the arrowheads in Figure 18-15. This is characteristic of:
A. Electrocardiogram artifact
B. Electrode "pop" artifact
C. Eye blink artifact
D. Respiratory artifact

16. A 60-year-old patient with a history of hypertension is referred to the sleep laboratory for evaluation of witnessed apneas and daytime sleepiness. What is the most likely cause of the unusual N/O signal demarcated by the stars in Figure 18-16?
A. The N/O lead has a fast-frequency artifact attributed to the patient's snoring.
B. The N/O lead has been dislodged, causing it to pick up electrocardiogram artifact.
C. The N/O signal's low-pass frequency has been adjusted incorrectly.
D. The N/O lead has a loose thermocouple connection.

17. A 59-year-old morbidly obese female undergoes a PSG for evaluation of possible sleep apnea. Her medical history includes hypertension, gastric reflux, and anxiety disorder. What activity is illustrated by the stars in Figure 18-17A?
A. Bi-metallic artifact
B. Electrode "pop" artifact
C. Electrocardiogram artifact
D. Intravenous drip artifact

18. Figure 18-18 demonstrates a 30-second epoch from a diagnostic PSG of a 44-year-old male who presents with morning headaches and waking up gasping for breath in the middle of the night. What is the artifact denoted by the stars?
A. Bruxism
B. Electrode "pop"
C. Swallowing artifact
D. Snore artifact

19. A 41-year-old man presented for a nocturnal PSG for possible obstructive sleep apnea. During the study, he was noted to produce unusual clicking sounds. An example from his study is shown in Figure 18-19. What is the artifact illustrated by the arrowhead?
A. Rhythmic movement disorder
B. Bruxism

C. Generalized seizure
E. Movement artifact

20. A 23-year-old overweight man is referred for a nocturnal PSG for the evaluation of sleep apnea. During his study the monitoring technician noted an unusual signal in the thoracic belt. What is noted in the arrowheads in Figure 18-20A?
A. Sine wave artifact
B. Cardioballistic artifact
C. Loose respiratory effort belt
D. Hiccup artifact

For questions 21–25, please match the artifact with the corresponding figure.

21. Time delay artifact:
A. Figure 18-21
B. Figure 18-22
C. Figure 18-23
D. Figure 18-24
E. Figure 18-25

22. Right eye trauma artifact:
A. Figure 18-21
B. Figure 18-22
C. Figure 18-23
D. Figure 18-24
E. Figure 18-25

23. Rhythmic movement disorder artifact:
A. Figure 18-21
B. Figure 18-22
C. Figure 18-23
D. Figure 18-24
E. Figure 18-25

24. Hiccup artifact:
A. Figure 18-21
B. Figure 18-22
C. Figure 18-23
D. Figure 18-24
E. Figure 18-25

25. Suck artifact:
A. Figure 18-21
B. Figure 18-22
C. Figure 18-23
D. Figure 18-24
E. Figure 18-25

Text continued on p. 364

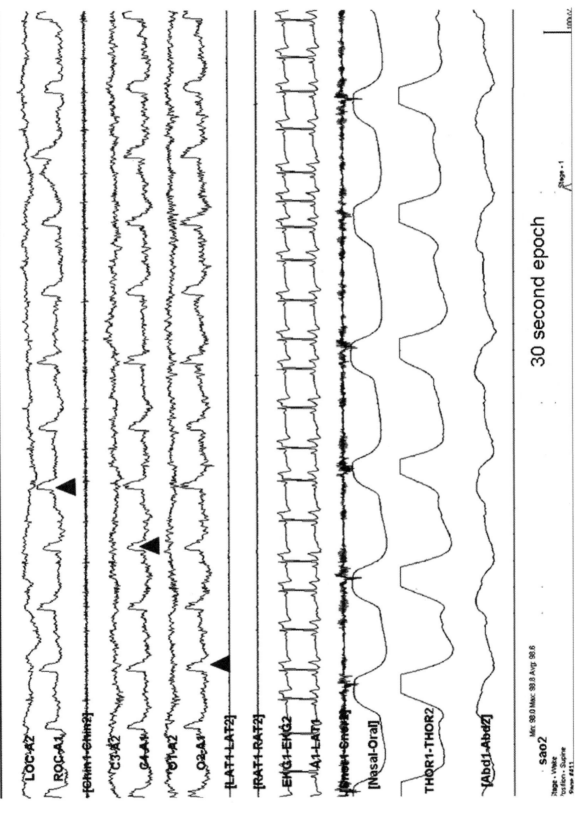

FIGURE 18-15 ■ Channels are as follows: electro-oculogram (left: LOC-A2, right: ROC-A1), chin electromyogram (EMG), electroencephalogram (left central, right central, left occipital, right occipital), two ECG channels, left and right limb EMG, snore channel, nasal-oral airflow, respiratory effort (thoracic, abdominal), and oxygen saturation (SaO2).

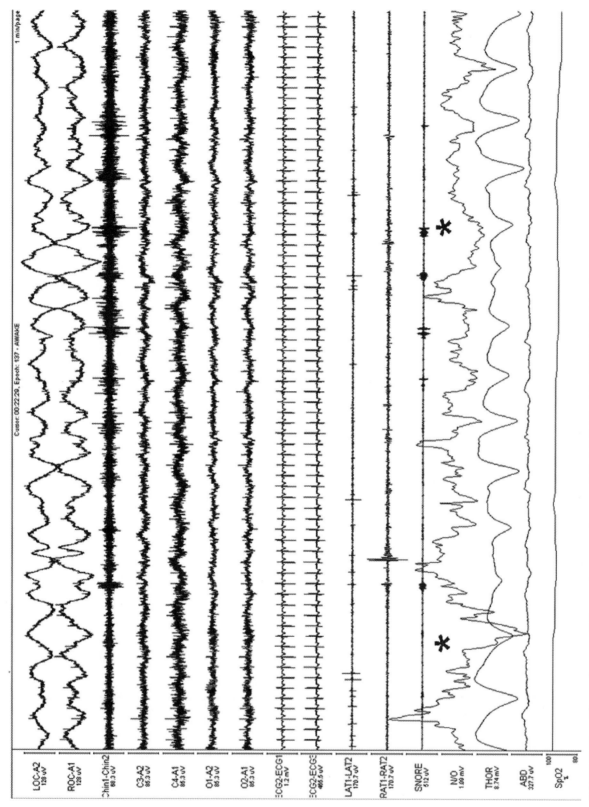

FIGURE 18-16 ■ Channels are as follows: electro-oculogram (left: LOC-A2, right: ROC-A1), chin electromyogram (EMG), electroencephalogram (left central, right central, left occipital, right occipital), two ECG channels, left and right limb EMG, snore channel, nasal-oral airflow, respiratory effort (thoracic, abdominal), and oxygen saturation (SpO₂).

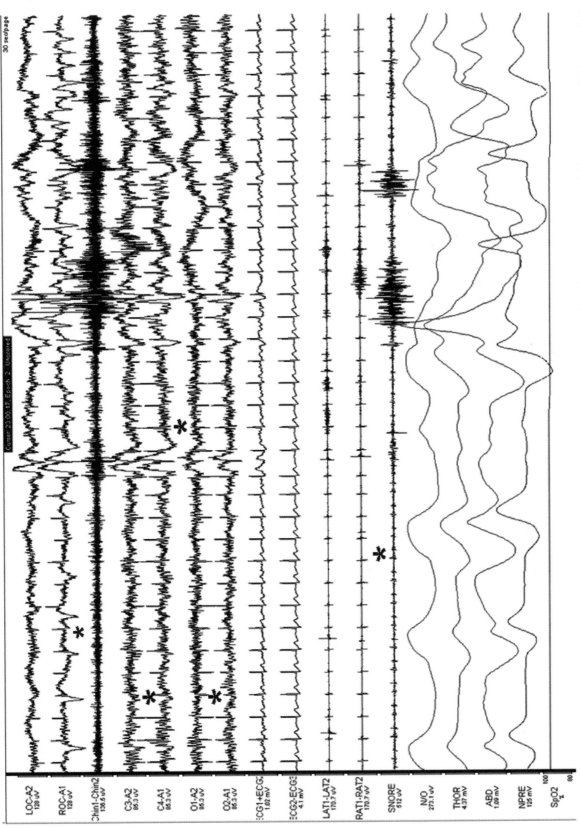

FIGURE 18-17A ■ Channels are as follows: electro-oculogram (left: LOC-A2, right: ROC-A1), chin electromyogram (EMG), electroencephalogram (left central, right central, left occipital, right occipital), two ECG channels, left and right limb EMG, snore channel, nasal-oral airflow, respiratory effort (thoracic, abdominal), nasal pressure (NPRE), and oxygen saturation (SpO₂).

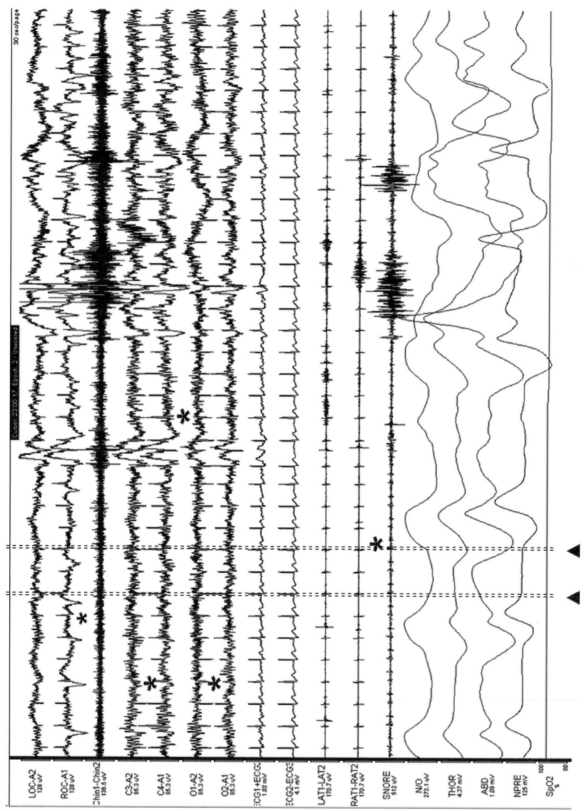

FIGURE 18-17B ■ Channels are as follows: electro-oculogram (left: LOC-A2, right: ROC-A1), chin electromyogram (EMG), electroencephalogram (left central, right central, left occipital, right occipital), two ECG channels, left and right limb EMG, snore channel, nasal-oral airflow, respiratory effort (thoracic, abdominal), nasal pressure (NPRE), and oxygen saturation (SpO₂).

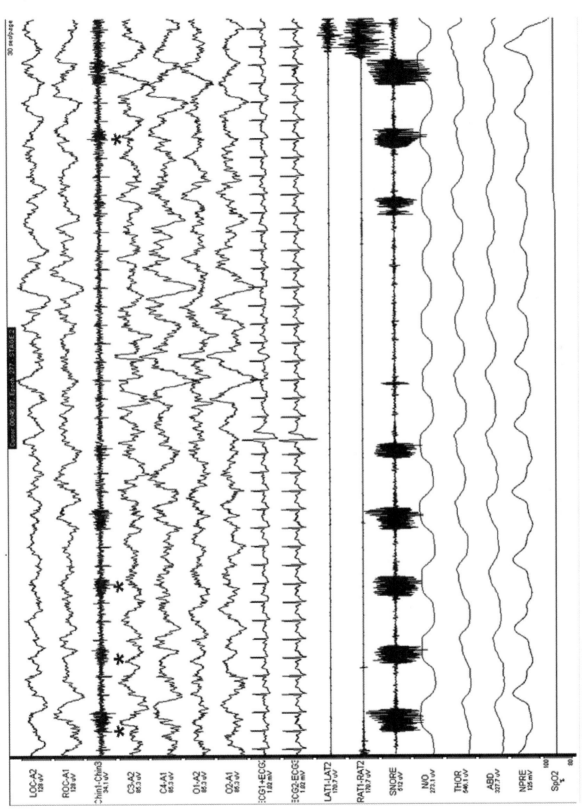

FIGURE 18-18 ■ Channels are as follows: electro-oculogram (left: LOC-A2, right: ROC-A1), electroencephalogram (left central, right central, left occipital, right occipital), two ECG channels, left and right limb EMG, snore channel, nasal-oral airflow, respiratory effort (thoracic, abdominal), nasal pressure (NPRE), and oxygen saturation (SpO2).

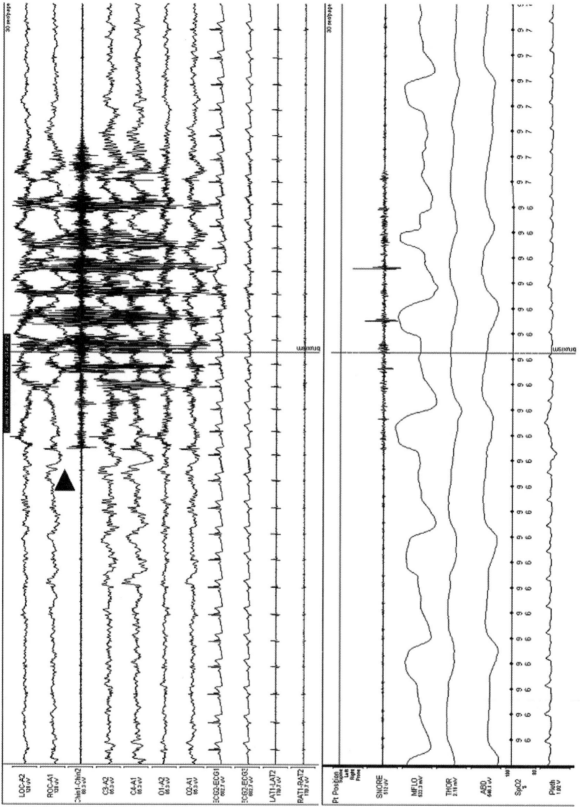

FIGURE 18-19 ■ Channels are as follows: electro-oculogram (left: LOC-A2, right: ROC-A1), chin electromyogram (EMG), electroencephalogram (left central, right central, left occipital, right occipital), two ECG channels, left and right limb EMG, position, snore channel, mask flow (MFLO), respiratory effort (thoracic, abdominal), oxygen saturation (SpO$_2$), and pleth wave.

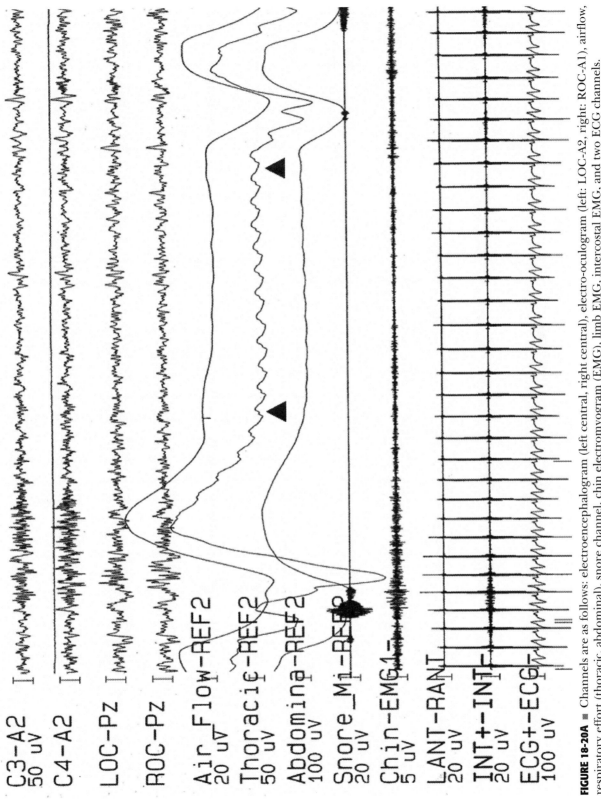

FIGURE 18-20A ■ Channels are as follows: electroencephalogram (left central, right central), electro-oculogram (left: LOC-A2, right: ROC-A1), airflow, respiratory effort (thoracic, abdominal), snore channel, chin electromyogram (EMG), limb EMG, intercostal EMG, and two ECG channels.

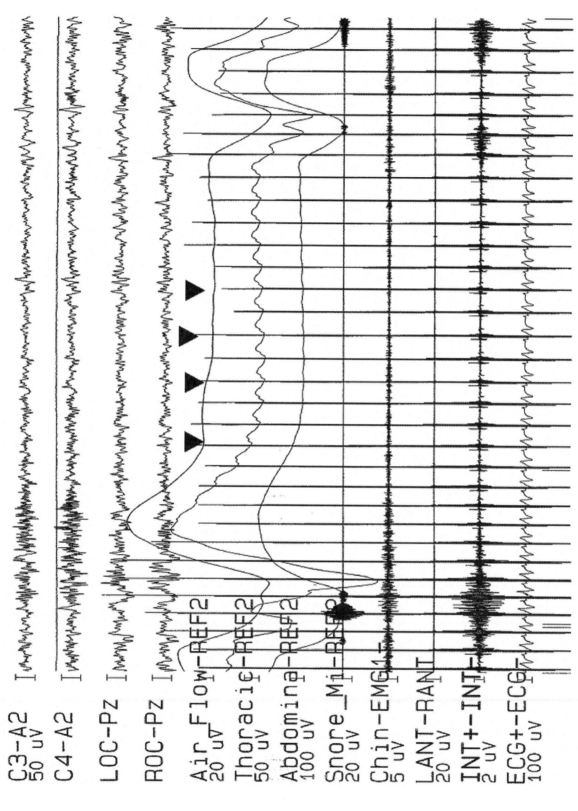

FIGURE 18-20B ■ Channels are as follows: electroencephalogram (left central, right central), electro-oculogram (left: LOC-A2, right: ROC-A1), airflow, respiratory effort (thoracic, abdominal), snore channel, chin electromyogram (EMG), limb EMG, intercostal EMG, and two ECG channels.

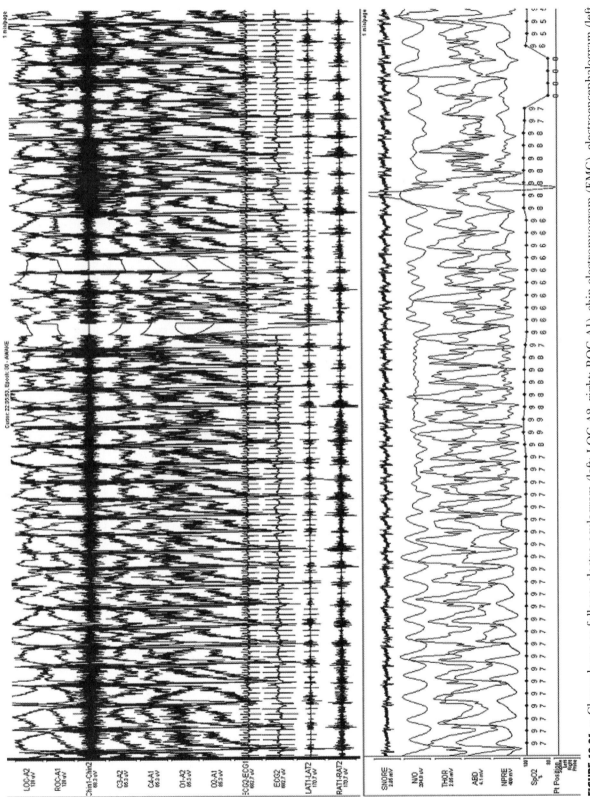

FIGURE 18-21 ■ Channels are as follows: electro-oculogram (left: LOC-A2, right: ROC-A1), chin electromyogram (EMG), electroencephalogram (left central, right central, left occipital, right occipital), two ECG channels, left and right limb EMG, snore channel, nasal-oral airflow, respiratory effort (thoracic, abdominal), nasal pressure (NPRE), oxygen saturation (SpO₂), and position.

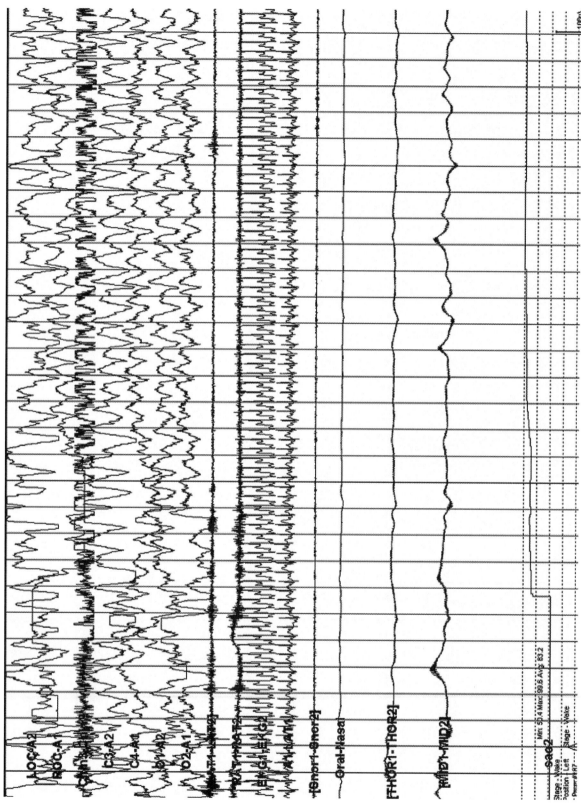

FIGURE 18-22 ■ Channels are as follows: electro-oculogram (left: LOC-A2, right: ROC-A1), chin electromyogram (EMG), electroencephalogram (left central, right central, left occipital, right occipital), two ECG channels, left and right limb EMG, snore channel, nasal-oral airflow, respiratory effort (thoracic, abdominal), and oxygen saturation (SaO₂).

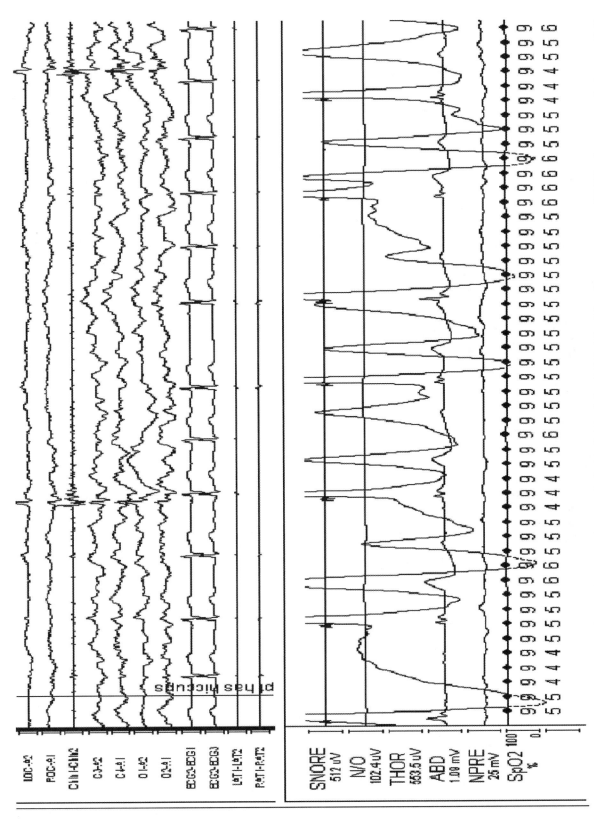

FIGURE 18-23 ■ Channels are as follows: electro-oculogram (left: LOC-A2, right: ROC-A1), chin electromyogram (EMG), electroencephalogram (left central, right central, left occipital, right occipital), two ECG channels, left and right limb EMG, snore channel, nasal-oral airflow, respiratory effort (thoracic, abdominal), nasal pressure (NPRE), and oxygen saturation (SpO2).

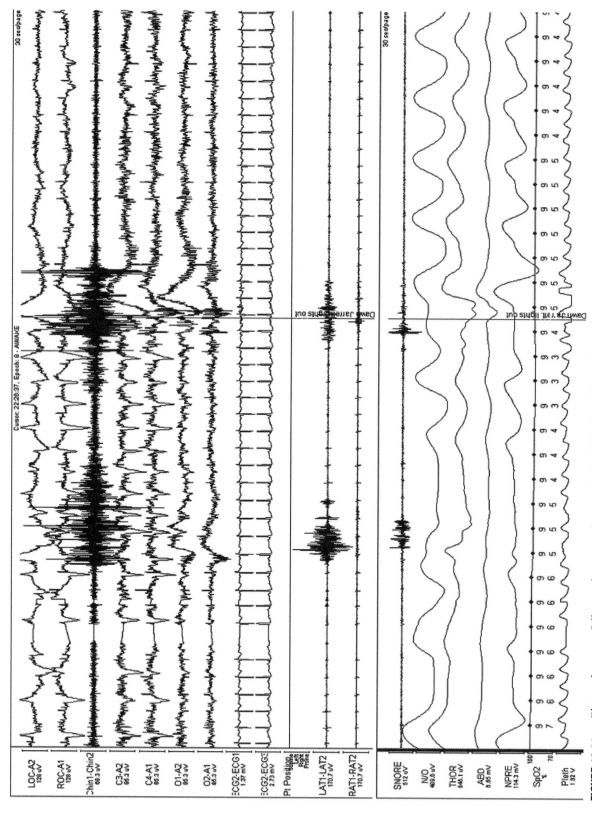

FIGURE 18-24 ■ Channels are as follows: electro-oculogram (left: LOC-A2, right: ROC-A1), chin electromyogram (EMG), electroencephalogram (left central, right central, left occipital, right occipital), two ECG channels, left and right limb EMG, snore channel, nasal-oral airflow, respiratory effort (thoracic, abdominal), nasal pressure (NPRE), oxygen saturation (SpO₂), and pleth wave.

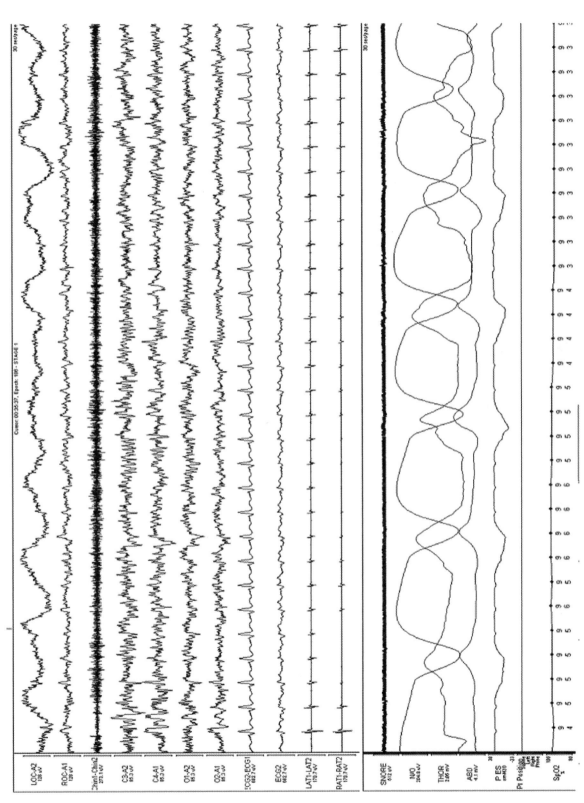

FIGURE 18-25 ■ Channels are as follows: electro-oculogram (left: LOC-A2, right: ROC-A1), electroencephalogram (left central, right central, left occipital, right occipital), two ECG channels, left and right limb EMG, snore channel, nasal-oral airflow, respiratory effort (thoracic, abdominal), esophageal pressure monitoring (PES), position, and oxygen saturation (SpO$_2$).

Answers

1. C. 60 Hz caused by environmental electrical interference

These figures display the characteristic "thick" black line associated with 60 Hz at 30 mm/sec epoch obscuring the desired physiologic signal. A measurement of 60 Hz can be caused by outside electrical interference such as outlets, power cords, and electrical ancillary equipment. Oftentimes it can be eliminated by engaging the "60 Hz notch filter" as long as the electrodes have been applied properly and the surrounding equipment is functioning correctly. In this case, the technicians discovered that the oximeter probe was faulty. When looking at Figures 18-1A and 18-1B, note the patient's position and the affected leads; the 60 Hz appears positional. The technician discovered that the patient had placed his finger, which was connected to the oximeter probe, under his head. The 60 Hz artifact did not persist in the EEG leads after the probe was replaced. If the reference and/or ground electrodes had been faulty, one would expect all of the leads to demonstrate interference. The ground lead is referenced to all alternating current (AC) electrodes, so if this lead was malfunctioning, one would expect to see the 60 Hz affecting all of the electrodes referenced to it as opposed to a more localized artifact, which is observed in these examples. Although it may be difficult to distinguish between muscle and 60 Hz artifact at an epoch of 30 mm/sec, 60 Hz artifact tends to have a more uniformed sinusoidal waveform. An additional method to differentiate between the two artifacts is to expand the time span to count out the frequency.

2. D. Muscle artifact in the A1 electrode

Muscle artifact is described as an irregular high-frequency signal that can be seen in the EEG and electrocardiogram (ECG) signals during movement. It is especially prominent in tense or anxious patients who obscure the EEG signal until they relax and fall asleep. One method to try to alleviate muscle artifact in this case is to readjust the position of the A1 and A2 electrodes so they are not picking up extraneous muscle signals. It is also helpful to ask the patient to open his/her mouth slightly or to put a pillow under their neck. Unlike muscle artifact, 60 Hz displays a sinusoidal high-frequency signal that can be differentiated when the page has been expanded from 30 seconds to 10 seconds (Figure 18-2B). It will not diminish when the patient relaxes or falls asleep. Muscle artifact in the EEG associated with bruxism tends to have a recognizable rhythmic signal that correlates with chin EMG burst, spreads to the other EEG electrodes, and typically does not affect one electrode alone.

Alpha intrusion is considered a sleep EEG phenomenon of wakefulness consisting of 8–12 Hz. Clearly, the EEG pattern here is affected by artifact and is not physiologic.

3. A. Movement artifact

Elements of respiratory, muscle, and electrode "popping" are illustrated in this example, but the entire picture is that of a movement artifact. Movement artifacts tend to encompass multiple artifacts owing to the instability of the electrodes or movement of the electrode wires during the movement. These conditions allow for further exaggeration of artifacts already present and may make it easier for new artifacts to take place. Movement artifacts are the result of changes in the electrode impedances causing deceptive waveforms, and they may cause misinterpretation of the EEG if the artifactual source is not immediately recognizable. The majority of artifacts encompassed in a movement artifact can be avoided with good electrode preparation and equipment maintenance.

4. C. Change the low-pass filter.

As the activity noted in the nasal pressure channel is a "fast activity," the low-pass filter, also known as the *high-frequency filter,* is most likely set incorrectly, allowing undesirable faster activity to manifest in the signal. The desirable signal of respiratory is a slow potential and should not be affected by an adjustment to the low-pass filter. Engaging the notch filter, also known as the *60 Hz filter,* would not eliminate this artifact, as it is a slower frequency. Changing the nasal cannula will not eliminate this artifact, which is most likely not physiologic.

5. D. Environmental artifact

Environmental artifacts are caused by objects, equipment, or activity other than physiologic or intrinsic to the patient (such as 60 Hz). The example provided in Figure 18-5A displays a slow potential signal in the C4-A1 channel that correlates directly (as shown by the dotted lines) with the patient's breathing, designating it as respiratory artifact, as can be illustrated in Figure 18-5B.

Respiratory artifact is considered a movement artifact caused by the movement of the electrode and/or wires as the patient breathes. It can be corrected or minimized by having the patient change position and/or by moving the wires in relation to the patient in an attempt to ease the applied tension on them. Along with respiratory artifact, this epoch displays a "sudden jump" in the signal at the apex of the slow potential signal (arrow in Figure 18-5A). This is most likely caused by the intermittent contact of the electrode associated with the movement of the patient's head, causing an electrode "pop." This type of artifact can also be caused by insufficiently applied conductive paste, intermittent contact of the electrode against the skin, or a faulty electrode cup.

6. B. Pacemaker artifact

These "sharp spikes" are characteristic of a paced rhythm caused by the firing of an implantable pacemaker. The patient's history should be referenced to confirm the presence of a pacemaker. Other artifacts can be ruled out by changing the input signal derivation and by verifying the integrity of the electrode and its application by checking the impedances. Bi-metallic artifact, which usually manifests as an abrupt high-voltage signal seen in the chin EMG and EEG channels, is thought to be caused by dissimilar metals in dental work. Finally, this is not the typical pattern of an electrode "pop" or poor electrode application.

7. D. 60 Hz resulting from a bad ground lead

In this example, the reader is asked to determine the type of artifact present and the affected electrodes and to decide whether the artifact is generalized or localized. The artifact shown in the figure is depicting a 60 Hz interference as indicated by the characteristic sinusoidal waveform occurring at 60 cycles per second (as noted in the 1-second box in Figure 18-7). The EEG, EMG, and ECG channels along with the snore sensor are all being affected, which identifies this as a generalized rather than a focal or localized artifact. As the ground is referenced to all alternating current electrodes, it can be concluded that the ground is the culprit. The 60 Hz interference signal is one of the most pervasive artifacts and will take any opportunity to manifest itself (for example, a detached electrode allows permeation of a signal). Muscle and chewing artifacts could be ruled out by noting the previously mentioned attributes of 60 Hz interference. In contrast, a muscle tends to be more of a mixed-frequency signal, and generally one would not expect to see muscle or chewing artifact in the snoring sensor. If the artifact were in fact chewing artifact, it would be expected to be seen in the chin EMG with corresponding rhythmic EMG artifact within the EEG.

8. B. The thermocouple is not picking up necessary temperature changes.

The N/O signal is derived from a thermocouple, which allows for recording of fluctuations in temperature change occurring during inspiration and expiration. It is important therefore that the sensor is secured directly under the nose and strategically positioned in the line of airflow from the mouth. Even with correct positioning, the thermocouple will have difficulty sensing temperature fluctuations if the expired air is being cooled by a fan. This can also be encountered if the patient places additional bedcovers over the head and mouth. One would expect to observe a more uniformed sinusoidal recording pattern in cases where snoring was interfering with the signal or in cases where the displayed sensitivity was reduced. A loose connection should usually produce an erratic, faster-frequency signal artifact.

9. B. Change the chin EMG configuration if additional input derivations are available.

This option would be the preferable next step in troubleshooting the cause of this sharp, high-amplitude signal indicative of electrode "popping." Whenever possible, the patient's study should not be disrupted by the technologist (i.e., by reapplying or repositioning the electrodes). If redundant leads are available, it is far less disruptive to reconfigure the derivation digitally at the computer rather than replacing or adding leads at the bedside. This option is of course easier with digital acquisition techniques. One might also confuse this artifact with bruxism, which is caused by the patient grinding the teeth. If this was the case, one would see a more rhythmic pattern with a corresponding characteristic spread to the EEG channels along with observations of teeth clenching by the technician.

10. C. Ocular artifact

The eye can be envisioned as a battery, with the positive pole at the cornea and the negative pole at the retina. As the eyes move during sleep, they produce corresponding changes in the electrical field, producing a correlating potential change in the EEG electrodes. This can be verified by noting corresponding movements in the electrooculogram channels. The sample does not have any movement; therefore movement artifact is an incorrect change. Sweat artifact is described as an undulating flow frequency movement that will affect all of the electrodes. The artifact present does not correspond with the breathing cycle; therefore respiratory artifact is an incorrect choice.

11. C. The ground lead is either faulty or detached from the patient's scalp.

The ground lead is referenced to all alternating current electrodes. Therefore, if it had come off the patient, it would be expected that all channels would be affected. Both answer A and B could be plausible, knowing that an output signal is the difference of two electrodes referenced to the "reference" lead put through a differential amplifier, known as *common mode rejection*. If the reference lead was included in a salt bridge or an averaging situation, it would cause the signal to be attenuated owing to many of the signals generated from all three electrode sites that are processed as identical and therefore rejected by the amplifier.

12. A. A chemical reaction in the conductive gel of the electrode cup

This condition corresponds to sweat artifact, which is associated with a characteristic slow wave signal activity with a wandering baseline, often mistaken as slow wave sleep. An electrode "pop" artifact would be associated with a higher amplitude and faster frequency. Respiratory artifact is characterized as a more rhythmic, slow-frequency signal correlating with the patient's breathing, unlike sweat. Sucking tends to be a more rhythmic artifact specifically depicted in the chin EMG corresponding to the rhythmic sucking movements of the infant patient.

13. C. Reattach electrode at next arousal.

It is evident the cardiac artifact dominates the O_2 channel. The prominence of extraneous artifact corresponds to the ECG activity in the O_2 lead. The lead has probably been dislodged from its original location, thus adjusting frequency filters (answer B) will not produce an accurate readable signal. As a general rule, when an artifact predominates in one channel, it typically indicates the problem lies with one lead. Therefore averaging the A1 and A2 leads is usually done when an ECG artifact is equally detectable in the EEG and electrooculogram signals. This indicates that the cardiac artifact is being brought into the signal via those reference leads and could be minimized by "double-referencing" them. The artifact present in Figure 18-13 is not a typical sweat artifact owing to the lack of low-frequency undulating sinusoidal pattern, and measures to alleviate the sweat artifact (answer D) will not be helpful here.

14. C. Instrumental artifact

This artifact is caused by malfunctioning or faulty equipment used in recording the PSG. This example in Figure 18-14 is indicative of a loosely connected head box, allowing for intermittent signal loss in all channels. Noise artifacts are also related to faulty or malfunctioning equipment, falling under instrumental artifacts. Any object, equipment, or activity with an electrical potential can cause an environmental artifact. Physiologic artifacts originate in the patient and consist of other sources of physiologic electrical potentials such as electrocardiogram, sweating, pulse, etc.

15. B. Electrode "pop" artifact

The artifact is most likely caused by an unstable A1 electrode. Instability may be related to insufficient conductive paste, intermittent contact of the electrode against the skin, and faulty electrode cup. The artifact could not be respiratory, eye blink, or ECG, as there is no correlation with the corresponding signals.

16. D. The nasal/oral (N/O) lead has a loose thermocouple connection.

This example showed a loose thermocouple connection that caused a fast-frequency artifact. The N/O lead should be replaced. Snoring and ECG artifact can be eliminated as choices, as neither demonstrates a consistent correlation.

17. C. Electrocardiogram (ECG) artifact

The ECG artifact is a common physiologic artifact and originates in the ECG electrical potential. This artifact can be encountered in any location of the body, but predominately in close proximity to large blood vessels. As can be seen in Figure 18-17A, the ECG artifact appears in the EEG, leg EMG, and snore sensor. The sharp activity in the EEG channels can be confirmed as originating in the ECG by visual correlation with the ECG channel (dotted line and arrows in Figure 18-17B).

The ECG artifact can be seen very commonly during sleep studies and is recognized by the characteristic sharp deflection at the time of the QRS complex.

The density of the cardiac field potential is maximal at close proximity to blood vessels, which enhance conduction of potentials. Choosing an electrical field farther from blood vessels (Cz-Oz derivation, posterior neck) helps prevent this.

The ECG artifact can be minimized by repositioning the ECG electrode via placement of the chin electrode away from the neck (i.e., over bony tissue).

The ECG artifact may be minimized by double-referencing, or "jumping" electrodes. The idea behind "jumping" electrodes, such as A1 and A2, is that the differential amplifier will receive the same ECG signal from both A1 and A2 and cancel out the like signal. The difficulty associated with jumping A1 and A2 is the potential exposure for additional generalized artifacts in the recording.

18. D. Snore artifact

The artifact depicted in the chin EMG corresponds with the snoring displayed in the snore sensor. The vibrations from snoring are picked up by the chin EMG electrodes. Sometimes this artifact can actually be helpful, as it can confirm the presence of snoring in cases when the snore sensor fails.

Bruxism artifact is associated with rhythmic EMG burstlike activity with an artifactual spread to the EEG electrodes.

19. B. Bruxism

Bruxism consists of repeated and rhythmical teeth grinding and clenching during sleep. It may be found in patients with an underlying stress and dental malocclusion. When it persists, it may cause further dental disease such as tooth decay. The PSG noted in the figure demonstrates the characteristic phasic increase in the chin masseter muscle tone. This produces the characteristic artifactual rhythmic EMG artifact in the EEG. The frequency of these EMG bursts is approximately 0.5–1.5 Hz. The other choice, rhythmic movement disorder, is excluded, as this is often not associated with an EEG artifact, which is indeed the case with bruxism. The EEG does not reveal an ictal pattern, and there is no evidence of movement to suggest a movement artifact.

20. B. Cardioballistic artifact (also known as *ballisto-cardiographic artifact*)

Figure 18-20A illustrates a central sleep apnea. The artifact noted in the thoracic belt is the cardioballistic artifact, which corresponds to cardiac pulsation artifact, as it becomes transmitted, via recoil movement, to the rib cage and becomes apparent in the thoracic channel. The artifact may also be picked up by the EEG electrodes and by esophageal pressure recording. Figure 18-20B illustrates exaggeration of the cardioballistic artifact (noted by the vertical lines and arrows). When the gain in the ECG lead is increased, QRS complexes become more apparent, and it becomes easier to comprehend the origin of this artifact. Please note that the airway is still occluded and the fluctuations in the thoracic lead *do not* correspond to airflow, a common mistake among new sleep trainees.

21. D. Figure 18-24

The figure illustrates time delay resulting from the lag time in saving PSG data into the computer's hard drive. This artifact was initially thought to be a cardiac conduction delay. The artifact is more general and goes further beyond the ECG channels.

22. E. Figure 18-25

Lack of unilateral electrooculogram movement can be related to trauma or surgical enucleation of the eye. Paralytic agents would affect the extraocular movements bilaterally. History taking about prosthetic eyes prior to the multiple sleep latency test (MSLT) or when suspected during the biocalibration may help to settle the question when the study is interpreted and questions arise regarding the existence of a unilateral rapid eye movement. Other explanations for a unilateral eye movement may be due to immobilization due to blepharcorneal adhesions. Loss of the normal corneoretinal dipole (the orbit, for all practical purposes, acts like a battery: the cornea is positive relative to the retina) owing to retinal damage or loss of the eye itself (as is the case here) is yet another reason.

23. A. Figure 18-21

Rhythmic movement disorder is a group of stereotyped, repetitive movements involving large muscles that typically occur immediately before sleep onset and are sustained into light sleep. The artifact is caused by the rhythmic movements of the torso and is rarely associated with EEG arousals.

24. C. Figure 18-23

Hiccup artifact is seen in the thoracic electrode as a series of rather abrupt high-amplitude and low-frequency activity, often exceeding the rate of spontaneous respiration.

25. B. Figure 18-22

Suck artifact is seen in the chin EMG electrode in this 3-year-old toddler. One notices a waxing and waning of the chin EMG tone corresponding to sucking and swallowing activities. Sucking behavior is seen in infants and toddlers when sucking on a pacifier or bottle or when breastfeeding. It is initially seen during wakefulness and persists into transitional sleep.

REFERENCES

1. Aldrich MS: *Sleep Medicine,* vol. 53. New York, Oxford University Press, 1999.

2. Berry RB: *Sleep Medicine Pearls*. Philadelphia, Hanley & Belfus, Inc., 1999.

3. Blume WT, Kaibara M: *Atlas of Adult Electroencephalography*. New York, Raven Press, 1995.

4. Butkov N: *Atlas of Clinical Polysomnography*, vol II. Ashland, OR, Synapse Media, Inc., pp 330–362, 1996.

5. Chokroverty S: *Sleep Disorders Medicine*, 2nd ed. Boston, Butterworth-Heinemann, 1998.

6. Kryger MH, Roth T, Dement WC: *Principles and Practice of Sleep Medicine*. Philadelphia, Elsevier/Saunders, 2005.

7. Geyer JD, Payne TA, Carney PR, Aldrich MS: *Atlas of Digital Polysomnography*. Philadelphia, Lippincott, Williams & Wilkins, 2000.

8. Rechtscaffen A, Kales A: *A Manual of Standardized Terminology, Techniques and Scoring System for Sleep Stages of Human Subjects*. Los Angeles, University of California, 1968.

9. Sheldon SH, Riter S, Detrojan M: *Atlas of Sleep Medicine in Infants and Children*. New York, Futura Publishing Company, Inc., 1999.

10. Shepard JW Jr, Harris C: Recording montage. In *The Atlas of Sleep Medicine*. Mount Kisco, NY, Futura Publishing Company, 1991.

11. Spriggs W: *Principles of Polysomnography: A Complete Training Program for Sleep Technicians*. Salt Lake City, UT, Sleep Ed, LLC, 2002.

12. Tyner FS, Knott JR, Mayer WB: *Fundamentals of EEG Technology*, vol 2. *Clinical Correlates*. Philadelphia, Lippincott, Williams & Wilkins, 1989.

Pediatric Sleep Medicine

CAROLYN M. D'AMBROSIO ■ ELIOT S. KATZ

Questions

1. Which of the following best describes the sleep-related rhythmic movement disorder in children?
   A. Incidence of less than 5% of infants in the first year of life. Movements include head banging, head rolling, and body rocking. Often associated with seizures in infancy.
   B. Incidence of less than 5% of infants in the first year of life. Episodes last several seconds to a few minutes and occur at a frequency of 0.5–2 Hz. Usually benign during infancy.
   C. Incidence of more than 50% of infants in the first year of life. Movements include head banging, head rolling, and body rocking. Often associated with seizures in infancy.
   D. Incidence of more than 50% of infants in the first year of life. Episodes last several seconds to a few minutes and occur at a frequency of 0.5–2 Hz. Usually benign during infancy.

2. The parents of a 7-month-old infant report that they observe episodes of irregular breathing in the infant during sleep. There is no apparent sleep disruption, discoloration, or respiratory distress associated with the irregular breathing. An overnight polysomnogram (PSG) demonstrated that the infant has 26 central apneas during the night. Most of the central apneas were less than 10–12 seconds long, but two of them were at least 15 seconds. Most of the central apneas followed sighs or movements. During REM sleep, one of the central apneas was associated with a decrease in the oxygen saturation to 90%. None of the central apneas terminated with electrocortical arousal. What do you advise the mother?
   A. This pattern of breathing is often life-threatening, and home infant apnea monitors have been shown to reduce the adverse outcomes.
   B. This history is typical for gastroesophageal reflux in infants and therefore you recommend use of an apnea monitor for the next 6 months.
   C. The child has an increased risk of dying of sudden infant death syndrome (SIDS).
   D. The central apneas and irregular breathing observed are a normal occurrence in infants, and no further intervention is necessary at this time.

3. Which of the following best characterizes the sleep architecture of term infants?
   A. The predominant sleep state at birth is rapid eye movement (REM). Spindles appear between 6 and 9 weeks of age. The sleep cycle is approximately 60 minutes.
   B. The predominant sleep state at birth is REM. Spindles appear at 1 year of age. The sleep cycle is approximately 90 minutes.
   C. The predominant sleep state at birth is non-rapid eye movement (NREM). Spindles appear between 6 and 9 weeks of age. The sleep cycle is approximately 60 minutes.
   D. The predominant sleep state at birth is NREM. Spindles appear at 1 year of age. The sleep cycle is approximately 90 minutes.

4. A 14-year-old child is brought to your office for evaluation of a 6-month history of excessive daytime sleepiness. He goes to bed between 11:30 P.M. and 4:00 A.M. and is awakened for school at 6:00 A.M. He falls asleep every morning in school and often needs a nap after school. On the weekends he sleeps until noon or later, as well as takes naps. Otherwise he is healthy appearing and has no medical history. He had previously been an excellent student but now his schoolwork is suffering. What elements of the sleep history are important to review in this patient?
   A. Caffeine, illicit drug or alcohol use
   B. Sleep diary
   C. Episodes of cataplexy, sleep paralysis, or hypnogogic hallucinations
   D. Presence of snoring
   E. All of the above

5. You are reviewing a PSG on a 3-year-old child who has been snoring for the past year and has recently been diagnosed with attention deficit hyperactivity disorder (ADHD). The PSG showed loud snoring, predominant mouth breathing, and paradoxical respirations. The overall apnea-hypopnea index (AHI) was only 1.5 events/hour (h), although the arousal index was elevated at 14.5 events/h. There were frequent obstructive hypopnea events less than 10 seconds long that were not counted in the overall AHI by your technician. There were no oxygen desaturations or periodic leg movements. The end-tidal CO_2 averaged 46 mm Hg and the peak was at 52 mm Hg. What diagnosis do you give?
   A. Primary snoring
   B. Primary snoring and ADHD
   C. Upper airway resistance syndrome
   D. Obstructive sleep apnea/hypopnea syndrome

6. Periodic breathing in healthy, term newborn infants is:
   A. Occasionally associated with oxygen desaturation
   B. A normal finding only up to 1% of the total sleep time
   C. A risk factor for SIDS
   D. Never normal, and its presence mandates home monitoring

7. A 13-year-old female is brought in complaining of a 2-month history of severe insomnia and excessive daytime sleepiness. She previously had no difficulty initiating or maintaining sleep and performed superbly in school. The family moved to this area 4 months ago in late spring. Previously they had been living in England. She is very tired when she goes to bed every night at 9:30 P.M. but wakes by 2 or 3 A.M. and cannot return to sleep. She does not take any naps and denies any specific anxiety or depressive symptoms. She does not drink any caffeinated beverages or smoke cigarettes. She is on the school swim team and works out in practice every day after school at 3 P.M. What is the likely precipitating cause of her insomnia?
   A. The psychological stress of moving to a new country and going to a new school
   B. Delayed sleep phase syndrome
   C. Illicit drug or alcohol use
   D. Poor sleep hygiene

8. A parent describes a disturbing pattern of awakening in their otherwise normal, nonsnoring 3-year-old child. Three times per week the child awakens after approximately 1.5 hours of sleep with eyes open, screaming, agitation, and confusion that last 5–10 minutes. The child subsequently falls back asleep and has no recollection of the event the next day. A complete history and physical examination are otherwise noncontributory. The most appropriate approach to the problem is:
   A. Obtain an overnight PSG with an extended electroencephalogram (EEG) montage
   B. Obtain a sleep-deprived EEG and refer to a neurologist
   C. Obtain a lateral neck radiograph to evaluate for adenotonsillar hypertrophy
   D. Reassure the family that this is a benign condition. Advise safety measures to prevent injuries during the episodes and good sleep hygiene.

9. A newborn infant is evaluated for a brief period of perioral cyanosis during sleep. The parents describe the infant's breathing as quiet but irregular. The history and physical examination is otherwise noncontributory. A 10-hour daytime PSG revealed the following: "6 hours of sleep; periodic breathing during 4% of the sleep period; four central apneas lasting 10–15 seconds, and a single central apnea of 19 seconds; baseline oxygen saturation was 97%, but there were four brief desaturations to 88% lasting 5–10 seconds associated with periodic breathing or central apnea; no obstructive apneas/hypopneas; no bradycardias." The most appropriate interpretation of these data and treatment is:
   A. Apnea of prematurity. Treat with caffeine.
   B. Apnea of prematurity. Treat with oxygen.
   C. Apnea of prematurity. Prescribe home apnea monitor only.
   D. Normal cardiorespiratory data.

10. A 9-year-old girl is sent to bed on school nights at 7:30 P.M. Every night the child denies sleepiness and she repeatedly gets out of bed, resulting in arguments with her parents. On average, she finally falls asleep at approximately 9:30 P.M. and sleeps through to 6:30 A.M. the next morning without further prolonged awakenings. There are no apparent daytime symptoms. On nonschool nights, the parents allow the child to stay up several hours later, which eliminates the difficulty with sleep onset. The most appropriate intervention based on this history is:
   A. Set up a positive reinforcement contract with the child that requires she go to sleep at 7:30 P.M. everyday, including nonschool nights.
   B. Enforce the 7:30 P.M. bedtime using "time-out" everyday, including nonschool nights.
   C. Put the child in bed an hour later on school nights.

D. Prescribe a short-acting benzodiazepine for 2 weeks only on school nights.

11. An 8-year-old male is brought in for evaluation of persistent bed-wetting. The child wets the bed 3–4 days per week and has never been dry for more than 1 week. The child does not snore and has no difficulty initiating or maintaining sleep. The parents eliminated fluids after 6:00 P.M. and initiated a positive reinforcement routine that failed to control the problem. The clinical history, physical examination, and urine analysis are otherwise noncontributory. The most appropriate next step is to:
    A. Obtain an overnight PSG, as bed-wetting is associated with obstructive sleep apnea syndrome (OSAS).
    B. Refer to an otolaryngologist for an adenotonsillectomy because bed-wetting has been shown to improve after treatment of sleep apnea.
    C. Reassure the family that enuresis is common and unlikely to be associated with a serious medical condition, and prescribe an enuresis alarm.
    D. Refer the patient to a urologist because persistent enuresis at this age is likely to be associated with an anatomical abnormality.

12. Which of the following statements are true regarding sleep in adolescents?
    A. Sleepiness increases in adolescents even if total sleep time remains the same.
    B. Slow wave sleep increases slightly throughout adolescence.
    C. Advanced sleep phase syndrome is the most common circadian disturbance in adolescents.
    D. REM sleep time decreases by 40% as adolescents pass through puberty.

13. Which of the following statements is true regarding sleep walking in children?
    A. Sleep walking is seen almost exclusively in males.
    B. Sleep walking is observed in less than 5% of children between 5 and 15 years old.
    C. Sleep walking is primarily seen during the first third of the night.
    D. Sleep walking is common but is always safe for the child.

14. What is the most common cause of sleepiness in adolescents?
    A. Narcolepsy
    B. Behaviorally induced insufficient sleep syndrome
    C. Idiopathic hypersomnia

D. Kleine-Levin syndrome

15. In addition to obstructive sleep apnea (OSA), a common PSG finding in children with Down syndrome includes:
    A. Frequent body movements
    B. Increased REM sleep
    C. Increased slow wave sleep
    D. Theta hypersynchrony

16. Epidemiological data indicate that there is an increased incidence of SIDS associated with:
    A. Pacifier use
    B. Supine positioning
    C. Maternal smoking
    D. Firm sleeping surfaces

17. Which of the following genetic conditions is associated with sleepiness independent of obesity or sleep apnea?
    A. Prader-Willi syndrome
    B. Crouzon's syndrome
    C. Duschenne's muscular dystrophy
    D. Achondroplasia

18. What percentage of obstructive apneas or hypopneas in children is associated with visible EEG arousals lasting at least 3 seconds?
    A. <10%
    B. 20%
    C. 50%
    D. 90%

19. A 7-year-old boy is sent to your sleep clinic complaining that he cannot fall asleep because his legs hurt. In the past 3 years, he claims that his legs hurt when he lies in bed but feel better when he gets up and moves around. His parents felt this was a behavioral issue and have been working on limit setting; however, the child continues to insist that he has pain. The boy does not experience leg pain at any other time of the day or after falling asleep. Once sleep is initiated, he appears to be normal. He is doing well in school and has no other behavioral issues. What is your leading diagnosis?
    A. Poor sleep hygiene
    B. Limit-setting behavior
    C. Delayed sleep phase syndrome
    D. Restless legs syndrome

20. The mother of a 3-month-old infant reports that her child had an episode of "holding her breath," becoming blue and limp while awake about 2 hours after a feeding. Paramedics were called, but the child had already responded to stimulation. The infant recovered spontaneously and is now acting

normally. The infant was full term, and there is no history of SIDS in the family. Assuming the physical examination is normal and you find no evidence of foul play, what diagnosis would be most likely?
A. Obstructive sleep apnea/hypopnea syndrome
B. Apparent life-threatening event (ALTE)
C. Central sleep apnea
D. Congenital central hypoventilation syndrome
E. Seizure

21. For the infant described in Question 20, what would be the most appropriate treatment plan?
A. Reassure the mother that this is a normal event, and send the infant home without further testing.
B. Treat empirically with medications for gastroespohageal reflux.
C. Schedule an overnight PSG for next week.
D. Admit the infant to the hospital for monitoring and further testing.
E. Send the child home with an apnea monitor for 2 weeks.

22. The peak incidence of snoring and OSA in children occurs at what age range?
A. From birth to 2 years old
B. Between 2 and 8 years old
C. Between 8 and 12 years old
D. Between 12 and 18 years old

23. When obtaining a history on a child, which of the following would *not* increase your suspicion for possible OSAS?
A. Secondary enuresis
B. Obesity
C. Mouth breathing
D. Difficulty arousing from sleep at night with no morning sleepiness
E. Daytime behavioral problems and attention deficits

24. In prepubescent children, the ratio of incidence of OSAS between boys and girls is approximately:
A. 1:1
B. 2:1
C. 4:1
D. 1:3

25. In an unselected population of school-age children, what is the prevalence of OSAS?
A. <1%
B. 1–2%
C. 7–8%
D. 9–10%
E. 11–12%

26. In an unselected population of school-age children, what is the prevalence of habitual snoring?
A. 1–2%
B. 2–4%
C. 8–12%
D. 18–25%

27. Comparing the PSG findings in adults with OSAS and children with OSAS, which of the following statements is true?
A. Children have fewer electrocortical arousals from obstructive hypopneas.
B. Children generally have a lower percentage of stages 3 and 4 sleep during the night.
C. Adults tend to snore, but children rarely snore.
D. Adults tend to have better preservation of REM sleep.

28. The percentage of slow wave (stages 3 and 4) sleep decreases dramatically:
A. Between 0 and 5 years of age
B. Between 5 and 10 years of age
C. Between 11 and 20 years of age
D. Between 21 and 30 years of age

29. A colleague asks you about his 8-year-old daughter. The child goes to bed around 9 P.M.and then at 10–11 P.M., she walks into her parents' room. She appears to be awake but does not respond when they speak to her. After about 5 minutes she responds, does not remember walking into the room, and goes back to bed uneventfully. She does this once or twice per month and has no other sleep problems. Your advice is to:
A. Start clonazepam (Klonopin), 0.5 mg four times a day by mouth, to prevent the sleep-walking.
B. Do nothing except prevent her from leaving the house or otherwise injuring herself; sleep-walking is normal in this age group.
C. Take her to a psychologist because there is some underlying psychological stress that is causing the problem.
D. Do a full-night PSG to look for abnormal sleep events.

30. A 12-year-old male is reported to awaken within 2 hours of sleep onset screaming at the top of his lungs and sweating. He is inconsolable for a few minutes and may become violent if approached. The episode lasts approximately 3 minutes, after which he calms down and returns easily to sleep. The following morning, he has no recollection of the event. The most likely diagnosis for these episodes is:

A. These are normal nightmares that happen when children approach puberty.

B. This represents a serious psychiatric disturbance, and professional counseling is indicated.

C. Medication should be started to help him sleep through the night.

D. These are sleep terrors, a normal phenomenon and common at this age.

31. OSAS is associated with the following genetic conditions:
    A. Prader-Willi syndrome
    B. Down syndrome
    C. Achondroplasia (dwarfism)
    D. Duchene's muscular dystrophy
    E. All of the above

32. A 3-year-old child is referred to you because of abnormal fear of sleeping. His parents state that he claims to be very frightened to be in his bed alone and wants them to sleep with him on the floor of the room. This started approximately 1 month ago when they bought him a toddler bed and removed the crib. The parents have tried to make him go to sleep on his own, but he screams and cries that he is having bad dreams. The mother says that the child claims to be having a bad dream while he is obviously still awake. Eventually one of them gives in and lies with him on the floor of his room until he falls asleep. They then place him in the bed, and he sleeps through the night. They deny any unusual stress or trauma in the child's life, and he has no other medical issues. Your diagnosis is:
    A. Sleep terrors
    B. Confusional arousals
    C. Behavioral insomnia of childhood
    D. Delayed sleep phase syndrome

33. A 10-year-old boy has a 1-month history of new-onset, secondary enuresis. He was fully toilet trained, including nights, at age 8 years old. Since then he has gained some weight and has started snoring. The potential causes of enuresis in this child include which of the following?
    A. Nocturnal seizures
    B. Obstructive sleep apnea syndrome (OSAS)
    C. Urinary tract infection
    D. All of the above

34. A 14-year-old boy is brought to you for evaluation of excessive daytime sleepiness. He reports falling asleep in class and often naps after school. On weekends he sleeps until noon and then does not need a nap. He has rare snoring, noted by his parents only during a viral illness. He completes his homework after dinner between 7:00 and 10:00 P.M. and is in bed by 11:00 P.M. His parents arouse him with great difficulty at 5:15 A.M. in order to arrive to swim practice at 6:00 A.M. Which of the following diagnoses is most consistent with this presentation?
    A. OSAS
    B. Delayed sleep phase syndrome
    C. Behaviorally induced insufficient sleep syndrome
    D. Behavioral insomnia of childhood

35. A 17-year-old girl comes to see you for evaluation of excessive daytime sleepiness. She states that she has difficulty staying awake in school and often needs a 90-minute nap after school. She is unable to resist the sleepiness at school and often just puts her head down on her desk in class. This is causing enormous problems with her teachers and peers. She typically goes to bed at 9:30 P.M. and wakes at 6 A.M. She does not snore and feels refreshed after sleeping. She denies illicit drug or alcohol use, is not pregnant, and keeps the same sleep hours on the weekends. This has started happening only in the past few months. There is no history of cataplexy. Which of the following additional symptoms would support a diagnosis of narcolepsy?
    A. Daily sleep paralysis
    B. A history of seizures with fever as a toddler
    C. Hypersexuality
    D. Suicidal thoughts

36. What percentage of children with OSAS will present with excessive daytime sleepiness?
    A. <25%
    B. 25–50%
    C. 50–75%
    D. >75%

37. Which of the following PSG characteristics would likely be found in a 2-year-old child but not a 2-week-old infant?
    A. Sleep-onset REM (active sleep)
    B. Ultradian cycle duration of 60 minutes
    C. Sleep spindles
    D. Periodic breathing pattern for 5% of the night

38. Risk factors for SIDS include which of the following?
    A. Sleeping in the supine position
    B. Nocturnal feeding
    C. Sibling with cystic fibrosis
    D. Exposure to passive cigarette smoke during pregnancy
    E. Cotton clothing

39. What percentage of children with OSAS do not have a return to normal breathing during sleep after a tonsillectomy and adenoidectomy?
A. 1–3%
B. 4–8%
C. 10–20%
D. 30–40%

40. What are the PSG risk factors in children with OSAS undergoing a tonsillectomy and adenoidectomy that predict perioperative complications?
A. Age >10 years old, apnea-hypopnea index (AHI) = 2/h, lowest saturation 90%
B. Age <3 years old, AHI = <5/h, lowest saturation 90%
C. Age <3 years old, AHI > 10/h, lowest saturation 80%
D. Age >10 years old, AHI > 10/h, lowest saturation 85%

41. Which of the following therapies have been shown to improve sleep apnea in children?
A. Rapid maxillary expansion
B. Nasal corticosteroids
C. Leukotriene antagonists
D. All of the above

42. A nonsnoring child with hyperactive behavior is referred for evaluation of sleep-disordered breathing. On a recent PSG, no apneas, hypopneas, or other respiratory events were observed despite 7 hours of total sleep time and an REM sleep percentage of 19%. The parents question whether their child may have simply had a good night in the laboratory and suggests repeating the study to diagnose OSA. A reasonable reply to this request would be:
A. A repeat sleep study is indicated because the frequency of respiratory obstructive events are highly variable in children.
B. A lateral neck radiograph would be a better choice for follow-up testing in this child.
C. A follow-up study is not indicated, as there is little significant variability in the frequency of respiratory obstructions in otherwise normal children.

D. A follow-up study should be performed on sedative medications to ensure sufficient sleep.

43. Which of the following patterns of respiration during sleep have been associated with daytime neurocognitive deficits in children?
A. Snoring alone
B. Apneas alone
C. Hypopneas alone
D. All of the above

44. A 13-year-old with myelomeningocele presents with a 3-year history of snoring, increasing daytime sleepiness, and new-onset morning headaches. There has been a gradual progression of scoliosis and weight gain over the past several years. There are no acute neurological findings, but her overnight PSG demonstrates an AHI of 6/h, desaturations below 80%, and carbon dioxide elevation to 72 torr. The most appropriate therapy at this point would be:
A. Scoliosis surgery
B. Nocturnal bilevel ventilation
C. Continuous positive airway pressure
D. Diaphragmatic pacing

45. Which of the following statements about pediatric OSA is true?
A. Obstructive sleep apnea syndrome (OSAS) can be accurately detected by clinical history without PSG.
B. Overnight oximetry alone is sufficient to rule out OSA.
C. Most children with OSA have excessive daytime sleepiness.
D. OSA may be diagnosed without gas exchange (oxygen, carbon dioxide) abnormalities.

46. The peak age at presentation of congenital central hypoventilation syndrome is:
A. From birth to 1 year old
B. Between 1 and 8 years old
C. Between 8 and 12 years old
D. Between 12 and 18 years old

Answers

1. D. Incidence of more than 50% of infants in the first year of life. Episodes last several seconds to a few minutes and occur at a frequency of 0.5–2 Hz. Usually benign during infancy.

Sleep-related rhythmic movement disorder is characterized by stereotyped repetitive movements of large muscle groups that often occur predominantly at sleep onset and NREM sleep. Occasionally, episodes have also been observed during REM sleep. Movements include head banging, head rolling, and body rocking. Episodes last several seconds to a few minutes and occur at a frequency of 0.5–2 Hz. Sleep-related rhythmic movement disorder often starts in the first year of life and is observed in more than two thirds of infants. The prevalence decreases to less than 10% of children at age 4 years. There is a male predominance, and movements may rarely persist in older children, particularly in those with ADHD or neurological impairment. Most cases are benign; however, traumatic injury has been reported.

2. D. The central apneas and irregular breathing observed are a normal occurrence in infants, and no further intervention is necessary at this time.

Central apneas, even as long as 20 seconds, are normally observed in infants, particularly after sighs or movements. Central apneas between 10 and 20 seconds are generally scored only if they are associated with a 4% oxygen desaturation or electrocortical arousal. Also, any central apnea lasting at least 20 seconds is scored, even without any associated findings. The presence of 10- to 20-second respiratory pauses on a PSG is not predictive of untoward outcomes. Although oxygen desaturation with 10- to 20-second central apneas are commonly seen in the first 6 months of life, it is rare after this time. If significant oxygen desaturation is observed in older children with central breathing pauses, consideration should be given for decreased oxygen reserve, including parenchymal lung disease.

3. A. The predominant sleep state at birth is REM. Spindles appears between 6 and 9 weeks of age. The sleep cycle is approximately 60 minutes.

At birth, infants spend approximately 60% of their sleep period in REM sleep. This decreases to 20% of the total sleep time by age 1 year. Sleep-onset REM periods are commonly observed in infants. Sleep spindles appear between ages 6 and 9 weeks. K-complexes usually develop by age 3 months. The sleep cycle is typically about 60 minutes at birth, compared with nearly 90 minutes in school-age children.

4. E. All of the above

Excessive daytime sleepiness most often will have a multifactorial etiology in children. Although poor sleep hygiene is usually an important contributor of sleepiness in this age group, the other causes, such as OSA, narcolepsy, delayed sleep phase syndrome, and drug use, must also be considered. A careful sleep diary including information on habits such as caffeine use, alcohol ingestion, smoking, and sleep habits would be important to help narrow the differential diagnosis. Although narcolepsy can present with sleepiness without cataplexy, children often have cataplexy early in the disease. The presence of snoring or restless sleep may increase suspicion of OSA or periodic limb movement disorder and necessitate PSG.

5. D. Obstructive sleep apnea/hypopnea syndrome

Many studies have now demonstrated that sleep apnea in the mild range can be associated with neurocognitive and behavioral impairment, including attention problems. An apnea index (AI) of 1/h is abnormal in children, particularly at this age. Although there are less data on hypopneas in children, they appear to be rare. Furthermore, obstructive apneas/hypopneas in children do not have to be 10 seconds long to be significant. Children have a faster resting respiratory rate, and therefore an obstructive apnea of greater than the duration of 2 normal breaths is considered abnormal. Thus, this child's AHI was much greater than 1.5 events/hour and has more significant disease than indicated by the AI reported. Another consideration is that children with adenoidal hypertrophy frequently breathe through their mouths, resulting in poor nasal pressure signals. In such instances, an oral thermistor may be the only available flow channel, resulting in a decreased sensitivity for identifying subtle obstructive events. The diagnosis of OSA in prepubescent children is based on an AI >1/h, peak PCO_2 >53 mm Hg, or if 60% of the night the PCO_2 is >50 mm Hg. There are no specific evidence-based guidelines for the diagnosis of OSA in adolescents.

6. A. Occasionally associated with oxygen desaturation

Periodic breathing is defined as three or more episodes of central apnea lasting at least 3 seconds, separated by no more than 20 seconds of normal breathing. It is usually observed in term infants up to 5% of the total sleep time, and up to 15% of the time in premature infants. Term infants spend approximately 6 seconds per hour of sleep with oxygen desaturations less than 90%. Most of these episodes of desaturation occur during periods of periodic breathing. Periodic breathing does not appear to be associated with SIDS, and generally no treatment or apnea monitoring is indicated.

7. A. The psychological stress of moving to a new country and going to a new city and school

Insomnia in children is most frequently related to underlying stress such as moving, trouble at school, divorce, stress in the home, deaths of loved ones, or sexual abuse. This child did not give any clues to point to illicit drug use or poor sleep hygiene. Her exercise is early enough in the evening that it would be unlikely to interfere with sleep. Delayed sleep phase is usually characterized by a progressively later bedtime, but not an early morning awakening. Moving and starting at a new school is a major psychological stress and is likely contributing to this child's insomnia.

8. D. Reassure the family that this is a benign condition. Advise safety measures to prevent injuries during the episodes and good sleep hygiene.

Confusional arousals and sleep terrors are part of a spectrum of disorders of arousal, with an incidence of approximately 25% in toddlers. The events described in this toddler are relatively brief and mild and therefore would be classified as confusional arousals. They are characterized by a typical onset within the first third of the sleep period with varying degrees of agitation and autonomic arousal. The child often appears fearful, flailing, confused, and crying. The events temporally occur at the transition out of slow wave sleep and thus may recur throughout the night. There is a strong familial predisposition toward confusional arousals and sleep terrors. Care should be taken to ensure that the child does not injure himself or herself during the episode, but treatment with benzodiazepines is rarely indicated. Nightmares, by contrast, typically occur in the latter third of the sleep period, during REM sleep. Children experiencing nightmares often have a detailed recollection of the dream and are awake and oriented immediately after the event.

9. D. Normal cardiorespiratory data

Perioral cyanosis is commonly observed in normal infants as is irregular ("periodic") breathing. Longitudinal data in infants have clearly documented that central apneas in the 10- to 15-second range are normally observed, particularly after movements or sighs. Even an occasional central apnea of 20 seconds may be seen in otherwise normal infants. These events may be associated with brief oxygen desaturations (see Question 3). These data should be considered as normal, and no treatment for these central apneas is indicated.

10. C. Put the child in bed an hour later on school nights.

Newborn infants may sleep 16–18 hours per day, 5-year-olds sleep 11 hours per night, and 9-year-old children sleep about 10 hours per night, on average; however, there is significant variability in the amounts of sleep an individual child needs. Some children in the prepubescent period require only 9 hours of sleep per night. These children may present with sleep refusal or insomnia if parents expect them to sleep longer. Parents must take this into account when setting an age-appropriate bedtime for older children. Gradually delaying their bedtime and observing their sleep pattern and daytime functioning is indicated in this setting.

11. C. Reassure the family that enuresis is common and unlikely to be associated with a serious medical condition and prescribe an enuresis alarm.

Approximately 15% of 7-year-old children will report bed-wetting, although only 2.6% do so at least twice per week. The spontaneous resolution rate is about 15% per year thereafter, leaving a residual prevalence of about 1% in adolescents. The prevalence of nocturnal enuresis in males is twice that of females. The principal treatments include alarms, tricyclics, desmopressin, and a variety of behavioral methods. Alarms are effective in approximately two thirds of patients and are generally first-line therapy. Tricyclics and desmopressin may work faster but are overall less effective and have a high recurrence rate after treatment ends. Children with OSAS have a high incidence of enuresis and an improvement in enuresis following treatment. Given the high incidence of enuresis in the general population and the low incidence of sleep apnea in nonsnoring children, however, screening tests for sleep apnea in enuretics are not indicated unless there is a compelling history consistent with sleep-disordered breathing.

12. A. Sleepiness increases in adolescents even if total sleep time remains the same.

Preadolescents are very alert and rarely fall asleep during the multiple sleep latency test (MSLT). During the second decade of life, the percentage of slow wave sleep decreases by 40%, and the mean MSLT times for sleep onset decrease into the adult range. Even when total sleep time remains the same, adolescents become sleepier between ages 13 and 18 years, which indicates that the sleep requirements may actually increase during this interval. Delayed sleep phase syndrome is the most common circadian rhythm disturbance observed in adolescents.

13. C. Sleep walking is primarily seen during the first third of the night.

Sleep walking is common in children, with more than 40% of children experiencing at least 1 episode between ages 6 and 16 years (Klackenberg 1982;71:495). There is no gender predisposition. Sleep-walking episodes tend to occur during the first third of the sleep period in the transition out of slow wave sleep. Although sleep walking per se is not harmful, serious injuries may occur, including falling down stairs, vehicle accidents, or drowning.

14. B. Behaviorally induced insufficient sleep syndrome

The most common cause of sleepiness in adolescents is insufficient sleep. Adolescents are challenged with earlier school start times, additional homework, and extracurricular activities that shorten their available sleep time. A short trial of improved sleep hygiene, including sleep extension, is generally successful in making the diagnosis of chronic insufficient sleep. Although one third of adult narcoleptics report that symptoms started before age 15 years, narcolepsy is nevertheless rare. Kleine-Levin syndrome is characterized by recurrent episodes of hypersomnolence that often begins in adolescence, but it is exceedingly rare.

15. A. Frequent body movements

Children with Down syndrome have consistently been observed to have increased body movements during sleep PSG. In addition, these children have neuromuscular weakness, midfacial hypoplasia, and enlarged tongues that predispose them toward sleep-disordered breathing.

16. C. Maternal smoking

The principal risk factor for SIDS is prone positioning during sleep. Other modifiable risk factors include excessively warm thermal environment, soft bedding, and maternal smoking. Pacifier use is associated with a lower risk of SIDS.

17. A. Prader-Willi syndrome

Patients with Prader-Willi syndrome (PWS) have excessive daytime sleepiness even without evidence of sleep-disordered breathing or obesity. The sleepiness in PWS may be continuous or intermittent and

may be associated with sleep-onset REM periods and cataplexy, as in narcolepsy. The other conditions may have excessive daytime sleepiness, which is mediated by sleep-disordered breathing.

18. C. 50%

Several studies in children have demonstrated that obstructive apneas/hypopneas are associated with visible 3-second EEG arousals in only about 50% of instances. By contrast, adults demonstrate EEG arousals after 70–83% of obstructive events. The relative lack of cortical arousals in children with OSAS may explain why some children have extended periods of obstructive hypoventilation characterized by snoring, paradoxical breathing, and elevated carbon dioxide, but few discrete obstructive apneas or hypopneas.

19. D. Restless legs syndrome

This is the classic presentation of restless legs syndrome (RLS). Initially the concept of limit-setting behavior should be considered, but the symptoms are most consistent with RLS. Although not that common in children, it does occur and can be disruptive to sleep and the family. There is nothing in the history to suggest poor sleep hygiene, such as late-night television viewing or video game playing. Delayed sleep phase syndrome would present with daytime sleepiness and inability to fall asleep at the normal bedtime; however, it should not consistently be associated with leg pain.

20. B. Apparent life-threatening event (ALTE)

The diagnosis of an ALTE includes a careful clinical history of an apnea (central, obstructive, or mixed) associated with skin color change and decreased muscle tone. An important component to the diagnosis is the observer and his/her reaction to the event (e.g., fear). Foul play must be ruled out, and the infant should be evaluated for signs of trauma. The differential diagnosis includes gastroesophageal reflux, seizures, and cardiac rhythm disturbances. OSAS, central sleep apnea, and congenital central hypoventilation syndrome present predominantly during sleep and are not usually associated with color changes and limp muscle tone during wakefulness. Infants often feed every 2–3 hours, so the history of feeding 2 hours previous is not particularly helpful.

21. D. Admit the infant to the hospital for monitoring and further testing.

Because the recurrence rate for ALTE is high, up to 68% in some studies, and because the parents may be extremely anxious, it is most appropriate to admit the infant to the hospital. This will allow some time for family education, a period of observation, and an evaluation for causes of ALTEs as indicated in the answer to Question 20. This infant in particular had a rather severe ALTE, and therefore further investigation is warranted. If the infant had a milder ALTE and it had been several days before seeing the pediatrician, then admission may not be necessary. A careful history for gastroesophageal reflux is important. Gastro-esophageal reflux can be demonstrated with esophageal pH or impedance monitoring.

22. B. Between 2 and 8 years old

The peak incidence of OSAS in children occurs between age 2 and 8 years. That is the time when the adenoids and tonsils are largest relative to the size of the airway. OSAS has also been reported in infants and adolescents.

23. D. Difficulty arousing from sleep at night with no morning sleepiness.

All of the other symptoms mentioned are reported in OSAS in children. It is normal for a child to be difficult to arouse from sleep, especially in the night-time. This is when they are likely in stage 3 or 4 sleep. Children tend to have a larger proportion of slow wave sleep than adults and therefore may be more difficult to arouse.

24. A. 1:1

For children before puberty, most studies have shown no gender predisposition to OSAS. Thus a 1:1 ratio is the closest to that observed in the population. After puberty, there is anecdotal evidence that the male predominant pattern observed in adults occurs. In adults, reports range from a 2:1 to 8:1 ratio of men versus women.

25. B. 1–2%

Current data are limited, but most studies indicate a prevalence of OSAS in children generally to be approximately 2%. There is a higher incidence in children with craniofacial syndromes, obesity, and neuromuscular weakness. As more subtle forms of sleep-disordered breathing have been associated with untoward neurobehavioral outcomes, the incidence of OSA may well be higher.

26. C. 8–12%

The incidence of habitual snoring in a population of normal school-age children is 12% by most studies. Habitual snoring is often defined as at least twice per week. Occasional snoring during viral illnesses is observed in a much higher proportion of children.

27. A. Children have fewer electrocortical arousals from obstructive apneas/hypopneas.

Children have fewer electrocortical arousals from sleep during obstructive respiratory events than adults. Both children and adults snore, and no differences between the groups have been noted in the literature on the quantity of snoring. It is well established that children on average have more stage 3 and 4 sleep than adults. In OSAS, children have a relative preservation of both slow wave sleep and REM sleep, compared with adults. That is, most children with even severe OSA will have a normal sleep state distribution, whereas adults with OSAS frequently lack slow wave and REM sleep.

28. C. Between 11 and 20 years old

Between ages 11 and 20 years, there does not appear to be a change in the total sleep requirement or REM sleep time; however, there is a 40% reduction in the amount of slow wave sleep as children pass through puberty. This parallels the increase in sleepiness (decreased sleep latency) observed during this interval.

29. B. Do nothing except prevent her from leaving the house or otherwise injuring herself; sleepwalking is normal in this age group.

Sleepwalking is common in this age group and usually does not present any problems. The child usually does not remember the event and will easily return to sleep if aroused. There may be a family history of sleepwalking. Most children outgrow this behavior without treatment, but care should be taken to ensure that injuries do not occur.

30. D. These are sleep terrors, a normal phenomenon and common at this age.

The episodes described are most consistent with sleep terrors. The age of onset of sleep terrors is generally before age 5 years, but these events may occur at any age, including adolescence. The events can be very dramatic, with the child giving a "blood-curdling" scream with diaphoresis and high autonomic activity. Children can hurt themselves or others if they get out of bed or if others try to console them. Sleep terrors last only a few minutes, and the child can often go back to quiet sleep without actually ever fully arousing. Treatment is generally not indicated, and the events are self-limited.

31. E. All of the above

Prader-Willi syndrome occurs because of a mutation on chromosome 15 and is associated with hyperphagia, perinatal hypotonia, hypogonadism, and learning disabilities. These children also have a high-arched palate and obesity that increases the risk

OSA after adenotonsillar removal include
seline OSA (AHI >10 events/h), craniofacial
ities, age less than 2 years, neuromuscular
, and obesity. These children often require
tinuous positive airway pressure or bilevel
n.

Age <3 years old, AI >10/h, lowest satura-

en with OSAS undergoing adenotonsil-
who are at the highest risk for perioperative
tions include children less than 3 years
hose with prematurity, craniofacial abnor-
obesity, neuromuscular weakness, cerebral
severe OSA (defined in children as an AHI
its/h).

All of the above

maxillary expansion, nasal corticosteroids,
otriene antagonists have all been shown to
improvement of sleep apnea in children.
axillary expansion is a dental procedure in
etainer device applies lateral pressure to the
olars over 3–6 months. Because the midline
ture has not yet fused in children, the lateral
results in a widening of the maxillary arch. As
there is an increase in the width of the nasal
d decreased nasal resistance. Rapid maxillary
n has been demonstrated to be an effective
t for OSA only in children with narrow baseline
dimensions. Both nasal corticosteroids and
ne antagonists are believed to improve OSA
asing inflammation of the nasal mucosa and
rway, resulting in decreased airway resistance.

A follow-up study is not indicated, as there is
ificant variability in the frequency of respira-
ructions in otherwise normal children.

parents express concern that their child's
g on the night of the sleep study was not
tative of its severity at home. Many studies,
, have shown that there is little night-to-night
y in the respiratory parameters, such as the
l oxygen saturation, during PSG in *otherwise*
hool-age children. Thus, as long as adequate
le and REM time were obtained on the first
follow-up study is generally not indicated un-
e has been a change in symptoms. One must
mind that studies of the night-to-night respi-
ariability data from infants and children with
ed medical conditions, such as craniofacial dys-
logy and neuromuscular weakness, have not
ne. Therefore it is possible that a single-night
dy may not be representative in all children.

43. D. All of the above

Several studies document neurocognitive impairment, including learning disabilities, attention
deficit, and mood disorders in children with mild
obstructive sleep apnea compared with children in
control groups. Further, even habitual snoring in the
absence of frank obstructive sleep apnea or hypopnea
has been associated with poor school performance and
behavioral disturbances. Thus, the threshold level
of sleep-disordered breathing sufficient to produce
symptoms in some children may be very low.

44. B. Nocturnal bilevel ventilation

Patients with myelomeningocele have several
factors that predispose toward sleep-disordered
breathing including (1) respiratory muscle weakness
depending on the level of their defect; (2) scoliosis,
which results in a mechanical disadvantage and ultimately hypoventilation; (3) obesity, which narrows the
upper airway and restricts the lungs, thus lowering lung
volumes and leading to hypoventilation; and (4) brainstem compression, which impairs upper airway motor
control and therefore predisposes to OSA. The key to
treating these patients is to recognize that hypoventilation is the principal problem, rather than just OSA.
Hypoventilation refers to the inadequacy of gas
exchange resulting in elevations of carbon dioxide.
Bilevel ventilation aims to enhance carbon dioxide
removal by increasing inspiratory pressures to enhance
the tidal volume. By contrast, continuous positive airway
pressure (CPAP) provides a steady pressure across the
respiratory cycle that serves to splint open the upper
airway. CPAP is very useful for OSA, but it has limited
value for hypoventilation in the absence of significant
upper airway narrowing. Thus bilevel ventilatory support is indicated during sleep to improve ventilation in
this child, as well as to control the OSA. Diaphragmatic
pacing is not indicated because the diaphragm is normally innervated and activated. Scoliosis surgery may
halt the progression of further spinal curvature, but it
will not improve the pulmonary function above the
current baseline.

45. D. OSAS may be diagnosed without gas exchange (oxygen, carbon dioxide) abnormalities.

Children will commonly present with subtle
increases in upper airway resistance leading to EEG
arousals but not gas exchange abnormalities. This
pattern of sleep-disordered breathing has been
termed the *upper airway resistance syndrome*. The introduction of nasal pressure measurements during pediatric PSG has resulted in the increased recognition of
small changes in the amplitude and/or the contour of
the flow signal. This has greatly facilitated the

of OSAS. Children with Down syndrome have midfacial and mandibular hypoplasia, macroglossia, and obesity, all of which increase the risk of OSAS. Achondroplasia is an autosomal dominant condition affecting endochondral bone formation. These children have craniofacial abnormalities such as midface hypoplasia and brainstem compression that increase the risk of OSAS. Duschenne's muscular dystrophy leads to weakness of the upper airway muscles and the respiratory muscles that eventually leads to obstructive apneas and hypopneas during sleep.

32. C. Behavioral insomnia of childhood

This is classic behavioral insomnia of childhood, previously referred to as *limit-setting disorder*, in which the parents allow the child to break the bedtime rules and not go to sleep quietly. It is important in making this diagnosis to confirm that the child is ready for sleep at the appropriate time and that the child falls asleep easily when the parents give in to the child's wishes.

Sleep terrors and confusional arousals occur after the child has fallen asleep. In this case, the child was clearly awake when describing the scary dreams and was easily consoled by having his wishes granted. Delayed sleep phase syndrome is a condition in which the child, usually an adolescent, cannot fall asleep until late night or early morning. This may occur as a result of improper limits set by the parents, but in delayed sleep phase syndrome, the child would not easily fall asleep once the parents stay in the room.

33. D. All of the above

This is a case of secondary enuresis because the boy was not enuretic for more than 1 year. Enuresis is associated with nocturnal seizures, urinary tract infections, and OSAS. The mechanism by which OSAS contributes to enuresis is unknown; however, treatment of OSAS has been shown to reduce enuresis in most children.

34. C. Behaviorally induced insufficient sleep syndrome

Adolescents often suffer from insufficient sleep as schoolwork, and other activities take time away from sleeping at night. Also, early start times at school impinge on the child's total sleep time. This child is obtaining no more than about 6 hours of sleep per night, which is well below the average requirement of about 9 hours per night. The history of rare snoring does not make OSAS likely, and children with OSAS rarely complain of sleepiness. Delayed sleep phase syndrome is a consideration, but usually the patient reports being unable to fall asleep until late at night or early in the morning. Behavioral insomnia of

childhood could also be c̶ indication that the child's p̶ the child's sleep habits or ar̶ child. Behavioral insomnia ̶ seen in younger children.

35. A. Daily sleep paralys̶

Narcolepsy is characteriz̶ sistible sleep attacks and ̶ associated features of sleep̶ hypnogogic hallucinations ̶ initially. Although sleep par̶ ally in otherwise healthy ch̶ ysis episodes were to occur̶ child's other symptoms, it w̶ of narcolepsy.

Suicidal thoughts would ̶ may be related to a moo̶ syndrome typically occurs ̶ male/female ratio) with fea̶ sodes of excessive daytime̶ and hypersexuality.

36. A. <25%

Only about 10% of chil̶ presenting symptom of exc̶ This is probably related to t̶ sleep architecture, includin̶ ved even in children with s̶ OSA are more likely to expe̶ tive deficits such as attent̶ learning disabilities, and agg̶

37. C. Sleep spindles

Sleep spindles start at ag̶ help define NREM sleep by ̶ sleep-onset REM cycles, an ̶ about 60 minutes, and frequ̶

38. D. Exposure to passiv̶ pregnancy

Passive cigarette smoke t̶ nant, overheating, and havin̶ all significant risk factors for̶ tion that infants sleep supine̶ the incidence of SIDS. Noctu̶ ciation with this disorder. ̶ fibrosis has not been specific̶

39. C. 10–20%

Approximately 10–20% o̶ still have sleep-disordered b̶ remove the tonsils and aden̶

persis̶ severe̶ abnor̶ weakn̶ nasal̶ ventila̶

40.
tion 8̶

Chi̶ lecton̶ comp̶ old, o̶ maliti̶ palsy,̶ >10 e̶

41.
Rap̶ and le̶ result̶ Rapid̶ which̶ upper̶ palata̶ pressu̶ a resu̶ cavity̶ expan̶ treatm̶ maxilla̶ leukot̶ by de̶ upper̶

42.
little s̶ tory o̶

Ma̶ breath̶ repres̶ howev̶ variab̶ AHI a̶ *normal̶ sleep ̶ study,̶ less th̶ keep i̶ ratory̶ *complic̶ morph̶ been ̶ PSG st̶ diagnosis of subtle sleep-disordered breathing. The history and physical examination have been shown to have a poor positive and negative predictive value in diagnosing pediatric OSA. Overnight oximetry has a good positive predictive value in diagnosing OSA, but if negative, it does not rule out the presence of OSA. Only 10–15% of children with documented OSA will have objective or subjective sleepiness.

46. A. From birth to 1 year

Congenital central hypoventilation syndrome (CCHS) usually presents in the first year of life, and often in the first few days of life. Cyanosis is typically the first sign of hypoventilation. CCHS has been shown to derive from a mutation of the PHOX2B gene. CCHS PSG findings include bradypnea and hypoventilation, principally during slow wave sleep, with relative sparing of REM sleep. There are also rare, late-onset central hypoventilation syndromes that may present in childhood, often with cor pulmonale.

REFERENCES

1. Ali NJ, Pitson DJ, Stradling JR: Snoring, sleep disturbance and behavior in 4–5 year olds. Arch Dis Child 68:360–366, 1993.

2. American Academy of Sleep Medicine: *The International Classification of Sleep Disorders. Diagnostic and Coding Manual.* Westchester, IL, American Academy of Sleep Medicine, 2005.

3. Arnulf I, Zeitzer JM, File J, et al: Kleine-Levin syndrome: a systemic review of 186 cases in the literature. Brain 128:2763–2776, 2005.

4. Brooks LJ, Topol HI: Enuresis in children with sleep apnea. J Pediatr 142:515–518, 2003.

5. Brouillette RT, Manoukian JJ, Ducharme FM, et al: Efficacy of fluticasone nasal spray for pediatric obstructive sleep apnea. J Pediatr 138:838–844, 2001.

6. Brouillette RT, Morielli A, Leimanis A, et al: Nocturnal pulse oximetry as an abbreviated testing modality for pediatric obstructive sleep apnea. Pediatrics 105:405–412, 2000.

7. Carroll J, McColley S, Marcus C, et al: Inability of clinical history to distinguish primary snoring from obstructive sleep apnea syndrome in children. Chest 108:610–618, 1995.

8. Carskadon MA: The second decade. In Guilleminault C (ed): *Sleeping and Waking Disorders: Indications and Techniques.* Menlo Park, CA, Addison Wesley, 1982, pp 99–125.

9. Carskadon MA, Dement W: Sleepiness in the normal adolescent. In Guilleminault C (ed): *Sleep and Its Disorders in Children.* New York, Raven Press, 1987, pp 53–66.

10. Curzi-Dascalova L, Peirano P, Morel-Kahn F: Development of sleep states in normal premature and full-term newborns. Dev Psychobiol 21:431–444, 1988.

11. Dyken ME, Lin-Dyken DC, Poulton S, et al: Prospective polysomnographic analysis of obstructive sleep apnea in Down syndrome. Arch Pediatr Adolesc Med 157:655–660, 2003.

12. Goldbart AD, Goldman JL, Veling MC, et al: Leukotriene modifier therapy for mild sleep-disordered breathing in children. Am J Respir Crit Care Med 172:364–370, 2005.

13. Gottlieb DJ, Chase C, Vezina RM, et al: Sleep-disordered breathing symptoms are associated with poorer cognitive function in 5-year-old children. J Pediatr 145:458–464, 2004.

14. Gottlieb DJ, Vezina RM, Chase C, et al: Symptoms of sleep-disordered breathing in 5-year-old children are associated with sleepiness and problem behaviors. Pediatrics 112:870–877, 2003.

15. Gozal D, Wang M, Pope DW: Objective sleepiness measures in pediatric obstructive sleep apnea. Pediatrics 108:693–697, 2001.

16. Guilleminault C, Pelayo R, Leger D, et al: Recognition of sleep-disordered breathing in children. Pediatrics 98:871–882, 1996.

17. Harris JC, Allen RP: Is excessive daytime sleepiness characteristic of Prader-Willi syndrome? The effects of weight change. Arch Pediatr Adolesc Med 150:1288–1293, 1996.

18. Hunt CE, Corwin MJ, Lister G, et al: Longitudinal assessment of hemoglobin oxygen saturation in healthy infants during the first 6 months of age. J Pediatr 134:580–586, 1999.

19. Katz ES, Greene MG, Carson KA, et al: Night-to-night variability of polysomnography in children with symptoms of sleep-disordered breathing. J Pediatr 140:589–594, 2002.

20. Katz ES, Marcus CL: Diagnosis of obstructive sleep apnea in infants and children. In Sheldon SH, Ferber R, Kryger MH (eds): *Principles and Practices of Pediatric Sleep Medicine.* St Louis, Elsevier Saunders, 2005, pp 197–210.

21. Klackenberg G: Rhythmic movements in infancy and early childhood. Acta Paediatr Scand 224(Suppl):74–82, 1971.

22. Klackenberg G: Somnambulism in childhood-prevalence, course, and behavioral correlates: a prospective longitudinal study (6–16 years). Acta Paediatr Scand 71:495–499, 1982.

23. Kohyama J, Matsukura F, Kimura K, et al: Rhythmic movement disorder: polysomnographic study and summary of reported cases. Brain Dev 24:33–38, 2002.

24. Levanon A, Tarasiuk A, Tal A: Obstructive sleep apnea syndrome in children with Down's syndrome. J Pediatr 134:755–760, 1996.

25. Louis J, Zhang JX, Revol M, et al: Ontogenesis of nocturnal organization of sleep spindles: a longitudinal study during the first 6 months of life. Electroenceph Clin Neurophys 83:289–296, 1992.

26. Manni R, Politini L, Nobili L, et al: Hypersomnia in the Prader-Willi syndrome: clinical-electrophysiological features and underlying factors. Clin Neurophys 112:800–805, 2001.

27. McColley SA, April MM, Carroll JL, et al: Respiratory compromise after adenotonsillectomy in children with obstructive sleep apnea. Arch Otolaryngol Head Neck Surg 110:203–210, 1992.

28. McGowen FX, Kenna MA, Fleming JA, et al: Adenotonsillectomy for upper airway obstruction carries increased risk in children with a history of prematurity. Pediatr Pulmonol 13:222–226, 1992.

29. McNamara F, Issa F, Sullivan C: Arousal pattern following central and obstructive breathing abnormalities in infants and children. J Appl Physiol 81:2651–2657, 1996.

30. Millman RP: Working Group on Sleepiness in Adolescents/Young Adults, and AAP Committee on Adolescence. Excessive sleepiness in adolescents and young adults: causes, consequences, and treatment strategies. Pediatrics 115:1774–1786, 2005.

31. O'Brien LM, Mervis CB, Holbrook CR, et al: Neurobehavioral implications of habitual snoring in children. Pediatrics 114:44–49, 2004.

32. Pirelli P, Saponara M, Guilleminault C: Rapid maxillary expansion in children with obstructive sleep apnea syndrome. Sleep 27:761–766, 2004.

33. Rosen GM, Muckle RP, Abboud FM, et al: Post-operative respiratory compromise in children with obstructive sleep apnea syndrome: can it be anticipated? Pediatrics 93:784–788, 1994.

34. Ruboyianes JM, Cruz RM: Pediatric adenotonsillectomy for obstructive sleep apnea. Ear Nose Throat J 75:430–433, 1996.

35. Stepanova I, Nevsimalova S, Hanusova J: Rhythmic movement disorder in sleep persisting into childhood and adulthood. Sleep 28:851–857, 2005.

36. Suen JS, Arnold JE, Brooks LJ: Adenotonsillectomy for treatment of obstructive sleep apnea in children. Arch Otolaryngol Head Neck Surg 121:525–530, 1995.

37. Thorpy M, Korman E, Spielman A, et al: Delayed sleep phase syndrome in adolescents. J Adolesc Health 9:22–27.

38. Tobias ES, Tolmie JL, Stephenson JB: Cataplexy in the Prader-Willi syndrome. Arch Dis Child 87:170, 2002.

39. Urschitz MS, Guenther A, Eggebrecht E, et al: Habitual snoring, intermittent hypoxia and academic performance in primary school children. Am J Respir Crit Care Med 168:464–468, 2003.

40. Weider DJ, Sateia MJ, West RP: Nocturnal enuresis in children with upper airway obstruction. Otolaryngol Head Neck Surg 105:427–432, 1991.

41. Younes M: Role of arousals in the pathogenesis of obstructive sleep apnea. Am J Respir Crit Care Med 169:623–633, 2004.

Sleep Pharmacology

TERI L. GABEL

Questions

1. Presynaptic enhancement of which neurotransmitter is currently thought to be key to the mechanism of action of amphetamines and methylphenidate in promoting wakefulness in narcolepsy?
   A. Adenosine
   B. Histamine
   C. Dopamine
   D. Glutamate

2. Carla is in clinic today with complaints of nausea, tremulousness, severe insomnia, irritability, and an increased heart rate. Four days earlier her primary care provider had started her on a 14-day course of ciprofloxacin for the treatment of a persistent respiratory tract infection. Concerned with these side effects, Carla had looked up theophylline in her *The Pill Book*, and these symptoms match the side effects listed for theophylline toxicity. Because the antibiotic was the only thing that had changed in her medication regimen, she immediately stopped taking the antibiotic and came to see you. Carla has been doing well on theophylline and has long been reticent to try the newer medications you have offered her to treat her asthma. Because of her wish to continue the theophylline, you give her a prescription for which of the following antibiotics, as it would be *least* likely to result in elevated theophylline levels?
   A. Clarithromycin
   B. Erythromycin
   C. Levofloxacin
   D. Pefloxacin

3. Maggie presents to the clinic with complaints of continuing episodes of depression and difficulty with midnight awakenings even with therapeutic doses and blood levels of divalproex. Maggie has been diagnosed with bipolar depressive disorder, recurrent, depressed type. The decision is made to switch her to lithium because of its successful track record in the treatment of bipolar depression. Lithium is also beneficial in restoring a normal sleep cycle in the patient with bipolar disorder.
   With which of the following changes in sleep architecture is lithium associated?
   A. Increased total rapid eye movement (REM)
   B. Decreased stage 2 sleep
   C. Increased slow wave sleep (SWS)
   D. Decreased SWS

4. Ronald is complaining of nightmares, insomnia, and hallucinations since starting betaxolol. Because he requires treatment with a beta-blocker, which of the following options would be the *best* choice for Ronald?
   A. Nadolol
   B. Metoprolol
   C. Pindolol
   D. Propranolol

5. Of the following benzodiazepines, which one has the shortest half-life?
   A. Estazolam
   B. Temazepam
   C. Quazepam
   D. Flurazepam

6. Arnold is having difficulty with being tired during the day. This is a new problem for him. Recently his ophthalmologist started him on a new treatment for his glaucoma. Which one of the following agents is most likely the reason for this new excessive daytime sleepiness (EDS)?
   A. Carbachol
   B. Dorzolamide
   C. Metipranolol
   D. Travoprost

7. Adenosine receptor antagonism is thought to be one of the mechanisms of action for promoting alertness in which of the following?
   A. Atomoxetine
   B. Caffeine

C. Modafinil

D. Methylphenidate

8. Jon is complaining of excessive morning sedation from the bedtime dose of trazodone that his health-care practitioner recently added to his regimen. Jon was started at a minimum dose of 50 mg. His other medications are fluoxetine, 40 mg, and fosinopril, 20 mg, every morning. Jon's enhanced response to this low dose of trazodone could be explained by:

A. Inhibition of cytrochrome P-450 (CYP) 1A2

B. Inhibition of CYP 2D6

C. Inhibition of CYP 3A4

D. Excessive agonism of alpha-2 receptors

9. Valerie uses herbal medications for most of her minor medical needs and to assist with health maintenance. She is having difficulty sleeping owing to stress at the office and has begun to use valerian in the evening. Data indicate that valerian can be useful in the treatment of insomnia. Valerian appears to have its sleep-enhancing activity because of its ability to affect brain levels of which of the following neurotransmitters?

A. Gamma aminobutyric acid (GABA)

B. Serotonin

C. Adenosine

D. Glutamate

10. Danni has been taking methylphenidate for her narcolepsy and has been doing well. At her annual physical exam, it was noted that her blood pressure was elevated. When she returned for follow-up evaluation, it was noted that her blood pressure was still high at 156/97, and her heart rate was also elevated. Because of concerns about methylphenidate's ability to cause hypertension and tachycardia, her physician wants to change the methylphenidate to a different agent. Which of the following would be most appropriate?

A. Amantadine

B. Modafinil

C. Duloxetine

D. Bupropion

11. Which of the following tricyclic antidepressant agents would be *least* sedating?

A. Trimipramine

B. Doxepin

C. Nortriptyline

D. Protriptyline

12. Mr. Patterson has been diagnosed with dementia of the Alzheimer's type. In the past week he has been having problems sleeping because of nightmares and insomnia, and he is more agitated than usual. His medication regimen is ranitidine 150 mg at bedtime, acetaminophen 500 mg twice a day for arthritis pain, and donepezil 10 mg at bedtime (recently increased from 5 mg/day). Vital signs: blood pressure 90/58, pulse 70, temperature 98.2° F. Which of the following interventions would be most appropriate for addressing his sleeping difficulties?

A. Add hydroxyzine at bedtime.

B. Add citalopram for depression.

C. Discontinue the ranitidine.

D. Change the donepezil dose to the morning.

13. Donna has difficulty with chronic pain and insomnia. Which of the following would be most likely to be helpful in assisting her with sleep, as well as her chronic pain issues?

A. Gabapentin

B. Topiramate

C. Lamotrigine

D. Levetiracetam

14. Paul is in clinic with complaints of excessive sweating, nausea, difficulty concentrating, tremulousness, and a rapid heartbeat. He denies any new medications in his regimen. He tells you that he has been having difficulty sleeping for several weeks, and he tried taking diphenhydramine but it was ineffective. Several years ago he had tried L-tryptophan at bedtime with success but was no longer able to find it. Paul admits that while perusing the aisle at the health food store, he had found some 5-hydroxytryptophan (5-HTP), the precursor to serotonin, so he decided to try it. The dose recommended on the bottle was 100–300 mg at bedtime. He found 300 mg only slightly effective, so he took 600 mg, then 900 mg. He has been taking 900 mg at night for about 1 week and is sleeping much better. You look over Paul's medication regimen and find that the cause of his new symptoms is obviously a drug interaction between 5-HTP and one of his medications. Which of the following medications on Paul's regimen was the problem?

A. Omeprazole

B. Citalopram

C. Lovastatin

D. Fosinopril

15. Doris is a 43-year-old schizophrenic who complains of having crawly feelings in her legs at night when she is trying to fall asleep. She ends up getting out of bed and doing stretching exercises. She denies having this restlessness in the daytime. Her current medication regimen includes quetiapine 650 mg at bedtime, atenolol 100 mg a day, and a multiple vitamin. Her

psychiatrist is confident that Doris is not experiencing akathisia because of the minimal ability of quetiapine to cause this side effect and the ability of atenolol to alleviate akathisia.

A sleep study is ordered, and it is diagnostic for restless legs syndrome. The resident begins Doris on pramepexole at bedtime. Several days later Doris is experiencing a worsening of her auditory hallucinations and goes in to see the psychiatrist. The psychiatrist stops the pramepexole.

Which of the following agents would be the most appropriate treatment for Doris's restless legs?
A. Acetaminophen
B. Clonazepam
C. Ropinirole
D. Risperidone

16. Methylphenidate has which of the following effects on sleep?
A. Decreases REM latency
B. Increases REM latency
C. Decreases sleep latency
D. Increases REM

17. Roger had gastrointestinal surgery 2 days ago and had been treated for postsurgical pain with morphine. This morning he reports bizarre vivid dreams that occurred during the night. Which of the following changes in sleep can be seen with morphine use and could be associated with Roger's dreams?
A. Increase in SWS
B. Decrease in REM sleep
C. Increase in sleep latency
D. Decrease in nocturnal awakenings

18. Albert has had a long and very rough day. He decides to kick back and have a beer or two to relax before going to bed. As he relaxes with his beer, what effect will his acute intake of alcohol have on his sleep?
A. Decrease in sleep continuity
B. Increase in sleep latency
C. Increase in total REM sleep
D. Increase in REM latency

19. Albert (in the previous question) fell asleep, but he awakens from a crazy dream, with a headache, in the early morning hours. What effects of alcohol consumption explain his early morning wakening?
A. Enhanced delta sleep
B. Further REM suppression
C. REM rebound
D. Enhanced stage 2 sleep

20. Lithium treatment can be associated with the development of which one of the following?

A. Somnambulism
B. Restless legs
C. Narcolepsy
D. Sleep apnea

21. A patient who has been dealing with depression and recurring nightmares since a tornado destroyed his home has been diagnosed with post-traumatic stress disorder (PTSD). His psychiatrist has prescribed mirtazapine. For the patient's hypertension, he wants to place the patient on an antihypertensive medication. Which of the following is the best choice for this patient?
A. Fosinopril
B. Metoprolol
C. Clonidine
D. Prazosin

22. Carlos is a 48-year-old male being treated with citalopram for resistant depression with associated anxiety. He still isn't sleeping well at night and finds his anxiety to be quite debilitating. Because of his continued difficulty sleeping and the development of sexual dysfunction, he was switched to nefazodone. Nefazodone is a good choice for Carlos owing to its ability to:
A. Block 5-HT1A receptors
B. Decrease REM sleep
C. Increase REM sleep
D. Increase stage 2 sleep

23. Which of the following is true regarding the mechanism of action of the new nonbenzodiazepine sleeping agents zaleplon, zolpidem, and eszopiclone?
A. They bind to the gamma subunit on the GABA-A complex.
B. They bind to the delta subunit of the GABA-A complex.
C. They bind to the benzodiazepine receptor on the GABA-B complex.
D. They bind to the omega subunit on the GABA-A complex.

24. Betty has been diagnosed with depression and irritable bowel disease and is currently having difficulty sleeping. Which of the following agents has the best profile for addressing all three of her problems?
A. Bupropion
B. Mirtazapine
C. Citalopram
D. Venlafaxine

25. Which tertiary tricyclic antidepressant has *not* been shown to suppress REM sleep?

A. Amitriptyline
B. Doxepin
C. Imipramine
D. Trimipramine

26. Melatonin has demonstrated benefits in the treatment of:
A. Restless legs syndrome
B. Narcolepsy
C. Circadian rhythm sleep disorders
D. Sleep apnea

27. Which of the following changes in sleep architecture is *not* seen with benzodiazepines?
A. Decrease in stage 2 non-rapid eye movement (NREM) sleep
B. Increase in total sleep time
C. Decrease in SWS
D. Increase in REM latency

28. Gamma hydroxybutyrate (GHB), also known as sodium oxybate (Xyrem), may be helpful for some patients with cataplexy caused by narcolepsy who do not respond to the usual antidepressant treatment. In patients treated with GHB for cataplexy, a slow improvement has also been noted in daytime alertness after the patient has used GHB for several weeks.

   This therapeutic benefit on alertness would most likely result from GHB's ability to:
A. Increase SWS
B. Block histamine-3 receptors
C. Increase stage 1 sleep
D. Block alpha-1 adrenergic receptors

29. Derek is requesting assistance with difficulty sleeping. He has no difficulty falling asleep but has been waking up in the middle of the night and very early morning hours. It doesn't happen every night, but it is very disruptive to him at work when it occurs. Derek used triazolam in the past when he awoke but had problems with vivid dreams and nightmares. He tried over-the-counter antihistamines, but they gave him a morning hangover. Because he falls asleep without difficulty, Derek only wants something to take on those occasions when he awakens around 2 A.M. and can't get back to sleep.

   Of the following, which would be the *best* option for Derek?
A. Zaleplon
B. Zolpidem
C. Eszopiclone
D. Estazolam

30. Robert is taking cetirizine for his seasonal allergies. He is surprised at how tired he is during the day. Which of the following reasons explains this situation?
A. Cetirizine has alpha-1 antagonist properties
B. Cetirizine is also a GABA
C. Cetirizine crosses the blood-brain barrier
D. Cetirizine has H-1 and H-2 blocking activity

31. Ramelteon is a selective melatonin (MT1) receptor agonist. Which of the following effects does ramelteon have on sleep parameters?
A. Increased sleep latency
B. Increased total sleep time
C. REM suppression
D. Decreased SWS

32. Sam abruptly discontinued his modafinil when he left for the Bahamas but his luggage went on a world cruise. What withdrawal effects will Sam notice while he waits for a new prescription to reach him?
A. Hypersomnolence
B. Gastrointestinal distress
C. Tremulousness and myoclonic jerking
D. Probably nothing

33. Thomas complains of difficulties at work resulting from EDS. He has had several reprimands because of napping on the job. A sleep study is negative for sleep apnea, periodic limb movements during sleep, and other causes of excessive daytime sedation. During the evaluation, Thomas describes excessive sleepiness and sleeping 10 or more hours on the weekend; he has no energy or interest to leave the house and spends most of his time watching TV and eating. He relates that he has gained 10 pounds over the last 3 months. His symptoms are suggestive of atypical depression. Thomas has a past history of alcohol abuse and is worried about relapsing with the stress of his current situation. His primary care provider has given him a prescription for trazodone, 50 mg, for his difficulty sleeping at night. He has taken this for a couple of weeks with little improvement.

   Which of the following interventions would be a next-best medication intervention for Thomas?
A. Increase the dose of trazodone and add amphetamine.
B. Increase the dose of trazodone and add bupropion.
C. Increase the dose of trazodone and add modafinil.
D. Discontinue the trazodone and add GHB.

34. Rachel is 85 years old and has been living in a nursing home for the past 5 years. In the last year she has developed increasing difficulty with her memory. Her physician started her on memantine, and it does seem to have helped her quite a bit over

recent months. Recently she has had trouble sleeping owing to the loss of her longtime roommate and trying to adjust to a new one. The physician wants to start a short-term sleeping aid for Rachel but wants one that will not disrupt her memory and cognition. Out of the following choices, which of the following agents is the *best* alternative for her?
A. Zolpidem
B. Ramelteon
C. Cyproheptadine
D. Temazepam

35. Schizophrenia is associated with specific polysmnographic (PSG) changes: impaired sleep onset and maintenance, reduced SWS, decreased REM latency, and decreased total REM. Several studies indicate no change in REM as well. Typical (e.g., haloperidol) and atypical antipsychotic medications, such as clozapine, olanzapine, and risperidone, have similar effects on PSG parameters. These effects are associated with response to treatment. Of the following, which PSG change is most consistently associated with the efficacy of these agents?
A. Improved SWS
B. Increased awakenings
C. Increase in stage 1 sleep
D. No change in sleep parameters

36. Andy is a 69-year-old with moderate Parkinson's disease (PD). He was sent to the sleep lab for evaluation of new-onset EDS and sudden daytime sleep episodes. His evaluation rules out sleep apnea, narcolepsy, and restless legs. A review of his history indicates that these sudden sleep episodes and the EDS developed after he was initiated on a higher dose of carbidopa-levodopa. Lowering the dose of Andy's carbidopa-levodopa is not currently an option. Other dopaminergic agents such as ropinirole and pramipexole can be associated with sudden sleep episodes in patients with PD, so changing to one of these agents is not possible. One dopaminergic option in the treatment of EDS in patients with PD is amantadine, but Andy has already failed a trial of this agent. While the neurologist works on the PD medications, he asks you for a suggestion to treat Andy's EDS

Which of the following interventions for EDS would be the *best* intervention at this time?
A. Adding an anticholinergic medication
B. Adding modafinil
C. Adding buspirone
D. Adding caffeine tablets

37. Linda has been taking lorazepam, 0.5 mg three times a day, and 1 mg at bedtime for anxiety for the past 6 months. On her last visit the physician discontinued the lorazepam because of concerns about dependence and started Linda on buspirone, 5 mg three times a day, for her anxiety. Four days later, Linda calls the office complaining of increased insomnia with vivid dreams, tremulousness, a rapid heart rate, and worsening anxiety. She says she doesn't like the buspirone and is asking to have her lorazepam back.

What is the most likely explanation for these complaints?
A. Benzodiazepine withdrawal
B. Medication seeking
C. Buspirone toxicity
D. The flu

38. Jim, the new patient in for detoxification, has been pacing the unit for the past few hours. He is very talkative and irritable. His urine drug screen came back positive for cocaine. What change in his sleep architecture would be expected tonight when he is in withdrawal?
A. Increased sleep latency
B. REM suppression
C. REM rebound
D. Decreased stage 3 sleep

39. Richard has obstructive sleep apnea. He also has active cirrhosis and is 50 pounds overweight. A consult to initiate continuous positive airway pressure (CPAP) has been sent. Currently Richard is having problems falling asleep at night owing to his anxiety about his health. The doctor has put him on buspirone for the anxiety and needs something to help with sleep because buspirone is not sedating. Which of the following would be the *best* option?
A. Temazepam
B. Triazolam
C. Eszopiclone
D. Diphenhydramine

40. Susan has a diagnosis of narcolepsy. She and her husband want to get pregnant. Currently she takes methylphenidate for her EDS. You explain that it is better to use no stimulants during pregnancy; however, she explains that she plans to continue employment. She is afraid the EDS on no medication will prevent her from maintaining work and wants a different, safer, agent to use when she is pregnant. Which of the following would be the safest option for Susan?
A. Modafinil
B. Dextroamphetamine
C. Imipramine
D. Pemoline

Answers

1. C. Dopamine

Amphetamines and methylphenidate affect presynaptic levels of the neurotransmitter dopamine by inhibiting of the dopamine reuptake transporter and enhancing the release of presynaptic dopamine. Although amphetamines and methylphenidate also block the reuptake and presynaptic release of norepinephrine, the magnitude of the effect on dopamine appears to be primary in their effectiveness in promoting wakefulness.

They do not have direct activity at the adenosine, histamine, or glutamate systems.

2. C. Levofloxacin

Theophylline can be associated with insomnia and agitation at blood levels within the therapeutic range. As theophylline levels rise, these symptoms can become evident or worsen. In patients with chronic obstructive pulmonary disease and other respiratory diseases, theophylline's ability to restore respiratory function generally seems to offset the sleep disruption seen in these disease states.

Theophylline is primarily metabolized via the cytochrome P450 isoenzyme 1A2. Antibiotic agents (e.g., quinolones and macrolides) vary in their inhibitory effect on 1A2. Inhibition of 1A2 could result in side effects as a result of elevated theophylline blood levels such as tremor, insomnia, agitation, and tachycardia. Hypotension, ventricular arrhythmias, and seizures can result at higher blood levels.

Levofloxacin has minimal effects on the clearance of theophylline and should not result in elevated blood levels. Carithromycin, erythromycin, and pefloxacin decrease the clearance of theophylline, and their use could result in increased side effects and potential toxicity.

3. D. Increased slow wave sleep (SWS)

According to the *Lithium Encyclopedia for Clinical Practice*, lithium causes a dramatic increase in SWS. It decreases time spent in stage 1 sleep and the duration of REM sleep and increases stage 2 sleep and REM latency. Although lithium use results in REM suppression, it is not associated with REM rebound. Total sleep time is unchanged, and with chronic use, improvement in sleep quantity and quality are reported. Sleepiness and fatigue are associated with lithium initiation but typically resolve over time. Once-daily dosing at bedtime (to a maximum one-time dose of 1200 mg) can maximize the benefit and minimize problems with this side effect.

4. A. Nadolol

Nadolol is a nonselective beta-blocker with low lipid solubility. Nadolol has minimal effects on sleep parameters, and in one report (Kales, 43:655, 1988), nadolol at doses of 80 mg a day improved sleep efficiency and enhanced REM sleep.

Metoprolol, a beta-1 selective beta-blocker, and pindolol, a nonselective agent, are moderately lipophilic, and the nonselective beta-blocker propranolol is highly lipophilic. Degree of beta selectivity is not associated with sleep disruption, but the extent of lipophilicity is. Metoprolol, pindolol, and propranolol are linked to multiple reports of disrupted sleep, including complaints of nightmares, vivid dreams, hallucinations, and insomnia.

5. B. Temazepam

Temazepam has a half-life of approximately 8–10 hours. Estazolam has a half-life of 12 hours, and quazepam and flurazepam can have half-lives over 72 hours when the active metabolites are considered. The duration of action of benzodiazepine is a function of its lipophilicity and the presence of active metabolites (Table 20-1).

6. C. Metipranolol

Metipranolol is a nonselective beta antagonist that is highly lipophilic and is readily absorbed into the bloodstream after topical administration. Metipranolol is associated with a high incidence of somnolence and fatigue. Anxiety and nervousness have also been reported. Insomnia is not a common side effect of metipranolol.

Travoprost is a prostaglandin-F2-alpha analog with similar agonist effectiveness to latanoprost. Daytime sedation and other sleep disturbances are not

TABLE 20-1 ■ Pharmacokinetic Parameters of Benzodiazepine Hypnotics	
Agent	**Kinetic Parameters**
Estazolam (ProSom)	Onset: rapid Insignificant active metabolites t1/2 = 12–24 hr
Flurazepam (Dalmane)	Onset: rapid 2 active metabolites t1/2 = 72+ hr
Quazepam (Doral)	Onset: rapid 2 active metabolites t1/2 = 72+ hr
Temazepam (Restoril)	Onset: intermediate Insignificant active metabolite t1/2 = 8–10 hr
Triazolam (Halcion)	Onset: rapid Insignificant active metabolite t1/2 = 4 hr

associated with the use of topical prostaglandin agonists. Carbachol is a direct-acting miotic. Systemic absorption results in symptoms related to cholinergic excess (nausea, salivation, urination, diarrhea). Dorzolamide is a carbonic anhydrase inhibitor with a propensity for allergic reactions because of its sulfonamide structure. Headaches are the most common neurological side effect for this agent.

7. B. Caffeine

Caffeine is thought to antagonize the sleep-promoting actions of adenosine. Accumulation of adenosine and activation of the adenosine system is associated with sedation and sleep; therefore antagonism of adenosine receptors enhances wakefulness. Caffeine is also thought to enhance the activity of cholinergic neurons and inhibit GABA neurons involved in wakefulness and sleep promotion, respectively. Caffeine may also indirectly affect dopamine transmission via action on the adenosine A_{2A} receptors on dopamine neurons, resulting in increased arousal.

8. B. CYP2D6 inhibition

Trazodone is metabolized to an active metabolite, meta-chlorophenylpiperazine (m-CPP), via n-dealkylation. Both trazodone and m-CPP are substrates for the cytochrome P450 isoenzyme 2D6. The CYP2D6 isoenzyme is subject to inhibition by multiple medications including fluoxetine. Inhibition would result in elevated blood levels of trazodone and cMPP, leading to EDS resulting from enhanced 5-HT2 and alpha-1 receptor blockade.

The 2D6 isoenzyme is also present in variable amounts in individuals. In some situations people may have relatively no functioning CYP2D6 (poor metabolizers), and others may have an abundance of CYP2D6 (rapid metabolizers). Poor metabolizers would have higher blood levels of compounds metabolized via 2D6. These elevated levels can result in problematic side effects from the same dose that normal or rapid metabolizers tolerate without difficulty. Jon's status is not known but could be contributory.

Trazodone is only slightly metabolized by the cytochrome isoenzyme 3A4, and inhibition of this isoenzyme would be unlikely to cause EDS. Trazodone is not metabolized via 1A2 and has only weak antagonist activity of alpha-2 adrenergic receptors.

9. A. Gamma aminobutyric acid (GABA)

The exact mechanism of action of valerian in the treatment of insomnia is yet fully elucidated. Research has identified several effects of valerian's many active constituents on GABA levels in the brain. Valerenic acid has been demonstrated to inhibit the breakdown of GABA, have agonist activity at GABA-A receptors, and may increase the release of presynaptic GABA. Other constituents have been shown to inhibit the reuptake of GABA. Research data support the concept that valerian exerts its sedative-hypnotic activity via pro-GABAergic activity.

Valerian has been reported to decrease sleep latency, increase SWS, and improve sleep quality. Reports on its effects on other sleep parameters are mixed. Valerian's ability to assist with sleep is dose related, with smaller doses being more anxiolytic and larger doses more helpful for sleep. There are also differing results for the ethanolic (more calming) and aqueous (more sedating) extracts. Use of the specific formulation for the desired effect, or even a whole-herb product, may be of more benefit on an individual basis. Some patients find it more helpful when taken on a consistent basis over a 2-week period than when taken acutely.

There is currently no evidence that valerian affects serotonin, adenosine, or glutamate levels.

10. B. Modafinil

Modafinil is the only agent on the list appropriate for substitution. Effective for EDS in narcolepsy, its mechanism of action has not been elucidated. Modafinil is less likely than methylphenidate to cause hypertension and an elevated heart rate and should still offer Danni an effective therapy for her daytime sedation.

The dopaminergic agent amantadine has shown effectiveness in decreasing fatigue associated with multiple sclerosis, but it is not reported to be effective in narcolepsy. Duloxetine blocks the reuptake of both serotonin and norepinephrine; it has demonstrated efficacy in depression and diabetic neuropathy (pain). Duloxetine has not been studied in narcolepsy. Bupropion inhibits the reuptake of norepinephrine and dopamine. Bupropion has demonstrated effectiveness in depression, attention deficit disorder, and fatigue associated with cancer and chronic fatigue syndrome. Bupropion has been shown to be effective for excessive sleepiness because of narcolepsy in one case report (Rye, 7:92, 1998), but the data are not robust. Bupropion therapy can result in increases in blood pressure.

11. D. Protriptyline

Protriptyline is a second-generation tricyclic with primarily noradrenergic activity relative to its effects on serotonin. Protriptyline has relatively little antagonistic effect on histaminergic receptors, which results in a minimal amount of sedation.

Tricyclic antidepressants have varying degrees of sedation and effects on sleep architecture. Other side

TABLE 20-2 ■ Receptor Activity of Tricyclic Antidepressants

Tricyclic Agents	Norepinephrine Reuptake	Serotonin Reuptake	Dopamine Reuptake	5-HT2 Antagonism	Alpha-1 Antagonism	M1 Antagonism	H1 Antagonism
Amitriptyline	+++	++++	0	+	++++	++++	++++
Imipramine	++	+++	0/+	0	++++	+++	++
Doxepin	++	+++	0	+	+++	+++	++++
Trimipramine	+/0	+/0	0	+	+++	++++	++++
Nortriptyline	+++	++	0	0	++	+++	++
Desipramine	++++	+	0/+	0	+++	++	++
Protriptyline	++++	+	0	0	+++	++	+

0, No activity; +, low activity; ++, mild activity; +++, modest activity; ++++, highest activity.

effects vary as well, depending on their activity at different receptors (Table 20-2).

Tertiary tricyclic agents are quite sedating with strong antagonism of alpha-1 and histaminergic receptors. The second-generation agents have differences in their ability to block reuptake of serotonin and norepinephrine, and all have less of an effect at alpha-1 and histaminergic receptors than their parent compounds and other tertiary agents.

12. D. Change the donepezil dose to the morning.

Donepezil and other acetylcholinesterase inhibitors have been associated with agitation, insomnia, and nightmares in some patients because of their procholinergic profile. Susceptible patients usually have resolution of these side effects when administration is changed to the morning.

Hydroxyzine's anticholinergic side effects could worsen memory, and antihistamines can be associated with morning hangover. A serotonin reuptake inhibitor, citalopram, is not indicated at this time because of the patient's lack of depressive symptoms. Ranitidine, a histamine-2 receptor antagonist, is inconsistently associated with alterations in the sleep cycle and may be associated with improved SWS with chronic use. Discontinuation is premature at this time.

13. A. Gabapentin

Gabapentin has been shown to cause somnolence and daytime fatigue when used in therapeutic doses. Its effects on sleep include increased stage 3 and 4 sleep, an increase in sleep quality, sleep consolidation, and fewer nocturnal awakenings.

Topiramate and levetiracetam are reported to cause fatigue, anxiety, and nervousness. Topiramate up to doses of 200 mg/day is not associated with daytime impairment. Lamotrigine is not commonly associated with fatigue.

14. B. Citalopram

Paul is most likely experiencing serotonin syndrome as a result of the combination of citalopram, a serotonin reuptake inhibitor, and the 5-HTP. Citalopram use results in higher concentrations of serotonin in the synaptic cleft after it is released from the presynaptic neuron. The use of 5-HTP results in greater amounts of serotonin being available for release from the presynaptic neurons into the synaptic cleft. The combined result is excessive stimulation of serotonin receptors, resulting in serotonin syndrome.

Orally 5-HTP is highly bioavailable. It easily crosses the blood-brain barrier and results in increased levels of serotonin, as well as norepinephrine, dopamine, and melatonin. In therapeutic doses, 5-HTP is typically well tolerated. Dose-related nausea is most commonly seen, and in higher doses, vivid dreams and nightmares have been reported.

15. B. Clonazepam

While clonazepam is no longer considered the treatment of choice, it has an established track record of usefulness in the treatment of restless legs syndrome. A small dose at bedtime should not be problematic for Doris. The lack of symptoms during the day rules out akathisia because of her antipsychotic quetiapine.

Acetaminophen does not have a role in the treatment of restless legs syndrome. Ropinirole, although indicated for the treatment of restless legs syndrome, would not be the first-line agent for Doris. Like pramepexole, its dopaminergic activity would worsen her primary problem of schizophrenia. Risperidone is not helpful in the treatment of restless legs, and adding another antipsychotic medication to Doris's regimen is not indicated.

16. Increase in REM latency

Methylphenidate, like amphetamine, is a potent REM suppressor; it also increases sleep latency and REM latency. Methylphenidate has been reported to increase stage 1 sleep; decrease stage 2 and either decrease or cause no change in the amount of SWS.

17. B. Decrease in REM sleep

Treatment with opioid analgesics has been associated with a decrease in SWS and REM sleep, a decrease in sleep latency, and an increase in nocturnal awakenings. Patients undergoing abdominal surgery are reported to experience an initial decrease in SWS and REM sleep followed by a significant degree of REM rebound in the following nights. Use of opioid analgesics can exacerbate these sleep alterations and may explain the increase in complaints of vivid nightmares and hallucinations postsurgery.

18. D. Increase in REM latency

Acute alcohol ingestion is associated with increases in REM latency, sleep continuity, and sleep quality, but decreases in sleep latency and total REM sleep.

19. C. REM rebound

Albert awoke as a result of the effects of alcohol withdrawal. Rapid metabolism of alcohol drops the blood alcohol level to zero by early morning, and reverse sleep changes can be seen. There is increased sleep latency, fragmented sleep with increased awakenings, vivid dreaming, and increased REM sleep. Decreases in total sleep time and delta sleep occurs.

20. A. Somnambulism

Lithium has been documented as the cause of new-onset somnambulism in patients treated with lithium for a variety of diagnoses. Lithium has not been associated with the development of restless legs, narcolepsy, and sleep apnea.

21. D. Prazosin

Studies indicate that high amounts of norepinephrine and increased postsynaptic adrenergic receptor responsivity may contribute to nighttime symptoms of PTSD. Excessive activation of alpha-1 adrenergic receptors results in an increase in the release of central nervous system corticotropin-releasing factor, causing disrupted sleep and impaired prefrontal cortex regulation of cognition. Prazosin, an alpha-1 adrenergic receptor antagonist, should treat elevated blood pressure, normalize sleep architecture, and decrease nightmares for this patient. Studies in patients with PTSD indicate that prazosin use is associated with a decrease in PTSD-related nightmares.

In one case report, metoprolol was reported to precipitate PTSD symptoms, possibly owing to its high lipophilicity and REM suppressant effects. Clonidine, an alpha-2 adrenergic agonist, is associated with a high degree of sedation, has been associated with reports of nightmares, and has been demonstrated to decrease REM sleep. Fosinopril, an angiotensin-converting enzyme inhibitor, is rarely associated with sleep changes.

22. C. Increase REM sleep

Nefazodone is an antidepressant with anxiolytic activity. Mechanistically, nefazodone has modest serotonin reuptake inhibition action, with a low ability to inhibit norepinephrine reuptake, and it has mild antagonistic action at alpha-1 and histaminergic receptors. Nefazodone has potent antagonist activity at 5-hydroxytryptophan (5-HT2) receptors. One of nefazodone's active metabolites, mCPP, is also a serotonin agonist and blocks 5-HT2 and 5-HT3 receptors.

Nefazodone's ability to antagonize 5HT2 receptors confers an extra ability to decrease anxiety and also decreases the incidence of sexual dysfunction, akathisia, and insomnia, often associated with serotonin reuptake inhibitors. Nefazodone has been reported to have stabilizing effects on sleep continuity. It decreases sleep latency and minimizes awakenings during sleep, and, unlike with other antidepressants, patients taking nefazodone have shown an increase in total REM sleep (Winokur, 14:19, 2001; Mayers, 20:533, 2005).

Because nefazodone has been implicated in hepatotoxicity in several case reports, while using nefazodone in this patient or any other, it is important to educate the patient regarding signs and symptoms of liver dysfunction and to monitor baseline and periodic liver function tests.

23. D. They bind to the omega (alpha) subunit on the GABA-A complex.

The new nonbenzodiazepine sleeping agents zaleplon, zolpidem, and eszopiclone bind with selectivity and differing binding affinities to the alpha subunit of the GABA-A receptor complex, which explains some of the differing effects of each agent. Ultimately their function, like that of GABA, is to enhance chloride conductance, resulting in inhibition of the system.

24. B. Mirtazapine

Mirtazapine is an antidepressant with multiple potential benefits for Betty. For initial assistance with sleep, low doses of mirtazapine are quite sedating because of antihistaminergic activity. As an antidepressant, mirtazapine increases both norepinephrine and serotonin, and with resolution of her depression, Betty's sleep should normalize. Mirtazapine also blocks the 5-HT2 receptor, which decreases serotonin-induced insomnia, anxiety, and akasthisia. Mirtazapine's 5-HT3 blockade decreases its ability to aggravate irritable bowel disease.

25. D. Trimipramine

Trimipramine appears to have no effect on total percentage of REM sleep. Other tertiary antidepressants—amitriptyline, doxepin, and imipramine—all appear to cause REM suppression. Other PSG effects seen with sedating tricyclic agents include increased sleep efficiency, reduced sleep latency, and reduced wakefulness during sleep.

26. B. Circadian rhythm sleep disorders

Melatonin has demonstrated rather consistent ability to assist with sleep disorders associated with circadian rhythm disruption (e.g., delayed sleep phase disorder, jet lag, shift work). When used for jet lag, 5-mg doses are recommended once daily, usually late in the day or at bedtime, for the first 5 days in the new time zone. This regimen was reported to result in less overall lag and a faster recovery of energy and alertness. Results of trials in shift workers were not numerically significant, but participants reported subjective improvement in sleep.

Melatonin has demonstrated a rapid onset of action, producing mild, short-lived, sleep-inducing effects. Melatonin lowers body temperature and alertness for roughly 3–4 hours after a low dose (0.5–5 mg) is given. Acute exposure to bright light has the opposite effects. Melatonin can advance or delay the internal clock depending on the timing of the dose. Giving a low dose (0.5–5 mg) approximately 8–13 hours before a person's lowest core temperature should result in phase advancement. Taking the dose 1–5 hours after the lowest core temperature should cause phase delay. Studies looking at phase shift adaptation and shift work demonstrate that melatonin given at bedtime (whether actually at night or during the day) is designed to delay sleep, improve sleep quality and duration, and decrease the number of awakenings during sleep.

Melatonin is not suggested for use in narcolepsy or sleep apnea and has been reported in isolated cases to worsen restless legs (Michaud, 55:372, 2004), but it may be of assistance in periodic limb movements during sleep (Patel, 8:498, 2002).

27. A. Decrease in stage 2 sleep

Use of benzodiazepines is associated with an increase in total sleep time, REM latency, and stage 2 NREM sleep. They are associated with a decrease in sleep latency, amount of time spent awake after sleep onset, and SWS. Benzodiazepines generally decrease REM density, especially with chronic dosing.

28. A. Ability to increase slow wave sleep (SWS)

GHB has been shown to induce central nervous system (CNS) depression and sleep, perhaps by its activity at the GABA-B receptor and its metabolism to GABA-enhancing gabaergic activity in the CNS. The CNS depressant effect of GHB is short lived, and GHB has differing dose-related effects. Low doses of GHB result in antianxiety and muscle relaxant effects, midrange doses increase SWS, and at higher doses it has the potential to be a useful adjunct to anesthesia and is used for this purpose in several European countries.

The exact mechanism behind GHB's effectiveness in catalepsy associated with narcolepsy is unknown. It has been theorized that it increases daytime alertness by increasing sleep continuity during the night by balancing NREM and REM sleep. Giving GHB at bedtime is associated with a decrease in the duration of stage 1 sleep, an increase in stages 3 and 4, and a decrease in REM latency. GHB's overall effect on the amount of total REM sleep is not fully understood. GHB has been reported to both increase (Wong, 54: S3, 2003) and decrease (Lemon, 40:433, 2006) the total amount of REM sleep. HGB has demonstrated effectiveness in decreasing hypnagogic hallucinations associated with narcolepsy.

Pharmacologic studies indicate that GHB may inhibit the release of dopamine, increase serotonin turnover, increase growth hormone release, and interact in undefined ways with opiate and cholinergic pathways. GHB has not been shown to have antihistaminergic or alpha-adrenergic blocking abilities.

29. A. Zaleplon

Zaleplon has a rapid onset of action and a short half-life of about 1 hour. Because of its short duration of action, it has not been shown to affect morning alertness when taken during nocturnal awakenings. Although they both have a rapid onset of effect, zolpidem and eszopiclone are reported to cause morning impairment when taken during nocturnal awakenings because of their longer half-lives and the associated longer duration of action (Table 20-3). The incidence of abnormal dreams with zaleplon and eszopiclone is reported to be similar to that of placebo. Zolpidem has been associated with nightmares.

Estazolam is a benzodiazepine with a longer half-life of about 12 hours. It would probably be effective for Derek's early morning awakening if given at bedtime but would be inappropriate for dosing when he awoke at 2 A.M.

TABLE 20-3 ■ Pharmacokinetic Variables of Nonbenzodiazepine Hypnotics

Agent	Kinetic Parameters
Zolpidem (Ambien)	Onset: rapid t1/2 = 4 hr No clinically significant active metabolites
Zaleplon (Sonata)	Onset: rapid t1/2 = 1 hr No clinically significant active metabolites
Eszopiclone (Lunesta)	Onset: rapid Tmax = 1–1.5 hr t1/2 = 6 hr No clinically significant active metabolites

30. C. Cetirizine crosses the blood-brain barrier.

Of the newer antihistamines, cetirizine has the greatest ability to cross into the brain and antagonize CNS histamine receptors. Although it should still be less sedating than the first-generation agents, it is more sedating than loratadine and fexofenadine.

Cetirizine has very low affinity for alpha-1 and H-2 receptors and is not GABAergic.

31. B. Increased total sleep time

In premarketing studies, ramelteon was noted to decrease sleep latency and increase total sleep time, but it did not alter sleep architecture. No withdrawal or REM rebound is associated with rapid cessation of this agent.

32. D. Probably nothing

Rapid discontinuation of modafinil has not been associated with withdrawal phenomenon. Unlike other stimulants, from which acute withdrawal would result in hypersomnolence, modafinil's lack of an effect on REM and other sleep parameters does not result in excessive sedation on discontinuation. Gastrointestinal distress and myoclonic jerking has not been reported with modafinil withdrawal.

33. B. Increase the dose of trazodone and add bupropion.

Bupropion is an antidepressant that has its primary effects via enhanced norepinephrine and dopamine levels. A potent inhibitor of the reuptake of both of these neurotransmitters, bupropion has a stimulating side effect profile and is associated with antidepressant activity, as well as the ability to enhance alertness in patients with attention-deficit hyperactivity disorder (ADHD) and Parkinson's disease. If Thomas's daytime sedation is related to depression, it should start to show improvement with the initiation of bupropion because of the side effects and continue to improve over time with resolution of his depression. Increasing the trazodone to a more therapeutic dose should also help regulate his sleep and augment the antidepressant activity of bupropion.

Amphetamine would counter the daytime sedation but would not be helpful with any underlying depression. It may also be a problem for Thomas with his history of alcohol abuse. Modafinil is a good alternative for the daytime sedation but is not effective in depression. Concerns about abuse would be less of an issue than with amphetamine. GHB is not an option for Thomas. He is not diagnosed with narcolepsy and has not failed other treatment options. In addition, GHB has a high addiction potential.

34. B. Ramelteon

Studies have demonstrated that ramelteon does not have a significant effect on cognition or on memory. Its parent compound, melatonin, has little effect on cognition and memory as well.

Although short acting and generally well tolerated, zolpidem can be associated with difficulties in memory and cognition, especially in the older population. Cyproheptadine is an antihistamine with anticholinergic properties that could interfere with memory and cognition in an older patient with dementia. Temazepam, as a benzodiazepine, would be potentially problematic. As a class, the benzodiazepines have varying degrees of effect on cognition and memory.

35. A. Improved slow wave sleep (SWS)

Normalization of sleep (improvement in sleep continuity and total sleep time) and an increase SWS and REM latency are observed as patients respond to treatment with most antipsychotic medications. Sleep latency is also shortened by most antipsychotic medications. Of interest, clozapine, the most effective of all antipsychotic medications, has been noted to increase NREM sleep by increasing stage 2 sleep but also has been reported to suppress SWS.

36. B. Adding modafinil

In Parkinson's disease, EDS can be a result of the disease process, disruption of the reticular activating system, and sleep disorders (sleep apnea, narcolepsy, REM sleep behavior disorder). It is also associated with medications used to treat Parkinson's disease. When altering Parkinson's disease therapy is not an option or does not affect the EDS, it is treated with alertness-promoting medications.

Modafinil may assist with alertness without aggravating the patient's Parkinson's disease. Its lack of robust dopaminergic activity would not increase the risk that Andy may develop hallucinations due to excessive dopaminergic activity. Modafinil appears to be well tolerated in patients with Parkinson's disease (Happe, 63:2725, 2003).

Adding an anticholinergic medication would not have a positive effect on the daytime sedation. Most of these agents have a high degree of sedation associated with their use. Caffeine might be helpful in the short term, but tolerance develops and caffeine can have its own disrupting effects on sleep. There is no evidence that adenosine antagonism is helpful in Parkinson's disease. Buspirone, an anxiolytic agent, may have a stimulating side effect profile but is not indicated for or shown to be effective for EDS in Parkinson's disease.

37. A. Benzodiazepine withdrawal

Cutting Linda's lorazepam cold turkey has triggered acute benzodiazepine withdrawal. Abrupt discontinuation of benzodiazepines results in withdrawal phenomenon even when the medication is taken as prescribed for several weeks. Benzodiazepine withdrawal has many of the same symptoms that alcohol withdrawal does but usually to a lesser intensity. Her insomnia and vivid dreaming are a direct result of the reverse of the effect benzodiazepines have on sleep parameters.

Medication-seeking behavior is realistic for a patient in withdrawal, but she is not seeking medication inappropriately; she wants the withdrawal to end. Buspirone is an effective anxiolytic, but it will not cross-cover benzodiazepine withdrawal. A dose of 5 mg three times a day is a typical starting dose, and she is not toxic. She may have the flu, but the time course makes this a highly unlikely answer.

38. C. REM rebound

Stimulant intoxication results in an increase in sleep latency and REM latency, and a decrease in REM sleep. Daytime sedation is decreased as well. Stimulant withdrawal results in decreased sleep latency and REM rebound.

39. D. Diphenhydramine

Diphenhydramine, an antihistamine, can be used to assist with sleep in patients with obstructive sleep apnea. Diphenhydramine decreases sleep latency, decreases REM sleep, and increases sleep continuity. It has no muscle-relaxing activity and no effect on airway dilator muscle tone. It is nonaddicting, is safe for use in cirrhosis, and will not interact negatively with buspirone. Diphenhydramine can have residual morning hangover and can negatively affect performance, and it may not continue to be successful with chronic use owing to the development of tolerance over time to its sedating action.

Triazolam and temazepam are benzodiazepines, and as a class they have the potential to depress respiratory function and worsen apnea. Eszopiclone is highly metabolized in the liver and may accumulate if the liver damage is bad enough. Eszopiclone is not recommended for patients with liver dysfunction.

40. D. Pemoline

Pemoline carries a pregnancy rating of B and can be used, if necessary, to treat hypersomnolence in narcolepsy. Because of the risk of elevated liver enzymes, baseline liver function studies and monitoring during therapy is recommended. Because of the risk of hepatotoxicity, however, its use should be discouraged. Modafinil and dextroamphetamine are both pregnancy category C agents. Imipramine is not especially recommended for hypersomnolence in narcolepsy, although useful for the REM effects of narcolepsy, and it is pregnancy category D.

REFERENCES

1. Arendt J: Jet-lag and shift work: (2) therapeutic uses of melatonin. J R Soc Med 92:402–405, 1999.
2. Attele AS, Xie J-T, Yuan C-S: Treatment of insomnia: an alternative approach. Alternative Medicine Review 5(3):249–258, 2000.
3. Ballard RD: Sleep and medical disorders. Prim Care Clin Office Pract 32:511–533, 2005.
4. Barone P, Amboni M, Vitale C, Bonavita B: Treatment of nocturnal disturbances and excessive daytime sleepiness in Parkinson's disease. Neurology 63(Suppl 3):S35–S38, 2004.
5. Becker PM: Pharmacologic and nonpharmacologic treatments of insomnia. Neurol Clin 23:1140–1163, 2005.
6. Birdsall TC: 5-hydroxytryptophan: a clinically-effective serotonin precursor. Altern Med Rev 3(4):271–280, 1998.
7. Boutrel B, Koob GF: What keeps us awake: the neuropharmacology of stimulants and wakefulness promoting medications. Sleep 27(6):1181–1194, 2004.
8. Broughton, RJ, Fleming JA, George CF, et al: Randomized, double-blind, placebo-controlled crossover trial of modafinil in the treatment of excessive daytime sleepiness in narcolepsy. Ovid Broughton Neurology 49(2):444–451, 1997.
9. Buysse DJ, Schweitzer PK, Moul DE: Clinical pharmacology of other drugs used as hypnotics. In Kryger MH, Roth T, Dement WC (eds): *Principles and Practice of Sleep Medicine*, 4th ed. Philadelphia, Elselvier Saunders, 2005, pp 452–465.
10. Bye DB, Dihenia B, Bliwise DL: Reversal of atypical depression, sleepiness, and REM-sleep propensity in narcolepsy with bupropion. Depression Anxiety 7:92–95, 1998.
11. Lee-Chiong TL: Parasomnias and other sleep-related movement disorders. Prim Care Clin Office Pract 32:415–433, 2005.
12. Conn DK: Cholinesterase inhibitors. Geriatrics 56(9):56–58, 2001.
13. De Feo V, Faro C: Pharmacological effects of extracts from valeriana adscendens trel. II. Effects on GABA uptake and amino acids. Phytother Res 17:661–664, 2003.
14. Diaper A, Hindmarch I: A double-blind, placebo-controlled investigation of the effects of two doses of a valerian preparation on the sleep, cognitive and psychomotor function of sleep-disturbed older adults. Phytother Res 18:831–836, 2004.
15. Dubocovich ML: Pharmacology and function of melatonin receptors. FASEB J 2:2765–2773, 1988.
16. Dykewicz MS, Fineman S, Skoner DP, et al: Diagnosis and management of rhinitis: complete guidelines of the Joint Task Force on Practice Parameters in Allergy, Asthma and Immunology. Ann Allergy Asthma Immunol 81:478–518, 1998.
17. Estelle F, Simons R: Comparative pharmacology of H_1 antihistamines: clinical relevance. Am J Med 113(9A):38S–46S, 2002.
18. Gardiner P, Kemper KJ: Insomnia: herbal and diet alternatives to counting sheep. Contemp Pediatr 2:69, 2002.
19. Guin Ting Wong C, Bottiglieri T, Snead OC: GABA, gamma-hydroxybutyric acid, and neurological disease. Ann Neurol 54(suppl 6):S3–S12, 2003.
20. Gyllenhaal C, Merritt SL, Peterson SD, et al: Efficacy and safety of herbal stimulants and sedatives in sleep disorders. Sleep Med Rev 4(3):229–251, 2000.
21. Happe S: Excessive daytime sleepiness and sleep disturbances in patients with neurological diseases: epidemiology and management. Drugs 63:2725–2737, 2003.
22. Hinze-Selch D, Mullington J, Orth A, et al: Effects of clozapine on sleep: a longitudinal study. Biol Psychiatry 42:260–266, 1997.
23. Hofstetter JR, Lysaker PH, Mayeda AR: Quality of sleep in patients with schizophrenia is associated with quality of life and coping. BMC Psychiatry 5:13, 2005.
24. Hoyt BD: Sleep in patients with neurologic and psychiatric disorders. Prim Care Clin Office Pract 32:535–548, 2005.
25. Jasinski DR: An evaluation of the abuse potential of modafinil using methylphenidate as a reference. J Psychopharmacol 14(1):53–60, 2000.
26. Jefferson JW, Greist JH, Ackerman DL, Carroll JA: *Lithium Encyclopedia for Clinical Practice*, 2nd ed. Washington, DC, American Psychiatric Press, 1987, pp 616–619.
27. Jellin JM, Gregory PJ, Batz F, et al: *Pharmacist's Letter/ Prescriber's Letter Natural Medicines Comprehensive Database*, 6th ed. Stockton, Therapeutic Research Faculty, 2004, pp 890–895, 146–148, 631–632, 664–667, 883–885, 1280–1282.
28. Jobert M, Jahnig P, Schulz H: Effect of two antidepressant drugs on REM sleep and EMG activity during sleep. Neuropsychobiology 39:101–109, 1999.
29. Kales A, Bixler EO, Vela-Bueno A, et al: Effects of nadolol on blood pressure, sleep efficiency, and sleep stages. Clin Pharmacol Ther 43(6):655–662, 1988.
30. Kelly RP, Yeo KP, Teng CH: Hemodynamic effects of acute administration of atomoxetine and methylphenidate. J Clin Pharmacol 45:851–855, 2005.
31. Keshavan MS, Reynolds CFIII, Miewald JM: Delta sleep deficits in schizophrenia. Arch Gen Psychiatry 55(5):443–448, 1998.
32. Krahn LE, Gonzalez-Arriaza HL: Narcolepsy with cataplexy. Am J Psychiatry 161(12):2181–2198, 2004.
33. Lemon MD, Strain JD, Farver DK: Sodium oxybate for cataplexy. Ann Pharmacother 40:433–440, 2006.
34. Linde K, Riet G, Hondras M, et al: Systematic reviews of complementary therapies: an annotated bibliography. Part 2: Herbal medicine. BMC Comp Alt Med 1:5, 2001.
35. Maixner S, Tandon R, Eiser A, et al: Effects of antipsychotic treatment on polysomnographic measure in schizophrenia: a replication and extension. Am J Psychiatry 155:1600–1602, 1998.
36. Mayers AG, Baldwin DS: Antidepressants and their effect on sleep. Hum Psychopharmacol 20(8):533–559, 2005.

37. Mendelson WB: Hypnotic medications: mechanisms of action and pharmacologic effects. In Kryger MH, Roth T, Dement WC (eds): *Principles and Practice of Sleep Medicine*, 4th ed. Philadelphia, Elsevier Saunders, 2005, pp 444–451.

38. McCurry SM, Israel SA: Sleep dysfunction in Alzheimer's disease and other dementias. Curr Treat Option Neurol 5:261–272, 2003.

39. Michaud M, Dumont M, Selmaoui B, et al: Circadian rhythm of restless legs syndrome: relationship with biological markers. Ann Neurol 55:372–380, 2004.

40. Mitler MM, Aldrich MS, Koob GF, Zarcone VP: Narcolepsy and its treatment with stimulants. Sleep 17(4):352–371, 1994.

41. Mitler MM, O'Malley MB: Wake-promoting medications: efficacy and adverse effects. In Kryger MH, Roth T, Dement WC (eds): *Principles and Practice of Sleep Medicine*, 4th ed. Philadelphia, Elsevier Saunders, 2005, pp 484–497.

42. Montplaisir J, Hawa R, Moller H, et al: Zopiclone and zaleplon vs. benzodiazepines in the treatment of insomnia: Canadian consensus statement. Hum Psychopharmacol Clin Exp 18:29–38, 2003.

43. Morin CM, Bastien CH, Brink D, Brown TR: Adverse effects of temazepam in older adults with chronic insomnia. Hum Psychopharmacol Clin Exp 18:75–82, 2003.

44. Neubauer DN: Chronic insomnia: current issues. Clinical Cornerstone 6(1C):S17–S22, 2004.

45. Nicholson AN, Pascoe PA, Stone BM: Histaminergic systems and sleep: studies in man with H1 and H2 antagonists. Neuropharmacology 24(3):245–250, 1985.

46. Niederhofer H: Atomoxetine also effective in patients suffering from narcolepsy? Sleep 28:9, 2005.

47. Nishino S, Mignot E: Wake-promoting medications: basic mechanisms and pharmacology. In Kryger MH, Roth T, Dement WC (eds): *Principles and Practice of Sleep Medicine*, 4th ed. Philadelphia, Elsevier Saunders, 2005, pp 468–981.

48. Nishino S, Mao J, Sampathkumaran R, et al: Increased dopaminergic transmission mediates the wake-promoting effects of CNS stimulants. Sleep Res Online 1(1):49–61, 1998.

49. Orzechowski RF, Currie DS, Valancius CA: Comparative anticholinergic activities of 10 histamine H$_1$ receptor antagonists in two functional models. Eur J Pharmacol 506:257–264, 2005.

50. Onen SH, Onen F, Courpron P, Dubray C: How pain and analgesics disturb sleep. Clin J Pain 21:422–431, 2005.

51. Pagel JF, Parnes BL: Medications for the treatment of sleep disorders: an overview. Primary care companion. J Clin Psychiatry 3:118–125, 2001.

52. Pagel JF, Helfter P: Drug induced nightmares—an etiology based review. Hum Psychopharmacol Clin Exp 18:59–67, 2003.

53. Pagel PF: Medications and their effects on sleep. Prim Care Clin Office Pract 32:491–509, 2005.

54. Patel S: Restless legs syndrome and periodic limb movements of sleep: fact, fad, and fiction. Curr Opin Pulm Med 8:498–501, 2002.

55. Peskind ER, Bonner LT, Huff DJ, Raskind MA: Prazosin reduces trauma-related nightmares in older men with chronic posttraumatic stress disorder. J Geriatr Psychiatry Neurol 16:165–171, 2003.

56. Poyares D, Pinto LR Jr, Tavares S, Barros-Viera S: Sleep promoters and insomnia. Rev Bras Psiquiatr 27(Supl 11):2–7, 2005.

57. Raskind MA, Peskind ER, Kanter ED, et al: Reduction of nightmares and other PTSD symptoms in combat veterans by prazosin: a placebo-controlled study. Am J Psychiatry 160:371–373, 2003.

58. Reeves RR, Liberto V: Precipitation of PTSD with metoprolol for hypertension. Psychosomatics 44(9–10):5, 2003.

59. Roth T, Zorick F, Sicklesteel J, Stepanski E: Effects of benzodiazepines on sleep and wakefulness. Br J Clin Pharmacol 11:31S–35S, 1981.

60. Rush AJ, Armitage R, Gillin JC, et al: Comparative effects of nefazodone and fluoxetine on sleep in outpatients with major depressive disorder. Biol Psychiatry 44:3–14, 1998.

61. Rye DB, Dihenia B, Bliwise DL: Reversal of atypical depression, sleepiness, and REM-sleep propensity in narcolepsy with bupropion. Depress Anxiety 7(2):92–95, 1998.

62. Salin-Pascual RJ, Herrera-Estrell M, Galicia-Polo L, Laurrabaquio MR: Olanzapine acute administration in schizophrenic patients increases delta sleep and sleep efficiency. Biol Psychiatry 46:141–143, 1999.

63. Santiago JR, Nolledo MS, Kinzler W, Santiago TV: Sleep and sleep disorders in pregnancy. Ann Intern Med 134:396–408, 2001.

64. Sauer JM, Ring BJ, Witcher JW: Clinical pharmacokinetics of atomoxetine. Clin Pharmacokinet 44(6):571–590, 2005.

65. Scammell TE, Estabrooke IV, McCarthy MT, et al: Hypothalamic arousal regions are activated during modafinil-induced wakefulness. J Neurosci 20(22):8620–8828, 2000.

66. Sharma A, Goldberg MJ, Cerimele B: Pharmacokinetics and safety of duloxetine, a dual-serotonin and norepinephrine reuptake inhibitor. J Clin Pharmacol 40:161–167, 2000.

67. Sharpley AL, Cowen PJ: Effect of pharmacologic treatments on the sleep of depressed patients. Biol Psychiatry 37:85–98, 1995.

68. Shinomiya K, Fujimura K, Kim Y, Kamei C: Effects of valerian extract on the sleep-wake cycle in sleep disturbed rats. Acta Med Okayama 59(3):89–92, 2005.

69. Singer C, Bahr A: Assessing and treating sleep disturbances in patients with Alzheimer's disease. Geriatric Times 5(6): 2004. Accessed November 28, 2005 from http://geriatrictimes.com/g041221.html.

70. Song JC, Nguyen NN, Yu SS: Ramelteon: a novel melatonin receptor agonist for the treatment of insomnia. Formulary 40:146–155, 2005.

71. Stahl SM: *Essential Psychopharmacology. Neuroscientific Basis and Practical Applications*, 2nd ed. Cambridge, Cambridge University Press, 2000, pp 199–296, 297–334, 401–498, 499–539.

72. Sugden D, Pickering H, Teh MT, Garratt PJ: Melatonin receptor pharmacology: toward subtype specificity. Biol Cell 89:531–537, 1997.

73. Ting L, Malhotra A: Disorders of sleep: an overview. Prim Care Clin Office Pract 32:305–318, 2005.

74. Vignatelli L, D'Alessandro R, Candelise L: Antidepressant drugs for narcolepsy. Cochrane Database Syst Rev (3), CD003724, Jul 20, 2005.

75. Winokur A, Gary KA, Rodner S, et al: Depression, sleep physiology, and antidepressant drugs. Depress Anxiety 14(1):19–28, 2001.

76. Yamadera H, Nakamura S, Suzuki H, Endo S: Effects of trazodone hydrochloride and imipramine on polysomnography in healthy subjects. Bipolar Clin Neurosci 52:439–443, 1998.

77. Zammit GK, McNabb LJ, Caron J, et al: Efficacy and safety of eszopiclone across 6 weeks of treatment for primary insomnia. Curr Med Res Opin 20(12):1979–1991, 2004.

Polysomnography Pearls

AMERICAN SOCIETY OF ELECTRONEURODIAGNOSTIC TECHNOLOGISTS, INC.

These questions were reprinted with permission from the publication *Review Questions in Polysomnography*, a 254-question study guide published by the American Society of Electroneurodiagnostic Technologists, Inc., www.aset.org.

Note: All references used to develop the *Review Questions in Polysomnography* are listed at the end of this chapter. After each question and reference citation is a reference number, which identifies the source on the accompanying Reference List.

Questions

Polysomnography (PSG) Preparation & Recording

1. The standard epoch length used in polysomnography recordings is:
   A. 30 mm/sec—10-sec epoch
   B. 15 mm/sec—20-sec epoch or 30 mm/sec—10-sec epoch
   C. 10 mm/sec—30-sec epoch or 15 mm/sec—20-sec epoch
   D. Either A or C

Chokroverty (2005), page 2

2. In addition to electroencephalography (EEG), electrooculogram, and electromyogram (EMG) (submental) monitoring, what is crucial for the interpretation of a polysomnographic recording in infants?
   A. Body temperature
   B. Behaviors and observation
   C. Physiological calibrations
   D. Limb movement (EMG) channel

Anders (1971), pages 2 to 5—reference #1

3. The minimum study duration for an accurate assessment of neonatal sleep is:
   A. 1 hour and/or 1 feeding
   B. 2 hours and/or 1 feeding
   C. 3 hours and/or 2 feedings
   D. 8 hours

Anders (1971), page 2—reference #1

4. At 10 mm per second, each epoch represents how many seconds?
   A. 10 seconds
   B. 20 seconds
   C. 30 seconds
   D. 40 seconds

Culebras (1996), page 102—reference #5

5. During instrumentation calibration, one pen deflection lagging behind the others requires correction of the:
   A. Mechanical baseline
   B. Time axis
   C. Electrical baseline
   D. Pen damping

Tyner (1983), page 124, Figure 9.5—reference #12

Scoring the Polysomnogram

The multiple sleep latency test (MSLT) study in Table 21-1 applies to questions 6 through 8. The numbers in the columns indicate epoch numbers of the MSLT study.

TABLE 21-1 ■ MSLT Summary Table					
	Nap 1	Nap 2	Nap 3	Nap 4	Nap 5
Lights out	160	200	280	340	400
Sleep onset	164	220	0	342	410
REM onset	170	0	0	344	412
End	194	260	320	372	440

REM, Rapid eye movement. Paper speed, 10 mm/sec; 30-second epochs.

6. What is the mean sleep latency, rounded to the nearest minute?
   A. 8 minutes
   B. 10 minutes
   C. 7 minutes
   D. 12 minutes

Carskadon (1986), pages 520–522—reference #4

7. What is the REM latency in Nap 1?
   A. 6 minutes
   B. 5 minutes
   C. 3 minutes
   D. 10 minutes

Carskadon (1986), pages 520–522—reference #4

8. When calculating mean sleep latency, how is Nap 3 scored?
   A. 0 minutes
   B. 20 minutes
   C. 15 minutes
   D. 40 minutes

Carskadon (1986), pages 520–522—reference #4

9. The formula for calculation of the periodic limb movement (PLM) arousal index is:
   A. The number of PLMs with arousal times 60 divided by total sleep time
   B. The number of leg jerks plus the number of arousals
   C. 100 times the number of PLMs divided by total sleep time
   D. The total sleep time minus arousal duration times total movement duration

Guilleminault (1982), page 273—reference #7

10. The scoring of a hypopnea requires:
    A. An amplitude reduction in respiratory channels
    B. Drop in O_2 saturation
    C. Both A and B
    D. A only

Butkov (1996), page 187—reference #2

11. In normal, healthy, young adults, sleep is entered through _____ sleep, whereas infants normally enter sleep through _____ sleep.
    A. Non-rapid eye movement (NREM), REM
    B. REM, NREM
    C. NREM, NREM
    D. REM, REM

Sheldon (2005), page 52—reference #9

Special Procedures

12. What is the minimum number of naps to be performed during the MSLT?
    A. 3
    B. 4
    C. 5
    D. 6

Carskadon (1986), page 520—reference #4

13. Epileptiform activity during the PSG is:
    A. Frequently observed in relation to oxyhemoglobin desaturation
    B. Adequately displayed on standard PSG montages
    C. Best displayed using additional EEG channels
    D. Indicated by any sharp-appearing activity

Butkov (1996), page 121—reference #2

14. MSLT studies performed after nocturnal recording should begin:
    A. 1.5–3 hours after the end of the nocturnal recording
    B. Immediately after the nocturnal study
    C. 6 hours after the nocturnal study
    D. 45 minutes after the nocturnal study

Carskadon (1986), page 520—reference #4

15. When snoring affects sleep onset during the MSLT, what monitors should be used?
    A. Intercostal EMG
    B. Oximetry
    C. Measures of respiratory flow/respiratory sounds
    D. Tracheal microphone exclusively

Carskadon (1986), page 521—reference #4

16. Continuous positive airway pressures (CPAPs) set too high may cause:
    A. Increased hypoventilation
    B. Intolerance of the treatment and triggering of central apneas
    C. Better patient compliance and tolerance of the treatment
    D. An increase in obstructive events

Butkov (1996), page 240—reference #2

17. Drugs known to affect sleep latency or REM latency should be:
    A. Withdrawn 2 weeks before the MSLT study
    B. Appropriately noted on the MSLT report
    C. Discontinued 2 nights before the scheduled MSLT study
    D. None of the above

Sleep (2005), page 119—reference #11

18. One of the contraindications for the use of CPAP is:

A. Chronic obstructive pulmonary disease
B. Congestive heart disease
C. Communication between the nasal pathway and cerebrospinal fluid (i.e., pneumocephalus)
D. All of the above

Kryger (2005), page 1071—reference #6

19. Which of the following instrumentation changes should be made when recording nocturnal seizures?
   A. Increase paper speed.
   B. Decrease paper speed.
   C. Lengthen time constant.
   D. Shorten time constant.

Chokroverty (1999), pages 155–156—reference #8

Clinical Correlations

20. Lorazepam, a benzodiazepine, generally affects sleep by:
   A. Increasing slow wave sleep and total sleep time
   B. Suppressing slow wave sleep but has no consistent effect on REM sleep
   C. Producing REM suppression early in the night, followed by PLMs
   D. Consistently increasing REM sleep

Kryger (2005), page 21—reference #3

21. Sleep-onset REM episodes during an MSLT can indicate:
   A. Fragmented nocturnal sleep, narcolepsy, and sleep apnea
   B. Sleep apnea, disturbed initiation and maintenance of sleep, and hallucinations
   C. Excessive somnolence, dream disturbance, and drug dependence
   D. A REM behavior disorder

Carskadon (1986), page 521—reference #4

22. Consistent asymmetry of sleep spindles is considered:
   A. A normal variant
   B. Abnormal
   C. A sign of nonrestorative sleep
   D. None of the above

Tyner (1993), page 245—reference #12

23. A patient history of episodic, uncontrollable screaming and amnesia during the first third of the night suggests:
   A. A dreaming state
   B. Sleep apnea
   C. Sleep terrors
   D. REM sleep behavior disorder

Kryger (2005), page 599—reference #13

24. *Hypnic myoclonia* is a term used to describe generalized or localized involuntary muscle contractions that may occur during the transition from wakefulness to sleep. These hypnic jerks are:
   A. Often associated with altered perceptions or images of falling
   B. A normal occurrence
   C. May appear more frequently during times of stress and altered or irregular sleep-wake schedules
   D. All of the above

Sheldon (2005), page 308—reference #10

Instrumentation and Technical Concerns

25. The electrode pair C4–A1 represents a:
   A. Referential montage
   B. Bipolar montage
   C. Phase reversal
   D. Cancellation effect

Tyner (1983), page 164—reference #12

Answers

Polysomnogram Preparation & Recording

1. C
2. B
3. C
4. C
5. B

Scoring the PSG

6. A
7. C
8. B
9. A
10. C
11. A

Special Procedures

12. B
13. C
14. A
15. C
16. B
17. A
18. C
19. A

Clinical Correlations

20. B
21. A
22. B
23. C
24. D

Instrumentation and Technical Concerns

25. A

REFERENCES

This reference section is reproduced from *Review Questions in Polysomnography* by the American Society of Electroneurodiagnostic Technologists, Inc. For updated information, please contact the corresponding publisher, library, or bookstore.

1. Anders T, Emde R, Parmelee A: *A Manual of Standardized Terminology, Techniques and Criteria for Scoring of States of Sleep and Wakefulness in Newborn Infants*. Los Angeles, CA: Brain Information Service, Brain Research Institute UCLA, 1971.
2. Butkov N: *Atlas of Clinical Polysomnography,* vol 1 and 2, Medford, OR, Synapse Media, Inc., 1996.
3. Carskadon MA, Dement WC: Normal human sleep: an overview. In Kryger MH, Roth T, Dement WC (eds): *Principles and Practice of Sleep Medicine*, 4th ed. Philadelphia, Elsevier Saunders, 2005, pp 13–23.
4. Carskadon MA, Dement WC, Mitler MM, et al: Guidelines for the multiple sleep latency test (MSLT): a standard measure of sleepiness. Sleep 9:519–524, 1986.
5. Culebras A: *Clinical Handbook of Sleep Disorders*. Woburn, MA, Butterworth-Heinemann, 1996.
6. Grunstein R: Continuous positive airway treatment for obstructive sleep apnea-hypopnea syndromes. In Kryger MH, Roth T, Dement WC (eds): *Principles and Practice of Sleep Medicine*, 4th ed. Philadelphia, Elsevier Saunders, 2005, pp 1066–1080.
7. Guilleminault C: *Sleep and Waking Disorders*. Woburn, MA, Butterworth-Heinemann, 1982.
8. Keenan SA: Polysomnographic technique: an overview. In Chokroverty S (ed): *Sleep Disorders Medicine, Basic Science, Technical Considerations and Clinical Aspects*. Woburn, MA, Butterworth-Heinemann, 1999, pp 151–174.
9. Sheldon SH: Polysomnography in infants and children. In Sheldon SH, Ferber R, Kryger MH (eds): *Principles and Practice of Sleep Medicine*. Philadelphia, Elsevier Saunders, 2005, pp 49–71.
10. Sheldon SH: The parasomnias. In Sheldon SH, Ferber R, Kryger MH (eds): *Principles and Practice of Sleep Medicine*. Philadelphia, Elsevier Saunders, 2005, pp 305–315.
11. Standards of Practice Committee of the American Academy of Sleep Medicine. Practice parameters for clinical use of the Multiple Sleep Latency Test and the Maintenance of Wakefulness Test. Sleep 28(1):113–121, 2005.
12. Tyner FS, Knott JR, Mayer WB Jr: *Fundamentals of EEG Technology, vol 1: Basic Concepts and Methods*. New York, Raven Press, 1983.
13. Vaughn BV, D'Cruz OF: Cardinal manifestations of sleep disorders. In Kryger MH, Roth T, Dement WC (eds): *Principles and Practice of Sleep Medicine*, 4th ed. Philadelphia, Elsevier Saunders, 2005, pp 594–601.

Polysomnography and Cases

Section I
Polysomnography Techniques

SHARON A. KEENAN

Reprinted with permission from The School of Sleep Medicine™, Inc.

1. Brief, single-administration afternoon nap studies are contraindicated as a screening technique for sleep apnea because:
   A. Inappropriate estimation of severity is possible.
   B. False–negative results are possible.
   C. A and B are true.

2. The most appropriate filter setting for recording electroencephalography (EEG) in polysomnography (PSG) is:
   A. High-frequency filter = 70 Hz, low-frequency filter = 0.03 Hz
   B. High-frequency filter = 35 Hz, low-frequency filter = 0.03 Hz
   C. High-frequency filter = 35 Hz, low-frequency filter = 0.3 Hz

3. Sensitivity can be associated with which of the following statements?
   A. Sensitivity = signal deflection/voltage
   B. Voltage = sensitivity/signal deflection
   C. Sensitivity = voltage/signal deflection

4. The most appropriate filter setting for recording electromyography (EMG) is:
   A. High-frequency filter = 30 Hz, low-frequency filter = 10 Hz
   B. High-frequency filter = 70 Hz, low-frequency filter = 5 Hz
   C. High-frequency filter = 70 Hz, low-frequency filter = 0.05 Hz

5. What two laboratory signs on the multiple sleep latency test (MSLT) are diagnostic of narcolepsy?
   A. Mean sleep latency >15 min and one sleep onset REM period (SOREMP)
   B. Mean sleep latency <5 min and no SOREMPs
   C. Mean sleep latency >20 min and two SOREMPs

   D. Mean sleep latency <8 min and two or more SOREMPs
   E. Mean sleep latency >15 min and no SOREMPs

6. Studies using the MSLT show that physiologic sleepiness in normal human adults is:
   A. Greatest in the morning
   B. Greatest in the afternoon
   C. Greatest in the evening
   D. Constant throughout the day with little variation
   E. Not measurable with the MSLT

7. The low-frequency filter is most closely related to the:
   A. High-frequency filter
   B. Time constant
   C. Sensitivity of the amplifier

8. One of the main differences between an alternating current (AC) and a direct current (DC) amplifier is:
   A. A DC amplifier cannot record variable signals such as respiration.
   B. An AC amplifier has better low-frequency filtering capabilities and can record higher frequencies.
   C. An AC amplifier cannot record very slow signals such as respiration.

9. An acceptable calibration setting for recording breathing during sleep is:
   A. High-frequency filter = 35 Hz, low-frequency filter = 5 Hz
   B. High-frequency filter = 15 Hz, low-frequency filter = 0.1 Hz
   C. High-frequency filter = 15 Hz, low-frequency filter = 1 Hz

10. In electrophysiology, the preferred type of amplifier for recording bioelectric potentials is:
    A. Single ended

B. Differential
C. Multifrequency

11. The polarity convention for electrophysiology states that when Input 1 is relatively more negative than Input 2, the signal:
A. Will not deflect
B. Will go up
C. Will go down

12. The electro-oculogram (EOG) is based on recording:
A. The corneoretinal potential difference
B. EMG activity from the muscles surrounding the eye
C. The potential difference between the eye and the brain

13. The recommended impedance level for scalp electrodes is less than:
A. 20,000 ohms
B. 5 ohms
C. 5000 ohms

14. What will the signal deflection be if the sensitivity is 10 μV/cm and the input voltage is 75 μV?
A. 75 mm
B. 10 cm
C. 75 cm

15. What is the sensitivity if the signal deflection is 1.5 cm and the input voltage is 75 μV?
A. 5 μV/mm
B. 50 μV/mm
C. 5 cm/μV

16. What is the voltage if the sensitivity is 5μV/cm and the signal deflection is 10 cm?
A. 500 μV
B. 5 μV
C. 50 μV

17. Active sleep in infants is characterized by all of the following except:
A. Facial movements
B. Limb movements
C. Rapid eye movements
D. Regular respirations

18. Quiet sleep in infants is defined by the following:
A. Closed eyes
B. Smiles
C. Sucking
D. Limb movements
E. None of the above

19. In monitoring infant sleep, the following observations are not recommended:
A. Facial expressions
B. Body movements
C. Caregiver interventions
D. Restraints

20. The minimum duration of an hypopnea in an adult is:
A. 10 seconds
B. 15 seconds
C. 20 seconds
D. The duration of two breaths

21. How many seconds of preceding sleep are needed to score an arousal?
A. 5 seconds
B. 8 seconds
C. 10 seconds
D. 12 seconds
E. 15 seconds

22. In addition to an increase in EEG frequency for 3 seconds, arousals in REM must include an increase in which of the following?
A. EEG amplitude
B. EMG amplitude
C. EOG amplitude
D. Ponto-geniculo-occipital amplitude

23. Tracé alternant pattern is characteristic of:
A. High-voltage slow waves mixed with fast low-voltage waves
B. Active sleep
C. Indeterminate sleep
D. Infant stage 1–2
E. Infant stage 3–4

24. What is the voltage requirement for high-voltage slow pattern in full-term infants?
A. 50 μV (frequency 0.5–4.0 Hz)
B. 75 μV (frequency 0.5–4.0 Hz)
C. 100 μV (frequency 0.5–4.0 Hz)
D. 125–175 μV (frequency 0.5–4.0 Hz)
E. 50–150 μV (frequency 0.5–4.0 Hz)

25. What is the average total sleep time during a 24-hour period for a term infant?
A. 10–12 hours
B. 13–15 hours
C. 16–18 hours
D. 19–21 hours

26. Airflow can be recorded using all but the following:

A. Thermocoupler
B. Thermistor
C. Capnograph
D. Breath sounds

27. Which of the following might cause 60-Hz interference?
    A. A faulty ground
    B. An open circuit
    C. Equipment plugged in near the patient
    D. A patient cable near the power cord
    E. All of the above

28. Which are the three most important parameters for sleep stage scoring?
    A. EEG, EOG, SaO_2
    B. EEG, EMG, electrocardiogram (ECG)
    C. EEG, EOG, EMG
    D. EEG, ECG, SaO_2

29. In newborn infants, which stage of sleep accounts for the majority of total sleep time?
    A. Quiet sleep
    B. Active sleep
    C. Active and quiet sleep are equally distributed.
    D. Indeterminate

30. The recommended protocol for the maintenance of wakefulness test (MWT) is:
    A. 5 trials of 20 minutes, 1.5–3 hours after PSG
    B. 4 trials of 40 minutes, 1.5–3 hours after final wake
    C. 4 trials of 40 minutes, 1.5–3 hours after PSG
    D. 5 trials of 20 minutes, 1.5–3 hours after final wake

31. Sleep onset for the MWT is defined as:
    A. First of three consecutive epochs of stage 1
    B. First 10 seconds of sleep
    C. First epoch of greater than 15 seconds of cumulative sleep in a 30-second epoch
    D. First epoch of greater than 10-second epoch

32. MWT trials are ended:
    A. If no sleep occurs
    B. After unequivocal sleep, defined as three consecutive epochs of stage 1 sleep
    C. After one epoch of any stage of sleep other than stage 1
    D. All of the above

33. A PSG is:
    A. Required before MSLT, recommended before MWT
    B. Required before MWT, recommended before MSLT
    C. Required before MSLT, at discretion of clinician before MWT
    D. Not required before MSLT, not recommended before MWT

Answers

1. C
2. C
3. C
4. B
5. D
6. B
7. B
8. B
9. B
10. B
11. B
12. A
13. C
14. A
15. A
16. C
17. D
18. A
19. D
20. A
21. C
22. B
23. A
24. E
25. C
26. D
27. E
28. C
29. B
30. B
31. C
32. D
33. C

REFERENCES

1. American Academy of Sleep Medicine: *The International Classification of Sleep Disorders: Diagnostic & Coding Manual*, 2nd ed. Westchester, IL, American Academy of Sleep Medicine, 2005.
2. American Academy of Sleep Medicine Standards of Practice Committee: Practice parameters for clinical use of the multiple sleep latency test and the maintenance of wakefulness test. Sleep 28(1):113–121, 2005.
3. Anders, T, Emde R, Parmelee A (eds): *A Manual of Standardized Terminology, Techniques and Criteria for Scoring of States of Sleep and Wakefulness in Newborn Infants.* Los Angeles, BRI Publications, 1971.
4. Arand D, Bonnet M, Hurwitz T, et al: The clinical use of the MSLT and MWT. Sleep 28(1):123–144, 2005.
5. Carskadon MA, Dement WC, Mitler MM, et al: Guidelines for the multiple sleep latency test (MSLT): a standard measure of sleepiness. Sleep 9(4):519–542,1986.
6. Doghramji K, Mitler MM, Sangal RB, et al: A normative study of the maintenance of wakefulness test (MWT). Electroencephalogr Clin Neurophysiol 103(5):554–562, 1997.
7. Kryger MH, Roth T, Dement WC (eds): *Principles and Practice of Sleep Medicine*, 4th ed. Philadelphia, Elsevier Saunders, 2005.
8. Kushida CA, Littner MR, Morgenthaler T, et al: Practice parameters for the indications for polysomnography and related procedures: an update for 2005. Sleep 28(4):499–521, 2005.
9. Mitler MM, Gujavarty KS, Sampson MG, Browman CP: Multiple daytime nap approaches to evaluating the sleepy patient. Sleep 5:S119–S127, 1982.
10. Rechtschaffen A, Kales A (eds): *A Manual of Standardized Terminology, Techniques and Scoring System for Sleep Stages of Human Subjects.* Los Angeles, BRI Publications, 1968.
11. Tyner F, Knott JR, Mayer WB: *Fundamentals of EEG Technology, Volume 1: Basic Concepts and Methods.* New York, Raven Press, 1983.

Section II
Cases

STUART G. HOLTBY ■ BRIAN H. FORESMAN ■ SHARON A. KEENAN ■ ROY SMITH

Reprinted with permission from The School of Sleep Medicine™, Inc.

Instructions: There are four cases labeled A through D. For each of the following cases, read the history and answer the questions. Remember to answer the questions as if you were a sleep specialist (and not another specialist, such as a neurologist).

CASE A

History: A 40-year-old male taxi driver is referred to your sleep disorders center from a urologist because of new-onset enuresis. The patient's symptoms began approximately 12 months before your evaluation. The urologist ruled out an identifiable pathology to explain these symptoms. The enuretic episodes now occur 1–2 nights each week, usually between Tuesdays and Thursdays; however, they may not occur for a few weeks at a time. Compared with 6 months ago, the occurrences are more frequent. He is unsure when or how he urinates during the night, but he awakens in the morning feeling very groggy and the bed is wet.

He usually goes to bed about 3 A.M. and arouses about 11:30 A.M. feeling unrefreshed. On days off he sleeps from 1–2 A.M. until 10–12 A.M. and generally feels the same as on workdays. The patient does not awaken during the night. He usually sleeps alone, but girlfriends over the past 15 years have told him he snores and moves "a lot" at night. There is no history of witnessed apneas or nocturnal awakenings. He reports awakening with a dry mouth (occasionally), morning headaches (often), and with the sheets on the bed in disarray (usually).

The patient denied any sleepwalking, cataplexy, hypnagogic hallucinations, sleep paralysis, symptoms of restless legs, or other parasomnias. During the day he is often drowsy. He naps several times a day between fares and feels somewhat better if he can sleep 15–20 minutes. His Epworth sleepiness score is 12.

Social history (SH): He reports driving a taxi for a living and working irregular hours. However, the most common time to work is from 4 P.M. to 2 A.M., and he usually has Sunday and Monday off. He denies any cigarette smoking but admits to drinking heavily on the weekends.

Past medical history (PMH) includes multiple minor fractures from falls and injuries, as well as chronic low back pain treated with Tylenol 3 (1–4/day). He smokes 1 pack per day and has a productive cough most mornings. He drinks 8–24 beers on Sunday and Monday night, his usual days off.

Family history (FH): is unknown (he is adopted).

Physical examination (PE): Physical exam reveals an unkempt and anxious obese man: 120 kg; 172 cm, BP 140/86, RR-22, HR 92; 45 cm neck. He is edentulous with a small, crowded posterior oropharynx and an old displaced nasal fracture with patent nasal airway. He has an "unusual" odor on his breath. His head and neck are otherwise normal. His lungs have wheezes throughout. No crackles or other abnormal breath sounds are noted. The heart rate and rhythm are regular without S3 or S4. Chest wall examination also reveals multiple spider nevi. The abdomen is soft and nontender. The liver span was percussed at 15 cm. The liver margins were palpable; however, the spleen was not palpable.

Neurological evaluation (NE): Pupils equally round and reactive to light and accommodation (PERRLA); extraocular movements intact (EOMI); and deep tendon reflexes (DTRs) are hyper-reflexic in the upper and lower extremities. Five-beat clonus was noted in the lower extremities. Cerebral and cerebellar function was unremarkable. Memory and mentation were intact.

Additional data: Urology reports normal physical findings, normal intravenous pyelogram (IVP) normal cystoscopy and cystometrogram, and no response to anticholinergic drugs. He has had no other neurological investigation. Pulmonary function tests (PFTs) done in the office show forced expiratory volume in 1 second (FEV1), 2.1 L and functional vital capacity (FVC) 4.0 L.

CASE A QUESTIONS

Using only the history and physical data, formulate a differential diagnosis for sleep disorders that may be contributing to this man's main complaint, and briefly state the support for each differential option.

1. List the differential diagnoses that might account for his nocturnal enuresis.
2. Give the key PSG findings that might be expected for each diagnosis listed.
3. Provide nine points of technical description (parametric analysis) regarding the study.

TABLE 22-1 ■ PSG Findings

A PSG was performed on the evening of your examination, a Monday night. A standard montage was used. The patient did not fill in the presleep questionnaire items re: alcohol intake before the study.

Frequent interruptions of all stages of sleep were noted, especially REM sleep. He snored, but no respiratory events, snoring arousals, or cyclical desaturations were noted. There was an absence of any epileptiform discharges. There were minor limb movements of 8–10 seconds' duration that accompanied arousals. The technologist noted only minor movements with arousals and did not report any enuresis. The patient awoke spontaneously and requested that the study end. Overall, the patient felt that his sleep that night was slightly better than his usual night's sleep.

Lights out	11:58 P.M.
Total study time	582 minutes
Sleep latency	87.5 minutes
Sleep efficiency	67%
REM latency	252 minutes
Stage 1	37%
Stage 2	24%
Slow wave	6%
Stage REM	33%
Low saturation	91%

4. The findings for the PSG are listed in Table 22-1. Discuss how these findings support or refute your working diagnoses.

5. List your initial recommendations to the patient after the sleep study.

CASE B

History. Chief complaint (C/C): A 22-year-old college student is referred to you because of excessive daytime somnolence. He notes a recent decline in daytime performance.

The patient reports that his symptoms began after a severe rollerblading incident that occurred approximately 10 months before evaluation. The patient was not wearing a helmet and fell about 6 feet from a railing and struck his head while attempting a trick. He was comatose for 2 days before regaining consciousness. Subsequent neurological examinations failed to reveal any focal deficit, and the computed tomography (CT) evaluations did not reveal any anatomical changes. The patient's symptoms of fatigue and sleepiness developed approximately 1 month after the initial accident. Over the subsequent months the symptoms have gradually worsened. Most recently, the patient has noted a dramatic dropoff in his grades this term, falls asleep in class, and complains that he can't concentrate. In addition, the patient also reports a significant level of fatigue that occurs regardless of the amount of sleep. He also reports depression.

He falls asleep promptly and doesn't rouse until an alarm at 8 A.M. Typically, he maintains a regular sleeping pattern and goes to bed at 10 P.M. In the past, he slept from 11 P.M. to 7 A.M. weekends and weekdays without any sensation of sleepiness or fatigue. As a child he had frequent sleepwalking episodes and still does on occasion. The last episode occurred about 7 or 8 months ago.

He is unsure if he snores, but his family and bed partners have never mentioned it. He is not restless at night and can make his bed just by pulling up the covers.

SH: He is a nonsmoker/nondrinker who denies drug use. He has no other medical history, except for a history of migraines, and no psychiatric history.

FH: Positive for sleepwalking in both parents.

PE: Physical exam reveals a slender, quiet individual who appears to be in no distress. He is alert and answers questions without difficulty or hesitation. Vital signs: 80 kg; 193 cm. BP 120/66, RR 12, HR 72; 38-cm neck. The oropharynx is patent and without evident abnormalities. Nasopharynx was unremarkable. The thorax was symmetrical. Lungs were clear to auscultation. No crackles or other abnormal breath sounds were noted. The heart rate and rhythm are regular without S3 or S4. The abdomen was soft with intact bowel sounds. Extremities were intact.

NE: The patient was oriented times three. His affect was somewhat flat. CN II-XII were grossly intact. There were no gross deficits of motor, cerebral, cerebellar, or sensory function. There was no evidence of short- or long-term memory loss. Deep tendon responses were 2/4 and symmetrical.

Additional data: A standard EEG was performed and showed mild slowing in the left frontal and temporal areas. No spike-and-wave activity was noted.

CASE B QUESTIONS

6. Formulate a differential diagnosis list and support your options very briefly from the history.

7. What findings in the PSG and MSLT data in Table 22-2 are the most pertinent to identifying the diagnosis in this patient?

8. Based on the results presented, what additional tests are indicated? What initial therapy is indicated?

CASE C

History. C/C: Witnessed apneas reported by a nurse when the patient was in the hospital.

This is a 63-year-old man with a history of witnessed apneas noted by a nurse when he was in the hospital 4 months ago for a right total hip replacement 4 months ago. He recalls that 2 days post-op he was awakened by a concerned nurse because she heard him stop breathing. During his hospitalization his blood pressure was noted to be quite high, and he was placed on

| | | **TABLE 22-2** ■ **MSLT Data Results** | | | |

The PSG was performed using a standard montage. No abnormalities on the EEG were noted and no abnormal movements were reported. The sleep architecture was unremarkable. There were infrequent awakenings and arousals. No diffuse or asymmetrical slow wave activity or spike and wave activity was noted. No other abnormalities were noted. No respiratory events, snoring arousals, or arterial desaturations were noted. The patient awoke spontaneously. Overall, the patient felt that his sleep that night was no worse than his usual night's sleep. A five-nap MSLT was performed.

	Nap 1	Nap 2	Nap 3	Nap 4	Nap 5
Lights out	10:31	12:28	14:33	16:30	18:31
Sleep latency	10 min	18 min	20 min	15 min	16 min
REM latency	None	None	None	None	None

antihypertensives. He lives alone and says he knows nothing about snoring. The patient reports a history of always being "tired and sleepy" but says that he can't sleep at night. On closer evaluation he reports difficulty getting to sleep and remaining asleep. These symptoms have been present for the past 15 years.

His usual sleep pattern is to go to bed at about 9:00 P.M. He works in bed or watches TV until turning out the lights at 10:00 P.M. The TV is set to turn off with a timer 1 to 2 hours after turning out the lights. After turning out the lights, he falls asleep around 10:45 P.M. After sleep onset the patient awakens four to six times on a typical night. The patient returns to sleep after 5–30 minutes. He gets up for the day by using an alarm that is set for 4:45 A.M. On days off from work, he arises spontaneously by 5:30 A.M. He estimates his average accumulation of sleep at 3–4 hours per night.

The patient reports that he is always worried and can't quiet his mind when he tries to sleep. Despite being sleepy in the late evening, he cannot fall asleep easily when he goes to bed. He generally remains in bed annoyed, trying to sleep and watching the clock. He denies falling asleep on the couch and does not travel.

SH: He is a 2-pack per day smoker with a chronic cough. He drinks several rye-and-Cokes in the early evening.

PMH: He has mild rhinitis for which he takes pseudoephedrine, and he is on atenolol for his blood pressure. He has been under treatment for hypertension for 4 months. He also has degenerative joint disease primarily affecting his hips. The disease is severe enough that he is planning to have the left hip replaced in 2 weeks. He describes a numb, tingly, somewhat painful sensation localized to the upper outer left thigh that comes on when he lies down. He also reports occasional cramps in his calves that are relieved with stretching and movement.

PE: On examination he is obese: 110 kg/172 cm and he has a 45-cm neck. His blood pressure is 180/104. He has full dentures and a shallow oro-/hypopharynx. His nose is normal. He has no other findings except for a mildly wheezy chest. His legs are neurologically normal.

CASE C QUESTIONS

9. List differential diagnoses for this patient's apparent difficulty sleeping. Briefly justify each of your responses.
10. The standard montage in the sleep laboratory includes the following: central and occipital EEG, EOG, chin EMG, one channel for leg EMG (both legs on one channel), respiratory effort and airflow, ECG, and oxygen saturation. Write any special instructions for the tech for the sleep study that should be undertaken based on this patient's history.
11. Briefly comment on the PSG fragments in Figure 22-1.
12. Based on the PSG fragments in Figure 22-1, detail your plan for the further evaluation and treatment of this patient.

CASE D

History. C/C: Insomnia.

This is a 51-year-old female who presents with a history of difficulty maintaining sleep. These symptoms have been present for the past 15 years, and now the patient is noting some general worsening of her symptoms.

The patient reports routinely going to bed at 11 P.M., reading for 5 to 10 minutes, and then turning out the light to go to sleep. She feels that she falls asleep within 5–10 minutes. After about 60–90 minutes the patient wakes, goes to the kitchen, and eats a large snack. Shortly thereafter, she returns to bed. During the remainder of the night, she may awaken two to four more times. Each time, she is able to return to sleep after 5–10 minutes. On weekdays, she arises at about 7 A.M. with the use of an alarm clock. On the weekends, she awakens spontaneously at about 8 A.M. There is no history of snoring; however, the patient has no bed partners to verify this impression. Her bed is not mussed in the morning.

Typically, she awakens in the morning feeling fatigued. During the day she reports mild drowsiness

Patient
Test date: 04/16/97

ID CODE: KWE33A16

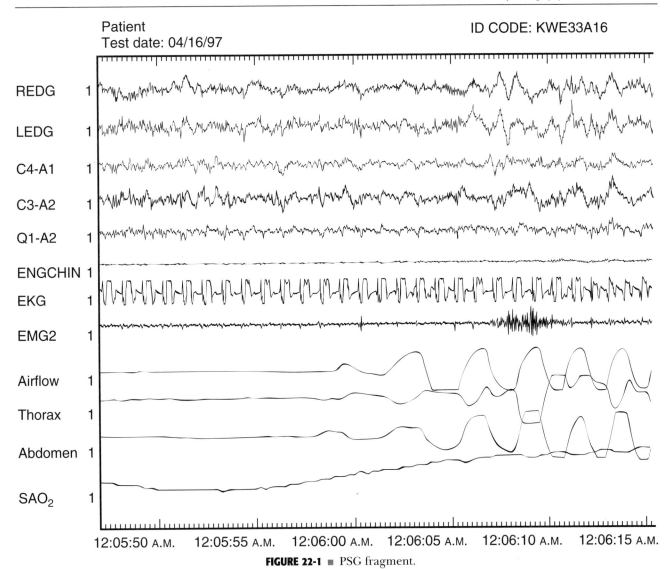

REDG 1

LEDG 1

C4-A1 1

C3-A2 1

Q1-A2 1

ENGCHIN 1

EKG 1

EMG2 1

Airflow 1

Thorax 1

Abdomen 1

SAO₂ 1

12:05:50 A.M.   12:05:55 A.M.   12:06:00 A.M.   12:06:05 A.M.   12:06:10 A.M.   12:06:15 A.M.

FIGURE 22-1 ■ PSG fragment.

and has an Epworth sleepiness scale score of 9. When she has attempted to nap during the day, she is unable to sleep.

In reviewing her history, the patient indicated that chronic nausea and upper abdominal pain started at the same time as insomnia. She says the pain came on abruptly when she was holding a very heavy textbook against her abdomen. She sought medical evaluations and underwent a significant amount of testing to determine the cause. As part of this evaluation she reports that the abdominal ultrasound was negative and that little else was identified. Five years ago an upper endoscopy suggested the presence of a mild hiatal hernia, and she was placed on therapy that included ranitidine and several other H₂-blockers and proton pump inhibitors. Little changed in her condition despite these interventions, except that her weight increased by 20 pounds over the 15-year period.

SH: She lives alone and is not sexually active. There is no childhood or young adulthood history of trauma or abuse. The patient works as a pharmacist at a nearby psychiatric hospital. She denies smoking or drinking alcoholic beverages.

PMH: Other than the hiatal hernia, the remainder of her past medical history is unremarkable. She denies taking medications other than those listed previously.

PE: This patient is in no apparent distress. Her vital signs are: weight 88 kg, height 170 cm, BP 124/78, RR 16, HR 84. The remainder of her physical examination is unremarkable.

CASE D QUESTIONS

13. List the major diagnostic considerations and identify the most likely cause of her insomnia. List the pertinent information that supports your conclusions.

14. Briefly discuss the diagnostic implications of the activity that the patient reports during her first nocturnal wakening.
15. A sample tracing from her PSG is shown in Figure 22-2.
    A. Qualitatively describe what is shown.
    B. Which of these findings has the most relevance in the diagnosis of the patient's insomnia, and what is suggested by this finding?
    C. Assuming that the main finding in this epoch is also seen during REM sleep and wakefulness, and that nothing else was seen on the PSG, give your first three choices for her diagnosis.

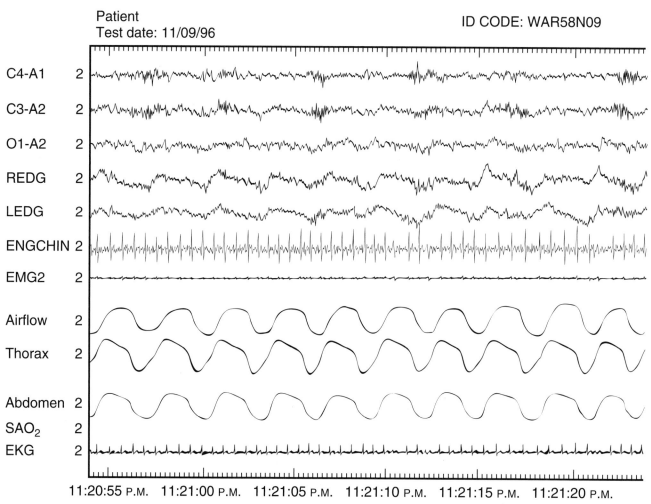

FIGURE 22-2 ■ PSG fragment.

Answers

CASE A

1. List the differential diagnoses that might account for his nocturnal enuresis:

Short answer: New-onset enuresis without identifiable urological findings suggests a number of possible diagnoses, including *sleep-related epilepsy, obstructive sleep apnea (adult)* (OSA), *alcoholism,* and *sleepwalking parasomnia.*

Discussion

Sleep-related epilepsy is suggested by the absence of any urological disease; heavy and intermittent alcohol use (with withdrawal over the interval when he reports peak event occurrence); amnesia for events and grogginess in the morning (postictal state); decreased personal hygiene (frequently seen with causes of seizures such as alcoholism as well as with focal brain lesions, hepatic or other metabolic disease); and abnormal deep tendon reflexes, which go along with these and also alcohol withdrawal. Moving a lot at night is not specific and doesn't help with the diagnosis. (Possible risk of chronic subdural hematoma as a cause of seizures or and/or seizures secondary to hypoxemia.)

OSA usually is not associated with enuresis unless it is very severe. OSA does not usually cause seizures but may exacerbate an underlying seizure disorder. The patient's presentation strongly suggests the presence of OSA: snoring with daytime somnolence, higher prevalence in men, obesity and large neck, alcoholism, smoking, and codeine usage.

Alcoholism is suggested by his history of alcohol usage and his appearance and social circumstances. With intoxication he might have enuresis, but the nights he experiences enuresis are not usually the nights he reports drinking heavily.

Sleepwalking or another disorder of arousal might lead to incontinence. His age and the lack of any prior history make it unlikely that a new-onset disorder of arousal could account for these findings. However, a change in his neurological status resulting from some other medical problem might alter the patient's pattern of arousal.

2. Give the key PSG findings that might be expected for each diagnosis you listed.

Sleep-related epilepsy:
Spike-and-wave activity epileptiform discharges or seizure activity might be seen, but absence of such activity does not rule out a seizure disorder even with an extended EEG montage (which should be used).

Generalized slowing or triphasic waves would suggest encephalopathy (such as hepatic encephalopathy) that might be associated with seizures.

EEG asymmetry would suggest a focal brain lesion, such as a chronic subdural (but more extensive montage would be needed to increase confidence).

Sleep-related breathing disorders:
Obstructive respiratory events should be seen if sleep-disordered breathing is the problem, although it might be underestimated in the study if he did not drink his usual alcohol intake or if the technology used was of limited sensitivity and/or qualitative in nature.

Abnormal oxygen saturation related to respiratory disease.

Alcoholism:
Increased muscle activity, sweating, and sleep-onset insomnia if he is in withdrawal.

Sleep fragmentation, particularly in the last half of the night.

Alterations in REM timing: early REM onset for withdrawal and delayed REM onset with fragmented REM late in the study if he drinks just before the study.

Sleepwalking parasomnia
Abrupt arousals from stage 2 or slow wave in the first third of the night.

3. Provide nine points of technical description (parametric analysis) regarding the study.

Lights out at 11:58 P.M. differs from stated bedtime usually at 1–2 A.M. (Monday, second day off; usual sleep onset at 1–2 A.M., other days 3 A.M.)

Sleep latency at 87.5 minutes possibly secondary to change in habitual schedule

Decreased sleep efficiency secondary to increased sleep latency

Prolonged REM latency

Increased stage 1

Decreased stage 2

Slightly elevated REM at 33%

No respiratory events reported, but question remains regarding limits of sensitivity of technology (temperature versus pressure versus Piezo)

No episodes of enuresis noted (presenting complaint)

4. The findings for the PSG are listed in Table 22-1. Discuss how these findings support or refute your working diagnoses.

Epileptiform discharges were not seen but may not be visible because of episodic occurrence and the limited montage used for the study. The study neither supports nor refutes this diagnostic possibility.

Sleep apnea syndrome is unlikely to be the cause of his enuresis. He could have significant sleep-disordered breathing on nights when he drinks heavily, and we do not have enough information on his alcohol use just before this study to draw a conclusion. The absence of events in this study, however, argues against OSA on the nights he has enuresis.

The sleep fragmentation and changes in REM sleep would be consistent with alcoholism with sleep fragmentation, and in particular withdrawal with increased REM sleep. Sleep fragmentation may also be seen in patients who are anxious in the lab environment.

The absence of abrupt arousals neither supports nor refutes sleepwalking parasomnia, which remains an unlikely diagnosis.

The long sleep latency is not unexpected given his typical sleep pattern.

The absence of enuresis during the study decreases the study's ability to reach a conclusion.

5. List your initial recommendations to the patient following the sleep study.

Decrease (preferably stop) alcohol.

Stop driving until a clear diagnosis is reached.

Discuss other safety issues in the setting of a possible seizure disorder, such as swimming/bathing alone, roof/ladder safety, etc.

Arrange a full montage EEG to assess for epileptiform activity.

Obtain complete blood count (CBC), thyroid-stimulating hormone (TSH), comprehensive metabolic profile (i.e., sequential multiple analysis [SMA] and lung function tests [LFTs]).

Refer to a neurologist with an interest in seizures.

Review his sleep hygiene and make any improvements possible.

Show him how to use sleep logs.

Book a follow-up after the EEG and blood work in ~2 weeks.

(Consider: if no results emerge, repeat the PSG on a Tuesday or Wednesday night.)

CASE B

6. Formulate a differential diagnosis list and support your options briefly from the history.

The C/C is mainly one of nonrestorative sleep and daytime drowsiness in a 22-year-old that started *after* a traumatic event (*not before*). The history is incomplete and there is no history available to assess for an environmental sleep disorder.

Hypersomnia resulting from a medical condition; subtype post-traumatic hypersomnia is suggested by excessive daytime sleepiness (EDS) (lasting more than 3 months) after head trauma; the long lag until symptoms could suggest secondary complications.

Secondary complications: chronic subdural hematoma, hygroma, hydrocephalus, chronic meningitis, seizures or medication side effects (seizure meds). EDS with asymmetry on the EEG might suggest one of these complications, but there is a lack of supporting symptoms or neurological findings.

Depression is common after serious head trauma.

Occult drug use not suggested by the history, but should be considered, especially after a long hospitalization; potential painkiller use.

OSA (obstructive sleep apnea) unrefreshing sleep, the lack of snoring or witnessed apneas and the patient's age makes this unlikely.

Idiopathic hypersomnia, without long sleep time, idiopathic recurring stupor or recurrent hypersomnolence unlikely, as there was no history before the traumatic event and these do not occur after trauma.

Sleepwalking history of occasional sleepwalking; this probably does not contribute to the current symptoms.

Hint: Do not answer a question such as this based on the PSG results. That would prematurely limit the scope of your differential diagnoses. If you read through the PSG, however, and you think of an additional (and reasonable) differential diagnosis to include, then add it to your answer.

7. What findings in the PSG and MSLT data in Table 22-2 are the most pertinent to identifying the diagnosis in this patient?

PSG

Assess presence of EEG asymmetry.

Determine if epileptiform activity occurs.

Confirm PSG features consistent with hypersomnia due to a medical condition; subtype post-traumatic hypersomnia.

Rule in or out a sleep-related breathing disorder and periodic limb movement disorder (PLMD)

MSLT

Assess the degree of sleepiness.

Determine whether SOREMPs are occurring—seeking evidence of narcolepsy.

Summary

We are curious to see whether the previously reported EEG asymmetry is demonstrated in this study and are looking carefully for possible epileptiform activity. This activity is most common during slow wave sleep (SWS) and transitions into and out of sleep. The PSG is needed to confirm that the sleep architecture is consistent with a diagnosis of hypersomnia because of a medical condition; subtype post-traumatic hypersomnia. Because of the prevalence of OSA and other disorders that disrupt sleep, sleep-related breathing disorders, and PLMD need to be ruled out. It may be reasonable, however, to note that periodic limb movements (PLMs) can be highly variable from night to night.

In the MSLT we seek evidence of narcolepsy and an assessment of sleepiness: two or more naps with SOREMPs is highly suggestive of narcolepsy in the absence of other disorders and in the presence of an appropriate history.

PSG Results

The latency to sleep onset was within normal limits. REM onset occurred 70 minutes after sleep onset. The sleep architecture was appropriate for the patient's age and consistent with the reported sleep pattern in the patient's history. There appeared to be a slight slowing of the EEG waveform throughout the study, with findings similar to the previous EEG. No epileptiform activity was evident during the study, and there were no reports of gross motor movements consistent with seizure activity.

MSLT

The mean sleep latency was 15.75 minutes. The MSLT data do not meet the criteria of a mean sleep latency of less than 8 minutes. No SOREMPs occurred on any nap. The PSG did not reveal any abnormalities; however, we do not have data about total sleep time, which must be greater than 6 hours. A clinically significant complaint of EDS should be addressed in absences of abnormal PSG or MSLT.

8. Based on the results presented, what additional tests are indicated? What initial therapy is indicated?

Additional history is needed.

Assess the sleeping environment.

Assess sleep times and obtain sleep logs.

Needed testing

CT or magnetic resonance imaging (MRI) of the head.

Sleep-deprived EEG

Neuropsychiatric testing to assess higher neural functions and for depression

If subjective sleepiness/drowsiness is a concern, then a vigilance test or driving evaluation should be included.

Referrals to consider

Psychiatry, especially if screening (interviews/questionnaires, etc.) suggests an increased probability of depression.

Interventions

Scheduled naps with follow-up evaluation to assess their effect.

Therapy with stimulants is not indicated (mean sleep latency >15 min) and should not be used, especially if a seizure disorder is being considered.

Treatment with nonsedating or activating antidepressants might be considered.

Communicate findings and recommendations to all appropriate individuals.

Safety

Instruct patient on safety measures with regard to sleepwalking.

Address concerns regarding driving or work-related activities.

Educate: Discuss and counsel the patient regarding the findings and the plan for intervention and follow-up.

Follow-up: Arrange for follow-up, anticipating that therapeutic interventions and re-evaluations may be necessary depending on the response of the patient.

CASE C

9. List differential diagnoses for this patient's apparent difficulty sleeping. Briefly justify each of your responses.

(*Major complaints:* Excessive sleepiness with witnessed apneas, sleep-onset and maintenance insomnia; anxiety; painful left hip)

Differential Diagnoses

OSAS, particularly supine predominant sleep apnea syndrome, witnessed apneas, EDS, presence of hypertension (consider central sleep apnea, but this is less likely, as there is no congestive heart failure [CHF] or obvious neurological disease)

Inadequate sleep hygiene syndrome—works in bed, watches TV in bed, monitors clock time

Insomnia due to drug or substance—caffeine use and pseudoephedrine; side effects of antihypertensive agents (atenolol), alcohol

Psychophysiologic insomnia—bedtime routines, pattern of remaining in bed annoyed

Insomnia resulting from a medical condition—arthritic pain that arouses the patient

Insomnia resulting from a mental disorder—anxiety and concerns that surround the patient's sleep; probably a generalized anxiety disorder (dysthymia or major depressive disorders could be present but are unlikely)

Insomnia resulting from drug or substance (alcohol-dependent sleep disorder)—regular use of alcoholic beverages at bedtime to assist with sleep onset

Paradoxical insomnia (formerly referred to as *sleep state misperception*)—the time in bed is 7 hours, but the patient relates only 3–4 hours of sleep.

Summary

Data support diagnoses of sleep-disordered breathing and several types of insomnia in this patient's history. The initial referral was made because of a concern regarding sleep-disordered breathing. A nurse noted apnea when the patient was forced to sleep supine after the surgery on his right hip. This suggests the possibility of *supine-dependent obstructive sleep apnea*, or sleep apnea induced by anesthetics, analgesics, and hypnotics used in the hospital. The presence of hypertension increases the chance that he has significant OSA. Although OSA is usually associated with EDS, approximately 10% of patients with OSA present with associated complaints of insomnia. *Inadequate sleep hygiene* is evident from his sleep environment, with the TV running most of the night, his time to bed, and his clock watching. His caffeine intake may contribute to his insomnia, as may his pseudoephedrine or beta-blockers. His vague leg pain may be a significant cause of insomnia. The symptoms are more suggestive of *neuralgia paresthetica* than *restless legs syndrome* (RLS), but RLS is a common syndrome and many patients with it do not recognize it as a main contributor to their symptoms. The patient awakens early in the morning and with "constant worries;" therefore, both *generalized anxiety disorder* and mood disorders (*dysthymia* or *major depressive disorder*) are considerations. He likely has *insomnia resulting from drug or substance (alcohol) abuse*, as suggested by the history of taking alcohol regularly for more than 3 months in the evening for its hypnotic effect. Although the patient goes to bed at 9 P.M., his reports suggest that he does not fall asleep until much later. *Paradoxical insomnia* may be present; he is very unsure of his sleep onset and claims only 3–4 hours of sleep despite spending 7 or more hours in bed. If the patient is suffering from paradoxical insomnia, then he may have sleep phase advance rather than some other cause of his early morning wakening.

10. The standard montage in the sleep laboratory includes the following: central and occipital EEG, EOG, chin EMG, one channel for leg EMG (both legs on one channel), respiratory effort and airflow, ECG, and oxygen saturation. Write any special instructions you would have for the tech for the sleep study that should be undertaken based on this patient's history.

Maintain patient's current routine for sleep study.

Watch sleep onset carefully, looking for subtle causes that might disrupt it, such as periodic limb movements during sleep or disordered breathing.

Attempt to have patient sleep in a supine position; if the patient has not slept on his back by ~2 A.M., then turn him onto his back.

Document reasons for arousals, specifically addressing issues of pain, cramping and behaviors on arousal. On awakening, ask if he was asleep.

11. Briefly comment on the PSG fragments in Figure 22-1.

The PSG shows sleep-onset insomnia with a moderate degree of alpha intrusion, and quite severe OSA.

If the patient's history is correct, there is a strong supine component to the OSA.

12. Based on the PSG fragments in Figure 22-1, detail your plan for the further evaluation and treatment of this patient.

Intervention for OSAS

Discuss the findings of the PSG, the implications/risks with regard to the upcoming operation, and treatment options.

Initiate therapy for OSA; initiate continuous positive airway pressure (CPAP) and titrate to ensure adequate control of the OSA before proceeding to surgery.

Communicate findings and concerns to his physicians; this should include the anesthesiologist and the surgeon, as this may affect when surgery is done, as well as preoperative preparation and postoperative management.

The patient is at risk for postoperative complications related to OSA; limit sedative use, monitor closely after, arrange for CPAP/BiPAP (bilevel positive airway pressure) in the hospital.

Safety issues: the patient may be at risk for accidents and should be counseled appropriately, documentation of sleepiness may be needed (i.e., MSLT, MWT, or vigilance testing).

General Medical Issues

Address rhinitis and its effect on sleep. The rhinitis needs more appropriate treatment: possibly nasal steroids, nonsedating antihistamines, and/or ear-nose-throat evaluation. This will help with treating the OSA.

Reduce or stop smoking. If this is accomplished immediately, surgery should be delayed for 8 weeks or more to prevent associated postoperative complications.

Evaluate pulmonary functions and obtain a chest x-ray; wheezing may require further evaluation and treatment.

Intervention for Insomnia

Address sleep hygiene issues (e.g., stop working in bed, do not watch TV in bed) and do a detailed assessment of the morning routine.

Address his sleep behaviors: establish regular sleep times and use stimulus-control and sleep restriction measures.

Address his anxiety or mood disorder, then initiate appropriate behavioral and psychological interventions. This should include consideration of a psychiatric consultation. Consider sedating agents only after completing the evaluation and treating the underlying OSA.

Address medication effects: stop the use of stimulants (caffeine and pseudoephedrine). Consider changing atenolol if insomnia appears temporally related to its use.

Follow-up

Arrange for close follow-up in the hospital, especially in the postoperative period.

Arrange for outpatient follow-up evaluation and monitoring of OSA and insomnia.

CASE D

13. List the major diagnostic considerations and identify the most likely cause of her insomnia. List the pertinent information that supports your conclusions.

Problem list

Sleep maintenance insomnia—rule out occult drug use, anxiety disorders, mood/affective disorders, OSAS, PLMs

Nocturnal eating/drinking—rule out sleep walking parasomnia, sleep-related eating disorder

Nocturnal awakening—rule out OSA, gastroesophageal reflux disorder (GERD), periodic limb movement disorder, mood/anxiety disorders

Daytime fatigue—rule out OSA, may be secondary to insomnia or nocturnal arousals

Chronic nausea and abdominal pain—rule out GERD, anxiety disorder

Obesity—rule out OSA

Hints

Do not expand the problem list beyond the history provided. You can say that certain disorders such as insomnia are more likely to be associated with psychiatric problems, but do not extend this beyond the available history. For example, don't include inadequate sleep hygiene syndrome as a problem. There is no suggestion from the history that this is present. You could reasonably include this under sleep maintenance insomnia as a disorder to be ruled out.

Summary

The sleep and psychiatric history are incomplete. The patient sought attention because she can't stay asleep: sleep maintenance insomnia. From the history provided, however, the interruptions in her sleep are relatively brief. She does not feel rested in the morning but has only "mild" daytime drowsiness and doesn't sleep if she lies down. Overall, it seems more likely that more than one disorder is contributing to her complaints. Her actual complaint needs to be clarified, and a more detailed history obtained with regard to the duration of the events and any progression of symptoms. There are no reported causes for several of the reported interruptions in her sleep. She seems fully aware of the nocturnal eating events, so it is unlikely that they represent a form of sleepwalking. Sleep-related eating disorder should be considered until other sleep disorders are ruled out as producing the awakenings. Without a partner she may not be aware of significant snoring or witnessed apneas. Because of her age, weight, body mass index (BMI), and recent worsening, OSAS needs to be considered; up to 10% of patients with OSA present with insomnia. The fact that she doesn't fall asleep if she lies down argues weakly against OSA. The absence of a mussed bed does not support or refute OSA or PLMD as a cause of nonrestorative sleep; both are common disorders. RLS is also a common disorder that causes sleep onset and maintenance insomnia and may not be recognized by the patient. She doesn't report features of inadequate sleep hygiene, and the history doesn't suggest environmental sleep disorder. Although there is limited data to suggest the possibility of mood disorders or anxiety disorders, these are extremely common in patients with chronic insomnia and are more common in middle-age women who live alone. Her chronic abdominal pain and nausea could be the primary problem inducing insomnia; however, prior treatment and evaluations have been unrewarding and would suggest that this symptom is secondary to another problem. The history is not clear enough to comment, except to note that the abdominal symptoms coincide with the onset of the sleep complaint.

14. Briefly discuss the diagnostic implications of the activity that the patient reports occurring during her first nocturnal wakening.

Sleep maintenance insomnia

Additional history involving the course and progression of the insomnia including details about the recent worsening in her condition, and factors that make it worse or better; prior interventions that have been tried, possible occult drug use

Obtain a more thorough psychiatric history, consider specific testing for mood and anxiety disorders.

Sleep logs

Nocturnal Eating/Drinking

Additional history is needed to determine how it developed and to clarify details such as: Does she awaken while she is eating? What awakens her? Why does she choose to eat?

Any other history of parasomnias

Nocturnal awakening

Additional history is needed to determine how it developed and to clarify details such as the reason she awakens.

Fatigue

Screen for metabolic causes of fatigue such as TSH, glucose, creatinine, hemoglobin, and calcium.

PSG to rule out OSA

Chronic nausea and abdominal pain

Additional history is needed to determine whether pain or reflux or other GI symptoms awaken her, and to determine whether eating is associated with GI complaints.

Obesity

Obtain PSG to rule out OSAS.

15. A sample tracing from her PSG is shown in Figure 22-2.

Introduction

The time of awakening is regular; this needs to be confirmed; however, it suggests a behavioral issue rather than other problems.

Routine eating of large amounts suggests *sleep-related eating disorder*; other reasons for eating need to be excluded, particularly GI symptoms.

The exact events need to be reviewed; this could be a form of *sleepwalking* or *REM behavior disorder (RBD)* from which she arouses and only remembers eating.

Endocrine issues such as *diabetes mellitus* are unlikely, as these normally present much later in the sleep period.

A. Qualitatively describe what is shown.

Epoch is stage 2.

There is a high density of spindles.

Respiration is unremarkable.

There is an occasional irregularity in the ECG.

B. Which of these findings has the most relevance in the diagnosis of the patient's insomnia, and what is suggested by this finding?

The history doesn't list any medications, but the large number of spindles suggests that the patient has used or is using medication, especially benzodiazepines. The use may be legitimate, but as a pharmacist, she has ready access to medication, and drug abuse is common in pharmacists.

Normal sleep spindles are seen primarily in stage 2, but may be seen in SWS, and isolated spindles may occur in REM sleep. The frequency is 12–14 Hz, with a waxing/waning "spindled" appearance. "Drug spindles" reflect overall increased beta activity. They have a higher frequency, typically 14–18 Hz, a higher density/epoch, and may be seen in all stages of sleep and in wake.

C. Assuming that the main finding in this epoch is also seen during REM sleep and wakefulness, and that nothing else was seen on the PSG, give your first three choices for her diagnosis.

The sleep study demonstrated a mild reduction in SWS and REM sleep. There were frequent sleep stage changes, and "pseudo-spindles" were reported to occur during the study. No arterial desaturations were noted, and no respiratory events occurred. Give the three most likely causes of the patient's disrupted sleep and include your rationale.

Insomnia Due to Drug or Substance—"pseudo-spindles" were seen throughout the study; patient is a pharmacist, and the history would be consistent with the diagnosis.

Sleep-Related Eating Disorder—routine eating at night after awakening, no other evident disorders.

Insomnia Due to Mental Disorder—most common cause of chronic insomnia, associated with self-administered but unreported hypnotic use.

REFERENCES

1. American Academy of Sleep Medicine: *The International Classification of Sleep Disorders: Diagnostic and Coding Manual*, 2nd ed. Westchester, IL, American Academy of Sleep Medicine, 2005.
2. Chokroverty S (ed): *Sleep Disorders Medicine: Basic Science, Technical Considerations and Clinical Aspects*, 2nd ed. Stoneham, MA, Butterworth-Heinemann, 1999.
3. Chokroverty S, Thomas RJ, Bhatt M: *Atlas of Sleep Medicine*. Philadelphia, Elsevier Butterworth Heinemann, 2005.
4. Lee-Chiong TL, Sateia M, Carskadon MA: *Sleep Medicine*. Philadelphia, Lippincott, Williams & Wilkins, 2001.
5. Kryger MH, Roth T, Dement WC (eds): *Principles and Practice of Sleep Medicine*, 4th ed. Philadelphia, Elsevier Saunders, 2005.

Clinical Case Studies I

CHARLES BAE ■ NANCY FOLDVARY-SCHAEFER

Questions

Case 1

A 22-year-old white male with no significant medical history presents with a history of excessive daytime sleepiness (EDS) for 5 years that has been getting worse with time. It started at the end of his junior year of high school after he had viral meningitis. He falls asleep in minutes by midnight and wakes up at 7 A.M. He has a difficult time waking up in the morning. On weekends, he wakes up around 9 A.M. on his own, and even if he slept longer he does not feel less sleepy.

He does not snore or wake up during the night, and his body mass index (BMI) is 25 kg/m². He was often late to his early morning class in high school and scheduled his classes in the afternoon or evening at college. He takes two 30- to 60-minute naps daily that help him get through the day but are not necessarily refreshing. He denies episodes of loss of muscle tone associated with strong emotion and hallucinations or paralysis as he is falling asleep or waking up.

Questions 1–6 are based on case #1:

1. What is the most likely diagnosis?
   A. Circadian rhythm sleep disorder, delayed sleep phase type
   B. Narcolepsy with cataplexy
   C. Narcolepsy without cataplexy
   D. Kleine-Levin syndrome
   E. Idiopathic hypersomnia

2. What test will confirm the diagnosis?
   A. Overnight polysomnogram (PSG) followed by a multiple sleep latency test (MSLT)
   B. MSLT
   C. Human leukocyte antigen (HLA) typing
   D. Cerebrospinal fluid hypocretin level

3. The overnight PSG showed sleep fragmentation and a total sleep time of 7 hours and 10 minutes. There was no evidence of sleep-disordered breathing or periodic movements during sleep. The MSLT showed the following results:

Trial	Sleep Latency	REM Sleep Latency
1	6.5 min	–
2	8.0 min	–
3	5.5 min	–
4	5.0 min	10.0 min
5	9.5 min	–

REM, Rapid eye movement.

What is the most likely diagnosis?
A. Narcolepsy without cataplexy
B. Narcolepsy due to a medical condition
C. Kleine-Levin syndrome
D. Idiopathic hypersomnia
E. Hypersomnia due to a medical condition

4. What would be your initial treatment recommendation?
   A. Amphetamine
   B. Methylphenidate
   C. Sodium oxybate
   D. Modafinil

5. What is a proposed mechanism of action of modafinil?
   A. Increased release of dopamine
   B. Decreased release of dopamine
   C. Increased reuptake of dopamine
   D. Decreased reuptake of dopamine
   E. Adenosine receptor antagonism

6. The patient develops cataplexy 2 years after the diagnosis of hypersomnia resulting from a medical condition. He is experiencing episodes of "head bobbing" when he laughs, particularly when he tells a joke. Which of the following is the most appropriate treatment option?
   A. Increase modafinil.
   B. Add an additional wake-promoting agent, such as an amphetamine.
   C. Add a tricyclic antidepressant or a selective serotonin reuptake inhibitor.
   D. Start sodium oxybate.

Case 2

A 45-year-old man presents with EDS that has worsened over the past year. He nearly fell asleep behind the wheel last week while driving home from work. His wife is threatening to sleep in another bedroom because of his loud snoring and leg movements in bed, and she thinks that he occasionally holds his breath during sleep. He wakes up three to four times per night but is not sure why. He has been gaining weight since he started a new desk job and has recently experienced episodes of feeling "paralyzed" upon wakening. His Epworth Sleepiness Scale score is 13/24.

Questions 7–10 are based on case #2:

7. What is the most likely diagnosis?
   A. Upper airway resistance syndrome
   B. Obstructive sleep apnea syndrome
   C. Narcolepsy without cataplexy
   D. Periodic limb movement disorder (PLMD)

8. What tests(s) would be helpful to confirm the diagnosis?
   A. Nocturnal oximetry
   B. Attended (laboratory) PSG
   C. Portable (home) PSG
   D. PSG with MSLT

9. What is the diagnosis, based on the PSG tracing shown in Figure 23-1?
   A. Obstructive sleep apnea (OSA)
   B. Central sleep apnea
   C. Cheyne-Stokes respiration
   D. Upper airway resistance syndrome

10. On physical examination, the posterior airway is crowded, demonstrating a Friedman tongue position 3 and grade 3 tonsils. There is also mild retrognathia. The neck circumference is 18 inches, and the BMI is 32 kg/m². The PSG revealed an apnea-hypopnea index (AHI) of 36 events/hour. The respiratory events were associated with oxygen desaturations as low as 70%.
    What would be the best initial treatment?
    A. Uvulopalatopharyngoplasty
    B. Continuous positive airway pressure (CPAP)
    C. Nocturnal oxygen
    D. Mandibular advancement device
    E. Weight loss

Case 3

A 30-year-old woman presents with EDS and difficulty falling asleep. She has been sleepy since high school and is surprised that she graduated because she fell asleep in every class. She has EDS independent of the number of hours she sleeps. She takes a short nap every day, but she is not fully refreshed after naps. She is not overweight, but she has been told that she snores and snorts occasionally during sleep. She calls herself a "night owl" and often stays up late because she is most productive after 10 P.M. Her typical sleep period during the work week is midnight to 7 A.M., although she often hits the snooze button and is late for work. On weekends, she goes to bed between 2 and 3 A.M. and sleeps until 11 A.M. She falls asleep instantly and sleeps through the night, waking feeling alert and refreshed.

Questions 11 and 12 are based on case #3:

11. What is the most likely diagnosis?
    A. Narcolepsy without cataplexy
    B. Sleep-onset insomnia
    C. Circadian rhythm sleep disorder, delayed sleep phase type
    D. Behaviorally induced insufficient sleep syndrome
    E. Obstructive sleep apnea syndrome

12. Which is the most cost-effective means of confirming the diagnosis?
    A. PSG
    B. MSLT
    C. Maintenance of wakefulness test
    D. Actigraphy

Case 4

A 55-year-old female presents with a chief complaint of difficulty falling asleep and daytime fatigue for the past 3 years. As a result, she has been taking short naps after lunch for the past year. Symptoms initially occurred once every 2 to 3 weeks but have recently increased to every night. She reports that the bed covers are "a mess" in the morning and states that she has difficulty falling asleep because her legs bother her at night. She describes an urge to move her legs in bed at night, which improves with stretching or repositioning.

Questions 13–16 are based on case #4:

13. What is the most likely diagnosis?
    A. Psychophysiologic insomnia
    B. Restless legs syndrome (RLS)
    C. Adjustment insomnia
    D. PLMD

14. What other clinical information can be helpful to make the diagnosis?
    A. Periodic limb movements during sleep
    B. Ability to nap during the day
    C. Presence of a significant stressor predating the difficulty falling asleep
    D. All of the above

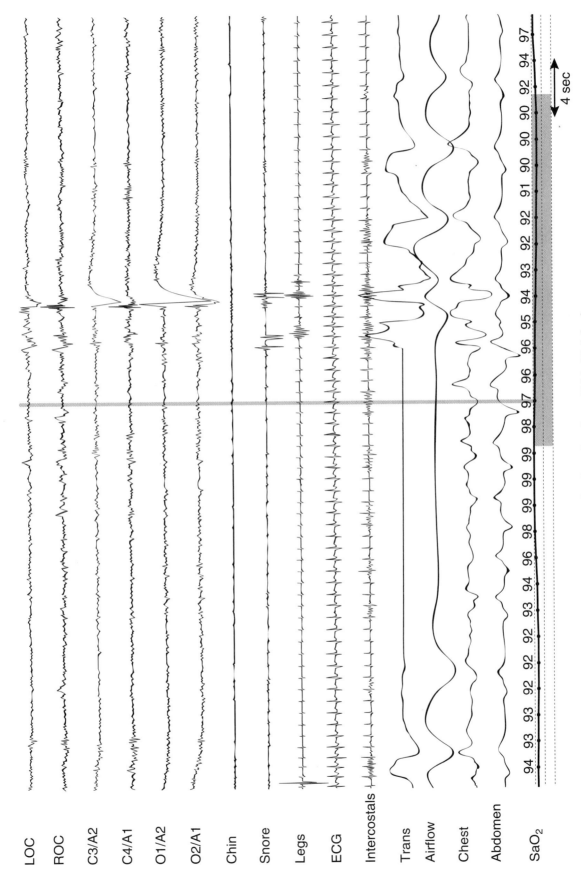

FIGURE 23-1 ■ For Question 9; see Table 23-1 for key.

TABLE 23-1 ■ Key for Figures	
Parameter	**Derivation**
EEG	C3-A2
	C4-A1
	O1-A2
	O2-A1
EOG	LOC-A1/A2
	ROC-A1/A2
EMG	Submentalis
	Tibialis anterior
	Intercostal
Respiration	Airflow
	Nasal transducer
	Thoracic/abdominal effort
Oximetry	———
ECG	V1-V5

EEG, Electroencephalography; EOG, electro-oculography; EMG, electromyography; ECG, electrocardiography; LOC, left outer canthus; ROC, right outer canthus.

15. What is the most useful test when making a diagnosis in this patient?
   A. PSG
   B. MSLT
   C. Suggested immobilization test (SIT)
   D. Serum ferritin
   E. Actigraphy

16. What would be the most appropriate first-line therapy for this patient?
   A. Counter-stimulation
   B. Levodopa/carbidopa
   C. Clonazepam
   D. Ropinerole
   E. Gabapentin

Case 5

A 20-year-old female presents for evaluation of episodes of paralysis on awakening. The most recent event occurred in the morning when she heard two of her roommates talking. She tried to get out of bed and yell for help, but she could not speak or move. She described this as a terrifying experience. She insists that she was awake and denies any associated confusion. The only other time this occurred was 1 month prior when she experienced a similar spell as she was falling asleep. She denies other sleep complaints including EDS.

17. What is the most likely diagnosis?
   A. Narcolepsy without cataplexy
   B. Panic attacks
   C. Isolated sleep paralysis
   D. Cataplexy

18. What would be a reasonable initial treatment option?
   A. Tricyclic antidepressant
   B. Selective serotonin reuptake inhibitor
   C. Modafinil
   D. Reassurance

Case 6

A 65-year-old male presents to your office at the urging of his wife. Over the past 2 years, he has punched or kicked the bed violently, nearly hitting his wife. He has had six episodes in total, all occurring in the second half of the night. These episodes are often accompanied by yelling and swearing, behavior that is very atypical for him. When his wife wakes him up after an episode, he remembers dreaming about being in a fight or being chased by an aggressor. He has gained 20 pounds over the past 5 years, and his wife reports worsening snoring, although she has not seen him stop breathing during sleep.

Questions 19–22 are based on case #6:

19. What is the most likely diagnosis?
   A. Obstructive sleep apnea syndrome
   B. Confusional arousal
   C. REM sleep behavior disorder (RBD)
   D. Sleep terrors

20. The 30-second epoch in Figure 23-2 is representative of this patient's REM sleep. What would be your initial treatment option?
   A. Reassurance
   B. CPAP
   C. Clonazepam
   D. Tricyclic antidepressant or selective serotonin reuptake inhibitor

21. What area of the brain is responsible for REM atonia?
   A. Tuberomammillary nucleus
   B. Laterodorsal and pedunculopontine tegmental areas
   C. Median and dorsal raphe nuclei
   D. Medial medulla
   E. Locus coeruleus

22. How would you counsel this patient?
   A. Explain that the condition is benign.
   B. Explain that patients with this condition have a higher chance of developing a parkinsonian disorder.
   C. Explain that the condition will get better over time.
   D. Explain that there is a high chance that his children will develop this condition.

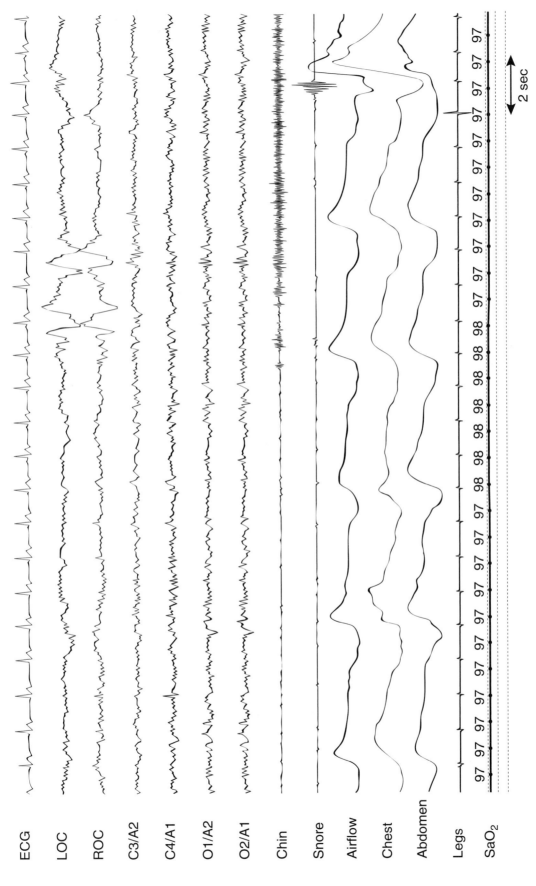

FIGURE 23-2 ■ For Question 20; see Table 23-1 for key.

Case 7

A healthy 40-year-old executive presents to the sleep clinic with a chief complaint of difficulty falling asleep for 3 weeks since he returned from a business trip. It takes him 1–2 hours to fall asleep, but once he is asleep he does not wake up during the night. His sleep problem started after he returned home to Denver from Los Angeles. On the third day of the trip, he learned that a major deal he had spent 6 months trying to finalize had fallen through. He has been worried about job security ever since and is using alcohol nightly to help fall asleep. He denies any other illicit drug use.

Questions 23–25 are based on case #7:

23. What is the most likely diagnosis?
    A. Circadian rhythm sleep disorder, jet lag type
    B. Circadian rhythm sleep disorder, delayed phase type

C. Adjustment insomnia
D. Idiopathic insomnia
E. Psychophysiologic insomnia

24. Which of the following is an appropriate first-line treatment?
    A. A benzodiazepine agent
    B. A nonbenzodiazepine hypnotic
    C. Sleep hygiene
    D. An antidepressant such as trazodone

25. Activity of which of the following nuclei is enhanced by benzodiazepines and nonbenzodiazepine hypnotics?
    A. Tuberomammillary nucleus
    B. Lateral and posterior hypothalamic nuclei
    C. Median and dorsal raphe nuclei
    D. Ventrolateral preoptic area (VLPO)
    E. Locus coeruleus

Answers

Case 1 answers

1. C. Narcolepsy without cataplexy

The patient has had daytime sleepiness for more than 3 months without episodes of cataplexy and has no other sleep disorder by history. Patients with narcolepsy typically report having short refreshing naps and persistent daytime sleepiness. This patient does not have delayed sleep phase syndrome as his sleep time is not delayed by 2 hours when compared with socially acceptable norms and he has daytime sleepiness despite getting adequate sleep. The diagnosis of Kleine-Levin syndrome is also not likely since the daytime sleepiness is not episodic. Patients with idiopathic hypersomnia typically report that naps are not refreshing. Idiopathic hypersomnia is a diagnosis of exclusion and requires a full sleep history to rule out other causes of daytime sleepiness.

2. A. Overnight PSG followed by an MSLT

An overnight PSG followed by an MSLT is required to confirm the diagnosis of narcolepsy without cataplexy. The overnight PSG provides information about sleep architecture and rules out other sleep disorders that may be contributing to the daytime sleepiness, such as sleep apnea or periodic limb movement disorder. On the MSLT, a mean sleep latency of less than 8 minutes with two sleep onset REM periods (SOREMPs) confirms the diagnosis of narcolepsy without cataplexy. In patients with narcolepsy with cataplexy, an overnight PSG and MSLT are not absolutely required to make the diagnosis but are recommended nonetheless. HLA typing is performed to identify the HLA DQB1*0602 allele that is seen in 85–100% of narcoleptics with cataplexy; however, HLA DQB1*0602 is not diagnostic of narcolepsy, because as many as 25% of the normal population has the allele. A cerebrospinal fluid hypocretin level less than 110 pg/mL is highly sensitive and specific for narcolepsy with cataplexy, but it lacks sensitivity for narcolepsy without cataplexy.

3. E. Hypersomnia resulting from a medical condition

The patient has a history of daytime sleepiness over 3 months that developed after a central nervous system infection and is not explained by another disorder. In addition, the patient takes naps that are not refreshing. The mean sleep latency is 6.9 minutes, and one SOREMP was present on the MSLT. This patient does not have narcolepsy because of a medical condition because he does not have cataplexy and had only one SOREMP on the MSLT. If the clinical suspicion for narcolepsy without cataplexy remains high, a repeat MSLT may be considered. This patient does not have Kleine-Levin syndrome because his sleepiness is not episodic with period of normalcy between episodes. This patient does not have idiopathic hypersomnia because his hypersomnia started after an episode of viral meningitis.[1,2]

4. D. Modafinil

The goal of treatment is to reduce the severity of daytime sleepiness. Modafinil is often an initial choice among the wake-promoting agents. It is effective in reducing daytime sleepiness and is well tolerated. The most common adverse effect is headache. Amphetamines and methylphenydate tend to have more adverse effects, including anxiety, nervousness, and hypertension. Sodium oxybate is indicated in patients with narcolepsy to treat EDS and cataplexy and is not a first-line therapy for EDS alone. Good sleep hygiene and strategic naps are important in the treatment of all patients with daytime sleepiness, regardless of etiology.

5. D. Decreased reuptake of dopamine

Modafinil is a novel wake-promoting agent. The mechanism of action is not entirely clear and believed to involve multiple neurotransmitters. A recent study demonstrated competitive binding of modafinil to the dopamine transporter responsible for dopamine reuptake, which is a proposed mechanism for promoting wakefulness. Amphetamines cause an increase in dopamine release. Caffeine acts by binding to adenosine receptors.

6. C. Add a tricyclic or selective serotonin reuptake inhibitor antidepressant.

Now that the patient has developed cataplexy, the diagnosis has changed to narcolepsy owing to a medical condition by International Classification of Sleep Disorders-2 (ICSD-2) criteria. Increasing the dose of modafinil or adding another stimulant may improve daytime sleepiness but will not significantly reduce cataplexy. Antidepressants have been traditionally used to treat cataplexy, but many tricyclic agents are associated with significant anticholinergic side effects. The selective serotonin reuptake inhibitors, including fluoxetine, are effective for treating cataplexy and have fewer adverse effects than tricyclic antidepressants. Sodium oxybate, which is the only Food and Drug Administration (FDA)-approved anticataplectic medication, is now also approved for EDS in the treatment of narcolepsy. Due to concerns of abuse potential, sodium oxybate is generally not considered as initial therapy in newly diagnosed cases. However, this agent is increasingly being used earlier in the course of treatment in patients with narcolepsy.

Case 2 answers

7. B. Obstructive sleep apnea syndrome

The history is highly suggestive of obstructive sleep apnea syndrome (loud snoring, witnessed apneas, daytime sleepiness). In *ICSD-2*, upper airway resistance syndrome is included under the obstructive sleep apnea syndrome, as they share a similar pathophysiology. The patient could have narcolepsy without cataplexy, but his history is much more suggestive of sleep apnea, which must be excluded. Diagnostic criteria for PLMD include a periodic limb movements during sleep index >5 in children or >15 in adults in association with a clinical sleep disturbance or complaint of daytime fatigue.

8. B. Attended (laboratory) PSG

An attended PSG is the gold standard test used to establish the diagnosis of sleep apnea. There is insufficient evidence to support the use of portable studies for this purpose. An MSLT is not indicated for the evaluation of sleep apnea alone. If the attended PSG fails to demonstrate evidence of sleep apnea and the patient has significant unexplained daytime sleepiness, an MSLT should be considered.[4]

9. A. Obstructive sleep apnea

Sleep is typically scored in 30-second epochs. The PSG tracing represents a 60-second period (Figure 23-1). Note the absent airflow and nasal transducer signals in the presence of continued thoracoabdominal effort with paradoxical breathing. The event culminates in an arousal. The oxygen desaturation is probably not directly due to the apnea on this epoch, but rather to an event on the prior epoch, as there is a lag time with desaturations recorded by finger-probe oximetry owing to circulation time.

10. B. CPAP

CPAP is the first-line treatment for most patients with OSA. Nocturnal oxygen will not prevent upper airway collapse in sleep. Uvulopalatopharyngoplasty effectively treats OSA in less than 50% of patients and is often used in cases of mild OSA. Similarly, mandibular advancement devices are typically reserved for patients with mild OSA or those who cannot tolerate positive airway pressure therapy. Weight loss is an important component of therapy for overweight patients with OSA; however, the severity of apnea and desaturation in this case warrants urgent treatment.

Case 3 answers

11. C. Circadian rhythm sleep disorder, delayed sleep phase type

The patient has a bedtime and wake time that is not compatible with her desired time or societal norms. On weekends she feels more awake after she is able to sleep according to her "usual" schedule. She has difficulty falling asleep earlier than her habitual bedtime. Delayed sleep phase syndrome is often misdiagnosed as sleep-onset insomnia or narcolepsy. During the week, insufficient sleep contributes to her daytime sleepiness and poor occupational and academic performance. The patient does not have any of the classical features of narcolepsy other than EDS. Her EDS is best explained by sleep deprivation accrued owing to an abnormal timing of the sleep-wake cycle.

12. D. Actigraphy

Actigraphy is a simple, noninvasive tool used to estimate bedtimes and wake times. If the actigraph is able to detect light, additional information about light exposure throughout the day could be obtained. A sleep diary completed by the patient can provide complementary information. The MSLT might be indicated to rule out narcolepsy in a patient with EDS in the absence of significant sleep deprivation. The maintenance of wakefulness test provides an objective measure of one's ability to stay awake and is not indicated in the initial assessment of suspected circadian rhythm sleep disorders. A PSG should be performed if the clinical history suggests sleep apnea or PLMD or if there were typical features of narcolepsy, in which case it should be followed by an MSLT.

Case 4 answers

13. B. Restless legs syndrome (RLS)

RLS is a clinical diagnosis that has four essential features. Patients have an urge to move the legs that may or may not be accompanied by uncomfortable sensations. The urge to move and accompanying sensations are made worse at rest and are partially or completely relieved by walking or moving the legs, at least temporarily. There is a circadian component in that the urge to move occurs exclusively or predominantly in the evening or at night. The patient may also have PLMD, but this diagnosis must be established by a PSG (some patients have both RLS and PLMD). This is not a case of psychophysiologic insomnia because the difficulty with sleep onset is due to leg discomfort and not from learned behaviors that interfere with falling asleep. This is not a case of adjustment insomnia because the difficulty falling asleep has been present for more than 3 months and the RLS symptoms predominate.

14. A. Periodic limb movements during sleep

Several supportive clinical features help establish the diagnosis of RLS. Supportive clinical features include a positive family history of RLS, periodic limb movements during sleep, and response to dopaminergic agents. Napping is not a universal feature of RLS. Identification of a stressor or inciting factor, often present in patients with adjustment insomnia, is not required to make the diagnosis of RLS.

15. D. Serum ferritin

A serum ferritin level less than 50 µg/L is associated with an increased severity of RLS symptoms and may predict a poor or incomplete response to dopaminergic agents. Other laboratory testing is not routinely required for the diagnosis of RLS. A PSG should be considered if there is a suspicion of underlying periodic limb movement disorder or sleep apnea. During the SIT, the subject is asked to lie for 1 hour before bedtime without moving the legs. The SIT may be helpful, although the sensitivity is only 81% and the test is typically reserved for research purposes. Actigraphy is not routinely indicated but can be helpful in assessing response to treatment.

16. D. Ropinerole

A dopamine agonist is a reasonable first choice in patients with daily RLS. Counter-stimulation (i.e., massage, wrapping the legs in bandages, using a vibrating device on the legs) may be effective in patients with intermittent symptoms. Levodopa/carbidopa is effective; however, long-term use is associated with augmentation (earlier onset of symptoms after an evening dose of medication). Benzodiazepines are not first-line therapy because of the higher likelihood of adverse effects and potential for tolerance. Gabapentin is a useful first-line therapy, particularly in patients with painful sensations in the legs, such as those with secondary RLS owing to peripheral neuropathy.[10]

Case 5 answers

17. C. Sleep paralysis

Isolated sleep paralysis can occur in patients without narcolepsy. Sleep deprivation and irregular sleep schedules are thought to be contributory factors. Panic attacks are not typically associated with an inability to move. Cataplexy is loss of muscle tone usually elicited by a strong emotional stimulus.

18. D. Reassurance

Reassurance and education are typically all that is required for isolated sleep paralysis. The patient should be informed that it could recur and made aware of the possible precipitating factors. This information should help to decrease the anxiety associated

with each episode of sleep paralysis. Complicated or unremitting cases may be treated with REM-suppressing medications.

Case 6 answers

19. C. REM sleep behavior disorder (RBD)

The history is highly suggestive for RBD, as the patient is an elderly male acting out violent dream content. Sleep terrors typically occur in children and tend to occur in the first third of the sleep period when slow wave sleep predominates. Sleep terrors are associated with intense autonomic activation, including pupillary dilation, tachycardia, and tachypnea. Patients with sleep terrors are typically hard to console, do not interact with the environment, and are confused or disoriented when awakened from an episode. Confusional arousals consist of confusion during an arousal from non-rapid eye movement (NREM) sleep or on waking in the morning or after a nap in the absence of intense autonomic activation. Patients with sleep apnea who also have confusional arousals during REM sleep may present as having pseudo-RBD.

20. C. Clonazepam

This epoch shows the loss of REM atonia (noted in the chin electromyographic channel), which is an abnormal characteristic of REM sleep and is the primary PSG finding of RBD. Low-dose clonazepam at bedtime is effective in 90% of cases. Patients should be advised to take safety precautions, including removing items from the bedroom (e.g., furniture, lamps) that could cause injury during an episode. Tricyclic antidepressants and selective serotonin reuptake inhibitors can provoke RBD and should be avoided.

21. D. Medial medulla

The laterodorsal and pedunculopontine (LDT/PPT) neurons are active during REM sleep, and the primary neurotransmitter is acetylcholine. Cholinergic projections from the LDT/PPT neurons activate the medial medulla. Projections from the medial medulla using glycine as a neurotransmitter inhibit brainstem and spinal motor neurons, which produce atonia during REM sleep. The tuberomammillary nucleus is the only source of neuronal histamine in the brain. The median and dorsal raphe nuclei are sources of serotonin, and the locus coeruleus is a source of norepinephrine.

22. B. Explain that patients with RBD have a higher chance of developing a parkinsonian disorder.

Up to two thirds of patients with idiopathic RBD develop a parkinsonian disorder. RBD is usually a progressive condition that does not remit spontaneously. There is not enough evidence to suggest a particular inheritance pattern.

Case 7 answers

23. C. Adjustment insomnia

The sleep difficulty in adjustment insomnia lasts for less than 3 months and is due to an identifiable stressor. Psychophysiologic insomnia is due to learned behaviors that prevent sleep, along with heightened arousal in bed that is present for at least 1 month. Idiopathic insomnia typically begins in infancy or childhood in the absence of an identifiable stressor. Patients with jet lag disorder have trouble falling asleep with daytime symptoms after traveling across at least two time zones. Patients with delayed sleep phase disorder syndrome have bedtimes and wake times that are incompatible with their desired time or societal norms.

24. B. Nonbenzodiazepine hypnotic

Benzodiazepines are effective in helping patients fall asleep, but they are associated with adverse effects such as prolonged sedation or grogginess, risk of tolerance and dependence, withdrawal symptoms, and rebound insomnia. The nonbenzodiazepine hypnotics such as zolpidem, zaleplon, and eszopiclone are effective for short-term insomnia resulting from stressors or jet lag. The risk of adverse effects such as dependence and abuse is less than those seen with benzodiazepines. Sleep hygiene should always be addressed but may not be adequate for patients who have had difficulty falling asleep for more than a few nights. The patient should be advised to stop using alcohol as a hypnotic and to ensure that the bedroom is conducive for sleep. Trazodone is an antidepressant that is commonly used for insomnia, but efficacy data for long-term use are lacking, and the drug has considerable associated adverse events (orthostatic hypotension, priapism, sedation, and arrhythmias). The goal is to prevent acute insomnia from progressing into chronic insomnia.

25. D. Ventrolateral preoptic area (VLPO)

The neurons in the VLPO are active during sleep, particularly deep NREM sleep. Benzodiazepine receptor agonists act on the gamma aminobutyric acid (GABA) complex to enhance the activity of the VLPO. The other nuclei are involved in promoting wakefulness.

REFERENCES

1. Allen RP, Picchietti D, Hening WA, et al: Restless legs syndrome: diagnostic criteria, special considerations, and epidemiology. A report from the Restless Legs Syndrome Diagnosis and Epidemiology Workshop at the National Institutes of Health. Sleep Med 4:101–119, 2003.

2. American Academy of Sleep Medicine: *International Classification of Sleep Disorders, 2nd ed. Diagnostic and Coding Manual.* Westchester, IL, American Academy of Sleep Medicine, 2005.

3. Chesson AL Jr, Berry RB, Pack A: Practice parameters for the use of portable monitoring devices in the investigation of suspected obstructive sleep apnea in adults. Sleep 26:907–913, 2003.

4. Espana RA, Scammell TE: Sleep neurobiology for the clinician. Sleep 27:811–820, 2004.

5. Insomnia: assessment and management in primary care. National Heart, Lung, and Blood Institute Working Group on Insomnia. Am Fam Physician 59:3029–3038, 1999.

6. Littner M, Kushida CA, Anderson WM, et al: Practice parameters for the role of actigraphy in the study of sleep and circadian rhythms: an update for 2002. Sleep 26:337–341, 2003.

7. Littner MR, Kushida C, Wise M, et al: Practice parameters for clinical use of the multiple sleep latency test and the maintenance of wakefulness test. Sleep 28:113–121, 2005.

8. Montplaisir J, Boucher S, Nicolas A, et al: Immobilization tests and periodic leg movements in sleep for the diagnosis of restless leg syndrome. Mov Disord 13:324–329, 1998.

9. Practice parameters for the treatment of snoring and obstructive sleep apnea with oral appliances. American Sleep Disorders Association. Sleep 18:511–513, 1995.

10. Schenck CH, Mahowald MW: REM sleep behavior disorder: clinical, developmental, and neuroscience perspectives 16 years after its formal identification in SLEEP. Sleep 25:120–138, 2002.

11. Sher AE, Schechtman KB, Piccirillo JF: The efficacy of surgical modifications of the upper airway in adults with obstructive sleep apnea syndrome. Sleep 19:156–177, 1996.

12. Silber MH, Ehrenberg BL, Allen RP, et al: An algorithm for the management of restless legs syndrome. Mayo Clin Proc 79:916–922, 2004.

13. Wisor JP, Eriksson KS: Dopaminergic-adrenergic interactions in the wake promoting mechanism of modafinil. Neuroscience 132:1027–1034, 2005.

Clinical Case Studies II

TERI J. BARKOUKIS ■ ALON Y. AVIDAN

Questions

For questions 1–4: Please match the following cases with Figures 24-1 through 24-4.

(Adapted with permission from Avidan AY: Abnormal eye movements during sleep. J Clin Sleep Med 1[4]:429–432, 2005.)

1. Patient A

A 49-year-old woman presented for a nocturnal polysomnogram (PSG) for evaluation of apneic episodes at night and excessive daytime somnolence. She had a history of chronic insomnia and, before going to bed at night, she watched television or read a book in bed to try to relax.

2. Patient B

A 52-year-old man presented for evaluation of frequent episodes of dream-enactment behaviors. The video portion of his nocturnal PSG demonstrated flailing of both arms associated with shouting and screaming. He had had a previous left eye enucleation following blunt trauma.

3. Patient C

A 38-year-old woman with a past medical history of major depression presented for a sleep study for evaluation of daytime sleepiness and snoring. Her medications include fluoxetine (Prozac).

4. Patient D

A 41-year-old woman presented for evaluation of snoring, witnessed apneas, and daytime sleepiness. At the age of 20 she suffered a traumatic knife injury to her right orbit and face and subsequently had multiple surgeries for this injury. On cranial nerve examination, her extraocular movements were full on the left. On the right, she was found to have a third, fourth, fifth, and sixth cranial nerve damage, with some aberrant regeneration of the third and sixth cranial nerves.

5. A 57-year-old obese woman presented with a 30-year history of loud snoring initially noted by her children. Because she lives alone, she is not sure whether she has apneic pauses or snores every night. She also reports decreased short-term memory and increased irritability during the last 5–7 years. She complains of significant morning headaches and feels very sleepy during the daytime. Which of the following would be most helpful as a first step in evaluating this patient?

A. A nocturnal PSG
B. Magnetic resonance imaging (MRI) of the brain
C. Evaluation of baseline pulmonary status with an arterial blood gas, chest x-ray film, and pulmonary function test
D. No evaluation is needed. This condition is self-limited.
E. Formal psychiatric evaluation

6. An 82-year-old woman is bothered by the irresistible need to constantly move her legs and daytime sleepiness. Her friends note that she is unable to stay still during conversations without "moving her legs back and forth." During the night these symptoms become intolerable. She is observed to be engaging in vigorous stretching and flexing of her legs. She stated that many times she thought about wishing "to cut her legs off." Activities that reduce or alleviate these symptoms include getting out of bed, walking, and massaging her legs. During the night, her husband describes leg jerks that also severely disrupt his sleep. The patient consumes up to 20 cups of coffee per day. She remembers that 50 years ago, when she was pregnant; these symptoms were extremely severe. Her family physician prescribed 25 mg of Benadryl, which "had no effect other than to make me sleepy the next morning."

Figure 24-5 is a PSG sample from this patient's sleep study. Her diagnosis includes which of the following?

A. Periodic leg movement disorder of sleep (PLMD) and restless legs syndrome (RLS)
B. Myoclonic epilepsy
C. Hypnic jerks
D. Akathisia
E. Hyperexplexia

Text continued on p. 443

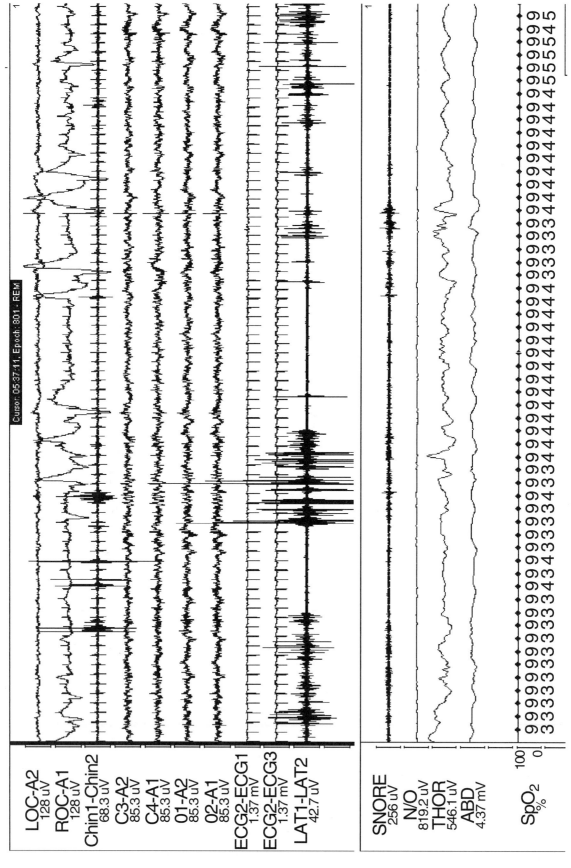

FIGURE 24-1 ■ Channels are as follows: Electro-oculogram (EOG) (left: LOC-A2, right: ROC-A1), chin electromyogram (EMG), electroencephalogram (EEG) (left central, right central, left occipital, right occipital), electrocardiogram (ECG2-ECG1, ECG2-ECG3), limb EMG, snoring, nasal-oral airflow, respiratory effort (thoracic, abdominal), and oxygen saturation.

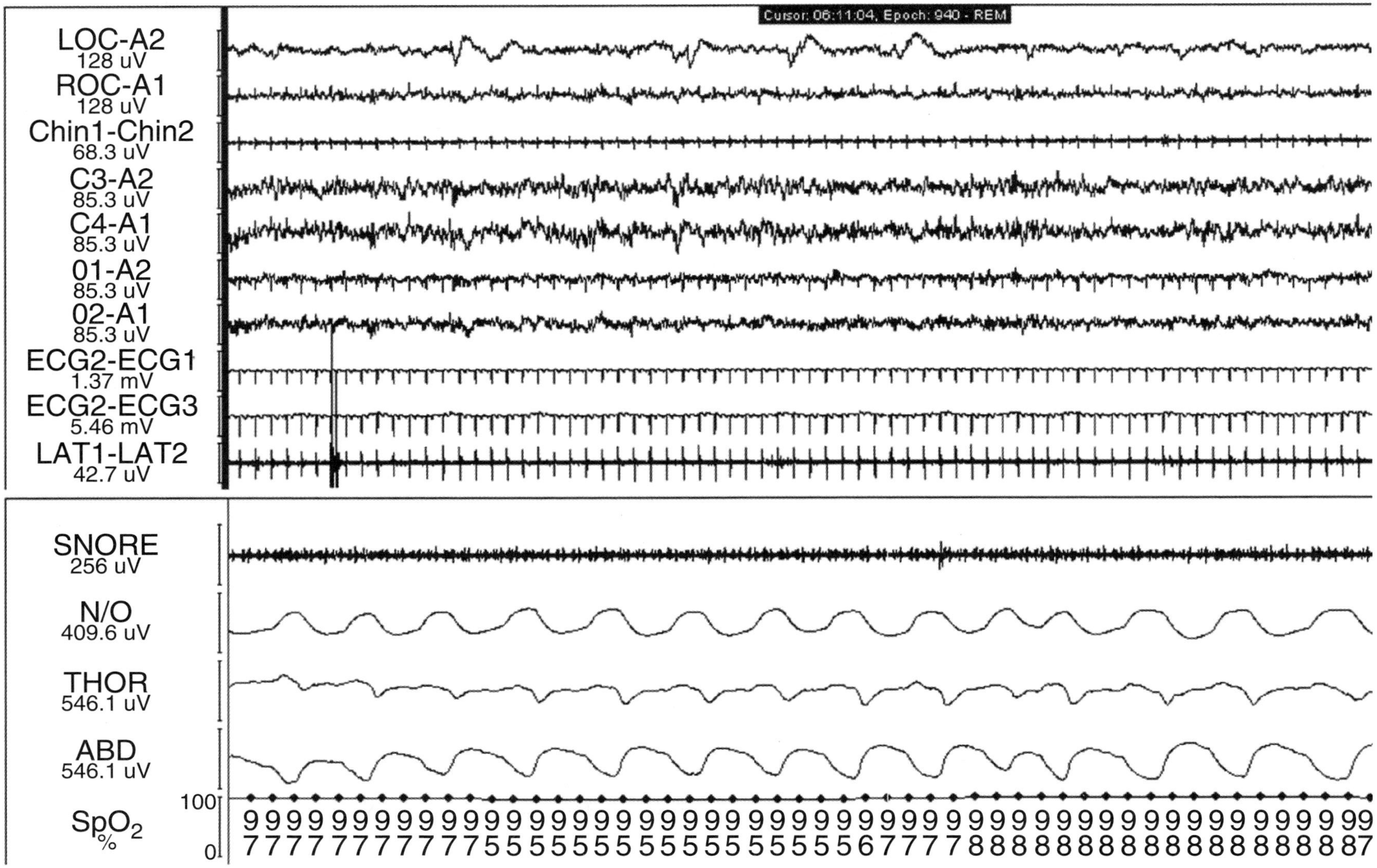

FIGURE 24-2 ■ Channels are as follows: EOG (left: LOC-A2, right: ROC-A1), chin EMG, EEG (left central, right central, left occipital, right occipital), ECG (ECG2-ECG1, ECG2-ECG3), limb EMG, snoring, nasal-oral airflow, respiratory effort (thoracic, abdominal), and oxygen saturation.

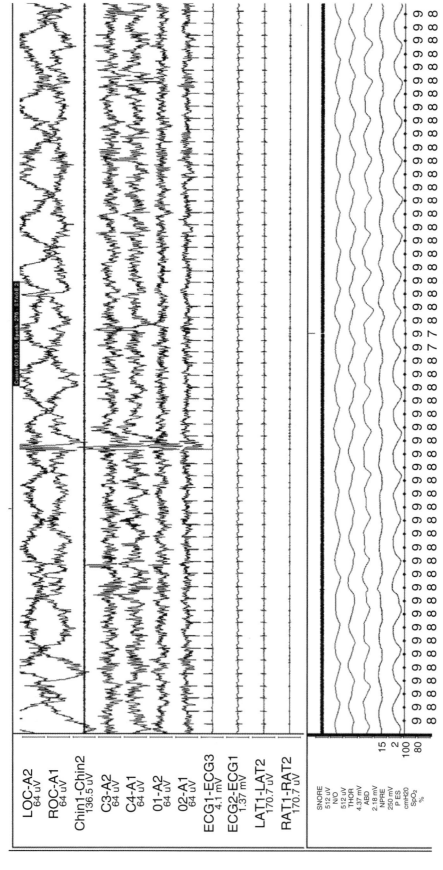

FIGURE 24-3 ■ Channels are as follows: EOG (left: LOC-A2, right: ROC-A1), chin EMG, EEG (left central, right central, left occipital, right occipital), ECG (ECG2-ECG1, ECG2-ECG3), limb EMG, snoring, nasal-oral airflow, respiratory effort (thoracic, abdominal), and oxygen saturation.

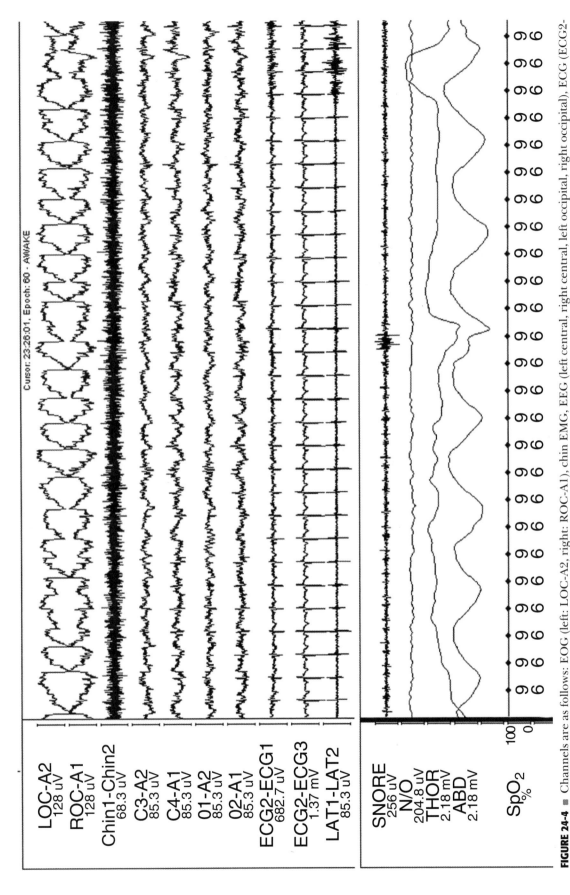

FIGURE 24-4 ■ Channels are as follows: EOG (left: LOC-A2, right: ROC-A1), chin EMG, EEG (left central, right central, left occipital, right occipital), ECG (ECG2-ECG1, ECG2-ECG3), limb EMG (left and right anterior tibialis), snoring, nasal-oral airflow, respiratory effort (thoracic, abdominal), nasal pressure, esophageal pressure monitoring, and oxygen saturation.

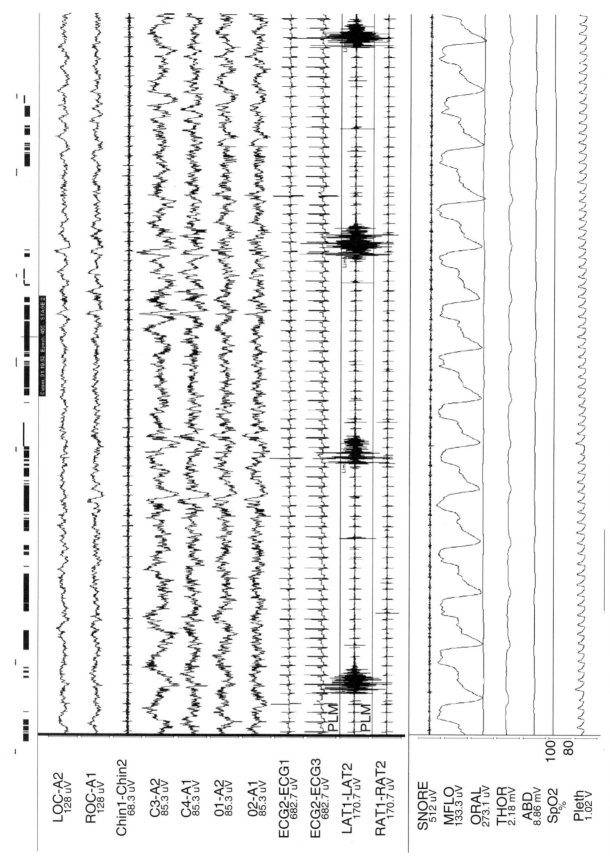

FIGURE 24-5 ■ Channels are as follows: EOG (left: LOC-A2, right: ROC-A1), chin EMG, EEG (left occipital, right central, left central, right occipital), ECG (ECG2-ECG1, ECG2-ECG3), limb EMG (left and right anterior tibialis), snoring, nasal-oral airflow, respiratory effort (thoracic, abdominal), nasal pressure, esophageal pressure monitoring, and oxygen saturation.

7. An 82-year-old man presents to the sleep disorders clinic complaining of a 6-year history of early morning awakening. He is usually in bed between 8:30 and 9:30 P.M. and has a sleep latency of 5 minutes. He wakes up at 3:00 A.M. and is unable obtain any further sleep. He lies in bed for 60–90 minutes and eventually gets up between 6:00 and 6:30 A.M. He takes 3-hour morning naps four to five times per week. His sleep log is illustrated in Figure 24-6.

What is the clinical diagnosis?
A. Delayed sleep-phase syndrome (DSPS)
B. Non–24-hour sleep-wake syndrome
C. Irregular sleep-wake syndrome
D. Sleep state misperception
E. Advanced sleep-phase syndrome (ASPS)

8. Which of the following treatments is most effective for the patient presented in Question 7?
A. Bright light therapy on awakening
B. Bright light therapy in the early evening
C. Scheduled 2-hour naps in the afternoon
D. Treatment with melatonin in the evening

9. A 73-year-old man is referred to the sleep disorders clinic because of violent movements during sleep, which have been present for the last 2 years. These spells are most commonly observed during the last third of the night and are heterogeneous varying from simple movement of the hand or leg to actual screaming, cursing, and fighting in bed. These episodes are somewhat more common after periods of sleep deprivation and after heavy alcohol ingestion. His wife requested that he seek medical attention after he hit her during one of these episodes. He was also diagnosed with Parkinson's disease 1 month ago by a neurologist. His sleep exam reveals evidence of bradykinesia and a parkinsonian tremor. A representative sample from his PSG is provided in Figure 24-7. What is the first treatment of choice?
A. Clonazepam (Klonopin)
B. Phenytoin (Dilantin)
C. Hydrochlorothiazide
D. Prednisone
E. Supplemental oxygen

10. A 45-year-old male in excellent health except for hypercholesterolemia was brought to his internist by his wife who says that, for the last few months, he has been screaming in his sleep and punching the walls of his bedroom. Once awakened, he recalls his dream and goes back to bed calmly. The next day he awakens refreshed and acts normally all day. Figure 24-8 demonstrates his brain MRI scan. A lesion in which of the following locations might help explain his sleep disorder?
A. Medial thalamus
B. Posterior hypothalamus
C. Cerebellum
D. Medial pons
E. Basal forebrain

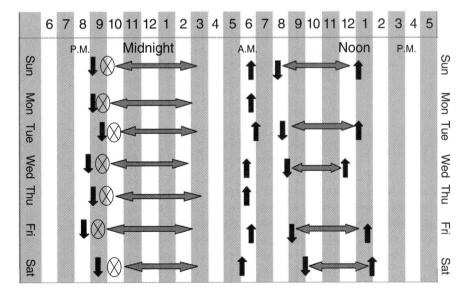

FIGURE 24-6 ■ Sleep log for Question 7.

| ↓ In bed | ↑ Out of bed | ⊗ Light out | ⟷ Asleep |

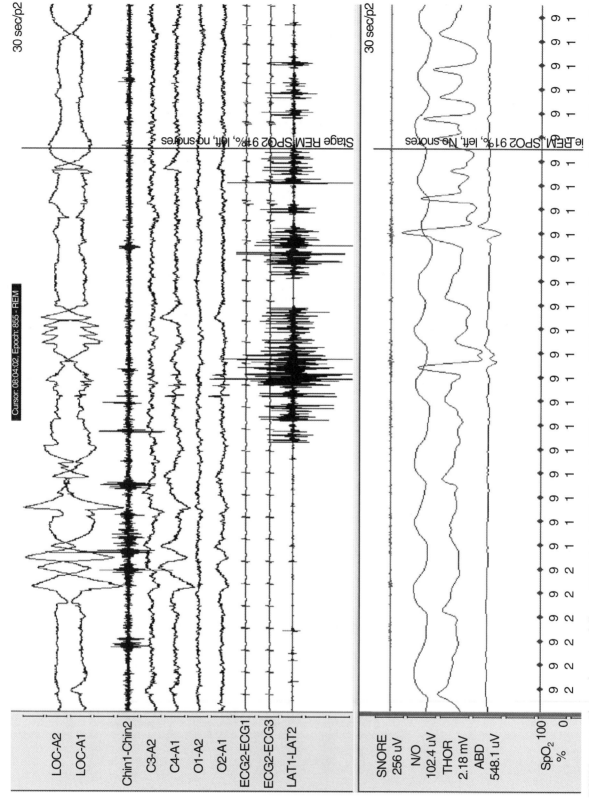

FIGURE 24-7 ■ Channels are as follows: EOG (left: LOC-A2, right: ROC-A1), chin EMG, EEG (left central, right central, left occipital, right occipital, ECG (ECG2-ECG1, ECG2-ECG3), limb EMG (left and right anterior tibialis), snoring, nasal-oral airflow, respiratory effort (thoracic, abdominal), nasal pressure, esophageal pressure monitoring, and oxygen saturation.

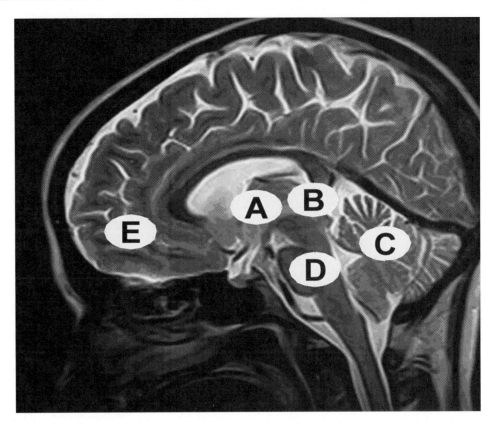

FIGURE 24-8 ■ MRI of the brain of a 45-year-old patient with dream enactment.

11. A 16-year-old high school student has been staying up until 2 A.M. accessing the Internet and then has difficulty making it to his 7:30 A.M. bus. On weekends, he sleeps in until 11 A.M. His parents have removed the computer from his room, but the boy is still awake at 1 A.M. every night complaining that he cannot fall asleep. During the day, he suffers from excessive daytime sleepiness (EDS). What is the most likely diagnosis?
A. Narcolepsy
B. ASPS
C. DSPS
D. Psychophysiologic insomnia
E. Non–24-hour sleep wake disorder

12. A 4-year-old girl was evaluated by her pediatrician for episodes of awakening with very loud screaming and severe sweating two to four times per week, usually before 3 A.M. According to her parents, the patient is very anxious during the episodes, sometimes short of breath, and very difficult to communicate with or to console. She is usually amnesic to these spells. The neighbors alerted police after they heard her screaming and suspected child abuse. Her examination is otherwise normal. What is the diagnosis?
A. REM nightmare
B. REM-sleep behavior disorder (RBD)

C. Confusional arousals
D. Night terror
E. Nocturnal agitation disorder of REM sleep

13. A 22-year-old female with a history of relapsing remitting multiple sclerosis (MS) presents for a sleep evaluation because of severe daytime sleepiness. Her MRI scan reveals multiple lesions described as small and irregular with high T2 signal intensities throughout the brain. Which of the neuroanatomical structures shown in Figure 24-9 would produce symptoms consistent with the patient's findings?

14. A 27-year-old woman came to see you for a second opinion for recent weight gain, fatigue, and unusual night behavior reported by her husband over the past year. He came with her and reported that he awakened to noise in the kitchen and saw her at the stove with a burner turned on over an unopened can of beans. She had no recollection of this event, but both of them became alarmed because of the seriousness of a potential fire. They reported that over the past 6 months, they were puzzled by finding empty candy wrappers in the morning, a buttered margarine lid, crumbs on the counter, and an occasional open refrigerator door. She had a history of somnambulism as a child, but

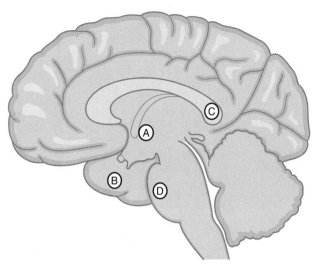

FIGURE 24-9 ■ Graphical representation of the brain sagital section.

these episodes appeared to stop by the time she was 12 years old. She was married at age 21 and had two children, now 2 and 4 years old. She has a happy marriage, although a very busy family life. About a year ago, she started a new job to help with the family income but has had a hard time adjusting to a very demanding boss and worries about her children being in daycare. She subsequently developed sleep onset and sleep maintenance insomnia about 2 months after starting this job. She enjoys working, despite the stress she is under, and went to her primary care provider who started her on zolpidem, 5 mg each night, which was later increased to 10 mg. She takes no other medication and is a nonsmoker. She does not have restless legs, but she started snoring about a month ago. Her past medical history is unremarkable. Physical exam is also unremarkable except for mild retrognathia. At 5′5″, she used to weigh around 120 pounds, but she has had a 25-pound weight gain over the last year. She had already been sent to an outside sleep lab by her physician, and the following epoch is representative of her PSG (Figure 24-10). Knowing the most likely diagnosis, what is the first therapy that you would advise this patient to pursue?

A. Start topiramate, 25 mg each night before bed

B. Refer this patient to a behavioral psychologist for stress management therapy.

C. Discontinue zolpidem and schedule a return visit in 1 month.

D. There is not enough information to recommend therapy at this time.

E. Schedule a dietitian appointment for a weight loss program.

15. A 20-year-old college student has EDS that is more predominant in his Monday afternoon lectures this semester. Recently he started to fall asleep in these afternoon classes when he had the sudden sensation that he was falling and jerked his arms and legs briefly. Because the somnolence was interfering with his Monday classes, he started drinking 3–4 cups of espresso coffee in the morning and switched to 4–5 cans of Mountain Dew from noon until his last class at 3 P.M. He did not experience daytime sleepiness before this semester. He would not have come to you except that he became concerned when he started to fall asleep in class 2 weeks ago and experienced a brief flash of very bright light. This occurred only once. He denies having any uncomfortable sensation in his limbs before this occurs or at night before bed. He denies cataplexy, snoring, or sleep paralysis. No one has ever said that he jerks his limbs in his sleep. He never had epilepsy. Before these symptoms started, he began to work a weekend job to help cover his costs that included a night shift on Sunday night at a 24-hour convenience store. Epworth Sleepiness Scale is 12. He denies drug or alcohol abuse. He is not overweight, and his physical exam is normal. You reassure him that the jerks during class are consistent with "sleep starts" but that he needs to schedule more sleep for his daytime somnolence. Only one of the following is *not* known to increase the incidence of sleep starts:

A. Excessive caffeine intake

B. Irregular sleep hours

C. Warm environment that is above 75° F

D. Alcohol intake

16. A 56-year-old morbidly obese patient came in with complaints of EDS, dyspnea on exertion, and ankle edema. His wife also reported loud snoring and shallow breathing. She became alarmed when he drifted out of his lane while driving her to a restaurant, but fortunately an accident did not occur. He had injured his back during a construction job about 5 years ago and could not return to work. He was obese, with a body mass index (BMI) of 32 kg/m² at the time of the accident, but over the past 5 years he has continued to gain weight to the point that his BMI is now 54 kg/m². His past medical history is significant for the discovery of coronary artery disease about 2 years ago, with recurrent angina now resolved after an angioplasty procedure. Recently he had gastroesophageal reflux symptoms and underwent an gastroesophageal endoscopy, where he

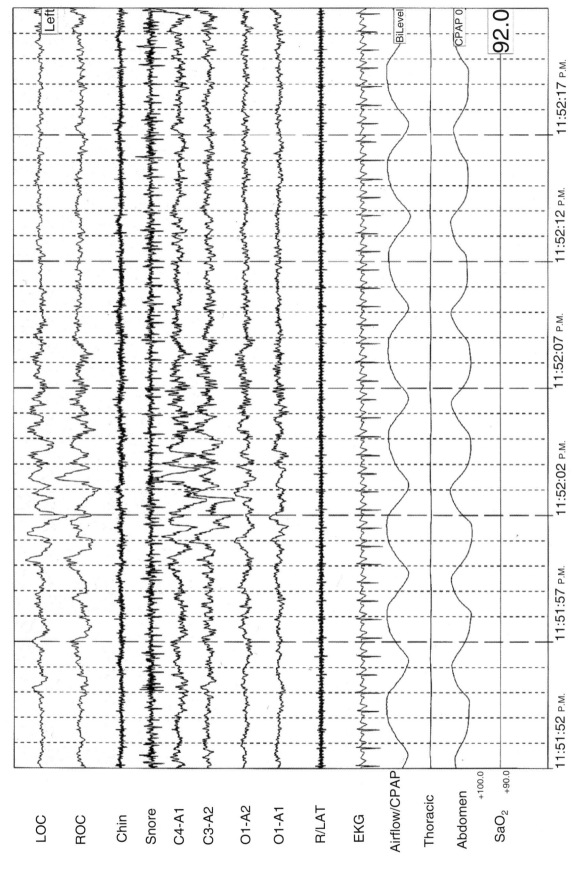

FIGURE 24-10 ■ 30-second epoch. LOC/ROC, Left/right oculogram; C4-A1/C3-A2, right/left central EEG leads; O1-A2/O2-A1, left/right occipital EEG leads; R/LAT, right/left leg EMG; "Airflow/CPAP" is only an airflow channel with no continuous positive airway pressure (CPAP) on this patient.

had severe desaturations into the 50s by pulse oximetry. Physical exam reveals a patient with a Mallampati Class IV airway, clear but decreased airflow to auscultation on pulmonary exam, a prominent S2 on cardiac exam, and 3+ pitting ankle edema. Epworth Sleepiness Scale is 21. The PSG was technically difficult to perform because of profuse sweating that started after sleep onset despite cooling the room and using a fan on the patient. The epoch in Figure 24-11 was typical of his sleep. His apnea-hypopnea index (AHI) was 4.7. Daytime arterial blood gas returned as pH 7.37, pCO_2 of 55, and pO_2 of 60 at sea level. Unless he agrees to therapeutic intervention, he has a high likelihood of developing which one of the following?

A. Pulmonary hypertension
B. Erythrocytosis
C. Right heart failure
D. All of the above

17. A primary care physician referred a 22-year-old man for management of narcolepsy. The referring medical records noted that this patient had EDS resulting in being placed on probation in his new job. He was sleeping through his alarm and was late to work several times. Because of the critical nature of his job as a railroad dispatcher, the employee health physician sent him for a PSG followed by a multiple sleep latency test (MSLT) with the following results:

PSG: Sleep efficiency 55%
Sleep latency (SL) 220 minutes
REM latency 95 minutes
AHI 0.4
Periodic limb movements during sleep index 1.0
MSLT: Nap #1 positive for stage REM; SL 0.5 minutes
Nap #2 positive for stage REM; SL 5 minutes
Nap # 3 no stage REM; SL 15 minutes
Nap # 4 no stage REM; SL 20 minutes
Nap # 5 no stage REM; SL 20 minutes

After your record review, the patient came in for his afternoon appointment on his day off and didn't appear sleepy at all, but he did add that this was his day off. When asked, he did admit that he was up until 4 A.M. and slept in until noon. He denies ever having cataplexy, sleep paralysis, or hypnogogic hallucinations. He started his current job only 6 months ago and is required to be at work by 7:30 A.M. Before this job, he took afternoon classes and worked a part-time evening job. His hypersomnolence started only around 6 months ago, with the exception of having a problem in his morning classes in high school. He also

has a great deal of difficulty with sleep-onset insomnia and feels that if he could just go to sleep, he would be fine. Today, his Epworth Sleepiness Scale is 7, compared with 15 on his last work day. Useful information for confirmation of this sleep disorder is:

A. Dim-light melatonin onset
B. Peak of the core body temperature rhythm
C. No further confirmation is necessary before starting modafinil, 200 mg each morning.
D. Laboratory evaluation for HLA DQB1*0602

18. A 45-year-old woman comes to your office for help with difficulty sleeping well. She has trouble with both initiating and maintaining sleep and awakens unrefreshed. She has had no snoring or witnessed apnea episodes. Her BMI is 24 kg/m². She has had gradually increasing fatigue over the past 7 years. She does complain of nonspecific muscle pain that has been gradually increasing over the past year. Her only medication is acetaminophen as needed for pain. On physical exam, she has a normal throat and soft palate, clear lungs, heart that is regular with no murmurs, and a normal neuromuscular exam, with the exception of 12 different tender points to palpation of her neck, upper back, and legs. If this patient were to have a PSG, you would most commonly find:

A. Pseudospindles
B. An increase in REM sleep
C. Recurrent alpha intrusions
D. An increase in delta sleep

19. A 19-year-old woman is troubled by three recent episodes of awakening with the sensation of being paralyzed. During one of these episodes, she saw her cousin sitting next to her talking to her about something at the end of her nighttime sleep, but she could not respond and was frightened to see her sitting there. She tried to move but could not. Eventually she was able to struggle out of this experience. She realized then that her cousin was not there, and the door to her dormitory room was indeed still locked. She relates that she just started college about 9 months ago. She had won an athletic scholarship for track and field and was required to attend a heavy workout schedule in addition to a full load of classes. She is staying up late studying and admitted to decreasing her sleep to fit in everything. Despite this routine, she is doing well in school and has won several medals in track meets. She has been hypersomnolent in an occasional class lately but still feels full of energy most of the time. She denies sleep attacks or cataplexy. She has never experienced anything

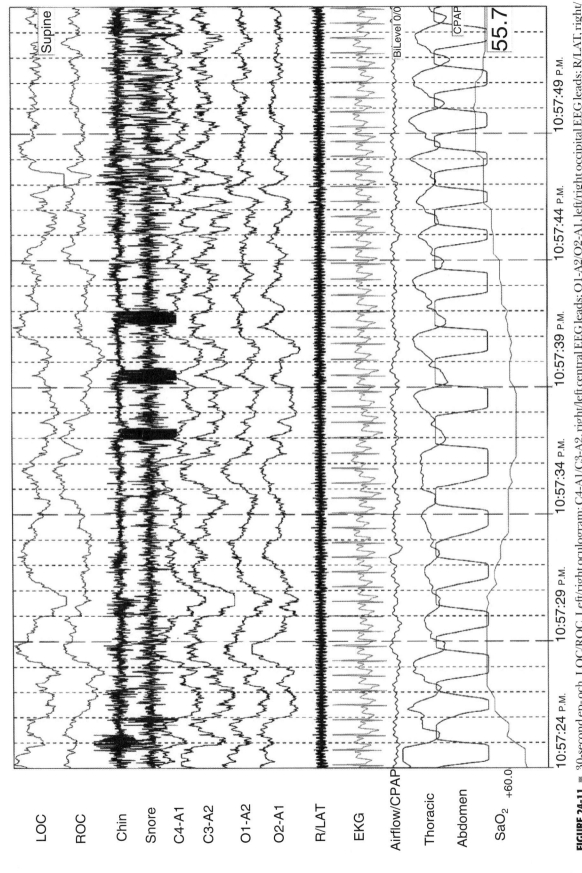

FIGURE 24-11 ■ 30-second ep- och. LOC/ROC, Left/right oculogram; C4-A1/C3-A2, right/left central EEG leads; O1-A2/O2-A1, left/right occipital EEG leads; R/LAT, right/left leg EMG; "Airflow/CPAP" is only an airflow channel with no CPAP on this patient.

LOC

ROC

Chin

Snore

C4-A1

C3-A2

O1-A2

O2-A1

R/LAT

EKG

Airflow/CPAP

Thoracic

Abdomen

SaO₂   +60.0

Supine

BiLevel 0/0

CPAP

55.7

10:57:24 P.M.   10:57:29 P.M.   10:57:34 P.M.   10:57:39 P.M.   10:57:44 P.M.   10:57:49 P.M.

like this hallucination before and does not use drugs. She has been drinking 4 or 5 cans of caffeinated soda each day. She has no physical complaints. She does not have any anxiety or depression. Her family history is unremarkable except for a cousin with bipolar disorder. The most likely predisposing factor to the sleep disorder that this patient has is:

A. Cerebrospinal fluid (CSF) that is hypocretin deficient
B. Inheritance of HLA subtype DR2
C. Family history of bipolar disorder
D. Chronic partial sleep deprivation

20. A 52-year-old man reluctantly came in after his wife insisted that he might have sleep apnea after seeing a television program during National Sleep Awareness Week. She noticed that the snoring occurred only in the supine position when he had an upper respiratory infection in the early years of their 22-year marriage. Over that last 10 years, he has gradually gained enough weight to achieve a BMI of 24 to 30 kg/m². He usually goes to bed after the 10 P.M. news and gets up with his alarm at 6 A.M. He denies ever being tired except when he drove 12 hours on a fishing trip last summer. He denies drowsy driving otherwise. He denies hypersomnolence and feels that his good energy level for his systems analyst job never changed. He tried over-the-counter aids such as strips to open his nares better and a throat spray for snoring patients without success. He insists that he has no sleep problems at all, and this "problem" only seems to bother his wife. She is concerned because the television show stated that medical risks increase in patients with undiagnosed obstructive sleep apnea (OSA). Physical exam shows a non–tired-appearing man who has slight leftward nasal septal deviation, nonenlarged tonsils, Mallampati Class 3 oropharyngeal airway, and predominant abdominal obesity. The remainder of the exam was unremarkable. A representative sample of the entire sleep time on his PSG is seen in Figure 24-12. This sleep disorder can increase the risk factor for:

A. Sustained ventricular tachycardia
B. Subarachnoid hemorrhage
C. Systemic hypertension
D. There are no cardiovascular risk factors with this disorder.

21. A physically fit 24-year-old man recently returned from a climbing expedition with a team of mountain climbers. They had camped at an elevation of 9000 ft. He felt great except for experiencing more dyspnea on exertion than at the base of the mountain. He had fragmented sleep and was noticed to have frequent pauses in his breathing by his tent-mate who was quite an early riser. Although this was his first trip to this elevation, he had no other problems on this entire adventure. He now loves mountain climbing but just wanted to be sure nothing else was wrong before he planned another climbing vacation. He denies EDS and has never been told that he snores. Physical exam is completely normal. Figure 24-13 is representative of his breathing pattern. You would expect the pathophysiology of this breathing pattern during sleep to be explained by:

A. Increasing hypoxic chemoresponsiveness primarily in REM sleep
B. Hyperventilation primarily in non-REM (NREM) sleep causing hypocapnic alkalosis
C. Carotid body stimulation by both hypoxia and hypercapnia
D. Elevation in PaO_2 and reduction in $PaCO_2$ during the initial apnea of stage 1 sleep

22. A 27-year-old woman in the beginning of her third trimester of pregnancy is being evaluated for fatigue that is much worse than during her previous pregnancy. She developed hypersomnolence and snoring. She had gained about 10 pounds more than the obstetrician recommended and started snoring at night, which was described by her husband as only mild. He has never witnessed apnea episodes. She is otherwise healthy. There is no family history of sleep disorders. Her review of systems and past medical history is unremarkable. Apparently a PSG was done because of concerns that she may have developed sleep apnea that could pose a risk to her baby. The results are as follows:

Sleep efficiency 78%
Sleep latency 63 minutes
AHI 0.7
Pulse oximetry range 93–98%
Snoring was present for only about 9% of total sleep time.

Periodic limb movements during sleep index was 34, of which at least 22 caused arousals not related to snoring After discussing these results with the patient and reassuring her that the evidence is against OSA, she recalls that she ran out of her prenatal vitamins about 6 weeks ago. During the initial recording, before sleep onset, Figure 24-14 is representative of why her sleep latency was prolonged, which is also a problem at home that she forgot to tell you about on the initial interview. Your advice to this patient is to do what *next*?

A. Resume her prenatal vitamins and reassure her that this disorder will likely resolve after delivery.

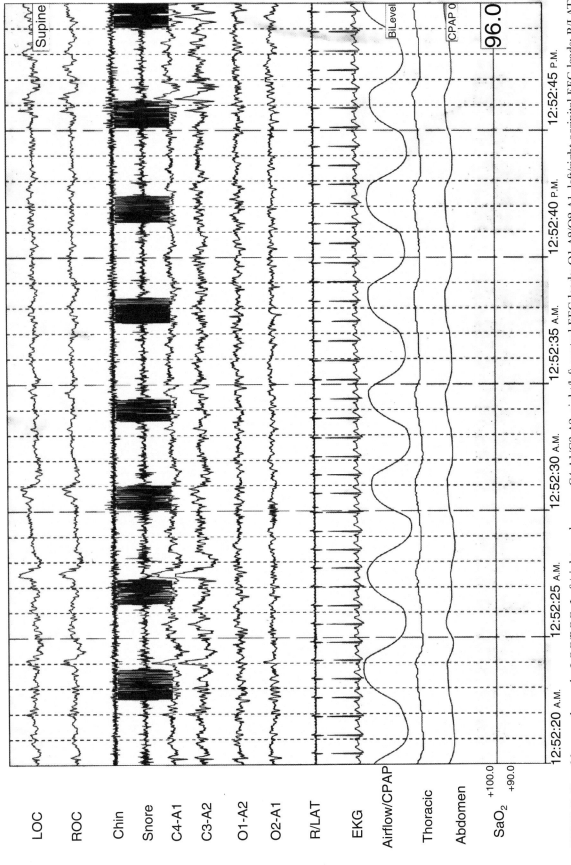

FIGURE 24-12 ■ 30-second epoch. LOC/ROC, Left/right oculogram; C4-A1/C3-A2, right/left central EEG leads; O1-A2/O2-A1, left/right occipital EEG leads; R/LAT, right/left leg EMG; "Airflow/CPAP" is only an airflow.

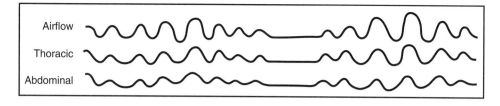

FIGURE 24-13 ■ Diagramatic representation of breathing pattern for the patient in Question 8.

B. Start gabapentin, 300 mg, a half hour before bedtime, as this is a Class A drug that is safe in pregnancy.

C. Start her on a stretching and massage program of her legs before bedtime each night.

D. Resume her prenatal vitamins and start ropinirole, 0.25 mg, each evening after delivery.

23. A 37-year-old man came in for help with his EDS since starting a new job about 4 months ago. He had been on a military mission in a combat zone when a surprise attack left him totally blind about 3 years ago. He was a determined man who underwent extensive blind rehabilitation, finished college, and started on a hopeful new career. He feels that the sleepiness is interfering with his ability to perform his work at peak efficiency. This is the first time he had to follow a regular work schedule since the accident, with an 8:00 A.M. to 5 P.M. job. He said that he tries to go to sleep on time each evening but cannot seem to fall asleep on most nights and thought that he might be suffering from insomnia. He tracked his actual sleep schedule on his voice-activated computer and brought in a printout for you to review, as follows:

Monday	Alarm 6:30 A.M.	Work 8–5	To bed 12 A.M.	To sleep 11:30 P.M.
Tuesday	Alarm 6:30 A.M.	Work 8–5	To bed 11 P.M.	To sleep 12 A.M.
Wednesday	Alarm 6:30 A.M.	Work 8–5	To bed 12 A.M.	To sleep 1:00 A.M.
Thursday	Alarm 6:30 A.M.	Work 8–5	To bed 11 P.M.	To sleep 1:30 A.M.
Friday	Alarm 6:30 A.M.	Work 8–5	To bed 10 P.M.	To sleep 2:30 A.M.
Saturday	Up at 9:30 A.M.	Off work	To bed 12 A.M.	To sleep 3:00 A.M.
Sunday	Up at 10:30 A.M.	Off work	To bed 11 P.M.	To sleep 3:30 A.M.

Fortunately, he's off work next week to work on a project in his home office. You would recommend effective therapy for his situation as:

A. Fix his sleep hours as 11 P.M. to 6:30 A.M., 7 days a week.

B. Obtain at least 2 weeks of actigraphy and sleep log data before prescribing treatment.

C. Start light therapy at 6:30 A.M. each morning for at least 30 minutes.

D. Start melatonin, 0.5 mg, at 9 P.M. when his free-running rhythm approaches his preferred bedtime of 11 P.M.

24. A 28-year-old businessman came in complaining of fatigue and headaches on awakening. He said that these symptoms have been present for only about 6 months, although he remembers similar problems as a child. His wife said that she awakened from a grinding noise but has never heard him snore or have irregular breathing. Social history is significant for a promotion in his sales job and, as a salaried employee, he has been working in excess of 70 hours per week under high stress to make sales quota and train new sales personnel. On physical exam, his BMI is 24 kg/m^2 with a normal oral exam except for mild teeth wear. The remainder of his physical is normal. Epworth Sleepiness Scale is 7. After the exam, he recalls that he will occasionally awaken with a sore jaw.

According to the 2005 edition of the *International Classification of Sleep Disorders* (ICSD), you inform this couple that:

A. You cannot make a final diagnosis based on the presentation without a standard PSG.

B. Audio recording with a masseter muscle EMG must be completed for a final diagnosis.

C. The presentation in this case is sufficient for a diagnosis.

D. A dental consultation is needed to finalize confirmation of the diagnosis.

E. A neurological consultation and head computed tomography (CT) will be necessary.

25. A 27-year-old woman came to see you because of great concern after the loss of her uncle while she was in another country working on postgraduate research in neuroanatomy. She explained that her uncle was only 52 years old at his death. She was having a great deal of difficulty understanding how he could have been healthy the last time she saw him about 18 months ago and died so suddenly. She learned from her aunt that his symptoms began with the initial onset of insomnia with complaints of trouble initiating and maintaining sleep. Preceding his death was a progressive and relentless course of insomnia, hyperhydrosis, tremors, tachycardia, and dyspnea. He developed

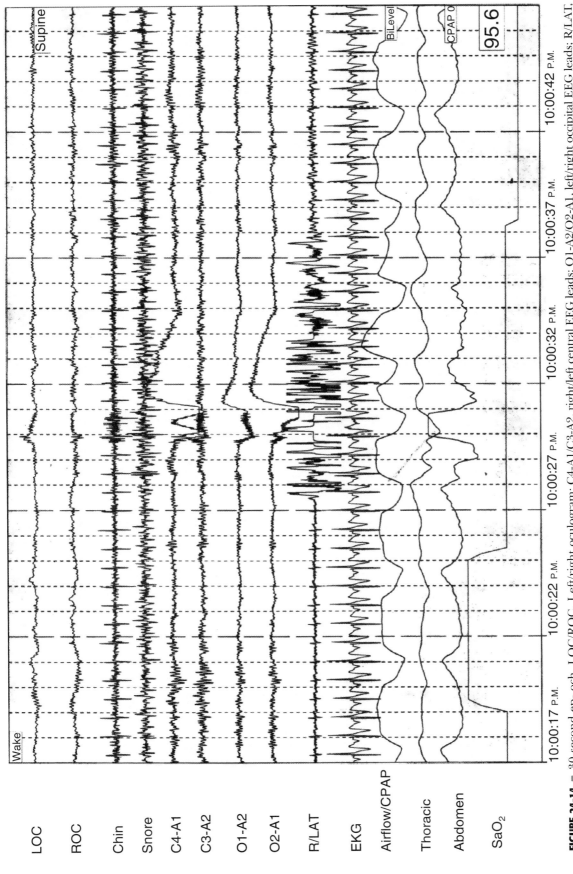

FIGURE 24-14 ■ 30-second ep- och. LOC/ROC, Left/right oculogram; C4-A1/C3-A2, right/left central EEG leads; O1-A2/O2-A1, left/right occipital EEG leads; R/LAT, right/left leg EMG; "Airflow/CPAP" is only an airflow channel with no CPAP on this patient.

daytime somnolence with occasional jerks during brief dreamlike episodes. He eventually developed progressive motor impairment, became bedridden, lapsed into a coma, and died, all within 12 months from the start of insomnia. Because of the woman's science background, she doesn't mind if you explain to her in technical terms what is known about the pathophysiology of this disease. You tell her that there is:

A. A severe loss of neurons in the anterior and dorsomedial thalamic nuclei and inferior olivary nuclei

B. An increase in Purkinje and granule cells in the cerebellum

C. A total loss of neurons in the median raphe nuclei

D. A severe loss of neurons in the anterior cerebral cortex and extending into the hypothalamus

Answers

1. Patient A: Figure 24-4
2. Patient B: Figure 24-1
3. Patient C: Figure 24-3
4. Patient D: Figure 24-2

Discussion for Questions 1–4

Patient A's PSG (Figure 24-4) demonstrates the typical eye movements associated with reading signal. Noted in the EOG channels are the repetitive rhythmic pattern consistent with reading at the rate of 30 lines per minute.

Patient B had left eye enucleation, which registers as loss of the left EOG signal (Figure 24-1). The recording takes place during REM sleep during one of his characteristic dream-enactment episodes. The EMG tone of the anterior tibias muscle is also abnormally augmented, consistent with his underlying diagnosis of REM sleep behavior disorder.

Patient C's tracing reveals the "Prozac eyes" noted in the EOG channels (Figure 24-3). Noted are prominent eye movements during stage 2 NREM sleep. Prozac eyes have been described in patients taking selective serotonin reuptake inhibitors such as fluoxetine. The effect of fluoxetine on NREM is postulated to derive from potentiation of serotonergic neurons that inhibit brainstem "omnipause neurons," which in turn inhibit saccadic eye movements, thus resulting in disinhibited release of saccades.

Patient D's tracing (Figure 24-2) is similar to that of patient B in that there is only a single REM during REM sleep (absence of the right EOG signal), consistent with her underlying right oculomotor cranial nerve dysfunction.

5. A. Nocturnal PSG

The patient presented in case 5 has many factors associated with OSA including loud snoring, apneic spells, obesity, and daytime sleepiness. In fact, in a study by Pillar et al looking into the specificity and sensitivity of several risk factors, signs, and symptoms in predicting OSA, self-reporting on apnea, increased neck circumference, older age, and a tendency to fall asleep unintentionally were all significant positive predictors of OSA, explaining 41.8% of the variability (J Sleep Res 3:241, 1994). The other choices are generally not appropriate, as in the initial evaluation of this patient. An MRI scan of the brain may help in the assessment of central sleep apnea in the context of an abnormal neurological examination (i.e., brainstem pathology). Evaluation of baseline pulmonary status with arterial blood gases, chest x-ray study, and pulmonary function testing is vital in the context of underlying cardiopulmonary disorders but does not have

a role in the initial confirmation of sleep apnea. Sleep apnea is not a limiting condition, and the condition is not self-limiting: Sleep-disordered breathing is associated with a wide spectrum of cardiovascular disorders, most notably hypertension, congestive heart failure, and coronary heart disease. Sleep apnea has also been shown to be a risk factor for stroke. A formal psychiatric evaluation is not needed at this time.

6. A. Periodic leg movement disorder (PLMD) of sleep and restless legs syndrome (RLS)

Both PLMD and RLS consist of nocturnal involuntary limb movements causing sleep disruption. Unlike PLMD, which is diagnosed by PSG, the diagnosis of RLS is made by meeting established clinical criteria. In addition, PLMD can occur in RLS and with other sleep disorders, as well as in normal patients, and is therefore a nonspecific finding. *RLS is characterized by a tetrad of* (1) disagreeable leg sensations that usually occur before sleep onset associated with an (2) irresistible urge to move the limbs, (3) partial or complete relief of the discomfort with leg movements, and the (4) return of the symptoms on cessation of leg movements, all symptoms depicted in this case. PLMD is a PSG finding characterized by periodic episodes of repetitive and stereotyped limb movements that occur during sleep. As in this patient, the movements, usually occur in the legs and consist of extension of the big toe in combination with partial flexion of the ankle, knee, and sometimes hip. The movements are often associated with a partial arousal or awakening; however, the patient is usually unaware of the limb movements or the frequent sleep disruption. Between the episodes, the legs are still. Patients experience symptoms of frequent nocturnal awakenings and unrefreshing sleep. Patients who are unaware of the sleep interruptions may have symptoms of excessive sleepiness. It is probable that the nature of the patient's complaint is affected by the frequency of the movement, as well as the associated awakenings. PLMD appears to increase in prevalence with advancing age. Individuals with RLS usually have PLMD detected during polysomnographic monitoring.

Myoclonic epilepsy may appear as abrupt stereotyped focal limb movements resembling PLM but may be associated with an epileptiform EEG discharge that generally accompanies the movement. Nocturnal leg cramps are painful muscular tightness usually involving the calf, but occasionally the foot, that occur during sleep. The symptom may last for a few seconds and remit spontaneously. The cramp often results in arousal or awakening from sleep. Patients with nocturnal leg cramps will often experience one to two episodes nightly, several times a week. Leg cramps can occur in some patients primarily during the daytime, and sleep disturbance is usually not a feature in these patients. Akathisias are described as a "whole body sensation" rather than centered only in limbs. Unlike RLS, akathisias do not improve with movement. Finally, *hyperreflexia* is defined as overactive or overresponsive reflexes. Examples of this can include twitching or spastic tendencies, which are indicative of upper motor neuron disease such as in amyotrophic lateral sclerosis, as well as the lessening or loss of control ordinarily exerted by higher brain centers of lower neural pathways.

7. E. Advanced sleep-phase syndrome (ASPS)

ASPS is defined by a abnormal advancement of the major sleep period, characterized by habitual and involuntary sleep onset and wakeup times that are several hours earlier relative to conventional and desired time. Patients with ASPS usually report sleep onset of 6 to 9 P.M. and wake time of 2 to 5 A.M., similar to the sleep pattern shown in the sleep log of the patient presented. Patients with ASPS may present with complaints of early morning awakenings, sleep maintenance insomnia, and sleepiness in the late afternoon or early evening. Non–24-hour sleep-wake syndrome is characterized by a steady drift of the major sleep period by 1–2 hours each day, which is not a pattern seen here. Irregular sleep-wake syndrome is characterized by the absence of a clear circadian rhythm of sleep-wake. Patients may present with a complaint of insomnia and excessive sleepiness, depending on the timing of the sleep-wake episode. Although the total amount of sleep per day may be normal, there are typically several sleep episodes (minimum of three). These sleep episodes vary in length, and duration and napping may be prevalent. Finally, DSPS is characterized by bedtimes and wake times that are 3–6 hours later than the desired or conventional sleep/wake times. Patients typically report difficulty falling asleep before 2 to 6 A.M. and waking up earlier than 10 A.M. to 1 P.M.

8. B. Bright light therapy in the early evening

Bright light and melatonin administration are useful agents to improve adaptation of circadian rhythms in shift workers by matching the circadian rhythm of sleep propensity with desired sleep time. Management of patients with ASPS includes chronotherapy, timed bright light exposure in the evening, and pharmacotherapy with hypnotics to maintain sleep during the early morning. Chronotherapy was one of the initial treatment approaches proposed for ASPS. Attempts to delay sleep times were unsuccessful, however, and only a 3-hour advance in sleep time every 2 days

resulted in a shift to the desired sleep schedule. The most commonly used treatment for ASPS is bright light therapy for 2 hours in the evening, typically between 7 and 9 P.M. Although bright light exposure improved sleep efficiency and delayed the phase of circadian rhythms, patients had difficulty complying with the treatment regimen. There are few data relating to the usefulness of melatonin administration to delay circadian rhythms and successfully treat ASPS. To advance circadian rhythms, theoretically, melatonin should be taken in the early morning; however, in addition to its phase resetting effects, melatonin also has sedative effects. Therefore early morning administration of melatonin may impair daytime function. Short, strategically planned scheduled naps can help improve fatigue. When naps are longer than 15–20 minutes, however, they run the risk of worsening ASPS.

9. A. Clonazepam

The PSG fragments depict RBD. Figure 24-7 demonstrates an example from this patient's PSG showing the abnormal augmentation of limb EMG tone. The nocturnal PSG and particularly video recordings may be especially important if the actual spells are demonstrated during the study. Environmental safety is prudent in every patient with likely RBD. Pharmacotherapy for RBD may be in the form of clonazepam (0.25–1 mg by mouth at bedtime), which is effective in 90% of cases with little evidence of tolerance or abuse. Treatment with this drug has little or no effect on the characteristic elevated limb-EMG tone during the night, but it acts to prevent the arousals associated with the REM-sleep disassociation. Clonazepam's safety for use during pregnancy has not been established. Caution should be exercised when using it in patients with chronic respiratory diseases (chronic obstructive pulmonary disease) or impaired renal function, and it is contraindicated in patients with documented hypersensitivity, severe liver disease, or acute narrow-angle glaucoma. Abrupt discontinuation of clonazepam can precipitate withdrawal symptoms. None of the other agents listed as choices (phenytoin, prednisone, oxygen, or hydrochlorothiazide) have been evaluated or found to be helpful for the treatment of RBD.

Besides clonazepam, other agents that may be helpful include imipramine (25 mg by mouth at bedtime) or carbamazepine (100 mg by mouth at bedtime), as well as pramipexole or levodopa, in cases where RBD is associated with Parkinson's disease. Recent studies have also demonstrated improvement with the use of melatonin, which is believed to exert its therapeutic effect by restoring REM-sleep atonia. One study reported that melatonin was effective in 87% of patients taking 3–9 mg at bedtime (Takeuchi et al, Psych Clin Neurosci 55:267, 2001), whereas a later study reported resolution in those taking 6–12 mg of melatonin at bedtime (Boeve B, Sleep 24:A35, 2001).

10. D. Medial pons

The normally generalized muscle atonia during REM sleep results from pontine-mediated perilocus coeruleus inhibition of motor activity. This pontine activity exerts an excitatory influence on medullary centers (magnocellularis neurons) via the lateral tegmentoreticular tract. These neuronal groups, in turn, hyperpolarize the spinal motor neuron postsynaptic membranes via the ventrolateral reticulospinal tract. In RBD, the brainstem mechanisms generating the muscle atonia normally seen in REM sleep may be disrupted. The pathophysiology of RBD in humans is based on the cat model. In the cat model, bilateral pontine lesions result in a persistent absence of REM atonia associated with prominent motor activity during REM sleep, similar to that observed in RBD in humans. The pathophysiology of the idiopathic form of RBD in humans is still not very well understood but may be related to reduction of striatal presynaptic dopamine transporters. The other structures (medial thalamus, posterior hypothalamus, cerebellum, and basal forebrain) have not been implicated in RBD.

11. C. Delayed sleep phase syndrome (DSPS)

DSPS is characterized by bedtimes and wake times that are 3–6 hours later than the desired or conventional sleep/wake times. As in this case, patients with DSPS typically report difficulty falling asleep before 2 to 6 A.M. and waking up earlier than 10 A.M. to 1 P.M.

12. D. Night terror

Night terror or sleep terror (Table 24-1) is the most dramatic disorder of arousal. It is characterized by a sudden arousal from slow wave sleep (SWS) with a piercing scream or cry and extreme panic, accompanied by severe autonomic discharge (i.e., tachycardia, tachypnea, diaphoresis, mydriasis, and increased muscle tone) and behavioral manifestations of intense fear. The typical spells demonstrate that the patient sits in bed, is unresponsive to external stimuli, and, if awakened, is disoriented and confused. The episodes are sometimes followed by prominent motor activity such as hitting the wall or running around or out of the bedroom, or even out of the house, resulting in bodily injury or property damage. Night terrors are characterized by amnesia for the episode, which may be

TABLE 24-1 ■ Characteristics Differentiating Sleep Terrors from REM Nightmares

Characteristics	Sleep Terror	REM Nightmare
Stages of sleep	Slow wave sleep	REM sleep
Timing during the night	First third	Last third
Recall	Rare	++++
Autonomic discharge	++++	Rare
Agitation and violence	++++	Rare
Ambulation	++	Very rare
Vocalization	+++	Rare

incomplete, accompanied by incoherent vocalizations. Sometimes attempts to escape from bed or to fight can result in harm to the patient or parents responding to the child. Mental evaluations of adults indicate that psychopathology may be associated with sleep terrors. Night terror episodes may become violent and may result in considerable injury to the patient and bedpartners, at times with forensic implications. Psychopathology is rare in affected children but may play a role in adult sufferers. Night terrors typically resolve spontaneously during adolescence. Precipitating factors include fever, sleep deprivation, or the use of central nervous system–depressant medications. The PSG shows episodes emanating out of SWS, usually in the first third of the major sleep episode; however, episodes can occur in SWS at any time. The recordings demonstrate episodes of tachycardia and other signs of increased sympathetic activation. Differentiating between sleep terrors and sleep-related epilepsy (temporal-lobe epilepsy) is sometimes difficult, and the use of an EEG with nasopharyngeal leads may be helpful. REM nightmares (choice A) also occur during the last third of the night but, unlike night terrors, are confined to REM sleep. Associated with a vivid recollection and normal cognition, nightmares usually lack the sympathetic activation and confusion that is frequent with sleep terrors. Confusional arousals are awakenings from SWS without terror or ambulation. RBD occurs in older individuals out of REM sleep and is associated with dream enactment and recollection. Finally, nocturnal agitation disorder of REM sleep is not a diagnosis.

13. A.

Option A points to the location of the wake-promoting hypocretin/orexin system activity within the anterior hypothalamus. This region, when destroyed (by a MS demyelination), can produce symptoms that can be indistinguishable from that of narcolepsy. The other regions (B, basal forebrain; C, corpus callosum; D, ventral pons) have not been implicated in narcolepsy.

Sleep disturbances in MS are common but are poorly recognized. Common sleep disorders in patients with MS include sleep-onset and sleep-maintenance insomnia, RLS, narcolepsy, and RBD. Although the incidence of OSA in patients with MS is not higher than in the general population, central nervous system– and brainstem-related nocturnal respiratory abnormalities such as central sleep apnea, paroxysmal hyperventilation, hypoventilation, respiratory muscle weakness, and respiratory arrest have all been described in MS and should be considered in this patient population if clinical suspicions arise. Certain neurovegetative symptoms are differentially associated with depression, fatigue, and physical disability in MS, and careful assessment for these symptoms when encountering depression in MS patients may be warranted. Sleep disruption in this cohort may result in hypersomnolence, increased fatigue, and a lowered pain threshold. An increased clinical awareness of sleep-related problems is therefore warranted in this patient population because they are extremely common and have the potential to negatively affect overall health and quality of life.

Patients with MS have been shown to have narcoleptic symptoms and, in fact, a genetic link between narcolepsy and MS has also been predicted for many years. Narcolepsy, as well as MS, is strongly linked to similar HLA expression, suggesting that similar autoimmune factors may play a role in the development of both disease states and may play a role in the symptoms of fatigue and hypersomnolence. MS plaques in the bilateral hypothalamus in association with low CSF hypocretin-1 level produced hypersomnia. These findings suggest that the hypothalamic hypocretin (orexin) system may be crucial to maintaining the arousal level and that lesions in the system can cause hypersomnia in MS. Methylprednisolone pulse treatment improved the hypothalamic lesion, normalized the hypocretin-1 level in the CSF, and ultimately resolved the hypersomnia. Modafinil, a novel wake-promoting agent, has been shown to significantly improve hypersomnia associated with narcolepsy and effectively manage fatigue associated with MS. Preclinical trials have demonstrated that modafinil can selectively activate lateral hypothalamic neurons that produce wake-promoting hypocretin-1, thus suggesting that the symptoms of hypersomnolence and fatigue seen in patients with both narcolepsy and MS may have a common or overlapping immunopathophysiologic mechanism.

14. C. Discontinue zolpidem and schedule a return visit in 2 weeks.

This patient fits the diagnostic criteria of sleep-related eating disorders (SRED). The current guidelines for diagnosis include eating or drinking during the sleep period associated with at least one other sign of unusual foods or items, nonrestorative sleep, injury, morning anorexia, or health complications from sleep-related eating. SRED involves involuntary eating during partial arousals and is often associated with somnambulism with little or no recall of the event the next day. Patients will often, but not always, have a past history of sleepwalking in childhood. Triggers can include stress; schedule changes; insufficient sleep; discontinuation of alcohol, street drugs, or tobacco products; certain medical conditions such as a brain injury; and certain medications. Sleep disruption from any other cause such as periodic limb movements during sleep or OSA can also exacerbate somnambulism in the susceptible patient. Medications that have been described to trigger sleepwalking episodes include zolpidem, bupropion, lithium, paroxetine, and others (see Table 24-2).

The 30-second epoch pictured in Figure 24-10 shows a partial arousal during stage 2 sleep within 1 hour of sleep onset. Partial arousals in the early portion of sleep are associated with these episodes. This epoch is consistent with a cyclic alternating pattern of K-complexes followed by alpha waves. Apneas or desaturations were not noted. Somnambulism was not noted during this study. Parasomnias are often not actually caught on a single-night PSG. Also noted here are ECG interference in the chin, snore, and R/LAT channels, as well as alternating current (AC) interference in the R/LAT channel.

Although stress management therapy can help with the original stress-related consequences of insomnia, which was her initial sleep disorder, this may not immediately resolve the SRED. Topiramate, starting

---

TABLE 24-2 ■ Sleep-Related Eating Disorders (SREDs) and Somnambulism Triggers

Precipitating Factors of SRED	Medications That Can Trigger Somnambulism
Acute and chronic stress	Anticholinergic agents
Daytime dieting	Bupropion
Sleep breathing disorders	Lithium carbonate
RLS or PLMS	Olanzapine
OSA	Paroxetine
Irregular sleep-wake scheduling	Phenothiazines
Smoking cessation	Triazolam
Alcohol cessation	Zolpidem
Substance abuse cessation	
Autoimmune hepatitis	
Encephalitis	
Bulimia or anorexia nervosa	
Narcolepsy onset	

RLS, Restless legs syndrome; PLMS, periodic limb movements during sleep; OSA, obstructive sleep apnea.

at 25 mg before bed, has been used successfully as therapy for SRED; however, if the SRED is directly triggered by zolpidem, then the first plan of action is to discontinue the offending medication.

15. C. Warm environment that is above 75° F

The *ICSD* published in 2005 describes sleep starts, also known as *hypnic* or *hypnagogic jerks,* as brief jerks at sleep onset associated with a brief dream, "sensory flash," or sensation of falling not resulting from another sleep disorder. Sleep starts can begin or can be exacerbated by irregular sleep schedules, sleep deprivation or fatigue, excessive caffeine or stimulant intake, alcohol intake, intense exercise, excessive physical work, and stress. Temperature extremes have not been mentioned in the literature to trigger sleep starts.

Sleep starts are either generalized or localized sudden muscle contractions that may also be associated with vivid imagery. Some sleep starts have been described as hypnagogic imagery not necessarily associated with myoclonic jerks that include bright flashes of light, a brief visual hallucination, or a snapping noise. These sudden jerks occur just at the transition to sleep onset. The EEG during PSG has shown a drowsy state or stage 1 sleep at the time of the body jerk that triggers an arousal or awakening. Often there is a sensation of falling associated with the jerk. This is a benign disorder that is often part of the normal transition to sleep onset with unclear mechanisms and should not be confused with a seizure disorder.

Of course, in this particular patient, sleep deprivation is the major trigger, as his symptoms started only after he began a night job to help with school expenses. It will be important for him to try to increase his sleep hours because driving will be hazardous in a hypersomnolent state.

16. D. All of the above

This patient's history and evaluation are consistent with obesity-hypoventilation syndrome (OHS), a subcategory of hypoventilation syndrome. OHS, like other hypoventilation syndromes, is primarily defined by hypercapnia ($pCO_2 > 45$ mm Hg) with subsequent hypoxemia more pronounced during sleep that more profoundly drops during stage REM. Hypoxemia can result in eventual erythrocytosis, pulmonary hypertension, and cor pulmonale. Untreated patients can progress toward right heart failure as well as chronic respiratory failure. Most of these patients also have significant OSA syndrome. It is much less common to have OHS without significant apnea, but it has been reported. The *ICSD* defines this disorder under the heading of "sleep-related hypoventilation/hypoxemia due to neuromuscular and chest wall disorders." The

diagnostic criterion includes desaturations on a PSG of <90% to a low of at least 85% for >5 minutes, >30% of sleep <90%, or hypercapnia on a sleeping arterial blood gas not explained by another disorder.

This patient had evidence of OHS by many signs. The chief evidence is hypercapnia on arterial blood gases. He also has evidence of cor pulmonale with ankle edema and a prominent S2 that generally indicates an increased force of pulmonary valve closure under an increased pressure gradient. The PSG in Figure 24-11 shows shallow breathing in a prolonged hypopnea, paradoxical breathing, and significant desaturation. At first glance, this appears to be a complete apnea; however, snoring is noted, and snoring cannot occur in a closed airway. This was representative of most of his PSG, as well as recurrent arousals from sleep. This epoch also shows a good example of sweat artifact, with a wandering baseline seen in the ocular and EEG channels.

The basic pathology of morbid obesity developing into hypoventilation syndrome appears to be primarily a restrictive ventilatory defect resulting from the mechanics of a large load compressing the ability of the chest to maintain adequate minute ventilation during sleep. The diaphragm is rendered more ineffective at larger abdominal girths, thus explaining why these patients develop much more profound hypoxemia in stage REM sleep where ventilation depends on a functional diaphragm; however, not all morbidly obese patients develop hypoventilation syndrome. There is a mechanism not yet well understood that leads to a reduction in the central chemoresponsiveness of respiratory drive.

The mainstay of therapy is nocturnal positive pressure ventilation and weight reduction. Medication has been investigated and tried in OHS but without significant impact on the disease process. Medroxyprogesterone has been used as a respiratory stimulant that may decrease the hypercapnia that results from hypoventilation and improve hypoxemia. The results are inconsistent with a greater effect on awake ventilation than on abnormal breathing events during sleep. Theophylline may have an effect by central stimulation on the hypoxic drive and may improve cardiac function and subsequent oxygen delivery; however, these are weak and inconsistent changes. Nocturnal positive pressure ventilation remains the treatment of choice.

Treatment is aimed at improving the hypercapnia and hypoxemic consequences of OHS. This can be most effectively accomplished by nocturnal ventilation initially by noninvasive positive pressure ventilation. The simplest way of starting this therapy is bilevel positive airway pressure (BiPAP) delivered by a nasal mask. A streamlined view of this intervention is thought of as the expiratory positive airway pressure boosting the functional residual capacity, thus minimizing atelectatic areas of the lung and improving oxygen exchange to correct hypoxemia. The inspiratory positive airway pressure portion of the BiPAP effectively improves tidal volume, thereby halting or decreasing the progression of hypercapnia.

17. A. Dim-light melatonin onset

This is not a case of narcolepsy without cataplexy but is actually circadian rhythm disorder, delayed sleep phase type. Although there are two sleep-onset REM periods on the MSLT, there are specific aspects of this case that do not fit. The *ICSD* criteria for diagnosis of narcolepsy without cataplexy also require that the PSG on the preceding night of sleep be a minimum of 6 hours of actual sleep. The actual total sleep time was not given; however, at a sleep efficiency of only 55%, 6 hours would not have been possible unless the recording time were 10.9 hours, which is unlikely in a clinical sleep center. Furthermore, this patient's MSLT mean sleep latency is calculated as 12.1 minutes, which is over the current criteria of less than or equal to 8 minutes. The previous health physician's conclusion that the patient had narcolepsy strictly based on seeing 2 sleep-onset REM periods (SOREMPs) on his MSLT is erroneous. Because the information does not quite fit a narcolepsy diagnosis, the possible answers of starting modafinil or of further evaluation for HLA DQB1*0602 are not correct.

Clues to this patient actually having DSPD are that his "hypersomnolence" only started when he began a job that now requires he arrive by 7:30 A.M. Prior to this job, it appears that he controlled his own schedule to be up and awake in the afternoons and evenings. When off work the day of the clinical evaluation and given the opportunity to free-run his own circadian rhythm, he stayed up until 4 A.M. and slept until noon, which is 8 hours of sleep with no residual excessive sleepiness. His Epworth Sleepiness Scale was much different when he had the opportunity to run his own circadian rhythm rather than the higher score taken by his employee health office. The Epworth Sleepiness Scale is a useful, although is a *subjective* score and can range from 0–24, with normal control subjects described as having a range from 2–10, with a mean of 5.9 (Johns, Sleep 14:540, 1991).

Sleep study clues included an extraordinarily long sleep latency on his PSG. It is also possible for a phase-delay patient to record stage REM on the morning naps of an MSLT, which is simultaneous with the second half of sleep by the free-running circadian rhythm. In view of these pieces of evidence, confirmation is usually obtained by history that usually includes sleep logs for work days and days off. Sleep logs or actigraphy are recommended to be at least 7 days long. Other means of confirmation that have been described

are actual measurements of the intrinsic circadian rhythm either by recording the core body temperature or measuring the dim light melatonin onset (DLMO). Body temperature *minimum* rather than the peak is the most useful for evaluating phase delay because the temperature minimum correlates with the onset of sleep. DLMO can be measured by serum or saliva, which correlates with a peak after 10 P.M. in patients with phase delay.

18. C. Recurrent alpha intrusions

This patient's clinical presentation is consistent with the American College of Rheumatology criteria of fibromyalgia syndrome. This patient has two of the criteria of (1) musculoskeletal pain for at least 3 months and (2) tender points of at least 11 of 18 sites on physical exam. Originally described as *alpha-delta sleep*, recurrent alpha intrusions are commonly seen in various stages of NREM sleep and not just delta sleep alone. Alpha intrusions are often present in any fragmented sleep. Examples include any cause of chronic pain, nocturnal coughing, psychophysiologic insomnia, periodic limb movements during sleep, snoring, sleep apnea, and virtually any disorder that can fragment sleep.

Although the preceding criterion is enough for diagnosis of fibromyalgia syndrome, there are also sleep architecture changes that may be useful. Many of these patients have a prolonged sleep latency and reductions in sleep efficiency, slow wave (delta) sleep, and stage REM concentration. The fragmented sleep may be seen as alpha intrusions with an increased alpha density throughout NREM sleep, alpha-delta sleep as in phasic alpha sleep, and cyclical patterns of K-complexes followed by alpha waves.

19. D. Chronic partial sleep deprivation

The history for this patient is most consistent with *recurrent isolated sleep paralysis*. Sleep paralysis occurs at sleep onset (hypnagogic) or at sleep offset (hypnapompic) with or without associated dreamlike images. This is a disorder not explained by another sleep disorder such as narcolepsy. This is most commonly described in students under the age of 30. Precipitating factors include sleep deprivation, irregular sleep-wake schedules, stress, leg cramps that occur with sleep, bipolar disorder, depression, alcohol use, and anxiolytic medication use.

Family history of bipolar disorder is not a precipitating factor unless the patient has this disorder, which is not part of her history. CSF that is hypocretin deficient or inheritance of HLA subtype DR2 as possible answers are incorrect for this particular case, which does not historically fit a narcoleptic patient. In addition, these symptoms did not even start until she carried a heavy college schedule, which would be consistent with a combination of an irregular sleep-wake schedule and sleep deprivation as triggering factors for these three isolated episodes of sleep paralysis.

20. C. Systemic hypertension

No apneas or hypopneas were present in the representative epoch shown, and the background in the question stated that this was an example of this patient's sleep time. This epoch (Figure 24-12) shows snoring that appears to be fairly significant in a patient with no hypersomnolence. The *ICSD* defines *snoring* as being in an asymptomatic patient in which the snoring is reported by an observer. The potential medical complications of the simple snorer have been controversial in the past, and it has been stated that there are increased cardiovascular risk factors with OSA but not necessarily in the snoring patient without sleep apnea; however, studies have shown an increased incidence of systemic hypertension that develops in snoring patients over control subjects. Other potential cardiovascular risk factors in patients with OSA and possibly simple snorers include ischemic heart disease, congestive heart failure, and ischemic stroke but not hemorrhagic stroke.

21. B. Hyperventilation primarily in NREM sleep causing hypocapnic alkalosis

With the high elevations of mountain climbing, the drop in FiO_2 triggers hyperventilation experienced by the climber whether awake or asleep. Hypocapnia and respiratory alkalosis subsequently develop. Periodic breathing during sleep is more prevalent in the first few days of altitude sleeping, with most climbers developing more regular breathing later in the experience as acclimatization occurs. Sleep is often initially fragmented, with a reduction in sleep efficiency resulting from increased awakenings as a consequence of the periodic breathing. There is an increase in stage 1 and a reduction of stages 2, 3, and 4 sleep, whereas the total sleep time is relatively preserved. During NREM sleep, periodic breathing can be pronounced in the initial sleep periods at high altitude with a hyperpnea phase alternating with a hypopnea phase with central apneas. In REM sleep, periodic breathing tends to revert to regular breathing except at altitudes greater than 4200 meters. Although there is an increased hypoxic ventilatory response in NREM sleep, there is a decreased, not increased, hypoxic responsiveness in stage REM. Response C is incorrect because there is increased carotid body sensitivity secondary to hypoxia, not hypercapnia, as a contributing factor.

During the hyperpnea phase when tidal volume increases, pCO_2 decreases, thus losing the CO_2 ability to trigger ventilation and leading to a central apnea. As the pCO_2 starts to climb during the apnea, the CO_2 set point is reached and the hyperpnea phase resumes. This cycle then repeats. Periodic breathing in NREM sleep has been abated with the introduction of exogenous carbon dioxide in experimental studies. The carbonic anhydrase inhibitor, acetazolamide, is effective as prophylactic therapy for altitude-induced sleep-disordered breathing by causing metabolic acidosis and improved chemoresponsiveness for ventilation.

22. A. Resume her prenatal vitamins and reassure her that this disorder will likely resolve after delivery.

Figure 24-14 shows an epoch during the wake period before this patient was able to achieve sleep that shows leg movements on the combined left and right leg EMG seen in channel 9. A PSG is neither diagnostic nor necessary for a diagnosis of RLS. This patient did not indicate this in her history until she was satisfied that she did not have OSA. She had stopped her prenatal vitamins 6 weeks before this evaluation and had prolonged sleep latency resulting from restless legs, a reduction in sleep efficiency, and periodic limb movements during sleep that caused arousals not linked to snoring. Although it is not clear from the written question whether she had snoring arousals as well, clearly the *next* advice to this patient and the only viable option from the possible answers is to restart her prenatal vitamins and reassure her that the leg movements at night will likely resolve after delivery. She may need initial high-dose iron replacement therapy depending on the ferritin level. Instructing her to stretch and massage her legs before bed each night may help as well and is a correct choice as part of management but is not the *next* step in her management. Gabapentin is a pregnancy category C medication that is not safe in pregnancy.

RLS is often linked to iron deficiency. Both iron and folate are important during pregnancy, with a higher incidence of RLS, especially during the third trimester, in those patients who did not take these vitamins. Those who develop RLS during pregnancy usually reverse this disorder on delivery. A dopamine agonist, such as ropinirole, can be considered after delivery, with the exception of the breastfeeding mother, only if the symptoms of restless legs continue to be a problem.

23. D. Start melatonin, 0.5 mg, at 9 P.M. when his free-running rhythm approaches his preferred bedtime of 11 P.M.

This case is consistent with circadian rhythm sleep disorder, free-running (nonentrained) type. This is a circadian rhythm disorder that is more predominantly associated with blind subjects who have lost the ability for photic stimuli to entrain their circadian rhythm to the environmental day. This rarely occurs in sighted individuals. The diagnosis is a minimum of 1 week (preferably more) of a sleep log in combination with complaints of insomnia or excessive sleepiness relative to the inability to synchronize to a standard 24-hour day. These patients often show a gradually delayed bedtime, as this case represents. Entrainment by social cues alone has not been successful. The current recommended therapy is to take melatonin at the time of the measured DLMO or about 2 hours before the preferred bedtime *only after* the free-running rhythm approaches this preferred bedtime. Light therapy has more success in sighted individuals but may be a consideration in the blind subject with intact photic responses. Melatonin is the initial treatment of choice for blind subjects with this disorder.

24. C. The presentation in this case is sufficient for a diagnosis.

Sleep-related bruxism is defined in the 2005 *ICSD* by a patient either reporting or aware of tooth-grinding sounds or clenching in sleep in conjunction with either abnormal tooth wear or jaw discomfort or masseter muscle hypertrophy upon clenching that is not better explained by other disorders. Although an adequate test for sleep-related bruxism should ideally be done with an audio recording in conjunction with one or more masseter leads, it is not necessary if the presentation fits these recommendations for diagnostic criteria. Eventually a dental consultation would be helpful for construction of a mouth guard to protect from further damage. All of his fatigue, however, cannot be explained by simply sleep bruxism, as he is now working excessive hours. Both the hours and stress are likely primary factors in exacerbating sleep-related bruxism. Sleep-related bruxism is not thought to be a direct result of anxiety but rather the coping style in a task-oriented individual.

Sleep-related bruxism is most commonly seen in the lighter stages of sleep (stages 1 and 2) but has been reported in other stages as well. Bruxism during sleep has also been described during a cyclic alternating period on the EEG that is sometimes associated with a rise in heart rate. Both children and adults can experience this disorder, with a drop in prevalence with age. Bruxism has been reported to have a familial tendency. Symptoms have a range from none to temporomandibular joint discomfort, headaches, and less commonly daytime somnolence. A dental evaluation is important for the fitting of a dental guard to avoid unnecessary tooth wear. Some success with pharmacological therapy in the short term may be considered in severe cases, such as benzodiazepines, muscle relaxants, or dopaminergic agents; however, greater evidence-based studies are needed.

25. A. A severe loss of neurons in the anterior and dorsomedial thalamic nuclei and inferior olivary nuclei

Fatal familial insomnia (FFI) is a prion disease that is autosomal dominant. This disorder entails a defective chromosome 20 of the prion protein gene PRNP with a missense GAC to AAC mutation at codon 178. Phenotype expression is linked to the 129 codon for methionine. This disease is fatal, and patients can have a short course of less than 12 months to death, as in this case (methionine homozygous at the 129 codon), or a longer course of death up to 72 months (methionine-valine heterozygous at codon 129). The resultant pathology is a severe loss of neurons in the anterior and dorsomedial thalamic nuclei and inferior olivary nuclei with astrogliosis. There are less dramatic and variable changes with astrogliosis in the hypothalamus and periacqueductal gray matter in the midbrain and basal ganglia. There is also some loss (not increase) of Purkinje and granule cells in the cerebellum. The neurons of the median raphe nuclei appear to be relatively preserved.

Subsequent sleep-wake architecture changes on the EEG are consistent with a gradual reduction and eventual loss of sleep spindles and K-complexes, as well as SWS. Eventually the affected individual alters between wakefulness and oneiric stupor, a state of desynchronous EEG activity marked with REM bursts often marked with myotonic tremor-like limb activity. Late disease states show marked slowing of the EEG with reduced amplitude as a patient progresses to a flat line in death.

REFERENCES

1. Albin RL, Koeppe RA, Chervin RD, et al: Decreased striatal dopaminergic innervation in REM sleep behavior disorder. Neurology 55:1410–1412, 2000.

2. American Academy of Sleep Medicine: *The International Classification of Sleep Disorders: Diagnostic and Coding Manual*, 2nd ed. Westchester, IL, American Academy of Sleep Medicine, 2005.

3. Armitage R, Trivedi M, Rush AJ: Fluoxetine and oculomotor activity during sleep in depressed patients. Neuropsychopharmacology 12:159–165, 1995.

4. Auer RN, Rowlands CG, Perry SF, et al: Multiple sclerosis with medullary plaques and fatal sleep apnea (Ondine's curse). Clin Neuropathol 15(2):101–105, 1996.

5. Baker SK, Zee PC: Circadian disorders of the sleep-wake cycle. In Kryger MH, Roth T, Dement W (eds): *Principles and Practice of Sleep Medicine*. Philadelphia, Saunders, 2000, pp 606–614.

6. Benca RM, Schenck CH: Sleep and eating disorders. In Kryger MH, Roth T, Dement WC (eds): *Principles and Practice of Sleep Medicine*, 4th ed. Philadelphia, Elsevier Saunders, 2005, pp 1337–1344.

7. Boeve B: Melatonin for treatment of REM sleep behavior disorder: response in 8 patients. Sleep 24(suppl): A35, 2001.

8. Dander HW, Geisse H, Quinto C, et al: Sensory sleep starts. J Neurol Neurosurg Psychiatry 64(5):690, 1998.

9. Dawson D, Encel N, Lushington K: Improving adaptation to simulated night shift: timed exposure to bright light versus daytime melatonin administration. Sleep 18(1):11–21, 1995.

10. *Diagnostic and Statistical Manual of Mental Disorders*, 4th ed. Text Rev. ed. Washington, DC, American Psychiatric Association, 2000.

11. Eisehsehr I, Linke R, Tatsch K, et al: Increased muscle activity during rapid eye movement sleep correlates with decrease of striatal presynaptic dopamine transporters. IPT and IBZM SPECT imaging in subclinical and clinically manifest idiopathic REM sleep behavior disorder, Parkinson's disease, and controls. Sleep 26:507–512, 2003.

12. Fantini ML, Gagnon J-F, Filipini D, Montplaisir J: The effects of pramipexole in REM sleep behavior disorder. Neurology 61:1418–1420, 2003.

13. Fleming WE, Pollak CP: Sleep disorders in multiple sclerosis. Semin Neurol 25(1):64–68, 2005.

14. Gilman S, Koeppe RA, Chervin R, et al: REM sleep behavior disorder is related to striatal monoaminergic deficit in MSA. Neurology 61:29–34, 2003.

15. Hamilton GS, Solin P, Naughton MT: Obstructive sleep apnea and cardiovascular disease. Intern Med J 34(7): 420–426, 2004.

16. Harazin J, Berigan TR: Zolpidem tartrate and somnambulism. Mil Med 164(9):669–670, 1999.

17. Howard RS, Wiles CM, Hirsch NP, et al: Respiratory involvement in multiple sclerosis. Brain 115(Pt 2):479–494, 1992.

18. Johns MW: A new method for measuring daytime sleepiness: the Epworth sleepiness scale. Sleep 14(6):540–545, 1991.

19. Kahn E, Fisher C, Edwards A: Night terrors and anxiety dreams. In Ellman SD, Antrobus JS (eds): *The Mind in Sleep. Psychology and Psychophysiology*, 2nd ed. New York, John Wiley & Sons, 1991, pp 437–447.

20. Kato T, Kanbayshi T, Yamomoto K, et al: Hypersomnia and low CSF hypocretin-1 (orexin-A) concentration in a patient with multiple sclerosis showing bilateral hypothalamic lesions. Intern Med 42(8):743–745, 2003.

21. Kawashima T, Yamada S: Paroxetine-induced somnambulism. J Clin Psychiatry 64(4):483, 2003.

22. Khazaal Y, Krenz S, Zullino DF: Bupropion-induced somnambulism. Addict Bio 8(3):359–462, 2003.

23. Kolivakis TT, Margolese HC, Beauclair L, Chouinard G: Olanzapine-induced somnambulism. Am J Psychiatry 158(7):1158, 2001.

24. Krachman S, Criner GJ: Hypoventilation syndromes. Clin Chest Med 19(1):139–155, 1998.

25. Landry P, Montplaisir J: Lithium-induced somnambulism. Can J Psychiatry 43(9):957–958, 1998.

26. Lavigne GJ, Kato T, Kolta A, Sessle BJ: Neurobiological mechanisms involved in sleep bruxism. Crit Rev Oral Biol Med 14(1):30–46, 2003.

27. Lavigne GJ, Manzini C, Kato T: Sleep bruxism. In Kryger MH, Roth T, Dement WC (eds): *Principles and Practice of Sleep Medicine*, 4th ed. Philadelphia, Elsevier Saunders, 2005, pp 946–959.

28. Lesage S, Earley CJ: Restless legs syndrome. Curr Treat Options Neurol 6–3:209–219, 2004.

29. Lesage S, Hening WA: The restless legs syndrome and periodic limb movement disorder: a review of management. Semin Neurol 24–3:249–259, 2004.

30. Mahowald MW, Ettinger MG: Things that go bump in the night: the parasomnias revisited. J Clin Neurophysiol 7:119–143, 1990.

31. Mahowald MW, Rosen GM: Parasomnias in children. Pediatrician 17:21–31, 1990.

32. Mahowald MW, Schenck CH: REM sleep parasomnias. In Kryger MH, Roth T, Dement WC (eds): *Principles and Practice of Sleep Medicine*, 4th ed. Philadelphia, Elsevier Saunders, 2005, pp 897–916.

33. Manconi M, Govoni V, De Vito A, et al: Restless legs syndrome and pregnancy. Neurology 63(6):1065–1069, 2004.

34. Moldofsky H, Musisi S, Phillipson EA: Treatment of a case of advanced sleep phase syndrome by phase advance chronotherapy. Sleep 9(1):61–65, 1986.

35. Montagna P: Fatal familial incomnia: a model disease in sleep physiopathology. Sleep Med Rev 9:339–353, 2005.

36. O'Regan JK: Eye movements and reading. Rev Oculomot Res 4:395–453, 1990.

37. Pillar G, Peled N, Katz N, Lavie P: Predictive value of specific risk factors, symptoms and signs, in diagnosing obstructive sleep apnea and its severity. J Sleep Res 3(4):241–244, 1994.

38. Rammohan KW, Rosenberg JH, Lynn DJ, et al: Efficacy and safety of modafinil (Provigil) for the treatment of fatigue in multiple sclerosis: a two centre phase 2 study. J Neurol Neurosurg Psychiatry 72(2):179–183, 2002.

39. Randolph JJ, Arnett PA, Higginson CI, et al: Neurovegetative symptoms in multiple sclerosis: relationship to

depressed mood, fatigue, and physical disability. Arch Clin Neuropsychol 15(5):387–398, 2000.

40. Reid KJ, Zee PC: Circadian disorders of the sleep-wake cycle. In Kryger MH, Roth T, Dement WC (eds): *Principles and Practice of Sleep Medicine*, 4th ed. Philadelphia, Elsevier Saunders, 2005, pp 691–701.

41. Remulla A, Guilleminault C: Somnambulism (sleep-walking). Expert Opin Pharmacother 5(10):2069–2074, 2004.

42. Roux F, D'Ambrosio C, Mohsenin V: Sleep-related breathing disorders and cardiovascular disease. Am J Med 108(5):396–402, 2000.

43. Schenck CH, Mahowald MW, Kim SW, et al: Prominent eye movements during NREM sleep and REM sleep behavior disorder associated with fluoxetine treatment of depression and obsessive-compulsive disorder. Sleep 15:226–235, 1992.

44. Schenck CH, Mahowald MW: Polysomnographic, neurologic, psychiatric, and clinical outcome report on 70 consecutive cases with REM sleep behavior disorder (RBD): sustained clonazepam efficacy in 89.5% of 57 treated patients. Cleve Clin J Med 57(Suppl):S9–S23, 1990.

45. Schrader H, Gotlibsen OB, Skomedal GN: Multiple sclerosis and narcolepsy/cataplexy in a monozygotic twin. Neurology 30(1):105–108, 1980.

46. Shahar E, Whitney CW, Redline S, et al: Sleep-disordered breathing and cardiovascular disease: cross-sectional results of the Sleep Heart Health Study. Am J Respir Crit Care Med 163(1):19–25, 2001.

47. Shepard J, Harris CD, Hauri PJ: Miscellanous polysomnographic findings and nocturnal penile tumescence. In Shepard J (ed): *Atlas of Sleep Medicine*. Mount Kisco, NY, Futura Publishing, 1991, pp 215–240.

48. Silber MH: Sleep-disordered breathing. In Bolton CF, Chen R, Wijdicks EFM, Zifko UA (eds): *Neurology of Breathing*. Philadelphia, Butterworth Heinemann, 2004, pp 109–135.

49. Tachibana N, Howard RS, Hirsch NP, et al: Sleep problems in multiple sclerosis. Eur Neurol 34(6):320–323, 1994.

50. Takeuchi N, Uchimura N, Hashizume Y, et al: Melatonin therapy for REM sleep behavior disorder. Psychiatry Clin Neurosci 55–3:267–269, 2001.

51. Tan A, Salgado M, Fahn S: Rapid eye movement sleep behavior disorder preceding Parkinson's disease with therapeutic response to levodopa. Move Disord 11:214–216, 1996.

52. Weil JV: Respiratory physiology: sleep at high altitudes. In Kryger MH, Roth T, Dement WC (eds): *Principles and Practice of Sleep Medicine*, 4th ed. Philadelphia, Elsevier Saunders, 2005, pp 245–255.

53. Wolfe F, Smythe HA, Yunus MB, et al: The American College of Rheumatology 1990 criteria for the classification of fibromyalgia. Report of the Multicenter Criteria Committee. Arthritis Rheum 33(2):160–172, 1990.

54. Yang W, Dollear M, Muthukrishnan SR: One rare side effect of Zolpidem—sleepwalking: a case report. Arch Phys Med Rehabil 86:1256–1256, 2005.

Clinical Case Studies III

SARAH NATH ZALLEK

Questions

1. A 45-year-old male physician complained of difficulty initiating sleep. He slept well until a bout of nightly abdominal pain that typically awoke him at 4:00 A.M. for several weeks. He began to dread going to bed in anticipation of the pain. The pain resolved after cholecystectomy. Since the operation he still dreads going to bed for fear he will not sleep. The harder he tries to fall asleep, the more difficult it is. He worries about his sleep during the day. His "mind races" as he tries to fall asleep. He sleeps better when he is away from home, staying in a hotel. He feels fatigued and has trouble concentrating in the daytime. When he tries to nap in the daytime, he is unable to fall asleep. What is his current primary sleep diagnosis?
   A. Inadequate sleep hygiene
   B. Psychophysiologic insomnia
   C. Pain-related insomnia
   D. Generalized anxiety disorder
   E. Sleep-onset association disorder

2. A 6-year-old girl has a 3-year history of screaming out in her sleep most nights. Her mother goes to her bedside to find her crying inconsolably. She does not respond to her mother's questions and is sometimes combative. She returns to sleep after a few minutes and does not recall the events in the morning. Which of the following is also typical of this disorder?
   A. It occurs in the final third of the night.
   B. If the patient awakens just after the event, dream content is recalled.
   C. Urinary incontinence
   D. There is a family history of similar events.

3. Which of the following statements is true about the non-rapid eye movement (NREM) sleep arousal disorders and sleep-related epilepsy?
   A. NREM sleep arousal disorders do not have associated electroencephalographic (EEG) changes.

   B. Epileptic seizures consistently show ictal epileptiform activity on the typical polysomnogram (PSG) EEG recording.
   C. Epileptic seizures and NREM sleep arousal disorders commonly exhibit stereotyped behavior.
   D. Epileptic seizures and NREM sleep arousal disorders may both lead to physical injury.

4. A 3-year-old boy presented with nightly vomiting in sleep. He sleeps about 11 hours a night and does not have excessive daytime sleepiness (EDS) or daytime irritability. He has no spells of vomiting or abnormal behavior in the daytime. The following (Figure 25-1) is a 10-second sample of his PSG. What does this finding most likely represent?
   A. Benign epilepsy of childhood with occipital paroxysms
   B. A partial seizure
   C. Artifact from lying on O1
   D. Positive occipital sharp transients
   E. Benign epilepsy of childhood with centrotemporal spikes

5. Which of the following statements is correct regarding restless legs syndrome (RLS) and akathisia?
   A. RLS typically involves the urge to move; akathisia does not.
   B. RLS and akathisia are both relieved by movement.
   C. RLS exhibits circadian rhythmicity; akathisia does not.
   D. Akathisia has a motor manifestation in sleep; RLS does not.
   E. Akathisia and RLS are both relieved by levodopa.

6. A 4-year-old girl presented with difficulty initiating sleep and difficulty maintaining sleep. She had a regular evening family routine of dinner, playtime, and bath before bed at 8:00 P.M. Within 15 minutes of going to bed, she would get up and ask for a drink, which she would receive and then return to bed. A few minutes later she would

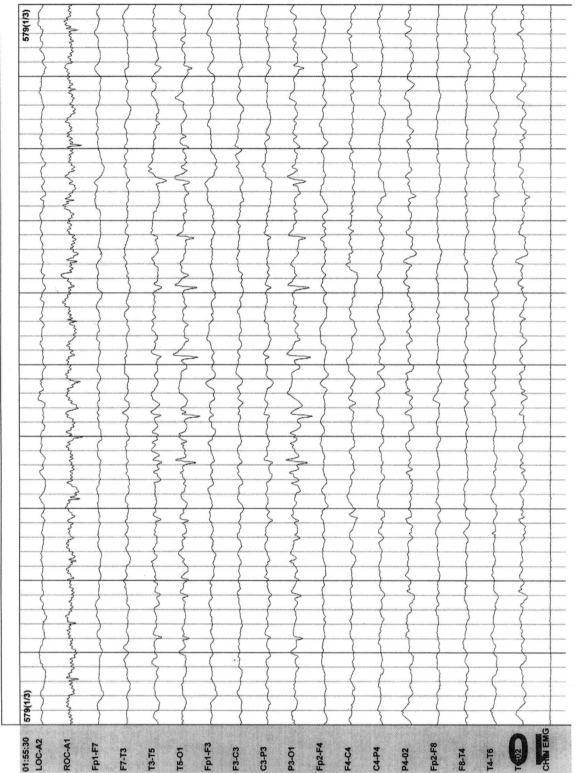

FIGURE 25-1 ■ 10-second PSG tracing sample.

arise again, saying she was lonely. She would then lie down on her mother's lap on the couch and fall asleep. Her mother would return her to bed, where she would sleep for another 2–3 hours. She would then awaken and go to her parents' bed to sleep for the remainder of the night. Her parents were aware she was there and knew she was aware of her actions. She consumed one caffeinated beverage a day. She has a television in her room and is allowed to watch it for 30 minutes before lights out for bedtime. What is the best treatment for this disorder?

A. Remove the television from the bedroom.
B. Discontinue caffeine.
C. Allow her to fall asleep in her parents' bed from the start each night and transfer her to her own bed once asleep.
D. Return her to her own bed with minimal interaction each time she gets up and allow her to fall asleep on her own.
E. Return her to her bed each time she gets up and lie down next to her until she falls asleep.

7. A 21-year-old college student complained of rocking in his sleep. He was embarrassed when he awoke one night to find his fraternity brothers standing at his bedside laughing at him for exhibiting body rocking while asleep. In retrospect, he recalls a habit of body rocking or rubbing his feet together to fall asleep at night or at a naptime during the day since early childhood. He denies any uncomfortable sensations that lead to the urge to move rhythmically in this manner. He has no seizure risk factors. What is his likely diagnosis?

A. Simple partial seizures
B. Complex partial seizures
C. Rhythmic movement disorder
D. Sleep starts
E. RLS

8. A 50-year-old woman presents with a several-year history of "sleepwalking" and eating in her sleep. She had gained 20 pounds without a perceived change in her caloric intake while awake. She does not recall her nighttime behaviors but has found remnants of food in her kitchen and bedroom on many occasions on awakening in the morning. She sought treatment after awakening distressed to find leftover pork chops in her bed in the morning. Which of the following would be the most appropriate treatment?

A. Topiramate
B. Clonazepam
C. Clonidine
D. Eszopiclone
E. Zolpidem

9. A 15-year-old boy presents with difficulty initiating sleep since age 13. He goes to bed at variable times (8:00 P.M. to 1:30 A.M.) depending on when he feels sleepy. He takes 30–120 minutes to fall asleep. Once asleep, he stays asleep and is difficult to awaken in the morning. He feels more fatigued than sleepy during the day and does not fall asleep inadvertently. He describes times when he falls asleep more easily for days at a time, but this does not persist. On one occasion he stayed up all night and started sleeping at a more "normal hour" for a few weeks. He would go to bed at 11:00 P.M. and awaken at 6:00 to 8:00 A.M. and felt less fatigued during that time.

When he cannot sleep he lies awake in bed for up to 2 hours before getting up to play computer games, watch television, or read. He currently denies depressed mood. He admits to chronic morning headaches. Past medical history is significant for diagnoses of "chronic fatigue syndrome" and depression. He was initially advised to stay awake 1 full night and then maintain a sleep schedule of 9:00 P.M. to 6:00 A.M. This was effective for approximately 1 week. He then went to sleep progressively later each night for several nights. When asked to sleep ad lib for 1 month and record sleep logs, he returned with the record shown in Figure 25-2 and reported feeling refreshed during his wakeful hours. What is his most likely diagnosis?

A. Nonentrained-type circadian rhythm sleep disorder (non–24-hour sleep-wake syndrome, or hypernychthemeral syndrome)
B. Delayed sleep phase type circadian rhythm sleep disorder
C. Inadequate sleep hygiene
D. Irregular sleep-wake type circadian rhythm sleep disorder

10. Treatment of the disorder in Question 9 may be best achieved with which of the following?

A. Eszopiclone
B. Good sleep hygiene
C. Stimulus control
D. Melatonin and bright light therapy
E. Chronotherapy

11. What would be an appropriate treatment for the finding in the following 30-second PSG (Figure 25-3)?

A. Oxcarbazepine

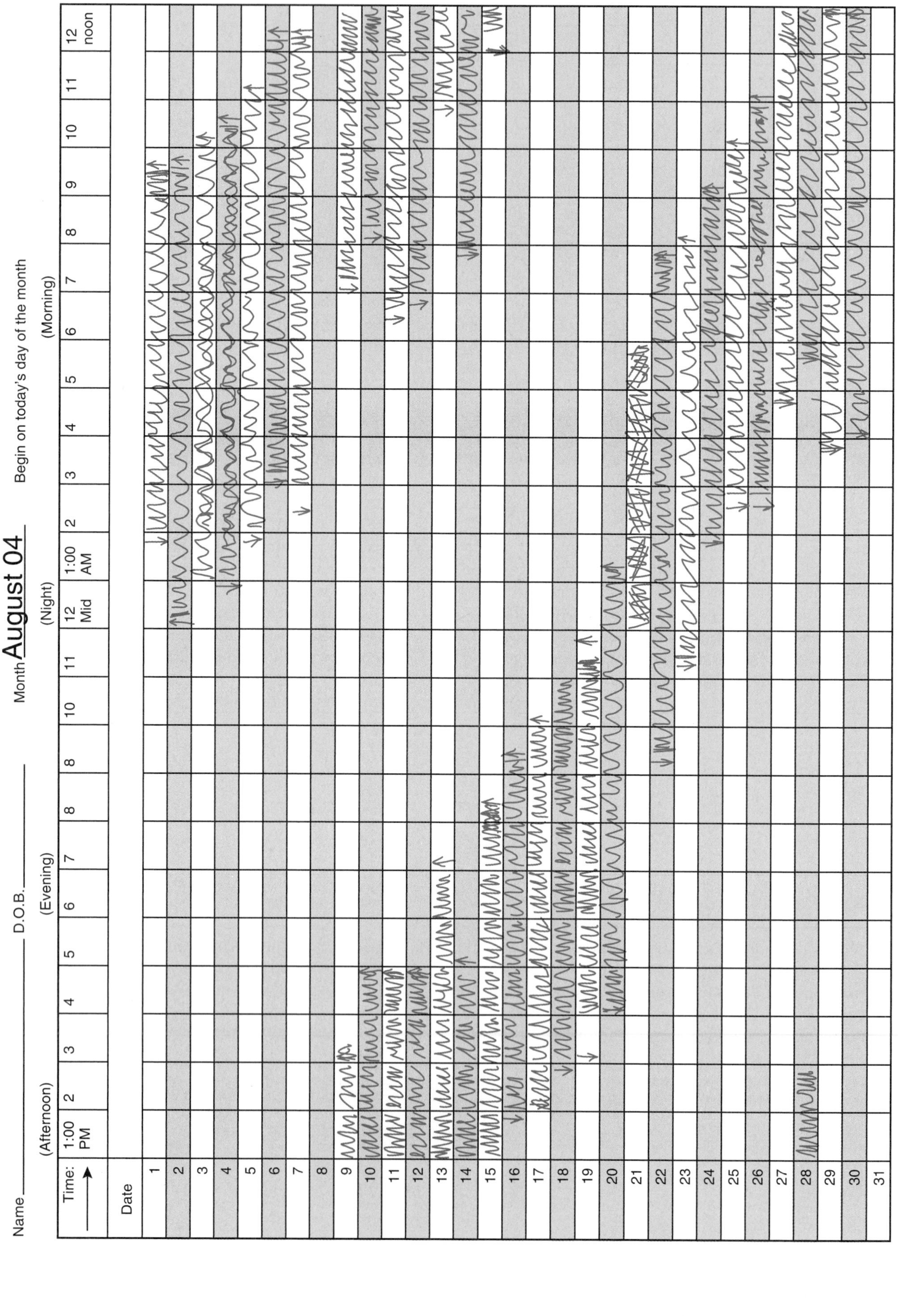

FIGURE 25-2 ■ Sleep log at baseline. Downward arrow marks time in bed. Filled areas indicate sleep. Upward arrow marks time up from bed.

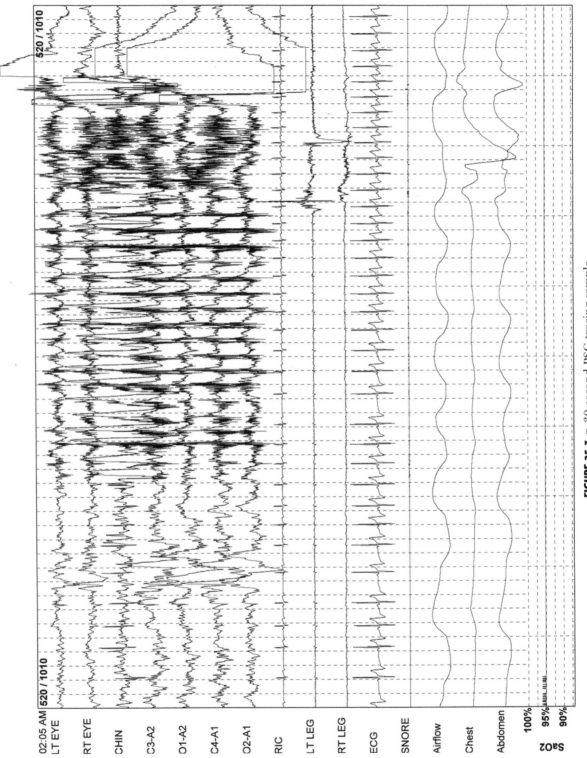

FIGURE 25-3 ■ 30-second PSG tracing sample.

B. Valproic acid
C. Ropinirole
D. Occlusal appliance

12. A 32-year-old nurse presents with difficulty initiating sleep. She works three to four nights a week on varying days in a hospital setting. On work nights, she starts work at 7:00 P.M. and feels alert. By 2:00 A.M. she feels sleepy and often dozes off at the nurses' station if she sits down. She has recently been disciplined by her supervisor as a result. Driving home she feels sleepy, but at 9:00 A.M. she is unable to initiate sleep. Once she does fall asleep, she awakens after 3 to 4 hours and cannot return to sleep. She may nap for an hour before going to work again but often does not have time. On her nights off, she sleeps at night and stays awake the next day.

What would be the most helpful *next* step?
A. Have the patient keep sleep logs for 1 month and return for follow-up evaluation.
B. PSG
C. PSG and multiple sleep latency test (MSLT)
D. Advise the patient to stop working nights and request day-shift work only.

13. A 53-year-old man presents with episodes of awakening with difficulty breathing for the last 2 years. He feels panicked when it happens and has a sensation of impending death. His heart races. He feels he is unable to breathe for about 15 seconds and then resumes breathing with stridor. His voice may be hoarse temporarily after episodes. Spells occur a few times a year. He denies a sensation of acidic fluid in his throat. His bed partner says he does not snore. He is not sleepy during the day. What is his *most* likely diagnosis?
A. Gastroesophageal reflux disease
B. Sleep-related abnormal swallowing
C. Sleep-related choking
D. Sleep-related laryngospasm
E. Obstructive sleep apnea (OSA)

14. A 44-year-old woman complained of not sleeping more than an hour or two each night for the last several months. She stated she would go to bed at 10:00 P.M. and lie awake most of the night. She may doze off for an hour or two and then lie awake until 6 A.M. She was fatigued during the day and had trouble focusing at work. She denied depressed mood, although she was feeling frustrated about her sleeplessness. She denied feeling anxious about sleep and did not tend to worry when lying in bed. She stated she consumes 2 cups of coffee each morning. You advise her not to lie awake in bed, stop drinking coffee, and keep sleep logs. On her return visit, sleep logs

showed mostly wakefulness at night and no daytime naps. Her bed partner stated she appeared to be sleeping through the night on most nights. What should you do now?
A. Prescribe a hypnotic.
B. PSG
C. Refer for a psychiatric evaluation for possible depression.
D. Stimulus control

15. A 71-year-old woman was evaluated for daytime fatigue. Her bedtime was midnight, and she would fall asleep in 5 minutes. She slept through the night and awakened at 5 A.M., which she related to the stress of caring for her ill husband. She snored sometimes, but neither nightly nor loudly. She drank 1 cup of tea each morning. Medications included clonazepam, 0.5 mg at bedtime, and tizanidine, 4 mg at bedtime, for shoulder pain that had resolved some time ago. On examination, body mass index (BMI) was 19, and retrognathia and a large uvula were noted. Which of the following might be the most beneficial *next* step?
A. PSG
B. Weight loss
C. Taper off clonazepam and discontinue tizanidine.
D. Discontinue caffeine.

16. Which of the following statements is true about normal sleep-related erections?
A. They mainly occur in the final 2 REM episodes of the night.
B. They are related to dreams with sexual content.
C. Reduction in testosterone reduces sleep-related erections without affecting REM sleep.
D. Depression does not affect sleep-related erections.

17. A 77-year-old man with probable Alzheimer's disease was brought to a sleep disorders center for evaluation of his "days and nights being mixed up." For the past several months his nighttime sleep had deteriorated, and he seemed to be awake more at night and often wandering. He napped frequently during the day. Sleep logs over the next 2 weeks revealed at least 3 bouts of sleep each 24 hours, day or night, usually less than 4 hours each. Before retirement 12 years ago, he used to work rotating shifts. What is his most likely diagnosis?
A. Advanced sleep phase syndrome
B. Nonentrained type circadian rhythm sleep disorder
C. Irregular sleep-wake rhythm
D. Shift work disorder

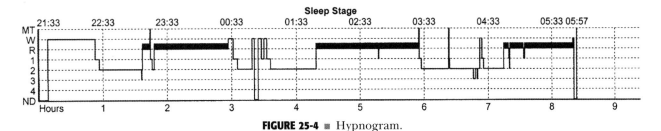

FIGURE 25-4 ■ Hypnogram.

18. At the end of her annual visit to her gynecologist, a 30-year-old woman told her physician she had become fatigued in the daytime and was having trouble concentrating at work. She denies EDS. Because she snored occasionally and had a BMI of 30, her physician referred her for a PSG. Figure 25-4 shows the resulting hypnogram; Figure 25-5 shows a 30-second sample of the PSG recording.

Sleep stage distribution:

Wake	13%
Stage 1	4%
Stage 2	34%
Stages 3 & 4	1%
REM	48%

Total sleep time = 428 minutes
Sleep latency = 44 minutes
REM latency = 44 minutes
Apnea-hypopnea index (AHI) 4 (using thermistor without nasal pressure transducer or esophageal pressure monitor [Pes])
What do the PSG results suggest?
A. Upper airway resistance syndrome (UARS)
B. Advanced sleep phase disorder
C. Mild OSA
D. Depression
E. Narcolepsy

19. For the past 15 years, a 50-year-old executive has traveled overseas several times per year. She sought medical attention after she traveled from Chicago (United States) to Frankfurt (Germany), arriving at 9:00 A.M., and falling asleep at the wheel of her rental car that morning. In her travels westward, she often had difficulty initiating sleep at night and awakening in the morning. She felt sleepy in morning meetings and alert in the evenings. Her trips to Europe generally lasted 3 or 4 days. On return home, she found it easier to initiate sleep but awakened early in the morning. Once home for a few days, she slept well at night, felt alert all day, and felt satisfied with her sleep. What is true about her diagnosis?
A. Gastrointestinal symptoms may be associated.
B. The condition can become permanent despite return to a routine schedule.

C. The rate of recovery is longer in younger adults.
D. PSG is usually helpful.

20. A child neurologist was consulted about a 3-week-old infant admitted for "seizures." The baby was born full term without complications to a healthy gravida 1, para 1 mother. The patient's parents described "massive repeated body jerks in sleep" that did not occur in wakefulness. All limbs were involved simultaneously. The clusters of rapid jerks ceased on awakening. Neurological examination, EEG, and biochemistry were normal. What is the *most* likely diagnosis?
A. Myoclonic seizures
B. Infantile spasms
C. Benign sleep myoclonus of infancy
D. Periodic leg movements
E. Sleep starts

21. A 10-year-old boy presents with sleep-related enuresis. He has never been dry at night for more than a few nights in a row. He has snored and had witnessed apnea since age 2 years. He is too embarrassed to go to sleepovers with his friends because of his snoring and bedwetting. What is true about OSA and enuresis?
A. OSA may predispose to enuresis by increasing atrial natriuretic peptide.
B. An AHI of >15 raises the risk of enuresis compared with an AHI of <15.
C. Enuresis is more common in girls.
D. Bladder pressure during sleep does not change during OSA events.

22. A 75-year-old woman presents with difficulty maintaining sleep. She describes worrying about her sleep and sleeping better when she is on vacation. She constantly checks the clock. Once she is in bed, her mind is constantly "playing like a movie and it won't stop." If she cannot sleep, she gets up and does housework. She does not snore. She denies sad or depressed mood. She snores and has a long uvula. She feels sleepy during the day but usually cannot sleep if she lies down. She denies caffeine or alcohol use. Her sleep log at presentation is shown in Figure 25-6.

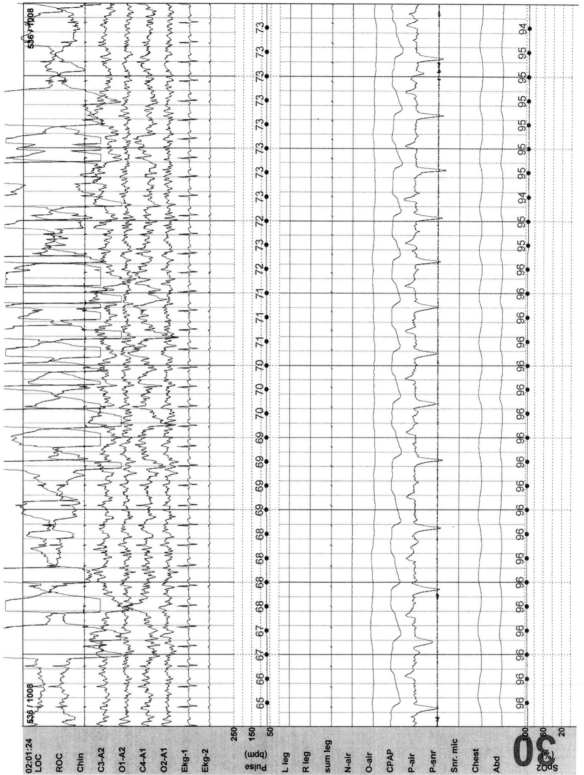

FIGURE 25-5 ■ 30-second sample of the PSG recording.

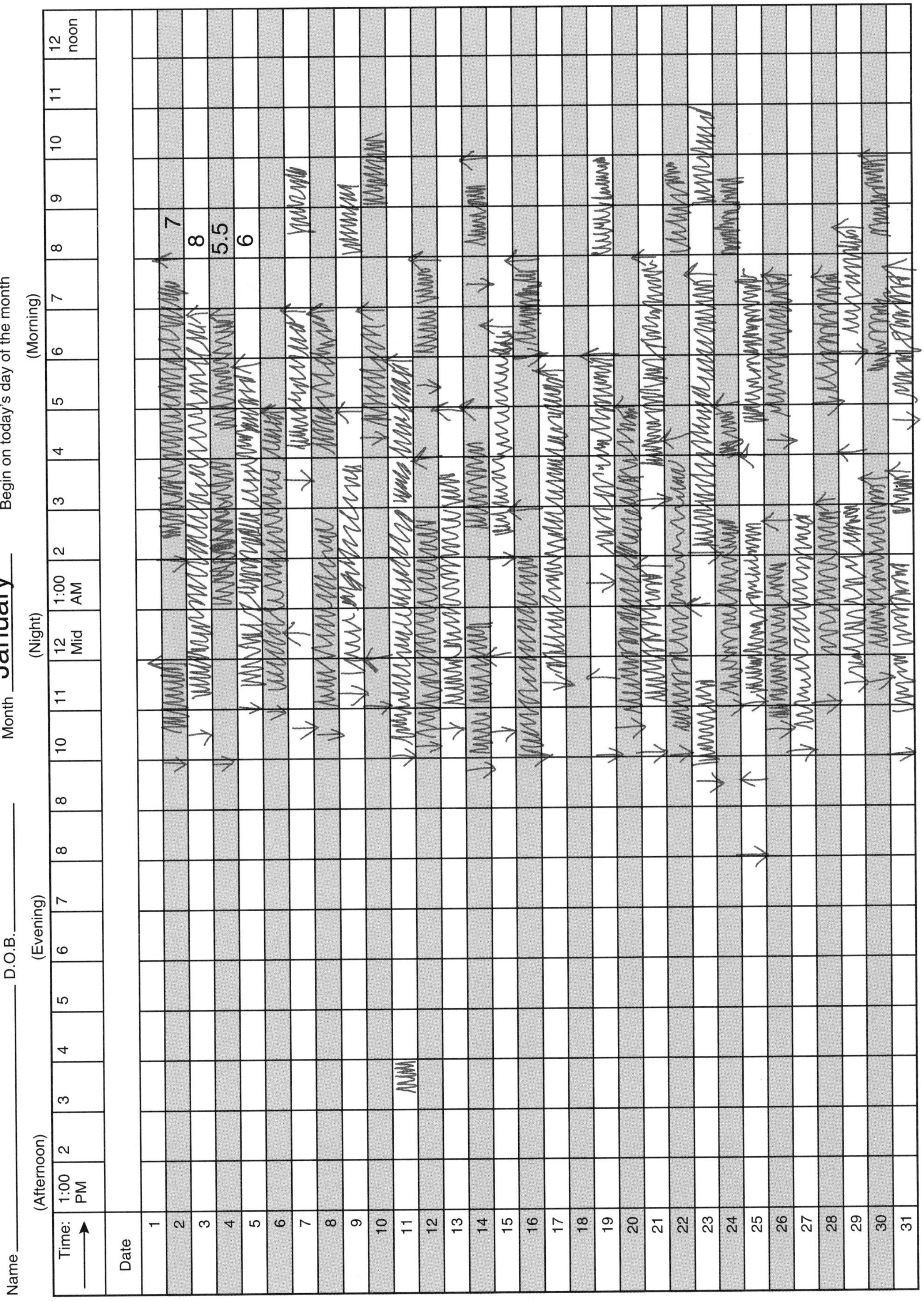

FIGURE 25-6 ■ Sleep log at presentation.

What intervention *most likely* led to the changes in her sleep log (Figure 25-7) on follow-up evaluation 1 month later?

A. Sleep restriction
B. If unable to return to sleep, she stays in bed and tries harder to sleep.
C. Eszopiclone
D. Fluoxetine
E. Psychotherapy

23. After 20 years of nightly alcohol consumption of 10–15 beers per night, a 48-year-old man is told by his wife that he must stop drinking or she will leave him. She asked him to enter an inpatient alcoholism treatment program, but he declined. He stopped drinking alcohol abruptly and did not seek treatment. When drinking, he felt he slept fine and felt alert most days. In the first few nights of abstinence, he slept little and awoke with vivid and disturbing dreams. Which of the following is characteristic of the acute effects of alcohol intake on sleep patterns?

A. Increased total sleep time
B. Increased sleep continuity
C. Decreased sleep latency
D. Increased REM sleep in the first half of the night

24. Which of the following is characteristic of withdrawal after chronic alcohol abuse?

A. Increased REM sleep (REM sleep rebound)
B. Sleep effects of withdrawal diminish by 1 month after last consumption of alcohol
C. Increased sleep continuity
D. Increased stages 3 and 4 sleep

25. A newly married 29-year-old dentist presents to a sleep clinic at the request of her husband who is concerned she does not sleep enough. She goes to bed at midnight and awakens at 5:00 A.M. to exercise. She works from 8:00 A.M. to 5:30 P.M. and feels alert all day until bedtime. She does not use caffeine or alcohol. She is fully satisfied with her sleep and wakefulness and has practiced this schedule since her teens. Her 30-year-old husband sleeps approximately 10 hours a night, from 10:00 P.M. to 8:00 A.M. He similarly has no sleep complaints and feels alert if he sleeps on his usual schedule. He works most days from 9:00 A.M. to 3:00 P.M. as a potter in his home studio. They have dinner together each night. After he goes to bed, she stays up to work on writing her third novel.

Which of the following is likely to be true about this couple?

A. She has EDS that she does not admit to; he is depressed, exhibiting sleep avoidance.
B. She is a *short sleeper* and he is a *long sleeper*.
C. An MSLT would show EDS for each of them.
D. She actively restricts sleep to get more accomplished in a day; he has enjoyed his sleep schedule all his life and has not found it to be interruptive of his educational or occupational goals.

Questions 9 and 10 are adapted with permission from:

Zallek SN: A teenager with insomnia and fatigue; habit or hard wiring? J Clin Sleep Med 2(1):92–93, 2006.

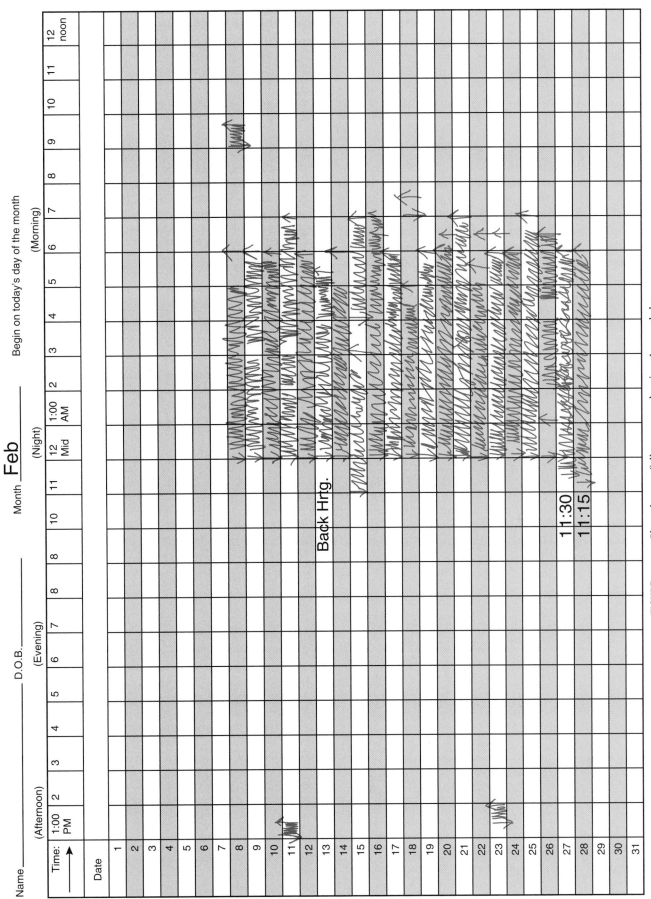

FIGURE 25-7 ■ Sleep log on follow-up evaluation 1 month later.

Answers

1. B. Psychophysiologic insomnia

Psychophysiologic insomnia often develops after a bout of insomnia triggered by a precipitating factor such as pain, as in this case. Sleep-preventing associations may develop, and the patient is then left with sleep-related worries and a "racing mind" at bedtime. Daytime dysfunction occurs, but napping does not lead to sleep. These patients typically sleep better elsewhere. In this case, although attempting to nap may not be good sleep hygiene, inadequate sleep hygiene is not his primary diagnosis. Sleep-onset association is a form of behavioral insomnia of childhood in which one is unable to initiate sleep without the presence of certain conditions. Although this began as pain-related insomnia, once the pain resolved, his difficulty initiating sleep was due to conditioning. His focus of worry on sleep rather than a broader range of concerns is a feature that distinguishes psychophysiologic insomnia from generalized anxiety disorder in this case.

2. D. There is a family history of similar events.

This patient has sleep terrors, a NREM sleep arousal disorder in which the patient usually arouses from stages 3 or 4 sleep with a loud cry or scream and is inconsolable. Intense autonomic symptoms and signs are commonly associated, including tachycardia, tachypnea, flushing, and diaphoresis. This parasomnia typically occurs in the first third of the night, as more NREM sleep occurs in the first third of the night than the latter two thirds. Onset is typically between the ages of 2 and 4, but it can occur at any age. It often runs in families. Dream recall is typical of nightmares, which occur in REM sleep. Bladder distention may precipitate an episode, but urinary incontinence is not typical.

3. D. Epileptic seizures and NREM sleep arousal disorders may both lead to physical injury.

The NREM arousal disorders include sleepwalking, sleep terrors, and confusional arousals. They typically begin in childhood and resolve spontaneously but may occur at any age. If an event is captured on PSG, an abrupt arousal from slow-wave sleep is seen, sometimes with associated high-amplitude synchronous delta frequency activity. These disorders vary on a spectrum of motor and autonomic activity: (1) sleepwalking involves a high level of motor activity (ambulation) and little autonomic activity; (2) sleep terrors exhibit high sympathetic activity (tachycardia, tachypnea, and diaphoresis) and little motor activity; and (3) confusional arousals exhibit little of either. Although epileptic seizures may have a typical ictal discharge visible on the routine four-channel EEG montage of a PSG, a focal seizure may be missed electrographically because the EEG leads do not record from the specific cortical area of discharge. This is especially true of frontal lobe seizures originating from the falcine cortex, where surface EEG leads cannot record.

Epileptic seizures commonly exhibit stereotyped behavior from one seizure to the next within the individual. The NREM arousal disorders are much less likely to be stereotypical. Both, however, can lead to physical injury to the patient and to others.

4. A. Benign epilepsy of childhood with occipital paroxysms

Benign epilepsy of childhood with occipital paroxysms is a localization-related epilepsy that typically begins between the ages of 3 and 6 years. Most seizures occur in sleep. Semiology often involves simple visual hallucinations. Blindness at seizure onset followed by migraine is common. More than 80% of patients have ictal vomiting. Secondary generalization (spread of the seizure to the entire cerebral cortex) occurs in half of cases. The characteristic EEG finding is runs of high-amplitude sharp and slow wave complexes in the occipital region, which may be bilateral or unilateral.

Benign epilepsy of childhood with centrotemporal spikes (also known as *rolandic epilepsy*) is a similar age-related, localization-related epilepsy, but the distribution of the interictal epileptiform activity is in the central leads. Onset is typically between the ages of 3 and 13 years, with a peak at 9–10 years. Semiology typically involves hemifacial twitching, drooling, speech arrest, and guttural vocalizations.

These interictal epileptiform discharges do not represent electrographic seizures; seizures are rhythmic discharges that evolve in amplitude and frequency.

Positive occipital sharp transients are a benign EEG variant that appears in the posterior region. They are synchronous but may exhibit as much as 60% asymmetry.

5. C. Restless legs syndrome (RLS) exhibits circadian rhythmicity; akathisia does not.

Both RLS and akathisia involve an urge to move, but RLS is relieved by movement. There is a circadian nature to RLS, for one of the diagnostic clinical criteria is onset or worsening of RLS symptoms in the evening or at night. Approximately 85% of patients with RLS have associated periodic leg movements in sleep, which can be seen on PSG. There is no sleep-related motor phenomenon for akathisia. Levodopa is thought to precipitate akathisia but alleviates RLS, as do dopamine agonists. Of note, in RLS, levodopa and dopamine agonists can lead to "augmentation" in which RLS symptoms develop or worsen at a time earlier than the dose of the medication is taken. This is particularly problematic with levodopa, occurring in up to 87% of cases. Dopamine agonists such as pramipexole and ropinirole are much less likely to cause augmentation.

6. D. Return her to her own bed with minimal interaction each time she gets up and allow her to fall asleep on her own.

This child has behavioral insomnia of childhood (limit-setting sleep disorder). Once behavioral limits are set, sleep occurs more easily. The repeated episodes of getting up from bed are the result of reinforcement of the behavior by parental response, even if the response is negative. Inconsistent enforcement of bedtime limits and unpredictable parental responses to the behavior perpetuate the problem. Treatment is accomplished by setting clear bedtime limits and consistently reinforcing them. If the child does get up, a return to bed with as little emotion (positive or negative) as possible, with reinforcement of the expectation that the child stay in bed and fall asleep on her own, is most effective. Having a parent lie down next to the child to fall asleep is likely to condition her to require a parent to be present for sleep initiation each time.

Caffeine can disturb a child's sleep and may be a factor in a case such as this one, but it is not the primary factor here. Similarly, having a television in a child's room is poor sleep hygiene but did not lead to this patient's difficulty initiating and maintaining sleep. The inability to initiate sleep without the television on at that time would be characteristic of sleep-onset association disorder.

7. C. Rhythmic movement disorder

Rhythmic movement disorder (RMD) is a parasomnia of the sleep-wake transition that involves stereotyped movements, usually of the large muscles. Typical movements include rubbing the feet together, head banging, and body rocking. Humming or chanting may also occur. Behaviors are exhibited before sleep onset and can last into all stages of sleep, most typically stage 2. Onset in infancy or early childhood is common. It tends to diminish with age. RMD is more common in developmentally delayed and autistic children but can occur in otherwise normal children. There have been no reports of systematic studies of pharmacological or behavioral treatment. Rhythmic movements before and during sleep are common in normal infants and children and do not necessarily constitute a disorder if there are no significant consequences. Interference with normal sleep, associated daytime dysfunction, or resultant injury would differentiate cases of rhythmic movement disorder from normally occurring rhythmic movements in sleep.

Stereotyped rhythmic movements may be the sole manifestation of a localization-related epilepsy, which should be considered in the differential diagnosis of RMD. Sleep starts are another parasomnia of the sleep-wake transition that involves a sudden body jerk rather than rhythmic movements. They may be associated with a sensation of falling or floating, or the feeling that one has heard a loud noise or seen a bright light flash. They are benign and not associated with epileptic phenomena.

RLS involves an urge to move, often related to an uncomfortable sensation that is better with movement. It begins or is worse in the evening or at night and at rest. The legs are typically involved, with more severe cases involving the arms and even torso.

8. A. Topiramate

This patient has sleep-related eating disorder (SRED), which consists of repeated episodes of involuntary eating and drinking during nighttime sleep with associated adverse consequences. Like sleepwalking, this parasomnia arises from NREM sleep and is not usually recalled by the patient. It can occur in isolation but is often associated with a primary sleep disorder, especially the arousal disorders such as sleepwalking and confusional arousal. The most common associated PSG finding is multiple confusional arousals arising from slow wave sleep, with or without eating at the time. Separate sleepwalking episodes without eating may occur in the same patients. Foods consumed may be unusual or even distasteful, such as cold or raw meats one would not eat in the same way while awake. Some patients report consumption of nonfood items, such as cigarettes or eggshells. High-calorie foods are often chosen, and weight gain is common.

Approximately 75% of patients with SRED are women. SRED is also more common in those with a primary sleep disorder, individuals undergoing acute or chronic stress, and after smoking cessation.

SRED differs from nocturnal eating syndrome, which involves overeating between the evening meal and bedtime, with full awakenings at night to eat foods one would normally eat. The majority of caloric intake occurs in the evening and nighttime hours in these patients.

Treatment may include control of other sleep disorders, if present. Topiramate has been reported to be of benefit in controlling SRED specifically. Benzodiazepines such as clonazepam and the nonbenzodiazepine hypnotic zolpidem have been associated with worsening of the sleep-related eating. Neither ezsopiclone nor clonidine has been reported to be beneficial.

9. A. Nonentrained type circadian rhythm sleep disorder (non–24-hour sleep-wake syndrome, or hypernychthemeral syndrome)

This patient has circadian rhythm sleep disorder, nonentrained type (also called *non–24-hour sleep-wake syndrome* or *hypernychthemeral syndrome*). This is well illustrated by his sleep logs (see Figure 25-2), which show a progressive delay in sleep onset. Delayed sleep phase type circadian rhythm sleep disorder (delayed sleep phase syndrome) would typically show a later sleep onset than desired but would not show a progressive nightly delay. Irregular sleep-wake type circadian rhythm sleep disorder manifests as three or more sleep periods throughout the 24-hour period without a major sleep period. Although the patient has some features of inadequate sleep hygiene, they are not the root cause of his difficulty initiating sleep.

The normal intrinsic period of the circadian pacemaker is slightly longer than 24 hours. Light is the strongest zeitgeber (time cue) to entrain the cycle in normal people. In nonentrained circadian rhythm sleep disorder, the circadian pacemaker is not in phase with the light-dark cycle and usually has a period of longer than 24 hours. Nonentrained circadian rhythm sleep disorder is common in blind people and is thought to be due to the lack of entrainment from light. It is much less common in sighted individuals, and the cause is not understood. A reduced sensitivity to light entrainment is one possible explanation.

This patient described periods of days when he could fall asleep more easily, which likely represents times in which his sleep phase is relatively in phase with the light-dark cycle.

Diagnosis of nonentrained circadian rhythm sleep disorder may be difficult, as the history may initially suggest delayed sleep phase type. Sleep logs, as in this case, can be very helpful. Actigraphy may provide more objective data. PSG is often not diagnostic and varies depending on the circadian phase at the time of testing.

10. D. Melatonin and bright light therapy

Treatment may include melatonin, administered in the evening starting at a time when the patient's free-running period most closely matches the desired sleep onset. Bright light therapy may also be helpful in the sighted and in blind individuals who respond to light by suppression of melatonin, although there is limited evidence in this particular disorder. If used, it should be administered at the core body temperature minimum in the morning.

Good sleep hygiene is appropriate in cases of inadequate sleep hygiene, but this circadian rhythm disorder is not likely to resolve with sleep hygiene alone. Similarly, stimulus control is appropriate for psychophysiologic insomnia but would not be an optimal choice for nonentrained circadian rhythm sleep disorder. Chronotherapy has been used to treat delayed sleep phase syndrome but requires strict adherence to maintain its effect.

This patient was eventually treated with melatonin and returned with the sleep log shown in Figure 25-8.

11. D. Occlusal appliance

The rhythmic activity shown here represents bruxism (grinding of the teeth or clenching of the jaw), which is a parasomnia that can occur in any sleep stage. The high-frequency component represents surface electromyographic (EMG) activity. These rhythmic bursts are distributed in all EEG electrooculographic (EOG), and chin EMG leads. Bruxism may be phasic, as in this case, or tonic. In phasic bruxism, bursts of muscle activity last 0.25–2.0 seconds. Tonic bruxism appears as a sustained EMG burst of >2.0 seconds. Treatment is commonly aimed at controlling the discomfort, if any, and dental wear associated with bruxism. Occlusal appliances are often used.

Oxcarbazepine would be an appropriate consideration for localization-related epilepsy, and valproic acid could be considered for a primary generalized epilepsy. There is no epileptiform activity in this sample. Sustained bruxism is a rare manifestation of epileptic seizures. The ictal discharge generally precedes the onset of bruxism in such cases. An expanded EEG montage may be helpful if seizures are clinically suspected. Ropinirole is a dopamine agonist indicated for RLS. Most patients with RLS have periodic limb movements in sleep (PLMS). PLMS are repetitive limb movements in NREM sleep that last 0.5–5 seconds, with a 5- to 90-second interval between them (typically 20–40 seconds) and occur in series of four or more movements in a row. They are recorded at the anterior tibialis muscle and would not be expected to appear in the EEG and EOG leads.

12. A. Have the patient keep sleep logs for 1 month and return for follow-up evaluation.

This patient most likely has shift work disorder with the typical features of difficulty staying awake while working during one's normal sleep period and difficulty sleeping during the day. This circadian rhythm sleep disorder is especially common in individuals working nights and early mornings. Total sleep time is reduced (average total sleep in 24 hours is approximately 5 hours), and sleep feels unsatisfactory to the patient. Work performance can suffer, and safety may be affected both on and off the job.

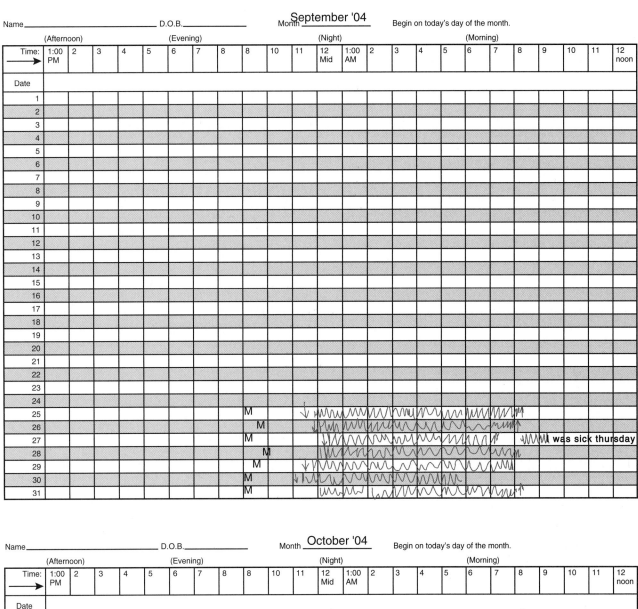

FIGURE 25-8 ■ Sleep logs of a patient once treated with melatonin. M indicates time melatonin was taken.

Workup does not require a PSG or an MSLT. History is sufficient. Sleep diaries can help clarify the pattern, and when caffeine, alcohol, and other environmental factors are included, they can aid in determining what other factors may influence sleep and wakefulness. Shift work disorder persists once environmental conditions for sleep have been optimized, but it is helpful to know what external and behavioral factors may be present for the particular individual.

Most shift workers are motivated to continue shift work because of higher pay or other significant reasons. Working with the patient to optimize sleep and wakefulness rather than abandoning the shift may be an important and realistic approach.

13. D. Sleep-related laryngospasm

Sleep-related laryngospasm is a capricious disorder that occurs less than once a week, often only a few times a year. The patient abruptly awakens from sleep with total or near total cessation of airflow, lasting 5–45 seconds, followed by choking and often stridor for several minutes. It causes a sense of panic and doom, as does sleep-related choking. Sleep-related choking, on the other hand, often occurs nightly and is not associated with stridor. Neither involves a feeling of acidic fluid in the throat, as gastroesophageal reflux disease might. In sleep-related abnormal swallowing, saliva pools in the upper airway, leading to coughing, choking, and arousal from sleep without stridor. Diurnal symptoms of abnormal swallowing may reflect an underlying neuromuscular or other disorder that affects deglutition.

None of these disorders is generally attributed to OSA, but in some cases sleep-related laryngospasm has comorbid sleep apnea.

14. B. PSG

This patient has paradoxical insomnia (sleep state misperception) in which one feels as if little or no sleep occurs when relatively normal sleep happens most nights. Daytime dysfunction is perceived as in other forms of insomnia. This relatively uncommon syndrome is present in only 5% of insomniacs, and the prevalence in the general population is not known. Initial improvement of any sleep hygiene issues may be appropriate but does not solve the problem. Most patients do not have associated psychopathology. Malingering is not common. Although hypnotics may improve the patient's perception of sleep, which can be helpful, a PSG is worth performing first for two reasons: it allows for investigation of sleep pathology not apparent by history, and it may provide helpful evidence of healthy sleep with which to confront the patient. Gentle but direct confrontation can be very effective alone in some cases. Stimulus control is appropriate for psychophysiological insomnia, which differs from this disorder in several ways, including that the patient's subjective impression of sleep more closely matches the amount of sleep obtained.

15. C. Taper off clonazepam and discontinue tizanidine.

This patient's fatigue is probably multifactorial, likely resulting from a combination of insufficient sleep syndrome, medication effect, and a possible mood disorder. She has some risk factors for sleep-disordered breathing, but addressing the other issues may lead to improvement or resolution of her symptoms, making a PSG a secondary consideration at the start. Weight loss is not appropriate for a patient with a BMI of 19 despite snoring. This patient was advised to taper off clonazepam and discontinue tizanidine as part of a multimodal initial approach. She also underwent counseling and started an antidepressant for a diagnosis of depression made on psychiatric consultation. She gradually increased her sleep time to 8 hours a night. She returned for follow-up evaluation with resolution of her daytime fatigue.

16. C. Reduction in testosterone reduces sleep-related erections without affecting REM sleep.

Sleep-related erections (SREs), also called *nocturnal penile tumescence*, normally occurs in almost every REM sleep period. They are not related to dreams of a sexual nature. Similarly, they are not affected by pre-sleep viewing of videos that are sexual in content, neutral, or dysphoric. While psychological factors may affect daytime erectile function, SREs are thought to be "insulated" from psychological factors. Depression, on the other hand, leads to several measurable changes in sleep, including greater variation of SRE even after being treated.

17. C. Irregular sleep-wake rhythm

Irregular sleep-wake rhythm is a circadian rhythm disorder in which sleep occurs in several (usually 3 or more) episodes throughout the 24-hour period. Episodes are often less than 4 hours long, and total sleep may be normal for age. It can be seen in older adults, particularly if they lack zeitgebers such as diurnal light and activity. Alzheimer's disease may predispose to it for these reasons in some, but may also involve a deterioration of the circadian rhythm.

Advanced sleep phase syndrome is also common in the elderly but involves an advance of the circadian sleep drive to an earlier than desired time, with sleepiness before desired bedtime and early morning awakenings. A single sleep period of normal length is typical. Nonentrained type circadian rhythm sleep disorder also involves a single sleep period, but with a perpetually later sleep onset time each night. Although this patient worked a rotating shift for many years, the sleep-associated disturbance would be expected to resolve when the patient no longer worked shifts.

18. D. Depression

PSG findings in depression include prolonged sleep latency, sleep disruption and increased wake time, decreased slow wave sleep, early morning awakening, reduced REM latency, high REM density (increased rapid eye movements per unit time during REM sleep), increased total REM time, and prolongation of the first REM period.

Several of those findings are featured in this study, including mildly prolonged sleep latency, decreased slow wave sleep, reduced REM latency, high REM density (increased rapid eye movements per unit time during REM sleep), increased total REM time, and prolongation of the first REM period.

An AHI of 4 is considered normal and does not constitute OSA. UARS is diagnosed with Pes, but a nasal pressure transducer can be suggestive of the pattern. Without these tools, this study does not suggest UARS.

A short REM latency is one of the characteristics of narcolepsy, but the other PSG findings in this case, along with her clinical history of fatigue rather than sleepiness, make depression much more likely.

19. A. Gastrointestinal symptoms may be associated.

Jet lag disorder, a circadian rhythm sleep disorder, is caused by a temporary mismatch between the timing of one's circadian rhythm and the desired sleep time after travel across at least two time zones. Insomnia at the desired sleep time and sleepiness at the desired wake time are typical. Gastrointestinal symptoms may be associated. Symptoms generally resolve after 1 day per time zone traveled; for example, it would take 7 days to adjust to travel across seven time zones. Older adults may take longer than younger individuals to adjust. PSG is generally not helpful unless other sleep disorders are being considered, for which testing would be indicated.

20. C. Benign sleep myoclonus of infancy

This disorder is characterized by clusters of myoclonic body jerks only in sleep, and it typically starts in the first month of life. It is unrelated to seizures and has no associated abnormalities on neurological examination at presentation or later in development. It may last only a few days or persist up to 1 year of age. It consists of clusters of four or five muscle jerks per second, mainly in quiet sleep, but it can occur in active sleep. Jerking resolves promptly upon awakening. There is no associated epileptiform activity on EEG.

Infantile spasms are epileptic seizures consisting of sudden neck flexion, arm extension, and leg flexion. EEG shows characteristic hypsarrhythmia (i.e., 0.5 to 3 Hz variable pattern of asynchronous slow waves with voltages >300 μV with multifocal spikes and sharp waves also present). Periodic leg movements can occur in infancy but have a different semiology. Rather than being myoclonic, they last 0.5–5 seconds and have an interval closer to 30 seconds. Myoclonic seizures occur in both sleep and wakefulness. Anticonvulsants may be helpful in myoclonic seizures but are of no known benefit in benign sleep myoclonus of infancy. Sleep starts occur at sleep onset and are generally not repetitive.

21. A. OSA may predispose to enuresis.

OSA may predispose to enuresis because of increased atrial natriuretic peptide (ANP) and decreased antidiuretic hormone, which results in greater than normal urine production in sleep, as has been seen in adults. Increased atrial volume from more negative intrathoracic pressure during an apnea may stimulate ANP production, leading to increased urine output. Acute hypoxemia may also stimulate ANP secretion.

Children with an AHI of <1 have a significantly lower prevalence of enuresis than those with an AHI of >1. There was no significant difference in prevalence of enuresis among children with an AHI of 1–5, 5–15, or greater than 15. Enuresis is more common in boys. Cystometrographic studies have shown bladder pressure as high as 60 cm H_2O (compared with normal pressures of 5 cm H_2O in wakefulness) associated with the respiratory effort during an obstructive apnea.

22. A. Sleep restriction

This patient with psychophysiological insomnia responded very well to sleep restriction. She was also instructed to get out of bed and, if unable to return to sleep, to read quietly until sleepy again, but she did not need this technique because her sleep improved so quickly with sleep restriction. Lying in bed and "trying harder" can be counterproductive in psychophysiological insomnia. Hypnotics may be helpful in some cases but are often not sufficient and does not address the underlying conditioning that perpetuates the insomnia. Fluoxetine and psychotherapy may be helpful in insomnia related to depression, but this patient had little evidence to suggest that diagnosis. Sleep disruption can be a feature of insomnia resulting from depression, but the associated symptoms in this patient and her lack of depressed mood make it less likely.

23. C. Decreased sleep latency

Alcohol is a sedative that has significant impact on sleep architecture. Acute effects include decreased sleep latency, decreased REM sleep in the first half of the night, and in some, REM sleep rebound in the second half of the night. Slow wave sleep may increase, but sleep is fragmented, and total sleep time is reduced.

24. A. Increased REM sleep (REM sleep rebound)

The acute effects of alcohol withdrawal include decreased total sleep time, sleep fragmentation, and a "lightening of sleep" with reduction of stage 3 and 4. REM sleep rebound may occur and may be associated with vivid and disturbing dreams. The sleep effects after alcohol cessation in a subject with history of chronic alcohol abuse can be long-lived, lasting up to 2 years.

25. B. She is a *short sleeper,* and he is a *long sleeper.*

Short sleepers obtain 5 hours or less sleep per 24 hours on a regular basis, without daytime effects. *Long sleepers* sleep 10–12 hours per 24 hours on a regular basis and feel refreshed during the day if they regularly obtain their usual amount of sleep.

Short sleepers do not volitionally restrict sleep and do not feel sleepy during the day despite their sleep length. They do not "catch up" with increased sleep on weekends or vacations, as a patient with insufficient sleep syndrome would. Most are psychologically normal, but some are described as hypomanic. *Short sleepers* are satisfied with their sleep, but they may be brought to medical attention by family members concerned about their sleep duration.

Long sleepers, by comparison, may have psychosocial impact from their sleep duration because of the need to curtail daytime activities to obtain adequate sleep. School, work, and social activities may be missed. Most patients are psychologically normal, but a trend toward introversion has been described. If their usual nighttime sleep need is met, there is no associated EDS. The pattern usually establishes itself in childhood and persists.

REFERENCES

1. American Academy of Sleep Medicine: *The International Classification of Sleep Disorders: Diagnostic and Coding Manual*, 2nd ed. Westchester, IL, American Academy of Sleep Medicine, 2005.
2. Ancoli-Israel S, Cole R, Alessi C, et al: The role of actigraphy in the study of sleep and circadian rhythms. Sleep 26:342–392, 2003.
3. Baertschi AJ, Adams JM, Sullivan MP: Acute hypoxemia stimulates atrial natriuretic factor secretion in vivo. Am J Physiol 255:H295–H300, 1988.
4. Brazil CW, Malow BA, Sammaritano MR: *Sleep and Epilepsy: The Clinical Spectrum*. Amersterdam, Elsevier Science, 2002.
5. Brooks LJ, Topol HI: Enuresis in children with sleep apnea. J Pediatr 142:515–518, 2003.
6. Chesson AL Jr, Littner M, Davila D, et al: Practice parameters for the use of light therapy in the treatment of sleep disorders. Standards of Practice Committee, American Academy of Sleep Medicine. Sleep 22:641–660, 1999.
7. Daly DD, Pedley TA: *Current Practice of Clinical Electroencephalography*, 2nd ed. Philadelphia, Lippincott-Raven, 1997.
8. Geyer JD, Payne TA, Carney MD, et al: *Atlas of Digital Polysomnography*. Philadelphia, Lippincott, Williams & Wilkins, 2000.
9. Krieger J, Follenius M, Sforza E, et al: Effects of treatment with nasal continuous positive airway pressure on atrial natriuretic peptide and arginine vasopressin release during sleep in patients with obstructive sleep apnea. Clin Sci 80:443–449, 1991.
10. Kryger MH, Roth T, Dement WC: *Principles and Practice of Sleep Medicine*, 4th ed. Philadelphia, Elsevier, 2005.
11. Lewy AJ, Emens J, Sack RL, et al: Zeitgeber hierarchy in humans: resetting the circadian phase positions of blind people using melatonin. Chronobiol Int 20:837–852, 2003.
12. McArthur AJ, Lewy AJ, Sack RL: Non-24-hour sleep-wake syndrome in a sighted man: circadian rhythm studies and efficacy of melatonin treatment. Sleep 19:544–553, 1996.
13. Meletti S, Cantalupo G, Volpi L, et al: Rhythmic teeth grinding induced by temporal lobe seizures. Neurology 62(12):2306–2309, 2004.
14. Sack RL, Brandes RW, Kendall AR, et al: Entrainment of free-running circadian rhythms by melatonin in blind people. N Engl J Med 343:1070–1077, 2000.
15. Sheldon SH, Ferber R, Kryger MH: *Principles and Practice of Pediatric Sleep Medicine*. Philadelphia, Elsevier, 2005.
16. Sheldon SH, Riter S, Detrojan R: *Atlas of Sleep Medicine in Infants and Children*. Armonk, Futura, 1999.
17. Watts RL, Koller WC: *Movement Disorders: Neurologic Principles and Practice*. New York, McGraw-Hill, 1997.
18. Yokoyama O, Amano T, Lee S, et al: Enuresis in an adult female with obstructive sleep apnea. Urology 45:150–154, 1995.
19. Zallek SN: A teenager with insomnia and fatigue; habit or hard wiring? J Clin Sleep Med 2(1):92–93, 2006.

Knowing Practice Parameters

SRINIVAS BHADRIRAJU

Questions

1. A 65-year-old male patient is referred to your sleep clinic for the evaluation of suspected obstructive sleep apnea (OSA). He has a history of loud snoring reported by his wife, who is worried about him as he seems to gasp for air and choke during his sleep. His medical history is significant for hypertension and diabetes. He has a 30-pack-year history of smoking. Physical examination was significant for a blood pressure of 160/90 mm Hg and a heart rate of 85 beats per minute. His weight was 210 lb, height was 61 inches, and the neck circumference was 17 inches. He had a Mallampati classification of 3 and narrow oropharyngeal airway. He had a class two molar malocclusion. His past medical history is significant for a left hemiparesis from a recent stroke.

   The most appropriate next step is:
   A. Perform polysomnography (PSG) because of the history of stroke.
   B. Perform PSG because of the history of snoring, witnessed apneas, and smoking.
   C. Perform PSG because of the history of snoring, witnessed apneas, hypertension, and stroke.
   D. Skip PSG and treat him with empiric continuous positive airway pressure (CPAP), as the risk of his having another stroke owing to untreated OSA is too high.

2. The indications for PSG in patients with systolic or diastolic heart failure include:
   A. Patients with ejection fraction less than 45%
   B. Patients with New York heart class 3 or 4 symptoms
   C. Patients with atrial fibrillation
   D. Patients not responsive to standard medical management of congestive heart failure

3. A 45-year-old nonobese female patient presents with the chief complaint of excessive daytime sleepiness (EDS), fatigue, and irritability. Her husband notes that he sleeps in a separate room, as she is a restless sleeper and kicks him repeatedly during sleep. She also complains of irritability during the daytime. She is restless during the night and has restless feelings in her legs, which she describes as painful. A PSG revealed an apnea hypopnea index (AHI) of 20 per hour and was significant for repetitive episodes of leg jerks, 0.5–5 seconds separated by an interval of 5–90 seconds.

   The next step in the management of this patient's EDS is:
   A. Modafinil
   B. Ropinarole and oral iron
   C. Pramipexole and oral iron
   D. CPAP titration trial

4. A 35-year-old female who is 6 months pregnant presents with the complaint of unpleasant sensations in her legs that started bothering her over the last month. The sensations are described as nonpainful and unpleasant sensations in both legs that occur close to her bedtime. Walking around or massaging the legs seem to give temporary relief only to recur when she returns to bed and tries to sleep. They occur about twice a week but when they occur, she has great difficulty initiating sleep and wakes up unrefreshed and feels tired all the next day. She has no other medical problems. Routine laboratory studies include normal chemistries. Hemoglobin was 12 g/dL, and her serum ferritin level was 35 μg/dL.

   A diagnosis of Restless legs syndrome was made. Initial approach in her management should be:
   A. Levodopa, leg massages, iron, and folate
   B. Pramipexole, leg massages, iron, and folate
   C. Gabapentin, leg massages, iron, and folate
   D. Leg massages, iron, and folate

5. A 40-year-old male presents with a chief complaint of EDS. He goes to bed around 10 P.M. and wakes up around 7 A.M. every day. He has no difficulty falling or staying asleep but has great

485

difficulty waking up. This has become a problem to the point that he lost his job. He remains sleepy during the rest of the day. He recalls a frightening experience of feeling completely paralyzed on awakening to the point of not being able to move even a finger on several occasions. He would "snap" out of the episodes when his wife would shake him to wake up. His wife reports that he snores during sleep. If he got "too excited" or laughed at a funny joke, he found himself getting very weak in his legs. His jaw would sag, and he would feel like he was paralyzed for a few minutes. Physical exam including the neurological examination was normal. Serum chemistries and complete blood count were all unremarkable. Narcolepsy is suspected in the differential diagnosis.

The appropriate next step in the diagnostic workup is:

A. Multiple sleep latency test (MSLT)
B. PSG
C. PSG followed by MSLT the next day
D. Polysomnography, followed by MSLT the next day; cerebrospinal fluid (CSF) analysis for hypocretin levels

6. Your cardiology colleague wants to obtain a curbside consult about a 55-year-old software consultant who emigrated from India 10 years ago and now complains of EDS and fatigue. His past medical history is significant for coronary artery bypass graft surgery 2 years ago, medication-controlled hypercholesterolemia, and hypertension. He recently had a pacemaker placement owing to symptomatic bradyarrhythmias.

The appropriate next step is:

A. PSG
B. Sleep clinic consultation
C. Nocturnal oximetry
D. Actigraphy

7. The following statements represent standard practice parameters provided by the American Academy of Sleep Medicine (AASM) *except*:

A. "Polysomnography is not indicated to diagnose chronic lung disease."
B. "Polysomnography, with additional EEG derivations and video recording, is indicated in evaluating sleep-related behaviors that are violent or otherwise potentially injurious to the patient or others."
C. "Polysomnography is not routinely indicated in the diagnosis of circadian rhythm sleep disorders."

D. "Common, uncomplicated noninjurious parasomnias, such as typical disorders of arousal, nightmares, enuresis, sleep walking and bruxism, can usually be diagnosed by clinical evaluation alone."

8. Pemoline is effective in the treatment of EDS in patients with narcolepsy. However, the use of pemoline is limited and currently discouraged by which of the following?
A. Renal failure
B. Seizures
C. Liver failure
D. Involuntary movements

9. A 45-year-old male truck driver was seen for the evaluation of EDS. His wife reported very loud snoring and interrupted sleep resulting from witnessed gasping with arousal episodes and nocturia. He frequently ground his teeth. His nocturnal symptoms worsened in the last year, coinciding with a 10-lb weight gain. He has had near-miss accidents on the road caused by sleepiness. Physical exam revealed a pleasant gentleman who was dozing frequently during the interview. His weight was 240 lb, and his height was 68 inches. His neck circumference was 17 inches. He had a crowded oropharynx with a Mallampati score of 3 and class two molar malocclusion. You schedule him for an overnight PSG.

The data from the report are given below:
Sleep latency: 4.5 minutes
Sleep efficiency: 85%
AHI: 65 episodes/h
Minimum oxygen desaturation: 75%
Based on a CPAP titration study, he was prescribed CPAP of 15 cm H_2O. At this setting the AHI was 4.5 per hour and oxygen saturation remained above 92%. This was tested both while supine and during REM sleep. He returns to see you in the sleep clinic 3 months after using CPAP and reporting to be compliant with its use. At this time he is very alert and gets at least 8 hours of uninterrupted sleep, and his daytime functioning has improved substantially. He does not feel sleepy or take any naps during the day. He wants to know if further testing is needed to assess his sleep apnea. The most appropriate response is:
A. Recommend follow-up PSG.
B. Recommend PSG followed by MSLT.
C. MSLT
D. Further testing is not required at this time.

10. Actigraphy is an experimental method used to study the evaluation of sleep-wake patterns and circadian rhythms by assessing for movement recorded on an accelerometer. All of the following statements are included in the AASM practice parameters *except*:
    A. Actigraphy is reliable and valid for detecting sleep in the normal healthy adult population.
    B. Actigraphy is routinely indicated for the diagnosis, assessment, and severity of RLS.
    C. Actigraphy should be conducted for a minimum of three consecutive 24-hour periods, but this length of time is highly dependent on the specific use in a given individual.
    D. Actigraphy may be useful in determining the rest and activity pattern during portable sleep apnea testing. However, the use of actigraphy alone in the detection of OSA is not currently established.

11. A 35-year-old female executive is seen in your sleep clinic for evaluation of insomnia. The patient is in bed by 9 P.M. but is unable to fall asleep before 2 or 3 A.M. and has to "drag" herself out of bed in the morning. She needs to be at work around 7:30 A.M. but finds herself increasingly sleepy during the day, especially during meetings and at times while driving. She reports feeling more irritable and snappy as the day goes by. Her husband says that she never snores. Her physical exam was unremarkable. Recently, she visited her sister in Los Angeles and for the first time in a long time she slept "normally, like everyone else."
    Which of the following recommendation(s) regarding light therapy as pertaining to this case is true?
    A. Light therapy may have a potential role in the treatment of this condition.
    B. Light therapy may also help in the treatment of hypomania.
    C. Light therapy should be used for a minimum of 6 months.
    D. Light therapy should be used for longer than 6 months.

12. All of the following are acceptable criteria for a split-night study *except*:
    A. An AHI of at least 40 is documented during a minimum of 2 hours of diagnostic PSG.
    B. CPAP titration is carried out for more than 3 hours.
    C. PSG documents that CPAP eliminates or nearly eliminates the respiratory events during REM sleep, NREM sleep, and REM sleep with the patient in supine position.

    D. A second night PSG with CPAP titration is performed to confirm the appropriate setting identified during the split-night study.

13. A 54-year-old male presents with the chief complaint of insomnia. He has slept well until a major setback in his family business 6 months ago, when he started experiencing difficulties initiating sleep. His business has recovered and is doing well, but he continues to have difficulty with insomnia. He has tried several treatments including zolipidem, diphenhydramine, alcohol, and yoga. He is very frustrated at his inability to sleep "normally" and watches the bedroom clock all night, keeping track of his sleep time to the minute. He has tried to "catch up" on his work while in bed. He also watches TV to see if it will lull him to sleep. His efforts remain unsuccessful. He feels sleepy during meetings in the office and drinks three to four cups of coffee during his afternoon meetings to be able to stay awake. His primary care physician has tried "everything possible" and is now referring the patient to your sleep clinic.
    Which of the following is correct regarding the management of his condition?
    A. PSG to rule out OSA and, if negative, institute stimulus control, sleep restriction, and sleep hygiene measures
    B. PSG followed by MSLT, and, if negative, institute stimulus control, sleep restriction, and sleep hygiene measures
    C. Sleep log and actigraphy followed by stimulus control, sleep restriction, and sleep hygiene measures
    D. Sleep log followed by stimulus control, sleep restriction, and sleep hygiene measures

14. All the following statements about the use of PSG in the evaluation of insomnia are true *except*:
    A. PSG is not useful in establishing a diagnosis of insomnia associated with fibromyalgia.
    B. PSG is not useful in the evaluation of insomnia.
    C. PSG is not useful in differentiating among different subtypes of insomnia.
    D. PSG is not useful except when the initial diagnosis is uncertain.

15. A 55-year-old male veteran is seen with symptoms of fatigue and EDS. His wife says that they have to sleep in different bedrooms because of his loud and heroic snoring. He frequently wakes up with a dry mouth and a headache. His symptoms have gotten worse along with increasing weight in the last 3–4 years. He is a current smoker and has a 40-pack-year history of smoking. Physical

examination reveals a pleasant gentleman who is obese with a body mass index (BMI) of 35 kg/m^2. His neck circumference is 18 inches. He has a large tongue and Mallampati IV airway classification. His pulmonary function studies reveal a forced expiratory volume in 1 second (FEV$_1$), which was 40% of predicted value, and a recent echocardiogram reveals estimated mean pulmonary artery pressure of 50 mm Hg. His arterial blood gas on room air revealed a pH of 7.3, PCO$_2$ of 55 mm Hg, PaO$_2$ of 55 mm Hg, and a bicarbonate level of 35 mm Hg. A PSG was performed, which revealed a sleep latency of 5 minutes, AHI of 35 events per hour of sleep, and an oxygen nadir of 65% compared with a baseline oxygen saturation of 92% on room air at rest. The sleep report states that the oxygen saturation remained persistently low, with a nadir of <80%, especially during REM sleep.

The appropriate next step in the management of this patient is:

A. Auto-titrating CPAP treatment
B. Unattended CPAP titration
C. Attended CPAP titration
D. Bilevel positive airway pressure (BiPAP) titration study

16. A 27-year-old female was referred to the sleep clinic for evaluation of EDS. The patient has always been a "sleepy kid" even as a child and has gotten into trouble for being tardy and not paying attention in class. On one occasion, when she was with a group of friends enjoying a joke, she suddenly felt weak in her limbs and dropped to the floor. She was conscious through this episode and quickly regained her strength. This episode has not since recurred. A few weeks earlier she woke up to find that she could not move at all except her eyes and only for a few minutes. Her husband says that she never snores. Physical exam demonstrates a weight of 130 lb and a height of 64 inches. Her neck circumference was 14 inches, and her oropharyngeal exam showed a Mallampati classification score of 1. The rest of her exam was unremarkable. She underwent a nocturnal PSG followed the next day by an MSLT. The PSG revealed an AHI of 2.1 events per hour of sleep, and her oxygenation nadir was 94%. Her MSLT revealed a mean sleep latency of 4.5 minutes and three sleep-onset REM periods. A diagnosis of narcolepsy was made.

In addition to adequate sleep hygiene and power naps, which of the following agents would you prescribe for this patient?

A. Methylphenidate, 30 mg/day
B. Pemoline, 37.5 mg/day
C. Baseline liver function tests followed by pemoline, 37.5 mg/day
D. Modafinil, 100–200 mg/day

17. A 30-year-old male software professional from India was seen after a recent motor vehicle accident in which he fell asleep at the wheel at a busy crossing. He and his wife emigrated from India and have lived in the United States for 15 years. His wife says she is worried about him because he feels unrested and sleepy during the day, even after getting a good night's sleep. His only medical problem is hypertension, for which he is on two different kinds of medications. She "envies" his ability to sleep anywhere and at any time. His sleep is associated with very loud snoring. The patient and his wife never thought that his symptoms were abnormal because his father and brothers also snored also and it was talked about as a family joke, rather than as a medical symptom. Recently, he has been unusually forgetful and irritable. His physical exam reveals a pleasant but tired-looking gentleman who weighs 140 lb and is 70 inches tall. His neck circumference was 16 inches. He had a retrognathic jaw with a Mallampati score of 3 and class two molar malocclusion. His blood pressure was 150/95 mm Hg, and his heart rate was 65 beats per minute. The rest of the exam was unremarkable. He underwent a PSG and his AHI was 85 events per hour and his oxygenation nadir was 65%. The patient and his wife were back in your clinic and wanted to discuss treatment options. The patient says that he prefers surgical treatment rather than the "mask" treatment so that the OSA can be cured permanently.

The next step in the management of this patient includes:

A. CPAP titration
B. Uvulopalatopharyngoplasty (UPPP) with tonsillectomy
C. UPPP without tonsillectomy
D. Bimandibular advancement surgery

18. Which of the following is an accurate statement regarding the role of PSG in patients with chronic obstructive pulmonary disease (COPD)?

A. PSG is routinely indicated in all patients with COPD to diagnose the "overlap syndrome."
B. PSG is routinely indicated in patients with severe COPD and cor pulmonale to diagnose the "overlap syndrome."
C. PSG is routinely indicated in patients with COPD and daytime hypoxemia and fatigue to diagnose the "overlap syndrome."

D. PSG is routinely indicated in patients with COPD who snore and are sleepy during the daytime to diagnose "overlap syndrome."

19. The beneficial effects of pramipexole in the treatment of RLS include all of the following except:
 A. Improvement in the sensory symptoms
 B. Improvement in the motor symptoms
 C. Improvement in sleep efficiency
 D. Improvement in periodic limb movements (PLMs)

20. A 50-year-old female was seen for evaluation of EDS. Her husband reports that she snores loudly and stops breathing and resumes breathing with a gasp. She is always tired and feels sleepy during periods of inactivity. Medical history is significant for hypertension and coronary artery disease. She has gained 50 pounds in the last 2 years. Her medications include hydrochlorothiazide, lisinopril, and aspirin. She doesn't smoke or use alcohol. She has no other complaints. On examination, she is obese, with a blood pressure of 145/90 mm Hg, and her heart rate was 64 beats per minute. She was afebrile and breathing comfortably at 16 times per minute. Oropharyngeal exam shows a Mallampati 3 airway classification and class two molar malocclusion. The rest of the exam was unremarkable. A PSG revealed an AHI of 24 events per hour and an oxygenation nadir of 85%. The study was also remarkable for periodic limb movements (PLMs), with a PLM index of 15/h.

 The next step in the management of this patient's PLMs is:

 A. CPAP titration alone
 B. Pramipexole alone
 C. CPAP titration along with pramipexole
 D. Check for iron levels and supplement if low.

21. PSG is routinely indicated as a diagnostic tool in all of the following conditions *except*:
 A. RLS
 B. Periodic limb movement disorder (PLMD)
 C. OSA
 D. Parasomnias

22. A 45-year-old female was referred for evaluation in the sleep clinic. She is being treated for a major depressive episode, and her psychiatrist wonders if a PSG can be performed to evaluate the effects of treatment of her depression. Her medical history is otherwise unremarkable, and she is currently not taking any medications except for the antidepressants prescribed by her psychiatrist. There is no history of snoring. She wakes up unrefreshed and feels tired all the time. Physical exam was unremarkable. Which of the following is true?
 A. PSG is routinely indicated in establishing a diagnosis of depression.
 B. PSG is routinely indicated to evaluate treatment response to depression.
 C. PSG is never indicated in either establishing a diagnosis or in follow-up evaluation of treatment response in depression.
 D. PSG may be indicated in the evaluation of patients with depression if a coexisting primary sleep disorder is suspected.

23. Which of the following statements is true with regards to sleep-monitoring devices in the diagnosis of OSA?
 A. Type 2 devices may be recommended in the preliminary screening of the general population for OSA in an attended setting.
 B. Type 2 devices may be recommended in the preliminary screening of the general population for OSA in an unattended setting.
 C. Type 3 devices may be recommended in the preliminary screening of the general population for OSA in an attended setting.
 D. Type 3 devices may be recommended in the preliminary screening of the general population for OSA in an unattended setting.

24. A 45-year-old male patient presents to your clinic with a history of loud snoring and apnea spells witnessed by his wife. He also complains of EDS. Physical exam is significant for a BMI of 31 kg/m^2 and neck circumference of 18 inches. He has a crowded oropharynx. The rest of the exam was unremarkable. He is a busy executive who could not find time for a sleep study and asks you if there are any other alternative tests that can be done to evaluate sleep at home. You use a portable monitoring device that is reported as negative for OSA with an respiratory disturbance index of less than five events per hour. Your next step should be:
 A. Reassure the patient that he does not have OSA.
 B. Repeat the sleep study since this could have been an atypical night.
 C. Repeat the sleep study using in-laboratory PSG.
 D. Reassure the patient that he has mild sleep apnea and recommend weight loss and positional treatment as options.

25. All of the following statements related to the use of actigraphy are true *except*:

A. Actigraphic studies should be conducted for a minimum of three consecutive 24-hour periods.

B. Interpretation must be done manually by visual inspection.

C. Actigraphy is an accepted modality for routine screening of patients with suspected circadian rhythm disorders.

D. Actigraphy is useful only for research purposes.

Answers

1. C. Perform PSG because of the history of snoring, witnessed apneas, hypertension, and stroke.

Option A is incorrect because a history of stroke by itself is not an indication for a PSG; however, it is an option in cases where clinical evaluation provides information that would make a diagnosis of OSA likely even in the absence of stroke. Evidence of an association between stroke and OSA is based on retrospective studies and case series. Similarly, option D is incorrect because it is not known whether a history of stroke and suspected OSA poses such a high risk for recurrent stroke as to warrant treatment without making a diagnosis first. Detailed clinical evaluation, which includes detailed sleep-wake cycles, history of snoring, witnessed apneas, and a physical examination, should be performed before obtaining a PSG. Option B is incorrect: Snoring and subjective sleepiness are common symptoms in the general population. The positive predictive value of snoring in one study was 0.63, with a negative predictive value of 0.56. The positive predictive value and negative predictive value for witnessed apneas were 0.40 and 0.60, respectively. Hence these symptoms cannot be relied on by themselves to rule in or rule out OSA. Routine use of an attended PSG is indicated in patients suspected of having sleep-related breathing disorders (SRBDs).

2. D. Patients not responsive to standard medical management of congestive heart failure

Some of the initial evidence for an association between sleep-disordered breathing and congestive heart failure was provided in a prospective evaluation of 45 patients with stable congestive heart failure (ejection fraction [EF] <45%) by Javaheri and colleagues. Almost 45% of these patients had OSA by PSG criteria of an AHI greater than 20 per hour. Another study by Chan et al found OSA in 55% of patients with an EF of greater than 45%, defined by an AHI greater than 10 per hour. The predictors of OSA in patients with congestive heart failure include a BMI >35 in men and age >60 years in women. Predictors of central sleep apnea (CSA) include male gender, presence of atrial fibrillation, and daytime hypocapnia or age >60. Among 46 consecutive patients who presented with pulmonary edema, 82% had SRBD, and of these, 75% had CSA and 25% had OSA. There is evidence of an association between heart failure and SRBDs, but the utility of using any of the criteria listed in options A, B, and C as an indication for PSG is not clear. At this time the standard indications for a PSG in patients with congestive heart failure include (1) patients who present with nocturnal symptoms suggestive of SRBDs, such as snoring, disturbed sleep, and EDS, and (2) patients who remain symptomatic despite optimal management of the congestive heart failure.

3. D. CPAP titration trial

Modafinil is a central nervous system stimulant that is indicated in the treatment of EDS in narcolepsy. Treating the symptom of EDS with a stimulant without treating the underlying cause is inappropriate. Hence option A is incorrect. Pramipexole and popinirole are dopaminergic agents used in the treatment of RLS. Oral iron supplementation may be indicated in patients with RLS whose serum ferritin level is less than 50 µg/dL. A diagnosis of RLS is made clinically based on the four criteria that are mandatory to make the diagnosis:

1. An urge to move the legs, usually accompanied by uncomfortable and unpleasant sensations in the legs
2. Uncomfortable sensations in the limbs that become worse during periods of rest or inactivity such as lying or sitting
3. The urge to move the legs or uncomfortable sensations that are partially or totally relieved by movement such as walking or stretching
4. The urge to move the legs or uncomfortable sensations that are worse in the evening or night than during the day (The symptoms may only occur in the evening or night.)

RLS is seen in about 10% of the general population. Part of the pathophysiologic basis for RLS is an abnormality in the body's use and storage of iron. Iron is needed in dopamine synthesis. The nadirs of iron and dopamine levels in the body correspond with the time of day when the RLS symptoms are at their worst. The anatomical sites in the brain involved in RLS are not clear, although there is some evidence for the involvement of the striatum (the putamen being a more likely site than the caudate nucleus). RLS can be seen in conditions associated with iron deficiency, including pregnancy, menstruation, chronic renal failure, gastrointestinal bleeding, etc. Evaluation of a patient with RLS should include measurement of serum ferritin levels and renal function. Treatment recommendations for RLS include the use of dopamine agonists (such as ropinirole and pramipexole) and dopamine precursors (carbidopa/levodopa). Options B and C are therefore incorrect because the patient does not have clinical criteria of RLS. The PSG description of leg movements in this patient meets the criteria for PLMs. Although 80% of patients with RLS have PLMs identified by PSG, only 20% of patients with PLMs also have RLS. The PLMs noted in this patient could be incidental associates of the respiratory disturbance, and her EDS is likely related to the OSA rather than the leg movements. The effect of CPAP treatment on PLMs may depend on the severity of OSA. In mild OSA the PLMs may resolve, and in cases of severe OSA the PLMs may actually be unmasked and become severe after CPAP treatment, in which case pharmacological treatment of PLMs may be indicated. Hence the appropriate next step is to perform CPAP titration, Option D.

4. D. Leg massages, iron, and folate

There is limited evidence for treatment of RLS in children and pregnant women. Iron and folate supplementation are reasonable approaches in pregnant women with RLS. Pharmacotherapy of RLS in pregnancy is problematic, as most of the effective therapies are category C drugs except for opioids. A more reasonable approach, given this patient's low iron storage, is to provide supplemental therapy with iron supplementation and folate, as well as conservative therapy with leg massages and a warm bath before bedtime. See explanation for question 3 also.

5. C. PSG followed by MSLT the next day

Narcolepsy is a neurological disorder that is characterized mainly by abnormalities in REM sleep. The estimated prevalence of narcolepsy in the general population is about 0.05%. The classic tetrad of narcolepsy includes hypersomnolence, cataplexy, hypnagogic hallucinations, and sleep paralysis. Human leukocyte antigen (HLA) DQB1–0602 marker is seen in more than 90% of individuals with narcolepsy, and a majority of them have abnormally low levels of hypcretin-1 (Orexin A) levels in the CSF. Objective evidence in the form of a mean sleep latency of less than 8 minutes and two or more sleep-onset REM periods (SOREMPs) on MSLT are useful in the diagnosis of narcolepsy. The sensitivity of two or more SOREMPs is 0.78 and specificity is 0.93 for narcolepsy. Reduced mean sleep latency and SOREMPs can occur in other sleep disorders such as OSA or severe sleep deprivation; hence it is important to perform PSG followed by MSLT the next day when evaluating for narcolepsy. The presence of cataplexy itself is diagnostic of narcolepsy and cataplexy, but sleep studies are still helpful in confirming the diagnosis. The HLA analysis and CSF analysis for hypocretin level may be used when there is no cataplexy or when all symptoms of narcolepsy are not present but is generally not indicated as an initial diagnostic option in patients with cataplexy as in this patient. Hence option D is incorrect. Options A and B are incorrect, as PSG or MSLT by themselves are less useful, as described previously.

6. B. Sleep clinic consultation

Recent studies have shown an association between tachyarrhythmias and bradyarrhythmias and SRBDs, both CSA and OSA. Kanagala and colleagues report that among patients with atrial fibrillation, a greater percentage of those with OSA had recurrence at the end of 12 months, and patients whose atrial fibrillation recurred spent more of their sleep-time in the hypoxic range. Similarly Fries and colleagues have shown that 40% of 40 patients had SRBD defined as an AHI of >10. Of patients with SRBD, 9 had CSA and 7 had OSA. At a 2-year follow-up evaluation, all of the patients with CSA and none with OSA died of various cardiac causes. Although these and other studies referenced show an association between SRBD and tachyarrhythmias and bradyarrhythmias, larger and longer studies are needed to draw more specific conclusions about a causal relationship. At this time PSG is recommended for patients with tachyarrhythmias or bradyarrhythmias if, after a clinical evaluation, it is found that they have symptoms of SRBD such as snoring, interrupted sleep, and EDS. Arrhythmia by itself is not an indication for PSG without the clinical evaluation. Hence option A is incorrect. Although this patient may need a PSG, it is not the first step. Nocturnal oximetry by itself has a limited utility in evaluation of suspected SRBD, and actigraphy has no role in the evaluation of SRBD; hence options C and D are incorrect.

7. B. "Polysomnography, with additional EEG derivations and video recording, is indicated in evaluating sleep-related behaviors that are violent or otherwise potentially injurious to the patient or others."

The AASM first published practice parameters for the performance of PSG for individual sleep disorders for the first time in 1997 and updated them in 2005 (Sleep 28:499, 2005). The Practice Parameters Committee reviewed the available evidence and categorized it as level I (randomized, well-designed trials with low alpha and beta error), level II (randomized trials with high alpha and beta errors), level III (nonrandomized, concurrently controlled studies), level IV (nonrandomized, historically controlled studies), and level V (case series). Based on the strength of the evidence, the recommendations are either:

- Standard: This is defined as generally accepted patient care strategy, which reflects a high degree of clinical certainty (usually level I or overwhelming level II evidence).
- Guideline: This is a patient care strategy that reflects a moderate degree of clinical certainty. It implies the use of level II or consensus of level III evidence.

- Option: This is a patient care strategy that reflects uncertain clinical use. This usually implies inconclusive or conflicting evidence or conflicting expert opinion.

Answers A, C, and D are standards, and Answer B is an option.

8. C. Liver failure

Pemoline is a central nervous system stimulant. Clinical uses include attention deficit disorder in children and narcolepsy. All the side effects listed in the question have been reported with the use of pemoline, but the one side effect that limits its usefulness is liver toxicity. Although uncommon, the liver toxicity can be lethal. The mechanism of hepatotoxicity is unknown, although autoimmune mechanisms and steroid responsiveness have been suggested. Careful risk-benefit analysis should precede the decision to use pemoline, and its use should be discouraged.

9. D. Further testing is not required at this time.

The appropriate follow-up evaluation of a patient diagnosed with OSA and treated with CPAP is clinical follow-up evaluation of symptom resolution. Repeating the PSG or performing an MSLT to assess for sleepiness is not routinely indicated. The appropriate use for MSLT is described next.

MSLT is a standard test for measuring sleepiness. It is based on the premise that sleep latency reflects the degree of sleepiness. The recommendations for conducting an MSLT are as follows:

- The test consists of five naps at 2-hour intervals. The initial nap begins 1.5–3 hours after termination of the nocturnal PSG recording.
- The MSLT should always be performed in conjunction with the nocturnal PSG, performed the previous night.
- Stimulant medications and REM-suppressant medications should ideally be stopped at least 2 weeks before the test.
- The conventional recording montage includes the following leads: Central and occipital electroencephalogram (EEG), electro-oculogram (EOG), mental and submental electromyogram (EMG), and electrocardiogram (ECG).
- Sleep onset for the clinical MSLT is determined from the time for lights out to the first epoch of any stage of sleep. The absence of sleep in a nap opportunity is counted as a sleep latency of 20 minutes. REM-sleep latency is determined by continuing sleep for 15 minutes after sleep onset. The duration of 15 minutes is determined by "clock time" and not by sleep time. REM-sleep

latency is also taken as the first epoch of sleep to the beginning of the first epoch of REM-sleep regardless of the intervening stages of sleep or wakefulness.

The AASM practice parameter statement regarding the indication for MSLT indicates that it is part of the evaluation of patients with suspected narcolepsy or idiopathic hypersomnia. It also states that the MSLT is *not* routinely indicated in the initial evaluation of OSA syndrome or in association in assessment of change after treatment with nasal CPAP. MSLT remains a poor discriminator of response to treatment. If the symptoms of EDS or impaired sleepiness persists despite adequate treatment of OSA with nasal CPAP, and inadequate sleep or other causes of sleepiness have been ruled out by clinical evaluation, and narcolepsy remains in the differential diagnosis, then the MSLT may have a role. But in this patient who has responded well to the treatment of OSA with nasal CPAP, further testing including MSLT is not routinely indicated.

10. B. Actigraphy is routinely indicated for the diagnosis, assessment, and severity of RLS.

Actigraphy is a method to study sleep-wake patterns. A device is worn on the wrist that uses an accelerometer, a portable device that records movement over extended periods of time.

Based on one level I and two level II studies, actigraphy is considered "reliable," and based on two level 1 and two level two studies, it is considered "valid." (Please refer to question #7 for explanation about the levels of evidence.) However, actigraphy is not indicated for the "routine" diagnosis and assessment of any sleep disorder. Hence option B is wrong (i.e., the correct answer to this question). Options A, C, and D are adapted from Sleep 26(3):337–341, 2003.

11. A. Light therapy may have a potential role in the treatment of this condition.

The diagnosis for the patient described in this question is compatible with delayed sleep phase syndrome (DSPS). DSPS is a circadian rhythm disorder in which difficulty waking up in the morning is the usual presenting complaint. Patients also complain of daytime sleepiness. A detailed history of the sleep-wake schedule reveals that they sleep normally over the weekends. Sleep log can be confirmatory. DSPS is generally seen in younger individuals. According to one theory proposed by Weitzman and colleagues, a few days of delayed sleep onset, resulting from late bedtime in college life, may result in phase delay, and the impaired phase-shifting capacity prevents resumption of normal schedule, resulting in DSPS. Phototherapy or light therapy is one of the potential options for the treatment of DSPS. Light exposure is generally recommended between 6 and 9 A.M., which corresponds with the body temperature nadir. The recommended light intensity is between 2000 and 2500 lux. The minimum or optimal duration of light therapy, at present, is unknown. Side effects of light therapy include eye irritation, headache, nausea, and dryness of eyes and the skin. In patients with bipolar disorder, light exposure may rarely provoke a hypomanic state.

12. D. A second-night PSG with CPAP titration is performed to confirm the appropriate setting identified during the split-night study.

Full-night PSG is generally indicated for CPAP titration in patients with OSA; however, in certain circumstances a split-night study may be indicated. Options A, B, and C are appropriate criteria justifying a split-night study. The fourth criterion is that a second-night study is indicated if criteria given in options B and C are not met, when CPAP titration was performed for less than 3 hours, or REM and supine positions were not evaluated.

13. D. Sleep log, followed by stimulus control, sleep restriction, and sleep hygiene measures

The clinical picture presented in this case is compatible with chronic insomnia in the form of psychophysiologic insomnia. The defining features with this type of insomnia are somatized tension or heightened arousal and learned sleep-preventing associations. The individual is generally preoccupied with the need to sleep "normally" and focuses excessively on sleeping. This results in a state of heightened arousal and anxiety that prevent sleep, and this becomes a self-perpetuating cycle. The patient may complain of difficulties with sleep initiation and EDS owing to the resultant sleep deprivation. Poor sleep hygiene also is frequently an associated factor, as is seen in this patient. Spielman provided a model to explain the basis for chronic insomnia in which he proposed that susceptible individuals predisposed to develop insomnia cross the "insomnia threshold" and present with insomnia when subjected to precipitating factors (i.e., life stress, as in this patient with business setbacks). The insomnia persists even after the precipitating factors have resolved. This is now a state of chronic insomnia and is sustained by perpetuating factors, which consist of futile efforts by the patients to improve sleep, poor sleep hygiene, heightened arousal, and excessive focus on sleeping and other learned sleep-preventing associations.

Recommendations for the nonpharmacological management of chronic insomnia include stimulus control (standard), sleep restriction, and sleep hygiene measures. Examples of good sleep hygiene include having regular sleep and wake times 7 days a week, using the bedroom for sleep or sex only, and avoiding stimulants such as caffeine or severe exercise close to bedtime. A sleep log, in which the patient documents the daily sleep and wakeup times and activities at times when unable to sleep, may be helpful in providing a measure of daily sleep routine. PSG or the MSLT is generally not indicated in the evaluation of primary insomnia unless there are symptoms suggestive of an underlying SRBD or other primary sleep disorders.

14. B. PSG is not useful in the evaluation of insomnia.

PSG is generally not indicated in the routine evaluation of chronic insomnia, but it is indicated when an SRBD or other primary sleep disturbances such as PLMs are suspected in the differential diagnosis. All the other options are acceptable recommendations by the practice parameters for the use of PSG to evaluate insomnia (Sleep 6:754, 2003).

15. C. Attended CPAP titration

CPAP is the most commonly used treatment option for patients with OSA. The standard of care at this time is to perform an attended CPAP titration, using full PSG to obtain a single fixed-pressure setting. Auto-titrating devices (APAP) use a new technology to continuously adjust the pressure within a defined range based on an algorithm that detects airflow limitation. Auto-titrating CPAP units can be used to obtain a single pressure setting or as self-adjusting devices. The recommendations of the Standards of Practice Committee for the use of APAP are as follows:

1. A diagnosis of OSAS must be established by an acceptable method.
2. APAP titration and treatment are not currently recommended for patients with congestive heart failure, significant lung disease (e.g. COPD), daytime hypoxemia and respiratory failure from any cause, or prominent nocturnal desaturation other than from OSA (i.e., obesity hypoventilation).
3. APAP devices are currently not recommended for split-night studies because of the lack of data and research studies examining this issue.
4. Certain APAP devices may be used during attended CPAP titration to identify by PSG a single pressure for use with standard CPAP for treatment of OSA.
5. Once an initial successful attended CPAP or APAP titration has been determined by PSG, certain APAP devices may be used in the self-adjusting mode for unattended treatment of patients with OSA.

6. The use of unattended APAP to initially determine pressures for fixed CPAP or self-adjusting APAP treatment in CPAP-naïve patients is not currently established.

7. Patients being treated with fixed CPAP on the basis of APAP titration or being treated with APAP must be followed to determine the effectiveness and safety.

8. A reevaluation and, if necessary, a standard attended CPAP titration should be performed if symptoms do not resolve or if treatment with CPAP or APAP otherwise appears to lack efficacy.

16. D. Modafinil, 100–200 mg/day

Narcolepsy is an uncommon disease whose clinical importance is in excess of its prevalence. Narcolepsy is characterized by the symptom of severe pathological EDS. It is considered to be a disease of abnormalities in the boundaries between the states of REM sleep and wakefulness. The intrusion of REM atonia into the wakeful state results in cataplexy, which this patient describes. Other symptoms include sleep paralysis and hypnogogic or hypnopompic hallucinations (i.e., hallucinations at sleep onset while awakening from sleep, respectively). Together these form the "narcolepsy tetrad." When making the diagnosis of narcolepsy, other causes of EDS should be carefully sought and excluded. A diagnostic PSG performed on the night before the MSLT helps in excluding SRBDs. With the discovery of neurotransmitters, orexin (hypocretin) system in the hypothalamus, it was shown that the deficiency of these neurotransmitters resulted in narcolepsy and provided a new understanding of the pathogenesis of narcolepsy. The management of this potentially disabling condition requires attention to sleep hygiene, social and occupational issues such as avoiding occupations that involve working with dangerous machinery or at heights and pharmacological treatment for the symptoms of EDS, as well as cataplexy when present.

The mainstay of treatment of EDS includes the use of stimulants.

The stimulants used traditionally include pemoline or cylert, methylphenidate (Ritalin), amphetamine, methamphetamine, and a newer agent, modafinil. Modafinil is perhaps safest of all the agents listed and is the preferred agent to treat narcolepsy. Its mode of action is probably via gamma-aminobutyric acid (GABA) receptors. Its interaction with oral contraceptives is an important issue, and patients given modafinil should be warned that oral contraceptives may fail. Unpredictable and lethal hepatotoxicity is the biggest limiting factor in the use of pemoline. With the availability of safer agents, it should never be a drug of first choice in the treatment of narcolepsy. The following paragraph is a direct quote of the current Food and Drug Administration (FDA) recommendations regarding the use of pemoline.

On October 24, 2005, the FDA concluded that the overall risk of liver toxicity from Cylert and generic pemoline products outweighs the benefits of this drug. In May 2005, Abbott chose to stop sales and marketing of Cylert in the U.S. All generic companies have also agreed to stop sales and marketing of this product. Cylert, a central nervous system stimulant indicated for the treatment of attention deficit hyperactivity disorder (ADHD), is considered second-line therapy for ADHD. Because of its association with life-threatening hepatic failure, health care professionals who prescribe Cylert, or any of its generics, should transition their patients to an alternative therapy. Cylert will remain available through pharmacies and wholesalers until supplies are exhausted. No additional product will be available thereafter. See the FDA website for more information.

17. A. CPAP titration

CPAP is the most efficacious mode of treatment for OSA. However, the compliance in the use of CPAP is generally low. In patients who are unable to tolerate CPAP or for those who are unwilling to use it, alternative treatment options may be considered. Several surgical options exist and are of variable efficacy. The location of pharyngeal narrowing or collapse in patients afflicted with OSA varies among patients. Patterns of airway narrowing or collapse can be classified into the following types: type I, narrowing or collapse in the retropalatal region; type II, narrowing or collapse in both retropalatal and retrolingual regions; and type III, narrowing or collapse in the retrolingual region only. Most of the surgical techniques for treating OSA modify either the retropalatal or retrolingual region of the pharyngeal airway.

UPPP enlarges the retropalatal airway. It involves trimming and reorienting of the posterior and anterior tonsillar pillars. The uvula and posterior portion of the palate are excised.

Laser midline glossectomy and lingualplasty are two procedures that enlarge the retrolingual airway size. Inferior sagittal mandibular osteotomy and genioglossal advancement with hyoid myotomy and suspension consists of two parts: inferior sagittal mandibular osteotomy and genioglossal advancement, and hyoid myotomy and suspension. The two components of the procedure create an enlarged retrolingual airway. In maxillomandibular osteotomy and advancement, the maxilla and mandible are simultaneously advanced through sagittal split osteotomies. Tracheotomy creates a direct percutaneous opening into the trachea. The diameter of the stoma is usually stented and maintained by means of a rigid or semirigid hollow tube that extends to the body surface.

The most important aspect of surgical treatment is that there should be adequate discussion with the patient about the options, known efficacy, and long-term outcomes, which are under investigation at present.

18. D. PSG is routinely indicated in patients who have chronic obstructive pulmonary disease (COPD) and in addition have symptoms of snoring and excessive daytime sleepiness.

At this time PSG is not routinely indicated in patients with COPD unless coexisting symptoms raise concern for OSA. The prevalence of OSA in patients with COPD is similar to that of the general population, although the coexistence of both disorders in the same patient can result in profound nocturnal hypoxemia, especially during REM sleep. This can potentially result in an accelerated course toward pulmonary hypertension and cor pulmonale. The coexistence of OSA and COPD has been termed the "overlap" REM sleep and is characterized by skeletal muscle atonia. Patients with emphysema who have dysfunctional diaphragms have to depend on the diaphragm as the sole source of respiratory effort. This can result in significant hypoventilation and hypoxemia.

19. C. Improvement in sleep efficiency

RLS is a clinical diagnosis that depends on four cardinal symptoms (Sleep 27[3]:560–583, 2004).

1. An urge to move the legs, usually accompanied or caused by uncomfortable and unpleasant sensations in the legs
2. The urge to move or unpleasant sensations begin or worsen during periods of rest or inactivity such as lying or sitting
3. The urge to move or unpleasant sensations that are partially or totally relieved by movement, such as walking or stretching
4. The urge to move or unpleasant sensations that are worse in the evening or night than during the day or only occur in the evening or night

The current understanding of the pathophysiology of RLS indicates an abnormality in the body's ability to store and use iron, which plays an important role in dopamine metabolism. Pramipexole is a dopaminergic agent that is a useful therapeutic option for the treatment of RLS.

20. A. CPAP titration alone

RLS is a sensory motor disorder characterized by abnormal and uncomfortable sensations in the limbs

that occurs or is worse when at rest and improves or resolves with exercise. PLMs, on the other hand, are limb movements with a characteristic pattern, observed during PSG while asleep. Almost 80% of patients with RLS can have PLMs at night, but only 20% of patients with PLMs have the daytime subjective counterpart of RLS. Treatment of RLS is generally recommended, but the indication for treatment of PLMs alone is less clear. When PLMs coexist with OSA, as in this patient, they may be considered an epiphenomenon, and treatment of the OSA is expected to help resolve the PLMs; hence the correct answer is CPAP titration alone.

21. A. RLS

RLS is a clinical diagnosis and relies on fulfilling the standard clinical criteria (described in the explanation for Question 19). PLMD is a PSG diagnosis; 80% of patients with RLS also have PLMs, but only 20% of patients with PLMs have RLS. PSG is indicated when a diagnosis of PLMD is considered.

Please also refer to the explanation provided for Question 20.

22. D. PSG may be indicated in the evaluation of patients with depression if a coexisting primary sleep disorder is suspected.

Depression can alter the sleep architecture, and antidepressant medications may result in changes in the sleep architecture. The changes related to depression may include paucity of slow wave sleep and reduced REM sleep latency. Similarly, antidepressant medications may result in changes to the sleep architecture. As an example, recovery from depression may result in increased slow wave sleep. However, none of these changes are specific enough to be helpful in either the establishment of depression or in the follow-up evaluation of treatment response. The fatigue and unrestful sleep may be seen in other primary sleep disorders such as SRBD, and hence a diagnostic PSG may have a role in patients with depression if there are symptoms suggestive of an underlying primary sleep disorder.

23. C. Type 3 devices may be recommended in the preliminary screening of the general population for OSA in an attended setting.

The gold standard for the diagnosis of OSA is an attended in-laboratory PSG using multiple channels. Because of the increasing demand for services and inadequate availability of the gold-standard procedure, there is ongoing discussion and debate about the utility of portable monitors for the screening or establishment of a diagnosis of OSA. Portable monitors can be classified into three categories: type 2, type 3, and type 4. The gold standard in laboratory PSG is referred to as a type 1 device. Type 2 has a minimum of seven channels, including EEG, EOG, EMG, ECG or heart rate, airflow, respiratory effort, and oxygen saturation. Type 3 has a minimum of four channels, including ventilation or airflow (at least two channels of respiratory movement, or respiratory movement and airflow), heart rate or ECG and oxygen saturation). Type 4 has a single parameter or two parameters that are generally measured. Using the in-laboratory PSG as a gold standard, these three types of portable monitors were reviewed for the ability to detect OSA when defined as an AHI <15 events per hour. The comparison was made both in attended and unattended settings. Type 3 portable monitors may be useful especially in an attended setting for the diagnosis of OSA. This device is not recommended in patients with cardiorespiratory co-morbidities such as congestive heart failure or COPD. Furthermore, when these devices are used, raw data should be carefully reviewed, and if there is a negative test in the presence of high clinical suspicion, this should be confirmed using a type 1 test.

24. C. Repeat the sleep study using in-laboratory PSG

The recommended gold-standard method for diagnosis of OSA is in-laboratory PSG. Any other alternative device, including a wide range of portable monitoring devices that are becoming available, must be compared against the gold standard. The basic point is that if a sleep study is conducted using a portable device that is reported as negative for OSA, in the presence of high pretest probability of having OSA as in this patient, the test has to be repeated using the gold standard (i.e., in-laboratory PSG); hence option B is the correct answer.

There is insufficient information in this question to be able to effectively compare the utility of the device used. However, the general principles and issues involved in making such a determination are discussed.

Sensitivity, specificity, and positive and negative predictive values are commonly used and are useful statistical measures when evaluating a test against an existing gold standard. This can be summarized using a 2 × 2 table where, by convention, the gold standard

reference measure is indicated at the top row, and the new test being evaluated is placed to the left of the table. What is of interest in this paradigm to the clinician is the probability that a patient with a positive test in fact has the disease (i.e., positive predictive value) and the patient that has a negative test truly does not have the disease (i.e., negative predictive value).

Several factors can influence the sensitivity and specificity of a test. For example, varying what constitutes a positive or negative test can change the sensitivity and specificity. Using a high threshold can increase specificity but will decrease the sensitivity. Conversely, lowering the threshold will increase the sensitivity but will diminish specificity. Thus, while evaluating the literature on the utility of a test or device against an accepted gold standard, the clinician should carefully take these factors into account. If a test is negative in the face of a high pretest probability, the test has to be repeated using the gold standard. Excluding a diagnosis of OSA solely based on the findings of the portable monitoring device is unacceptable. Similarly, saying that he has mild sleep apnea is also inappropriate. OSA is a disease with a wide spectrum of severity and using an arbitrary number such as respiratory disturbance index or AHI, which measures only one dimension of the disease, can underestimate the clinical significance of the disease.

25. C. Actigraphy is an accepted modality for routine screening of patients with suspected circadian rhythm disorders.

Actigraphy is a wrist-worn device that detects physical motion (accelerometer) and stores the resulting information. It has been used in sleep research as a tool to measure sleep disturbances including insomnia and circadian rhythm disorders. Actigraphy may be a useful adjunct, along with a thorough clinical evaluation, in the assessment of sleep disorders such as insomnia or circadian rhythm disorders. Actigraphy, however, is not recommended for "routine use" in the assessment of any sleep disorder; hence option C is the correct answer. Although actigraphy is generally accepted as a reasonable research tool, its routine clinical use at present is not clear and it may have an adjunctive role clinically.

REFERENCES

1. A review by the Restless Legs Syndrome Task Force of the American Academy of Sleep Medicine. An update on the dopaminergic treatment of restless legs syndrome and periodic limb movement disorder. Sleep 27(3): 560–583, 2004.

2. Allen RP, Pichietti D, Henning WA, et al: Restless legs syndrome: diagnostic criteria, special considerations and epidemiology. A report from the restless legs syndrome diagnosis and epidemiology workshop at the National Institute of Health. Sleep Med 4(2):121–132, 2003.

3. American Academy of Sleep Medicine: *International Classification of Sleep Disorders*, 2nd ed. *Diagnostic and Coding Manual*. Westchester, IL, American Academy of Sleep Medicine, 2005.

4. American Sleep Disorders Association Standards of Practice Committee: Practice parameters for the indications for polysomnography and related procedures. Sleep 20:406–422, 1997.

5. Baran AS, Richert AC, Douglass AB, May W: Change in periodic limb movement index during treatment of OSA with continuous positive airway pressure. Sleep 26(6):717–720, 2003.

6. Basetti C, Aldrich MS: Sleep apnea in acute cerebrovascular diseases: final report on 128 patients. Sleep 22(2):217–223, 1999.

7. Boetz MI, Lambert B: Folate deficiency and restless legs syndrome in pregnancy. N Engl J Med 297:670, 1977.

8. Bonnet M, Carley D, Carskadon M, et al: Recording and scoring leg movements. ASDA report. Sleep 16(8): 748–759, 1993.

9. Chan J, Sanderson J, Chan W, et al: Prevalence of sleep-disordered breathing in diastolic heart failure. Chest 111(6):1488–1493, 1997.

10. Deegan PC, McNicholas WT: Predictive value of clinical features for the obstructive sleep apnea syndrome. Eur Respir J 9(1):117–124, 1996.

11. Dyken ME, Sommers VK, Yamada T, et al: Investigating the relationship between stroke and obstructive sleep apnea. Stroke 27(3):401–407, 1996.

12. Exar EN, Collop NA: The association of upper airway resistance with periodic limb movements. Sleep 24(2): 188–192, 2001.

13. Ferber RA, Millman RP, Coppola MP, et al: ASDA standards of practice: portable recording in the assessment of obstructive sleep apnea. Sleep 17:378–392, 1994.

14. Flemons WW, Littner MR: Measuring agreement between diagnostic devices. Chest 124:1535–1542, 2003.

15. Fries R, Bauer D, Heisel A, et al: Clinical significance of sleep related breathing disorders in patients with implantable cardioverter defibrillators. Pacing Clin Electrophysiol 22(1 pt 2):223–227, 1999.

16. Good DC, Henkle JQ, Gelber D, et al: Sleep disordered breathing and poor functional outcome after stroke. Stroke 27(2):252–259, 1996.

17. Haram K, Nilsen ST, Ulvik RJ: Iron supplementation in pregnancy—evidence and controversies. Acta Obstet Gynecol Scand 80:683–688, 2001.

18. Hublin C, Partinen M, Kaprio J, et al: Epidemiology of narcolepsy. Sleep 17:S7–S12, 1994.

19. Javaheri S, Parket TJ, Wexler L, et al: Occult sleep-disordered breathing in stable congestive heart failure. Ann Intern Med 122(7):487–492, 1995.

20. Kanagala R, Murali NS, Friedman PA, et al: Obstructive sleep apnea and the recurrence of atrial fibrillation. Circulation 107(200):2589–2594, 2003.

21. Kushida CA, Littner MR, Morgenthaler T, et al: Practice parameters for indications for polysomnography and related procedures: an update for 2005. Sleep 28(4): 499–521, 2005.

22. Littner M, Hirshkowitz M, Kramer M: Practice parameters for using polysomnography to evaluate insomnia: an update. Sleep 6:754–760, 2003.

23. Littner M, Johnson SF, MacCall WV, et al: Practice parameters for the treatment of narcolepsy: an update for 2000. Sleep 24(4):451–466, 2001.

24. Littner M, Kushida CA, Anderson WM, et al: Practice parameters for the role of actigraphy in the study of sleep and circadian rhythms: an update for 2002. Sleep 26(3):337–341, 2003.

25. Littner M, Kushida CA, Wise M, et al: Practice parameters for clinical use of the Multiple Sleep Latency test and the Maintenance of Wakefulness Test. Sleep 28(1):112–121, 2005.

26. Mansfield DR, Gollogy NC, Kaye DM, et al: Controlled trial of continuous positive airway pressure in obstructive sleep apnea and heart failure. Am J Respir Crit Care Med 169(3):361–366, 2004.

27. Montplaisir J, Boucher S, Poirier G, et al: Clinical, polysomnographic, and genetic characteristics of restless legs syndrome: a study of 133 patients diagnosed with new standard criteria. Mov Disord 12(1):61–65, 1997.

28. Montplaisir J, Nicolas A, Denesle R, Gomez-Mancilla B: Restless legs syndrome improved by pramipexole: a double-blind randomized trial. Neurology 52(5):938–943, 1999.

29. Mooe T, Gullsby S, Rabben T, Eriksson P: Sleep-disordered breathing: a novel predictor of atrial fibrillation after coronary artery bypass. Coron Artery Dis 7(6):475–478, 1996.

30. Nicholas A, Lesperance P, Montplaisir J: Is excessive day time sleepiness with periodic leg movements during sleep a specific diagnostic category? Eur Neurol 40(1):22–687, 1998.

31. Nishino S, Ripley B, Overem S, et al: Hypocretin (Orexin) deficiency in human narcolepsy. Lancet 355(9197): 39–40, 2000.

32. Phillips B, Young T, Finn L, et al: Epidemiology of restless legs symptoms in adults. Arch Intern Med 160(14): 2137–2141, 2000.

33. Pien GW, Schwab RJ: Sleep disorders during pregnancy. Sleep 27(7):1405–1417, 2004.

34. Puliot Z, Peters M, Neufeld H, Kryger MH: Using self-reported questionnaire data to prioritize OSA patients for polysomnography. Sleep 20(3):232–236, 1997.

35. Review by the MSLT and MWT Taskforce of the Standards of Practice Committee of American Academy of Sleep Medicine. Sleep 28(1):123–144, 2005.

36. Rosh JR, Dellert SF, Narkewicz M, et al: Four cases of severe hepatotoxicity associated with pemoline: possible

autoimmune pathogenesis. Pediatrics 101(5):921–923, 1998.

37. Shahar E, Whitney CW, Redline S, et al: Sleep-disordered breathing and cardiovascular disease: cross sectional results of the Sleep Heart Health Study. Am J Respir Crit Care Med 163(1):19–25, 2001.

38. Spielman AJ: Assessment of insomnia. Clin Psychol Rev 6:11, 1986.

39. Standards of Practice Committee of the American Academy of Sleep Medicine: Practice parameters for clinical use of the multiple sleep latency test and the maintenance of wakefulness test. Sleep 28(1):113–121, 2005.

40. Standards of Practice Committee of the American Academy of Sleep Medicine: Practice parameters for the dopaminergic treatment of restless legs syndrome and periodic limb movement disorder. Sleep 27(3):557–559, 2004.

41. Standards of Practice Committee of the American Academy of Sleep Medicine: Practice parameters for the role of actigraphy in the study of sleep and circadian rhythms: an update for 2002. Sleep 26(3):337–341, 2003.

42. Standards of Practice Committee of the American Academy of Sleep Medicine: Practice parameters for the treatment of narcolepsy: an update for 2000. Sleep 24:451–466, 2001.

43. Standards of Practice Committee of the American Academy of Sleep Medicine: Practice parameters for the use of light therapy in the treatment of sleep disorders. Sleep 22:641–660, 1999.

44. Stegman SS, Burroughs JM, Henthorn RW: Asymptomatic bradyarrhythmias as a marker for sleep apnea: appropriate recognition and treatment may reduce the need for pacemaker therapy. Pacing Clin Electrophysiol 19(6):899–904, 1996.

45. Sun Er, Chen CA, HO G, Allen RP: Iron and the restless legs syndrome. Sleep 21(4):371–374, 1998.

46. Thorpy M, et al: Practice parameters for the treatment of obstructive sleep apnea in adults: the efficacy of surgical modifications of the upper airway. Sleep 19:152–155, 1996.

47. Tremel F, Pepin JL, Veale D, et al: High prevalence and persistence of sleep apnea in patients referred for acute left ventricular failure and medically treated for over 2 months. Eur Heart J 20(16):1201–1209, 1999.

48. Weitzman ED, Czeisler CA, Coleman RM, et al: Delayed sleep phase syndrome. A chronobiological disorder with sleep onset insomnia. Arch Gen Psychiatry 38:737, 1981.

Literature Review 2003–2006

DANIEL A. COHEN ■ JEAN K. MATHESON

Questions

1. A 54-year-old woman reports a several-year history of an uncomfortable sensation in her legs associated with an urge to move, occurring primarily at night when lying in bed. On the basis of current clinical diagnostic criteria for restless legs syndrome (RLS), which of the following is the most appropriate question to help confirm the diagnosis?
   A. Has anyone noticed your legs twitching during sleep?
   B. Is there a family history of similar symptoms?
   C. Are symptoms improved by moving your legs?
   D. Are symptoms exacerbated by caffeine?

2. When normal sleeping subjects are awakened from non-rapid eye movement (NREM) sleep, they often report very little conscious recollection. This is in contrast to the reports obtained after arousal from rapid eye movement (REM) sleep, which tend to be long and vivid in their description. Which of the following mechanisms may be responsible for the reduction in conscious recollection during NREM sleep?
   A. Decreased neuronal firing synchrony across distributed cortical networks
   B. Decreased effective connectivity across distributed cortical networks
   C. Increased global cerebral metabolism
   D. Complete blockade of sensory signals from reaching the cerebral cortex

3. A 35-year-old woman presents with a complaint of poor quality, nonrestorative sleep with prolonged awakenings. She has a remote history of unpleasant sensations in the legs while watching television at night, and she would frequently shift position of her legs to get comfortable. This symptom has resolved with iron supplementation. A polysomnogram (PSG) was notable for 186 leg movements, each greater than 25% of the calibration amplitude, occurring in long clusters every 15–20 seconds for the first 3 hours of sleep. The majority of movements immediately preceded arousals. Which of the following statements is *most* accurate?
   A. Continuous positive airway pressure (CPAP) is recommended to minimize respiratory-related movement arousals.
   B. Dopamine agonists are likely to substantially improve sleep quality.
   C. Benzodiazepine receptor agonists are the treatment of choice.
   D. Stimulus control therapy is recommended for her sleep-maintenance insomnia.

4. Which of the following best characterizes the physiologic differences between patients with insomnia and normal sleepers?
   A. Insomnia is associated with an increase in anterior cingulate metabolism during REM sleep.
   B. Insomnia is associated with a relative increase in prefrontal metabolism during wakefulness.
   C. Insomnia is associated with decreased whole brain metabolism during wakefulness.
   D. Insomnia is associated with increased thalamic metabolism during wake-sleep transitions.

5. Which of the following best characterizes the relationship between cerebrospinal fluid (CSF) ferritin subunits in patients with RLS?
   A. CSF H and L ferritin subunits are decreased in early-onset (age < 45) RLS.
   B. CSF H and L ferritin subunits are increased in early-onset (age < 45) RLS.
   C. CSF H and L ferritin subunits are decreased in late-onset (age ≥ 45) RLS.
   D. CSF H and L ferritin subunits are increased in late-onset (age ≥ 45) RLS.

6. Which of the following statements reflects the association between sleep-disordered breathing (SDB) and menopausal status in women?
   A. The decline in progesterone increases upper airway muscle tone and reduces collapsibility.

B. Postmenopausal status is independently associated with increasing risk of SDB.

C. Fat redistribution after menopause reduces abdominal fat and neck girth, conferring relative protection from SDB.

D. After controlling for age, there is no association between menopausal status and SDB.

7. Despite adequate treatment of severe obstructive sleep apnea-hypopnea syndrome with CPAP, excessive somnolence may persist. Which of the following is the most plausible explanation?

A. Oxidative damage to wake-promoting neurons secondary to intermittent hypoxia

B. Recurrent ischemia and lacunar infarction in diffuse neuronal regions

C. Chronic hypoventilation and hypercarbia

D. Secondary adrenal insufficiency

8. A 19-year-old college student complains of difficulty waking for classes this semester. Previously, she was able to schedule her first class at 11:00 A.M. but now must attend class at 8:30 A.M. 3 days per week. She generally finds her most productive study time to be 9 P.M. to midnight, and she has trouble falling asleep before 2:00 A.M. Which of the following treatment options is recommended?

A. Dark shades and an eye mask to minimize early morning sunlight

B. Melatonin administration on awakening to advance the circadian clock

C. Melatonin administration at 11:00 P.M.

D. Melatonin administration at 8:00 P.M.

9. Which of the following physiologic disturbances in obstructive sleep apnea (OSA) most strongly correlates with the degree of carotid intima-media thickness, a marker of preclinical atheroma?

A. Plasma homocysteine level

B. Arousal index

C. Mean nocturnal oxygen saturation

D. Sympathetic nerve activity

10. Which of the following statements best characterizes the association between sleep apnea and the inflammatory cytokines C-reactive protein (CRP) and interleukin-6 (IL-6)?

A. CRP and IL-6 levels are elevated in sleep apnea, and they correlate with the degree of sleep disruption as measured by the arousal index and percentage of stage 1 sleep.

B. CRP and IL-6 levels are elevated in patients with sleep apnea, but this association is explained by increased body mass index (BMI).

C. CRP and IL-6 levels are elevated in patients with sleep apnea and are lowered by treatment with nasal CPAP.

D. CRP and IL-6 levels are elevated in patients with sleep apnea, but there is no correlation with the severity of the SDB.

11. OSA is characterized by repeated upper airway collapse during sleep. Which of the following has been demonstrated in the upper airway of patients with sleep apnea relative to controls?

A. Inflammatory infiltrates restricted to the upper airway mucosa

B. Heightened responses to tactile and thermal stimuli to the upper airway

C. Hypertrophy and increased contractile force in pharyngeal muscles

D. Inflammatory infiltration and denervation of upper airway muscles

12. A 25-year-old anxious man presents with a complaint of disturbing dreams. These are described as images of snakes and various insects crawling over him. Within 2 hours of falling asleep, he suddenly jolts upright in bed, with a fearful expression and incoherent mumbling for a few seconds as he attempts to brush the animals away. Rarely he may get out of bed and wake to find himself near the bedroom door. These occur roughly three times per month, and he does not recall similar episodes as a child. He reports significant job-related stress, concerns over his current relationship, too little time to exercise, and recent weight gain. What is the most appropriate *next* step?

A. Referral to a psychotherapist

B. Prescribe clonazepam, 0.5 mg, before bed.

C. Order a PSG.

D. Order a sleep-deprived electroencephalogram (EEG) with mini-sphenoidal electrodes.

13. A 33-year-old accountant states that she has had trouble falling asleep for the past year. She finds herself lying in bed, desperately trying to fall asleep. She repeatedly looks at the clock and worries that she will not get the necessary 8 hours of sleep unless she falls asleep soon. She frequently changes position out of frustration. This process may span over an hour before she sleeps. If she wakes to go to the bathroom, which occurs every few nights, she finds it difficult to return to sleep. Which of the following treatments is recommended?

A. Ropinirole 0.25 mg

B. Paroxetine 20 mg

C. Zolpidem 10 mg

D. Cognitive behavioral therapy

14. Narcolepsy with cataplexy is associated with a deficiency of the hypothalamic neuropeptide orexin (hypocretin). Which of the following best describes the current evidence for the role of the orexin deficiency in the sleepiness of narcolepsy?
    A. Inadequate activation of arousal regions
    B. Low threshold for behavioral state transitions (REM, NREM, wake)
    C. Poor circadian control of sleep and wakefulness
    D. Increased sleep pressure secondary to abnormal sleep homeostasis

15. Which of the following statements is true regarding the efficacy of oral appliance therapy for OSA?
    A. A better success rate is seen in patients with more severe sleep apnea.
    B. The presence of positional sleep apnea (worse when supine) renders the oral appliance less effective.
    C. BMI should not be considered in the decision to use an oral appliance.
    D. Increased amounts of mandibular protrusion produce greater reductions in respiratory events.

16. Which of the following statements most accurately reflects the current evidence for the use of atrial overdrive pacing as treatment of sleep apnea syndrome?
    A. Atrial overdrive pacing is as effective as nasal CPAP in reducing obstructive events in patients with sleep apnea.
    B. Atrial overdrive pacing reduces vagal tone during sleep, prevents the withdrawal of efferent activation of the pharyngeal dilator muscles, and minimizes upper airway collapsibility in sleep apnea.
    C. Atrial overdrive pacing has no beneficial effects on sleep apnea.
    D. Atrial overdrive pacing may decrease the severity of sleep apnea in patients with symptomatic bradyarrhythmias, congestive heart failure, and mixed apneas.

17. A 71-year-old man presents with a history of falling out of bed. He recounts several dreams that have been associated with his ending up on the floor. His wife comments that he has slowed down over the past year, and his ability to pay attention to important conversations seems to significantly fluctuate throughout the day. She has had to take over the finances because of several significant mistakes. On examination, he has reduced verbal fluency, working memory, and visuospatial construction skills with relatively intact confrontation naming and memory. There is also mild cogwheel rigidity bilaterally without the presence of tremor. A PSG confirms the presence of REM without atonia. Which of the following is the best clinical diagnosis?
    A. Parkinson's disease
    B. Alzheimer's disease
    C. Dementia with Lewy bodies
    D. Frontotemporal dementia

18. Which of the following statements is true regarding sleep restriction?
    A. Healthy individuals require, on average, 6 hours of core sleep each day to prevent neurobehavioral deficits.
    B. Subjective sleepiness cumulatively increases over the course of chronic partial sleep deprivation, whereas cognitive decline quickly stabilizes.
    C. Throughout the course of sleep restriction, EEG delta frequency power declines, reflecting adaptation with a lower baseline homeostatic sleep drive.
    D. Neurobehavioral performance deficits increase in a near-linear fashion with cumulative increases in wakefulness during sleep restriction or deprivation.

19. Central apneas occur in heart failure in association with a Cheyne-Stokes (periodic) respiratory pattern. A recent study documented that acetazolamide administered before sleep to patients with heart failure resulted in improvement in the apnea-hypopnea index (AHI) and nocturnal oxygenation. Prior studies have demonstrated that acetazolamide is effective for idiopathic central sleep apnea (CSA) and high-altitude CSA. The mechanism of action is based on which of the following?
    A. Acetazolamide causes a metabolic alkalosis that increases respiratory drive.
    B. Acetazolamide causes a metabolic acidosis that increases respiratory drive.
    C. Acetazolamide results in a higher $PaCO_2$ that stimulates respiration.
    D. Acetazolamide raises the apnea threshold.

20. In adults, OSA is an established risk factor for hypertension. Even before the onset of clinical hypertension, there may be dysregulation of blood pressure (BP) indicative of autonomic or endothelial dysfunction. Evidence of BP dysregulation has been identified in children with OSA and includes which of the following?

A. Decreased BP variability during wake
B. Decreased BP variability during sleep
C. Decreased nocturnal BP dipping
D. Increased nocturnal BP dipping

21. A healthy 62-year-old woman with narcolepsy with cataplexy is currently prescribed modafinil for excessive daytime sleepiness (EDS). Despite lack of specific treatment for cataplexy, she has not had a cataplectic episode in years; however, daytime sleepiness is still a problem for her. Prior therapy with methylphenidate and amphetamines resulted in her feeling too jittery, and BP readings were borderline high. She has read about gamma hydroxybutyrate (GHB, sodium oxybate, Xyrem) and is interested in your opinion as to whether she should try it. Her insurance company will only cover medications for Food and Drug Administration (FDA)-approved indications. Which of the following would be the best response to this situation?
    A. GHB is FDA approved for cataplexy, but not for EDS.
    B. GHB is contraindicated at her age because of the possibility of confusional episodes.
    C. GHB is approved for both cataplexy and EDS and would be an appropriate medication to try.
    D. GHB is contraindicated because it has a high sodium content that may exacerbate her borderline hypertension.

22. An 80-year-old man complains of difficulty getting to sleep and difficulty returning to sleep after waking to urinate. He has a history of hypertension and has a mildly unsteady gait. Sleep lab evaluation showed only minimal SDB and no periodic leg movements (PLMs). In your discussions with him, you want to provide an effective therapy while not placing him at undue risk. He is most anxious for therapy, however, and asks for your assessments of his risks and benefits to help him make an informed decision. He is resistant to your recommendation to consider cognitive behavioral therapy (CBT). On reviewing recent literature on insomnia, which of the following statements do you find to be most accurate?
    A. CBT is known to have greater long-term efficacy than medications such as benzodiazepines or benzodiazepine-receptor agonists (BZRAs) in the elderly population.
    B. Benzodiazepines and BZRAs, although posing a modest risk, are more effective than CBT in the elderly population in the short- and long-term.
    C. A recent large meta-analysis of risks and benefits of hypnotics commonly used in the elderly

population showed that improvements in sleep quality were statistically more likely than adverse events.
    D. A recent large meta-analysis of risks and benefits of hypnotics commonly used in the elderly population showed that the benefits were statistically as likely as adverse events.

23. Narcolepsy is a disorder associated with loss of hypocretin (orexin)-containing neurons in the hypothalamus. Currently available treatments for narcolepsy do not target the hypocretin neuropeptide system. Which of the following statements best describe the reason that hypocretin is not currently used as a therapy for narcolepsy?
    A. Hypocretin has no effect in any animal models of narcolepsy.
    B. The blood-brain barrier is impermeable to hypocretin.
    C. Cell loss of hypocretin-containing neurons has been shown to be an epiphenomenon unrelated to the pathophysiology of narcolepsy.
    D. Administration of hypocretin results in unacceptable side effects.

24. Hypocretin-1 levels in CSF have been shown to be decreased in human narcolepsy. Which of the following best describes the measurement of CSF hypocretin-1 levels in clinical practice?
    A. Highly specific (97%) and sensitive (87%) in cases with typical cataplexy
    B. Highly specific (97%) and sensitive (87%) in cases without cataplexy
    C. No more specific than measuring the genetic marker HLA-DQB1*0602
    D. Should only be obtained if the genetic marker HLA-DQB1*0602 is not present

25. OSA has recently been shown to be an independent risk factor for the development of a composite end point of stroke and death (hazard ratio 1.97, 95% CI 1.12–3.48, $p = 0.01$) in a recently published observational cohort study (Yaggi HK et al: N Engl J Med 353[19]:2034–2041, 2005). Which of the following has been proposed as one explanation for the higher rate of stroke and death in patients with OSA compared with those without it?
    A. They have higher levels of low-density lipoprotein.
    B. They have an increase in cerebral blood flow.
    C. They have a higher rate of factor X deficiency.
    D. They have a higher risk of paradoxical embolization.

26. CSA occurs in 25–40% of patients with heart failure. Patients with heart failure have a variety of physiologic and neuroendocrine disturbances that suggest a potential beneficial role for CPAP to modulate these abnormalities. A recent large multicenter trial was designed to test the hypothesis that CPAP could improve survival rate without cardiac transplantation in patients with CSA and heart failure. The study demonstrated which one of the following?
    A. CPAP lowered mortality.
    B. CPAP lowered the levels of atrial natiuretic peptide.
    C. CPAP lowered norepinephrine levels.
    D. CPAP lowered the risk for rehospitalization.

27. It has been hypothesized that SDB is a risk factor for the development of type 2 diabetes. A recent population-based study demonstrated that 14.7% of subjects with an AHI of 15 or higher had a known diagnosis of diabetes compared with only 2.8% in those with an AHI of less than 5 (Reichmuth KJ et al: Am J Respir Crit Care Med 172[12]:1590–1595, 2005). Which of the following is the most accurate statement about the use of CPAP in patients with SDB and type 2 diabetes?
    A. CPAP delays the onset of type 2 diabetes in patients with impaired glucose tolerance.
    B. CPAP has no effect on the onset of type 2 diabetes in patients with impaired glucose tolerance.
    C. CPAP improves glycemic control in patients with type 2 diabetes.
    D. CPAP has no effect on glycemic control in patients with type 2 diabetes.

28. Diabetes mellitus (DM) and sleep apnea are two common disorders that share several risk factors. Several lines of evidence suggest in fact that SDB could be causal for DM. These include the fact that individuals with SDB and high AHIs have less sensitivity to insulin. Which of the following best summarizes recent epidemiological data on the association of SDB and DM?
    A. The association of SDB and DM is independent of body habitus.
    B. SDB is associated with DM, but this effect is negated when controlling for body habitus.
    C. Individuals with SDB who are not known to have DM are more likely than those with no SDB to develop DM over time.
    D. After adjusting for age, sex and body habitus, over time it is more likely that patients

with AHIs >15 will develop DM than those with AHIs between 5 and 15.

29. OSA is associated with collapse of the upper airway during sleep. Collapse of the airway is primarily promoted by intraluminal negative pressure generated by the diaphragm during inspiration, as well as extraluminal positive pressure resulting from bony and tissue elements surrounding the airway. Factors that act to oppose airway collapse include which of the following?
    A. A positive-pressure reflex in the airway that activates the genioglossus muscle
    B. Decreased pharyngeal dilator muscle activity at sleep onset
    C. Pharyngeal dilator muscle activity and increased lung volume
    D. Decreased longitudinal traction on the airway by decreased lung volume during sleep

30. Cheyne-Stokes respiration is a crescendo-decrescendo breathing pattern in which central apneas occur. The following is the most accurate statement concerning this type of breathing pattern:
    A. It is exacerbated by REM sleep.
    B. It shows a cycle length that is typically short, less than 45 seconds.
    C. It occurs because the CO_2 apnea threshold is lower at sleep onset than when awake.
    D. It is seen primarily in congestive heart failure because of long circulation times in that condition.

31. The Sleep Health Heart Study (SHHS) is a longitudinal cohort study that assesses the cardiovascular consequences of SDB and collected data on metabolic parameters including glucose intolerance as measured by glucose tolerance tests. Multiple mechanisms have been suggested as an explanation for the association of SDB and DM. Which of the following best summarizes data from the SHHS?
    A. The severity of SDB was not associated with glucose intolerance.
    B. Sleep-related hypoxemia was independently associated with glucose intolerance.
    C. The arousal index (average number of arousals per hour of sleep) was associated with glucose intolerance.
    D. A decrease in REM sleep was associated with glucose intolerance.

32. There are two main forms of hypertension. Isolated systolic hypertension (ISH) is primarily a disease of elderly individuals, whereas combined

systolic and diastolic hypertension (S/D hypertension) usually begins earlier in life and may extend into older age groups as patients age. Many studies have shown that SDB is associated with hypertension. Which of the following best describes the association of hypertension and SDB?

A. SDB is associated with S/D hypertension in patients <60 years.

B. SDB is associated with S/D hypertension in patients >60 years.

C. SDB is associated with ISH in patients <60 years.

D. SDB is associated with ISH in patients >60 years.

33. Which of the following statements best characterizes the association between the apolipoprotein E (APOE) ε4 genotype and obstructive sleep apnea-hypopnea (OSAH)?

A. APOE ε4 genotype is associated with reduced adiposity and confers a protective advantage for OSAH.

B. APOE ε4 genotype is associated with an increased risk of OSAH, particularly in individuals <65 years old.

C. The presence of an APOE ε4 allele in patients with OSAH minimizes the risk of future hypertension.

D. APOE ε4 is a risk factor for Alzheimer's dementia and cardiovascular disease, but there is no relationship to OSAH.

34. A 9-year-old boy is referred to you by his pediatrician for the question of SDB. He underwent a tonsillectomy and adenoidectomy at the age of 6 because of snoring and witnessed apneas. He is improved but continues to mouth breathe, snore intermittently, and complain of fatigue. His mother reports that because he is not active, he has gained weight. He is undergoing orthodontic evaluation for crowded teeth and a cross-bite. The child's otolaryngologist has noted a mildly deviated septum and mild allergic rhinitis. On examination you note a high arched hard palate, narrow maxilla, no retrognathia, and a BMI of 23 kg/m². PSG shows an AHI of 10 and lowest O_2 saturation of 79%. On the basis of current literature, your advice to the family is the following:

A. Weight loss and treatment of allergic rhinitis should be expected to provide adequate treatment for this degree of SDB in this child without adenotonsillar hypertrophy.

B. CPAP or bilevel positive airway pressure (BiPAP) is the only effective treatment for SDB of this degree.

C. Septoplasty is warranted if the child fails to respond to weight loss and treatment of allergic rhinitis.

D. Maxillary expansion is a good option that could result in significant improvement.

35. A middle-age woman with a long history of RLS is referred to the sleep clinic for your opinion as to the best pharmacological therapy for her condition. She complains of daily symptoms that significantly interfere with her ability to enjoy her evenings and initiate sleep. She has no other significant medical problems. You write back to her referring physician that, as recommended by a recent consensus statement of experts in the field, the first-line medication for patients requiring daily therapy for restless legs is which one of the following?

A. Low-dose opioids

B. Low-dose dopaminergic agonists

C. Gabapentin

D. Levodopa

36. Which of the following statements is most accurate regarding the regulation of sleep and wake?

A. Orexin neurons stimulate sleep-promoting neurons in the hypothalamus to foster consolidated sleep.

B. The tuberomammillary nucleus, composed of histamine-containing neurons, promotes sleep by inhibiting the ascending arousal system.

C. The locus coeruleus, containing serotoninergic projections, promotes REM sleep.

D. The ventrolateral preoptic nucleus promotes sleep by inhibiting the ascending arousal system via gamma aminobutyric acid (GABA) and galanin.

37. Which of the following statements best describes features of the delayed sleep phase syndrome (DSPS)?

A. DSPS likely reflects an abnormal phase relationship between the circadian system and the desired sleep-wake schedule.

B. DSPS is caused by abnormalities of the CLOCK gene, causing an inversion of the normal phase response curve to bright light and melatonin.

C. DSPS may be treated by bright light exposure of approximately 2500 lux from 5–7 A.M. in most patients.

D. DSPS is generally associated with an abnormally short intrinsic period of the circadian pacemaker.

38. A 30-year-old male has had a 19-year history of nocturnal spells. He suddenly arouses from sleep, with eyes open and a fearful expression, clears his throat, turns his head to the left, and then goes back to sleep. These may occur three or four times within a night. Occasionally the spells are longer, during which time he may sit up in bed or leave the bed. These are more likely to occur during times of stress. Which of the following findings is most likely on video-PSG?

A. REM periods with excessive chin tone and visible movements on video

B. Hypersynchronous high-voltage delta activity before the arousals

C. Hypopneas and arousal during stage 3 NREM sleep

D. Anterior low-voltage, fast activity with increased chin tone and tachycardia during the spells

39. Which of the following statements is true about adenosine?

A. Basal forebrain extracellular adenosine concentrations increase during prolonged wakefulness.

B. Adenosine increases the activity of brainstem monoaminergic and cholinergic neurons.

C. Caffeine and theophylline are potent adenosine receptor agonists.

D. Adenosine primarily serves to regulate the circadian timing of REM sleep.

40. Among the physiologic effects of photic stimulation are phase shifting of the circadian pacemaker; inhibition of melatonin production; and increased alertness, heart rate, and core body temperature. Recent evidence shows that these responses show a peak sensitivity to short wavelengths in the range of 443–483 nm. Which of the following statements adds support to these findings?

A. Short-wavelength light sensitivity is consistent with the fact that rods and cones are both required for circadian entrainment.

B. Short-wavelength light sensitivity is consistent with the fact that only cones mediate circadian entrainment.

C. Short-wavelength light sensitivity is consistent with the fact that only rods mediate circadian entrainment.

D. Short-wavelength light sensitivity is consistent with the fact that neither rods nor cones are required for circadian entrainment.

41. GABA is the major inhibitory transmitter in the brain. Gaboxadol is an agent in development as a hypnotic that has been described as a "super-agonist" of what type(s) of GABA receptors?

A. Extrasynaptic GABA-A receptors

B. GABA-B receptors

C. GABA-C receptors

D. All known GABA receptors

42. Melanopsin is a photopigment found in photoreceptive retinal ganglion cells. Most melanopsin-containing cells project to the suprachiasmatic nucleus and are known to be important for circadian entrainment. Recent work indicates that these cells also project to what sleep-regulating area?

A. Raphe nuclei

B. Locus coeruleus

C. Ventral lateral preoptic nucleus

D. Tubomammillary nucleus

Answers

1. C. Are the symptoms improved by moving your legs?

The International Restless Legs Syndrome Study Group has developed essential diagnostic criteria for RLS (Allen RP et al: Sleep Med 4[2]:101–119, 2003). These include the following:

1. An urge to move the legs usually accompanied by or caused by uncomfortable and unpleasant sensations in the legs
2. The urge to move or unpleasant sensations begin or worsen during periods of rest or inactivity such as lying or sitting
3. The urge to move or unpleasant sensations are partially or totally relieved by movement such as walking or stretching, at least as long as the activity continues
4. The urge to move or unpleasant sensations are worse in the evening or night than during the day, or occur only in the evening or night.

Supportive but not essential clinical features of RLS include (1) family history of RLS, (2) response to dopaminergic therapy, and (3) PLMs during wakefulness or sleep.

2. B. Decreased effective connectivity across distributed cortical networks

A recent transcranial magnetic stimulation (TMS) study demonstrated that during NREM sleep, the effective connectivity between distant cortical networks is reduced, and this may explain a reduction of conscious recollection (Massimini M et al: Science 309[5744]:2228–2232, 2005). *Effective connectivity* refers to the ability of a set of neuronal groups to causally effect the firing of other neuronal groups within a system. The effect of TMS during NREM sleep remains localized to the site of stimulation rather than affecting a distributed set of neurons, demonstrating reduced effective connectivity. Neuronal firing synchrony is actually increased, rather than decreased, during NREM sleep, and this explains the relative increase in EEG amplitudes as compared with wakefulness or REM sleep. Global cerebral metabolism is decreased, rather than increased, during sleep. Sensory signals in multiple domains, including tactile, auditory, visual, and painful stimuli, are transmitted to the cerebral cortex during NREM sleep.

3. B. Dopamine agonists are likely to substantially improve sleep quality.

In this setting the patient has a clear history of RLS that has been alleviated with iron supplementation.

The PSG revealed periodic limb movement disorder (PLMD) with frequent arousals. By the information given, it is likely that PLMD is the primary fragmenting process. A component of psychophysiologic insomnia may be an additional factor, but treatment of PLMD is the recommended next step. Treatment with a dopamine agonist has been shown to substantially reduce PLMs of sleep and PLM arousals, reduce sleep latency, and improve subjective measures of sleep adequacy (Allen R et al: Sleep 27[5]:907–914, 2004). Although BZRAs may minimize arousals from a variety of stimuli, they are not considered the treatment of choice for PLMD. CPAP would be suggested only if the PSG showed clear evidence of SDB.

4. D. Insomnia is associated with increased thalamic metabolism during wake-sleep transitions.

Insomnia is associated with nocturnal sleep disruption as well as impaired daytime functioning. Functional imaging has demonstrated an overall increase in waking and sleep whole brain metabolism in insomnia compared with normal sleepers (Nofzinger EA et al: Am J Psychiatry 161[11]:2126–2128, 2004), consistent with the concept of insomnia being a condition of hyperarousal. However, the relative metabolism in the prefrontal cortex during wakefulness is reduced in insomnia, possibly explaining some of the cognitive symptoms and associated daytime fatigue. Wake-promoting structures fail to decline in metabolism during the transition from wake to NREM sleep, including the ascending reticular activating system, hypothalamus, thalamus, and anterior cingulate regions. There is currently no evidence for differences in neuronal metabolism during REM sleep in patients with insomnia compared with normal sleepers.

5. A. CSF H and L ferritin subunits are decreased in early-onset (age <45) RLS.

Several lines of investigation, including magnetic resonance imaging (MRI), autopsy specimens, and CSF analysis, have implicated decreased brain iron in the pathophysiology of RLS. Low brain iron may play a role in decreased dopamine synthesis or receptor function. Ferritin molecules are composed of two subunits, H and L subtypes. H chains are involved in ferrous iron oxidation and increase as a result of inflammation. L-ferritin reflects long-term iron stores. Late-onset (≥45 years old) RLS is more often due to secondary causes such as iron deficiency anemia, and serum ferritin values may be low. However, CSF ferritin levels are normal for both subtypes in late-onset RLS compared with healthy control subjects. In contrast, early-onset RLS is more likely to be related to a primary problem with central nervous system iron acquisition, and both H and L ferritin subunits are decreased. Total body iron stores may be normal as reflected in normal serum ferritin values (Clardy SL et al: J Lab Clin Med 147[2]:67–73, 2006).

6. B. Postmenopausal status is independently associated with increasing risk of SDB.

The Wisconsin Sleep Cohort assessed the association between menopausal status and SDB. The study design incorporated both longitudinal and cross-sectional data. SDB was assessed with overnight PSG. Scoring of hypopneas required at least 4% oxygen desaturation, and the AHI was used to determine severity of SDB. Menopausal status included information on menstrual history, gynecological surgery, hormone replacement therapy, follicle-stimulating hormone levels, and vasomotor symptoms. When compared with premenopause, postmenopause was associated with an odds ratio of 2.6 for mild SDB (AHI >5) and 3.5 for moderate SDB (AHI >15) after adjusting for age, smoking status, BMI, and other measures of body habitus, hypertension, alcohol, education, exercise, and self-rated evaluation of health. Perimenopausal status was associated with an intermediate risk when compared with premenopausal and postmenopausal status. Therefore this study suggests an independent risk of SDB in the transition to menopause (Young T et al: Am J Respir Crit Care Med 167[9]:1181–1185, 2003).

7. A. Oxidative damage to wake-promoting neurons secondary to intermittent hypoxia

Obstructive sleep apnea-hypopnea syndrome (OSAHS) is associated with a variety of physiologic changes, including nocturnal arousals, autonomic disturbances, acid-base abnormalities, and intermittent hypoxia. Among these physiologic disturbances, oxygen desaturation is most strongly correlated with sleepiness. In a mouse model of long-term intermittent hypoxia (8 weeks), residual sleepiness persisted for at least 2 weeks after return to normoxic conditions. This was reflected in increased total sleep times per day, as well as reduced mean sleep latencies. Markers of oxidative injury were found in wake-promoting regions of the brain including areas of the basal forebrain, lateral hypothalamus, and dorsal raphe nuclei. Chronic oxidative injury to these cell groups from chronic intermittent hypoxia associated with severe OSAHS may be responsible for residual somnolence despite adequate treatment. Residual cognitive dysfunction may also represent a similar form of irreversible injury (Veasey SC et al: Sleep 27[2]:194–201, 2004).

Diffuse lacunar infarction would be expected to cause focal neurological signs and functional consequences beyond sleepiness alone. OSAHS is not generally associated with significant waking hypercarbia, and there is no evidence for a direct relationship between OSAHS and adrenal insufficiency.

8. D. Melatonin administration at 8:00 P.M.

This scenario describes a patient with DSPS. Treatment options include the use of melatonin or timed light exposure to advance the timing of the circadian clock. Melatonin administration in the evening before the dim light melatonin onset (DLMO) produces phase advances. The magnitude of the phase shift depends on the timing of melatonin administration relative to the DLMO. There is a significantly greater phase advance when melatonin is administered roughly 6 hours before DLMO when compared with 2 hours before DLMO, with a linear relationship within this range. Sleep onset generally occurs within 2 hours of DLMO in delayed phase subjects. In this case, the earlier time of administration, 6 hours compared with 3 hours before habitual sleep time, is expected to have a greater phase advance (Mundey K et al: Sleep 28[10]:1271–1278, 2005). Therefore the patient would be more likely to wake for her morning classes.

Light exposure in the evening before the core body temperature minimum produces phase delays, whereas morning light exposure after the core body temperature minimum causes phase advances. In this case, minimizing early morning sunlight may contribute to phase delays, depending on the timing of this patient's circadian clock in relation to environmental time.

9. C. Mean nocturnal oxygen saturation

OSA is recognized as a cardiovascular risk factor. Comorbid conditions such as hypertension, hyperlipidemia, insulin resistance, and obesity contribute to the atherosclerotic risk. In a recent study, mean sleep oxygen saturation was the strongest determinant of carotid intima-media thickness (IMT) after controlling for hypertension. Oxygen desaturation and resaturation leads to oxidative stress, free radical formation, and a cascade of metabolic processes that favor the formation of atheroma (Baguet JP et al: Chest 128[5]:3407–3412, 2005). High sympathetic output, which has been associated with OSA, may lead to insulin resistance, oxidative injury, and vascular remodeling, but it was not a critical determinant of carotid IMT in this study.

10. C. C-reactive protein (CRP) and interleukin (IL)-6 levels are elevated in patients with sleep apnea and are lowered by treatment with nasal CPAP.

There is increasing evidence of the role of inflammation in the development of atherosclerosis. CRP and IL-6 are markers of cardiovascular risk and may play a causal role in the development of atherosclerosis.

Levels of both inflammatory markers are elevated in patients with sleep apnea, and the increased levels are correlated with each other. In addition, IL-6 production by monocytes is elevated in sleep apnea. In addition to BMI, the severity of SDB (as measured by the AHI) is independently associated with elevated CRP, and oxygen desaturation is independently associated with elevated IL-6. A recent study using 1-month treatment with nasal CPAP demonstrated a significant reduction in both markers without a significant change in BMI. Reduction of these inflammatory markers may play a causal role in the cardiovascular benefit associated with CPAP treatment of SDB (Yokoe T et al: Circulation 107[8]:1129–1134, 2003).

11. D. Inflammatory infiltration and denervation of upper airway muscles

Repeated episodes of upper airway occlusion, large intraluminal pressure swings, and violent muscle contractions against an occluded airway may impose mechanical trauma to the upper airway in patients with sleep apnea. Recent work has demonstrated pharyngeal muscle inflammatory infiltrates in addition to adjacent mucosal inflammation, and the T lymphocyte profile was distinct. Therefore the inflammation detected in the muscles was unlikely to reflect extension of the adjacent mucosal inflammatory reaction and was a sign of intrinsic muscle injury. Histochemical markers of pharyngeal muscle denervation changes such as PGP9.5 and N-CAM immunoreactivity were present, as well as signs of axonal sprouting and regeneration. Inflammation in the muscles and degeneration of motor nerves may impair dilator muscle contractile strength, contributing to a vicious cycle of worsening upper airway collapse and recurrent trauma (Boyd JH et al: Am J Respir Crit Care Med 170[5]:541–546, 2004).

Pharyngeal sensory abnormalities have been previously demonstrated in patients with sleep apnea, including reduced ability to detect temperature changes, vibration, and two-point discrimination. Mucosal biopsies have demonstrated sensory nerve degenerative changes. Impaired sensory function may contribute to upper airway collapsibility as evidenced by topical anesthetic administration.

12. C. Order a PSG.

The most appropriate next step in this case depends on the interpretation of the clinical scenario. Although the patient complains of disturbing "dreams," this clinical scenario best represents night terrors. These occur during the first third of the night during slow wave sleep, and patients may report unpleasant imagery. There is generally a strong sense of fear. The patient also has episodes suggestive of sleepwalking, a related arousal phenomenon from slow wave sleep (SWS).

An American Academy of Sleep Medicine (AASM) practice parameter suggests that PSG is not routinely indicated in cases of typical, uncomplicated, and non-injurious parsasomnias when the diagnosis is clearly delineated (Kushida CA et al: Sleep 28[4]:499–521, 2005). However, there is an increased incidence of SDB in patients with SWS parasomnias (Guilleminault C et al: Pediatrics 111[1]:e17–25, 2003), and evidence suggests that treatment of SDB may be effective in minimizing these arousal phenomenon (Guilleminault C et al: Brain 128[Pt 5]:1062–1069, 2005). In this case, the lack of childhood history suggests a new triggering process, and recent weight gain may be associated with SDB. The most appropriate next step is a PSG to evaluate for the presence of a fragmenting process such as SDB.

REM behavioral disorder, which may be treated with clonazepam, tends to occur in older individuals, is more common in the last third of sleep, and has associated motor activity that corresponds to the contents of a dream. Nocturnal seizures tend to occur with greater frequency, may cluster within a night, and are characterized by stereotyped motor behavior.

13. D. Cognitive behavioral therapy (CBT)

This scenario describes psychophysiologic insomnia, a disorder in which associations form between bed or bedtimes and arousal. A recent study demonstrated that CBT was superior to zolpidem on improving sleep latency and sleep efficiency after 4 weeks of treatment, and zolpidem-treated patients trended toward baseline values after a 2-week medication washout. CBT was effective for the 12-month follow-up period after the treatment phase. CBT assists patients in recognizing, challenging, and changing distorted ideas about sleep that increase the heightened arousal. For example, excessive concern over getting 8 hours of sleep perpetuates this patient's insomnia. Sleep restriction therapy entails curtailing the time in bed close to the duration of actual sleep, as excessive time in bed has been demonstrated to perpetuate insomnia. Stimulus-control therapy entails getting out of bed after 20–30 minutes if unable to sleep, going to another room to perform a quiet, relaxing activity until drowsy, and repeating this as often as necessary. This serves to foster new associations between the bed and the ability to sleep (Jacobs GD et al: Arch Intern Med 164[17]:1888–1896, 2004).

Although this patient frequently changes position out of frustration, there is no clear unpleasant sensation in the limbs with an urgency to move in order to relieve the discomfort. Therefore treatment of RLS with a dopamine agonist is not appropriate. There is no clear history of generalized anxiety disorder or depression that would prompt treatment with a serotonergic reuptake inhibitor. The patient's worry may be restricted to sleep, and psychophysiologic insomnia does not imply a diagnosis of a mood disorder.

14. B. Low threshold for behavioral state transitions (REM, NREM, wake)

Recent work with orexin knockout mice has tested several hypotheses related to the sleepiness found in narcolepsy. The most striking difference between orexin-deficient and wild-type mice is a shorter duration of time in each behavior state (REM, NREM, wake) and increased number of bouts in each state. The evidence best supports the notion of behavioral state instability, with a low threshold for state transitions (Mochizuki T et al: J Neurosci 24[28]:6291–6300, 2004).

Orexin-deficient mice are able to maintain wakefulness in a novel environment for a normal duration, suggesting the ability to activate normal arousal mechanisms in this context. Orexin-deficient mice have essentially normal total amounts of REM, NREM, and wake across 12-hour light and dark periods. In constant darkness, the period of the free-running circadian clock was no different from wild-type mice, and there was no significant difference in the amplitude and timing of sleep-wake rhythms across the circadian cycle. When orexin-deficient mice were sleep deprived for 2, 4, or 8 hours, the increase in REM and NREM sleep pressure and the rate of recovery of the sleep deficit were not significantly different than for wild-type mice, demonstrating normal homeostatic sleep mechanisms. Therefore inadequate activation of arousal regions, poor circadian control of sleep and wakefulness, and abnormal sleep homeostasis may not be adequate explanations for the sleepiness found in narcolepsy.

15. D. Increased amounts of mandibular protrusion produce greater reductions in respiratory events.

The Standards of Practice Committee of the AASM recently reviewed the medical literature regarding oral appliance therapy in OSA (Ferguson KA et al: Sleep 29[2]:244–262, 2006). Four variables appeared to contribute to oral appliance efficacy: the severity of OSA, the degree of mandibular protrusion with a mandibular repositioning appliance (MRA), the presence of positional sleep apnea, and the BMI. Increased amounts of mandibular protrusion have been shown to increase the efficacy of oral appliances; the effect of vertical opening is less clear.

Methodological differences make comparisons across studies difficult, but overall oral appliances are more efficacious in mild and moderate OSA compared with severe OSA. A higher BMI was associated with lower efficacy of the MRA in several studies. Three

studies have demonstrated improved oral appliance efficacy in the setting of positional sleep apnea (worse in the supine compared with the lateral position). Overall, CPAP is more efficacious than oral appliances in terms of improving oxygenation and lowering the AHI, but oral appliances may be better accepted by patients.

16. D. Atrial overdrive pacing may decrease the severity of sleep apnea in patients with symptomatic bradyarrhythmias, congestive heart failure, and mixed apneas.

In a recent study, atrial overdrive pacing has been suggested as an effective intervention for patients with OSA and CSA (Garrigue S et al: N Engl J Med 346[6]:404–412, 2002). In this study, 15 patients with a previously implanted pacemaker for symptomatic bradycardia and sleep apnea were studied. Atrial overdrive pacing was set to increase the mean sleep heart rate by 15 beats per minute. The mean AHI in this population decreased from nine events per hour to three. In a recent randomized crossover trial in patients with purely obstructive sleep apnea, normal left ventricular function, and implanted pacemakers for symptomatic bradycardia, atrial overdrive pacing did not show any benefit on measures of sleep apnea compared with baseline. Nasal CPAP, in stark contrast, was extremely effective in minimizing the AHI, the arousal index, desaturation index (number of events with less than 90% oxygen saturation per hour), mean and low oxygen saturation, and Epworth Sleepiness Scale score (Simantirakis EN et al: N Engl J Med 353[24]:2568–2577, 2005).

There is currently no evidence for the direct effects of atrial overdrive pacing on upper airway collapsibility. In patients with mixed apneas and abnormal left ventricular function, the possibility remains that improved cardiac output and decreased circulation times reduce central apneas and possibly secondary obstructive events. Therefore there may be some beneficial effects of atrial overdrive pacing in selected patients with sleep apnea, but the role of this intervention remains unclear.

17. C. Dementia with Lewy bodies

This case illustrates REM behavior disorder (RBD) with episodes of movement from the bed to the floor associated with the contents of a dream. PSG confirms the presence of REM without atonia. RBD generally occurs in degenerative conditions associated with abnormal alpha-synuclein metabolism including Parkinson's disease, dementia with Lewy bodies (DLB), and multiple system atrophy, and rarely with other neurodegenerative disorders. The DLB Consortium has recently revised the diagnostic criteria to include RBD as a suggestive feature in the diagnosis of DLB. An *essential* feature of the diagnosis of DLB includes cognitive impairment of sufficient magnitude to interfere with routine functioning. This is usually in the form of poor attention and executive function and visuospatial skills, but memory may become affected as the illness progresses. *Core* features include fluctuations in arousal and attention throughout the day, parkinsonism, and recurrent, usually well-formed visual hallucinations. One core feature may diagnose possible DLB, and two core features are required for probable DLB. RBD is now considered a *suggestive* feature. If one core feature is present in the context of RBD (or other suggestive feature not discussed), a diagnosis of probable DLB may still be made. Therefore in that context the presence of RBD may confirm the clinical diagnosis. If only RBD is present in a patient with dementia but there are no diagnostic core features, a diagnosis of possible DLB is made (McKeith IG et al: Neurology 65[12]:1863–1872, 2005).

Differentiation of DLB from Parkinson's disease is generally based on the time course of cognitive deficits in relationship to the parkinsonism. In cases of Parkinson's disease with dementia, the parkinsonism generally is present for several years before the onset of dementia. Frontotemporal dementia is associated with poor planning and judgment as well as personality changes, but the underlying pathology reflects abnormal accumulation of hyperphosphorylated tau protein. Patients with disorders of tau and amyloid deposition such as Alzheimer's disease generally do not develop RBD.

18. D. Neurobehavioral performance deficits increase in a near-linear fashion with cumulative increases in wakefulness during sleep restriction or deprivation.

The construct of critical wake duration has been proposed to denote a postulated maximum period of stable waking neurobehavioral functions. Wake periods in extension of this critical wake duration would be expected to accumulate neurobehavioral performance deficits. Data from both total sleep deprivation over 3 days as well as 2 weeks of sleep restriction to 8, 6, or 4 hours per night have been integrated to estimate the critical wake duration as 15.84 hours per wake period. This would correspond to 8.16 hours of sleep per 24-hour sleep-wake cycle. Neurobehavioral performance deficits increase in a near-linear fashion with the cumulative duration of wakefulness in excess of this critical wake duration. The construct of critical wake duration parsimoniously accounts for data from both cumulative sleep restriction as well as total sleep deprivation (Van Dongen HP et al: Sleep 26[2]:117–126, 2003).

Neurobehavioral performance continuously declines across 2 weeks of partial sleep restriction to 4 or 6 hours per night, as well as during 3 days of total sleep deprivation. The magnitude of performance deficits over a 2-week course of chronic sleep deprivation to 6 hours or less may approximate the deficits seen over 1–2 days of total sleep deprivation. Therefore 6 hours of "core sleep" does not appear to be sufficient, on average, to preserve neurobehavioral performance. Across 3 days of total sleep deprivation, subjective sleepiness increases in a near-linear fashion. In contrast, subjective sleepiness in the setting of cumulative partial sleep restriction increases initially and then plateaus. Therefore in the setting of chronic sleep restriction, subjective reports of sleepiness do not accurately reflect neurobehavioral performance. EEG delta power tends to increase with increasing sleep loss, and this is considered a marker for increased homeostatic drive for sleep.

19. B. Acetazolamide causes a metabolic acidosis that increases respiratory drive.

Acetazolamide is a carbonic anhydrase inhibitor. Carbonic anhydrase is important in acid-base balance and respiratory control because of the following reaction:

$$CO_2 + H_2O \leftrightarrow {}^{ca}H_2CO_3 \leftrightarrow H^+ + HCO_3^-.$$

Over hours, acetazolamide administration results in metabolic acidosis because it induces HCO_3 wasting in the renal tubule. The resultant metabolic acidosis stimulates both the central and peripheral respiratory chemoreceptors, inducing increased ventilation. The apnea threshold is the partial pressure of CO_2 ($PaCO_2$) below which an apnea will occur. Lowering $PaCO_2$ through hyperventilation induced by a metabolic acidosis might intuitively be expected to increase the likelihood of an apnea. However, acetazolamide-induced metabolic acidosis also lowers the apnea threshold. In a study by Javaheri (Am J Respir Crit Care Med 173[2]:234–237, 2006), $PaCO_2$ dropped by a mean of 2.8 mm Hg as measured in the morning after administration of acetazolamide (3.5–4.0 mg/kg) once nightly for 6 nights. Despite this drop in $PaCO_2$, central apneas improved; the AHI dropped from a baseline of 55 ± 24 to 34 ± 20. These findings are consistent with prior studies showing that the net effect of acetazolamide-induced respiratory stimulation is a decrease in the apnea threshold (a lower pCO_2 is tolerated without apnea) that is greater than the fall in $PaCO_2$.

20. C. Decreased nocturnal blood pressure (BP) dipping

Amin et al (Am J Respir Crit Care Med 169[8]:950–956, 2004) studied ambulatory 24-hour ambulatory

BP in 60 children with OSA with a mean age of 10.8 years. Among three groups stratified for AHI, a dose-dependent increase in BP variability was seen with increasing AHI. Increased BP variability was noted during both wake and sleep. Nocturnal BP dipping was decreased in children with OSA and correlated best with the desaturation index (defined as number of events with at least 4% desaturation/h sleep). In adults, increased BP variability and decreased nocturnal dipping are risks for cardiovascular morbidity. This study did not demonstrate evidence of sustained elevation of hypertension in children with OSA, but other studies have shown elevated systolic or diastolic BP in children with OSA.

21. C. GHB is approved for both cataplexy and EDS and would be an appropriate medication to try.

GHB, also known as sodium oxybate (Xyrem), is an effective treatment for narcolepsy and cataplexy. The original FDA approval for sodium oxybate in 2002 was limited to cataplexy, but studies demonstrating efficacy for EDS resulted in FDA approval for that indication in 2005 (Group XIS: J Clin Sleep Med 1[4]:391–397, 2005). Revisions of labeling in November 2005 warned that Xyrem has been associated with the development of confusion. In clinical trials, at the maximum recommended dose of 9 g per night, confusion was reported in 17%, and the overall rate of confusion was 2.6% at doses of 6 to 9 g. Warnings regarding paranoia, agitation, hallucinations, depression, and suicidality were also added to the safety label. Sleepwalking and enuresis are established side effects occurring in a minority of patients. A 9-g dose of sodium oxybate provides a 1.6-g sodium load, which can exacerbate hypertension and/or heart failure. However, borderline hypertension would not be an absolute contraindication.

GHB is a unique medication with multiple side effects that need to be understood by both the patient and physician. Among other side effects, the patient should be warned of the possibility of confusion and the complications of sodium excess, including hypertension. With careful monitoring by the physician and patient, however, these side effects are not reasons to withhold therapy in the patient described.

22. A. Cognitive behavioral therapy (CBT) is known to have greater long-term efficacy than medications such as benzodiazepines or BZRAs agonists (BZRAs) in the elderly population.

A large meta-analysis of risks and benefits of commonly used sedative hypnotics in older people demonstrated a rather small effect on sleep quality while causing significant adverse events (Glass J et al: BMJ 331[7526]:1169, 2005). The medications studied were almost exclusively benzodiazepines and BZRAs. The data indicated that treatment was more than twice as likely to induce an adverse event as to improve measures of sleep quality. Falls and motor vehicle crashes were more likely in patients who took sedative hypnotics. A recent review of chronic insomnia (Silber MH: N Engl J Med 353[8]:803–810, 2005) summarizes relevant prior work that addresses the question of hypnotic versus behavioral treatment. Randomized controlled studies comparing CBT with hypnotics (benzodiazepines and BZRAs) have shown that CBT results in better long-term efficacy, even in the elderly population. In these comparisons, short-term efficacy in the hypnotic and CBT treatment groups has been reported as either similar or favoring CBT. CBT is a first-choice therapy, especially in an elderly patient at risk for falls.

23. B. The blood-brain barrier is impermeable to hypocretin.

In a review of emerging narcolepsy treatments, Mignot suggests, "The gold standard for narcolepsy treatment will one day likely be hypocretin replacement therapy." Hypocretin is a polypeptide. There are two forms, hypocretin-1, 33 amino acids, and hypocretin-2, 29 amino acids. Because of its size, hypocretin does not permeate the intact blood-brain barrier. Hypocretin interacts with arousal systems in the brain. Loss of hypocretin in the hypothalamus is the most likely explanation for the symptoms of narcolepsy and cataplexy. In animal models of hypocretin-deficient mice, intraventricular administration of hypocretin resulted in reversal of symptoms of narcolepsy and cataplexy. Intravenous administration of hypocretin to animals has been ineffective but has not resulted in unacceptable side effects (Mignot E, Nishino S: Sleep 28[6]:754–763, 2005).

24. A. Highly specific (97%) and sensitive (87%) in cases with typical cataplexy

Hypocretin-1 (Hcrt-1) levels are highly specific (97%) and sensitive (87%) in patients with typical cataplexy but not in patients without cataplexy. The specificity in patients without cataplexy remains high at 99%, but the sensitivity is low at 16%. Almost all cases of narcolepsy with low Hcrt-1 levels also demonstrate the genetic marker HLA-DQB1*0602. However, DQB1*0602 is present in 8–38% of the general population, and therefore a positive DQB1*0602 itself has low specificity for narcolepsy. On the other hand, if patients are negative for DQB1*0602 and have no evidence of cataplexy, it is estimated that the chance of finding a low Hcrt-1 level in CSF is less than 1%.

It would rarely be useful to obtain a CSF Hcrt-1 level in a DQB1*0602-negative patient. Most patients with low CSF Hcrt-1 levels without cataplexy are children with narcolepsy who have not yet developed cataplexy. CSF Hcrt-1 levels are most helpful in the diagnostic evaluation of DQB1*0602-positive patients with equivocal clinical evidence of cataplexy and in children with EDS (Mignot E et al: Sleep 26[6]:646–649, 2003).

25. D. They have a higher risk of paradoxical embolization.

Several factors are likely possibilities explaining the higher stroke and death risk in OSA including lower cerebral blood flow, hypercoaguability, and hypoxia-related cerebral ischemia. Right to left shunting through a patent foramen ovale with subsequent paradoxical embolization is one proposed mechanism for the higher risk of stroke in OSA. Factor X deficiency is a rare cause of bleeding and is not associated with hypercoaguability. An elevated low-density lipoprotein level is a risk for stroke but is not known to be associated with sleep apnea.

26. C. CPAP lowered norepinephrine levels.

The Canadian Positive Pressure CPAP Trial (CANPAP) randomly assigned patients with heart failure and CSA to CPAP or no treatment (Bradley TD et al: N Engl J Med 353[19]:2025–2033, 2005). The use of CPAP resulted in a variety of beneficial effects such as lowering the levels of norepinephrine, improving nocturnal oxygenation, improving left ventricular function, and improving distance walked in 6 minutes. Although CPAP lowered the AHI, its use in this population did not lower morbidity, mortality, rehospitalization rate, quality of life, or atrial natiuretic peptide. Whether this is true for patients with heart failure and OSA is not known.

27. C. CPAP improves glycemic control in patients with type 2 diabetes.

Babu et al, in a recent study, demonstrated that the use of CPAP resulted in a significant reduction in the level of the HgbA1C in diabetic patients who had HgbA1C values above 7 (Arch Intern Med 165[4]: 447–452, 2005). In addition, these authors noted that those subjects who used CPAP for more than 4 hours per night were the ones with the greatest reduction in the HgbA1C levels. To date, no specific study has as yet shown that CPAP is effective in delaying the onset of diabetes in patients with impaired glucose tolerance.

28. A. The association of SBD and diabetes mellitus (DM) is independent of body habitus.

The Wisconsin Sleep Cohort Study is a population-based longitudinal study of sleep disorders that has been carried out on 1387 participants. It offered a unique opportunity to study the association of diabetes and SDB in that it not only collected data on sleep habits and performed PSG, but it also collected data on a variety of health problems. In a cross-sectional analysis, self-reporting of diabetes was three to four times more prevalent in the cohort with AHI >15. This relationship was independent of age, sex, and body habitus (Reichmuth KJ et al: Am J Respir Crit Care Med 172[11]:1363–1370, 2005). However, it has not yet been established that patients with SDB are more likely to develop diabetes or that the severity of SDB correlates with the development of diabetes.

29. C. Pharyngeal dilator muscle activity and increased lung volume

Pharyngeal dilator muscle activity is the primary factor that opposes collapse of the upper airway. One component of pharyngeal dilator control is a negative-pressure reflex in the airway that promotes activity of the genioglossus muscle (a dilator), via laryngeal nerve afferent activity and increased hypoglossal nerve efferent activity. Most patients with OSA have anatomically small airways with augmented pharyngeal dilator muscle activity that maintains patency while awake. During sleep, pharyngeal dilator muscle activity decreases due to both a decrease in the "wakefulness" stimulus from medullary motor neurons and a reduction in the negative-pressure reflex. These decrements in pharyngeal muscle activity during sleep result in greater collapse of the upper airway. Lung volume also influences upper airway patency. Increased lung volume results in downward traction of the trachea and larynx that stiffens the airway and reduces collapse, whereas decreased lung volume during sleep promotes collapse (White DP: Am J Respir Crit Care Med 172[11]:1363–1370, 2005).

30. D. It is seen primarily in congestive heart failure because of long circulation times in that condition.

Cheyne-Stokes respiration occurs because of instability of ventilatory control that is induced by (1) prolonged circulation time, (2) relatively low partial pressure CO_2 ($PaCO_2$) at baseline, and (3) increased responsiveness to CO_2 (high gain). Prolonged circulation time in congestive heart failure results in delays in the feedback loop for ventilatory chemoresponsiveness to $PaCO_2$ in the carotid body and medulla. $PaCO_2$ tends to be maintained at a lower level in congestive heart failure because of lung edema. At sleep onset, the $PaCO_2$ at which ventilation ceases (apnea threshold) is higher than when awake. Therefore in patients who maintain a low $PaCO_2$, the $PaCO_2$ at sleep onset is often lower than the apnea threshold, and an apnea ensues. The slope of ventilatory response to change in $PaCO_2$ is a measure of CO_2 responsiveness. If CO_2 responsiveness is high, and there is also delay in the feedback loop to chemoreceptors because of prolonged circulation time, there is overshoot of corrective responses to the apnea. Hyperpnea induced by this high CO_2 responsiveness results in hypocapnia relative to the PCO_2 set point: an apnea ensues that begins another cycle of waxing and waning ventilatory response. Chemoresponsiveness is decreased during REM sleep, resulting in improvement in the Cheyne-Stokes respiratory pattern. Cycle length reflects the delay in circulation time and is usually more than 1 minute (White DP: Am J Respir Crit Care Med 172[11]:1363–1370, 2005).

31. B. Sleep-related hypoxemia was independently associated with glucose intolerance.

The SHHS included patients from several cardiovascular risk studies, giving the study the opportunity to correlate a number of PSG findings with metabolic abnormalities. One objective of a recent substudy of the SHHS was to determine whether SDB was related to glucose intolerance as measured by the glucose tolerance test. Secondary questions were whether hypoxemia and numbers of arousals predicted the degree of metabolic dysfunction. This study by Punjabi et al (Am J Epidemiol 160[6]:521–530, 2004) clearly showed that SDB was associated with glucose intolerance. The severity of SDB, as assessed by the respiratory disturbance index (defined as apneas and hypopneas each with at least 4% desaturation/h of sleep) was found to be independently associated with degree of insulin resistance in a linear fashion. Furthermore, the authors demonstrated that hypoxemia, but not arousal index, was associated with glucose intolerance. This study did not address the influence of sleep stages, and specifically REM sleep duration, on glucose intolerance.

32. A. SDB is associated with systolic and diastolic (S/D) hypertension in patients <60 years.

SDB is thought to exert its effect on hypertension by activation of the sympathetic nervous system. Loss of arterial compliance is an important mechanism in ISH and has not been shown to be a consequence of SDB. No association between SDB and ISH has been identified. A study by Haas and colleagues (Circulation 111[5]:614–621, 2005) provided insight into the association of SDB and hypertension by showing that the major impact of SDB is on S/D hypertension in patients less than 60 years old, but not a consistent relationship in those over 60. Because this was a cross-sectional study, it is possible that survival bias

and other factors may be at play in the explanation as to why SDB is a clear risk in younger as opposed to older individuals. Prospective studies are needed to answer this question.

33. B. APOE ε4 genotype is associated with an increased risk of obstructive sleep apnea-hypopnea (OSAH), particularly in individuals <65 years old.

APOE is a cholesterol transport protein, and the ε4 polymorphism has been associated with increased risk for atherosclerosis and amyloid plaque formation in Alzheimer's dementia. It is associated with increased total cholesterol and lower higher-density lipoprotein levels. The genetic basis of OSAH is largely unknown, but there is a heritable contribution independent of body habitus. Two large cohort studies, the Wisconsin Sleep Cohort Study and the SHHS, have demonstrated an increased risk of OSAH associated with the presence of the APOE ε4 allele. In the SHHS cohort, this effect was greatest in those <65 years old, which may explain the lack of association found in an older cohort in the Honolulu-Asian Aging Study. In the SHHS, there was a greater risk of OSAH in hypertensive subjects. The mechanism in which APOE ε4 plays a role in the causal pathway for the development of OSAH is not known (Gottlieb DJ et al: Neurology 63[4]:664–668, 2004).

34. D. Maxillary expansion is a good option that could result in significant improvement.

A study by Pirelli et al (Sleep 27[4]:761–766, 2004) was designed to evaluate the effect of rapid maxillary expansion (RME) in children with maxillary constriction and OSA. RME is an orthodontic procedure that uses a fixed appliance anchored to the teeth to expand the palatal suture. Abnormal maxillary development resulting in reduced cross-sectional size may be a developmental sequela of increased nasal resistance in early childhood. These patients demonstrate a narrow maxilla with high arched palate and cross-bite. In this study, 31 children ages 6–12 (mean 8.7 years) with these anatomical abnormalities, without adenotonsillar hypertrophy, with BMI less than 25 kg/m^2 and OSA by PSG, underwent RME. Marked improvements in PSG findings were noted at 4 months. AHI decreased from a mean of 12.18 ± 2.6 to 0.4 ± 1.1, and nadir SpO_2 at baseline of $78.5\% \pm 8.2\%$ increased to 95.3 ± 1.7. Weight loss and treatment of allergic rhinitis are important treatment recommendations, but untreated craniofacial abnormalities in children commonly result in persistent SDB. Positive pressure with CPAP or BiPAP is an effective treatment, but not the only effective modality, as demonstrated by this study. A mild septal deviation does not warrant surgery in childhood.

Expansion of the maxilla also increases the size of the nasal cavities and decreases airway resistance, thus decreasing the impact of septal deviation.

35. B. Low-dose dopaminergic agonists

The Medical Advisory Board of the Restless Legs Syndrome Foundation has published an algorithm for the management of RLS. Dopaminergic agonists are recommended as the drugs of choice in most patients with RLS, especially those with daily symptoms. Levodopa may be used in patients with intermittent symptoms, but daily use is associated with the development of augmentation. Silber et al (Mayo Clin Proc 79[7]: 916–922, 2004) noted that "Augmentation is defined as worsening of RLS symptoms earlier in the day after an evening dose of medication, including earlier onset of symptoms, increased intensity of symptoms, or spread of symptoms to the arms." Augmentation may occur with dopaminergic agonists, but less frequently. Gabapentin and low-dose opioids are alternative medications for daily restless legs symptoms.

36. D. The ventrolateral preoptic nucleus promotes sleep by inhibiting the ascending arousal system via GABA and galanin.

The regulation of sleep and wake is governed by a network of arousal- and sleep-promoting structures (Saper CB et al: J Comp Neurol 493[1]:92–98, 2005). The ascending arousal system is composed of cholinergic projections from the pedunculopontine and lateral dorsal tegmental nuclei, as well as monoaminergic projections from the dorsal and medial raphe nuclei (serotonin), locus ceruleus (norepinephrine), and tuberomammillary nucleus (histamine). These have a variety of targets including regions of the thalamus, lateral hypothalamus, basal forebrain, and the cortex. The monoaminergic neurons fire faster in wakefulness than in NREM sleep, and most stop firing during REM sleep. The ventrolateral preoptic nucleus (VLPO) of the hypothalamus contains neurons that fire twice as fast during sleep as during wakefulness and inhibit the ascending arousal system via GABA and the inhibitory neuropeptide galanin. There is mutual inhibition between the VLPO and components of the ascending arousal system, producing what has been called a "flip-flop" switch. This engineering principle describes a system with rapid state transitions and minimal time in a transition between states (such as a state between fully asleep and fully awake). State transitions may occur abruptly, and orexin projections promote activity of the ascending arousal system, stabilizing this "flip-flop" switch by promoting wakefulness. This may help explain the rapid state changes and hypersomnia in patients with narcolepsy.

37. A. Delayed sleep phase syndrome (DSPS) likely reflects an abnormal phase relationship between the circadian system and the desired sleep-wake schedule.

DSPS is a circadian rhythm disorder that is characterized by sleep and rise times that are later than desired. The patient therefore complains of sleep-onset insomnia as well as extreme difficulty rising in the morning at the desired wake time. Under ad lib circumstances, such as vacations, these patients may have normal sleep initiation, maintenance, and quality of sleep when allowed to change their sleep and wake times to a more biologically conducive schedule. The disorder is thought to reflect an abnormal phase relationship between the circadian system and the desired sleep-wake schedule (Wyatt JK: Sleep 27[6]:1195–1203, 2004).

Sleep and wakefulness are thought to be regulated by an interaction between the homeostatic and circadian systems. Alertness in the morning is typically due to reduced homeostatic sleep drive from the prior night's sleep. As the alerting mechanisms from this process decline over the day, the circadian system begins to promote wakefulness, with the maximal alerting effects of this system occurring several hours before habitual bedtime. Sleep in the early portion of the night is largely promoted by the homeostatic sleep drive, whereas the circadian system actively promotes sleep during the later portion of the habitual sleep episode. The intrinsic period of the circadian pacemaker is slightly longer than 24 hours, but the timing is reset or entrained to environmental time by a variety of cues such as light exposure, posture, and feeding behaviors. Without this resetting, the pacemaker would drift to a progressively later phase relationship to environmental time. An intrinsic period that is shorter than 24 hours would produce phase advances, with sleep and wake propensity occurring progressively earlier; therefore this is not the cause of DSPS.

The timing of the circadian drive for sleep and wakefulness may be modulated (with phase advances or delays) by melatonin and bright light with a characteristic phase response curve. Patients with DSPS do not have an inverted phase response curve. Bright light at the end of the subjective night produces phase advances. However, bright light prior to the core body temperature minimum produces phase delays. Although bright light in the morning may be used as treatment, the timing of 5–7 A.M. may be too early in relationship to the phase of the core body temperature minimum in some DSPS patients, and therefore caution must be used in phototherapy to avoid further phase delays.

38. D. Anterior low-voltage, fast activity with increased chin tone and tachycardia during the spells

The clinical phenotype strongly suggests nocturnal frontal lobe epilepsy. The onset in this case is age 11, which is typical. The description indicates that these are stereotyped with a fearful expression, throat clearing, and head turning to the left. Arousal phenomena from other parasomnias tend to be less stereotyped. The occurrence of multiple episodes within a night would be unusual for SWS parsasomnias. Limitations in scalp EEG recording may fail to show typical ictal features of spike and slow wave discharges owing to the typical midline frontal seizure focus. Ictal EEG may be normal, be obscured by muscle artifact, or show frontal low-voltage fast activity.

Although the spells tend to be highly stereotyped within an individual, several phenotypes have been described across large groups of patients. One notable classification scheme (Tinuper P et al: Neurol Sci 26[suppl 3]:S210–214, 2005) groups seizures into the following categories: (1) very brief motor seizures, which appear as paroxysmal arousal with eye opening and fearful expression; (2) hypermotor seizures with complex, often violent movements involving the trunk or limbs; these may include cycling, rocking, or other repetitive movements; (3) asymmetrical bilateral tonic movements (paroxysmal dystonia); and (4) more prolonged spells with ambulation and semipurposeful behavior (epileptic nocturnal wanderings); these are usually a continuation of one of the above patterns, a potential distinguishing feature from somnambulism. A fearful expression and stereotyped vocalization (in this case, throat clearing) are common. These seizures are often responsive to low-dose carbamazepine and may occur due to mutations in the gene for subunits of the neuronal nicotinic acetylcholine receptor. Nocturnal seizures generally occur in stages 2, 3, and 4 of NREM sleep.

REM without atonia occurs in REM sleep behavior disorder, which generally occurs in older individuals and is not stereotyped. Hypersynchronous high-voltage delta ("delta build-up") may be seen in SWS parasomnias, and hypopneas may be a potential triggering event for the arousal.

39. A. Basal forebrain extracellular adenosine concentrations increase during prolonged wakefulness.

Adenosine may play an important role in the regulation of sleep and wakefulness (for a review, see Basheer R et al: Prog Neurobiol 73[6]:379–396, 2004). Andenosine is a nucleoside that serves as a building block for nucleic acids and energy storage molecules. Extracellular adenosine has a modulatory effect on specific neuronal populations such as the cholinergic neurons in the basal forebrain and lateral dorsal tegmental nuclei. Sleep is thought to have an energy restoration function, and as a by-product of energy metabolism, adenosine may serve a key homeostatic function by promoting sleep. Extracellular adenosine concentrations increase in response to increased metabolic rate and neuronal activity. Animal experiments with extracellular dialysis techniques have demonstrated increases in the adenosine concentration in the basal forebrain and thalamus in response to prolonged wakefulness and a decline during recovery sleep. Adenosine has an inhibitory effect on wake-promoting neurons, fostering sleep as the extracellular concentration increases during wakefulness. In the basal forebrain, adenosine's effect on sleep and wakefulness is mediated via A1 receptors on the cholinergic neurons. Via a second messenger system, adenosine increases intracellular calcium stores and activates transcription factors. This may play a role in the long-term consequences of sleep deprivation and the molecular basis of the "sleep debt." Caffeine and theophylline act as competitive antagonists of adenosine at the A_1 and A_{2a} receptor subtypes, the mechanism by which these agents promote wakefulness. Adenosine is not implicated in the control of the circadian timekeeping system.

40. D. Short-wavelength light sensitivity is consistent with the fact that neither rods nor cones are required for circadian entrainment.

Short-wavelength light sensitivity is consistent with the fact that neither rods nor cones are required for circadian entrainment. Melanopsin is a photopigment with peak spectral sensitivity in the short-wavelength range found in intrinsically photosensitive retinal ganglion cells that have a major projection to the suprachiasmatic nucleus. On the other hand, neither rods nor cones show peak spectral sensitivity to short-wavelength light. Knock-out mice without rods and cones, as well as some humans without functional rods and cones, retain circadian entrainment to light. However, absence of rods, cones, and melanopsin abolishes all photic responses. Melanopsin is implicated as an important mediator of many nonvisual photic responses (Lockley SW et al: Sleep 29[2]:161–168, 2006).

41. A. Extrasynaptic GABA-A receptors.

GABA-A receptors exist at both synaptic and extrasynaptic sites. Benzodiazepines and nonbenzodiazepine hypnotics act to modulate subtypes of the GABA-A receptor complex by enhancing the flow of chloride ions in response to GABA, primarily at synaptic sites. Gaboxadol is a GABA agonist that acts as a "super agonist" (i.e., more potent than GABA) at extrasynaptic GABA-A receptors, and a weak agonist at synaptic sites that are sensitive to benzodiazepines. Extrasynaptic GABA-A receptors are found on axons, dendrites, and soma in cerebellum, thalamocortical relay neurons of the ventral basal complex and the neocortex. Stimulation of extrasynaptic GABA-A receptors results in tonic inhibitory conductance that makes the membrane less sensitive to excitatory stimuli (Lu J, Greco MA: J Clin Sleep Med 2[2]:S19–S26, 2006).

Gaboxadol is not a GABA-B agonist, whereas baclofen is a GABA-B receptor agonist. GABA-C receptors are found primarily in the retina and have a unique pharmacological responsiveness. Drugs that decrease reuptake of GABA, such as tiagabine, are capable of stimulating all GABA receptors by increasing endogenous GABA concentrations.

42. C. Ventral lateral preoptic nucleus (VLPO)

Recent work indicates that retinal ganglion cells (RGCs) containing the light-sensitive pigment melanopsin depolarize in response to light and send projections to the suprachiasmatic nucleus, as well as to other brain structures that are influenced by photic stimulation. These other structures include the VLPO, a structure in the anterior hypothalamus that is sleep activating and sleep promoting. Other targets of the melanopsin-containing RGCs include the subparaventricular zone and the intergeniculate leaflet of the lateral geniculate nucleus, which are both areas involved in circadian regulation, and the pretectal area, which influences the pupillary light reflex. The raphe nuclei, locus coeruleus, and the tuberomammillary nucleus are important components of the aminergic arousal system that are inhibited by the VLPO during sleep (see Question 36). None of these other cell groups is known to have projections from RGCs (Gooley JJ et al: J Neurosci 23[18]:7093–7106, 2003).

REFERENCES

1. Allen R, Becker PM, Bogan R, et al: Ropinirole decreases periodic leg movements and improves sleep parameters in patients with restless legs syndrome. Sleep 27(5):907–914, 2004.

2. Allen RP, Picchietti D, Hening WA, et al: Restless legs syndrome: diagnostic criteria, special considerations, and epidemiology. A report from the restless legs syndrome diagnosis and epidemiology workshop at the National Institutes of Health. Sleep Med 4(2):101–119, 2003.

3. Amin RS, Carroll JL, Jeffries JL, et al: Twenty-four-hour ambulatory blood pressure in children with sleep-disordered breathing. Am J Respir Crit Care Med 169(8): 950–956, 2004.

4. Babu AR, Herdegen J, Fogelfeld L, et al: Type 2 diabetes, glycemic control, and continuous positive airway pressure in obstructive sleep apnea. Arch Intern Med 165(4):447–452, 2005.

5. Baguet JP, Hammer L, Levy P, et al: The severity of oxygen desaturation is predictive of carotid wall thickening and plaque occurrence. Chest 128(5):3407–3412, 2005.

6. Basheer R, Strecker RE, Thakkar MM, McCarley RW: Adenosine and sleep-wake regulation. Prog Neurobiol 73(6):379–396, 2004.

7. Boyd JH, Petrof BJ, Hamid Q, et al: Upper airway muscle inflammation and denervation changes in obstructive sleep apnea. Am J Respir Crit Care Med 170(5):541–556, 2004.

8. Bradley TD, Logan AG, Kimoff RJ, et al: Continuous positive airway pressure for central sleep apnea and heart failure. N Engl J Med 353(19):2025–2033, 2005.

9. Clardy SL, Earley CJ, Allen RP, et al: Ferritin subunits in CSF are decreased in restless legs syndrome. J Lab Clin Med 147(2):67–73, 2006.

10. Ferguson KA, Cartwright R, Rogers R, Schmidt-Nowara W: Oral appliances for snoring and obstructive sleep apnea: a review. Sleep 29(2):244–262, 2006.

11. Garrigue S, Bordier P, Jais P, et al: Benefit of atrial pacing in sleep apnea syndrome. N Engl J Med 346(6): 404–412, 2002.

12. Glass J, Lanctot KL, Herrmann N, et al: Sedative hypnotics in older people with insomnia: meta-analysis of risks and benefits. BMJ 331(7526):1169, 2005.

13. Gooley JJ, Lu J, Fischer D, Saper CB: A broad role for melanopsin in nonvisual photoreception. J Neurosci 23(18):7093–7106, 2003.

14. Gottlieb DJ, DeStefano AL, Foley DJ, et al: APOE epsilon 4 is associated with obstructive sleep apnea/hypopnea: the Sleep Heart Health Study. Neurology 63(4):664–668, 2004.

15. Group XIS: A double-blind, placebo-controlled study demonstrates sodium oxybate is effective for the treatment of excessive daytime sleepiness in narcolepsy. J Clin Sleep Med 1(4):391–397, 2005.

16. Guilleminault C, Kirisoglu C, Bao G, et al: Adult chronic sleepwalking and its treatment based on polysomnography. Brain 128(Pt 5):1062–1069, 2005.

17. Guilleminault C, Palombini L, Pelayo R, Chervin RD: Sleepwalking and sleep terrors in prepubertal children: what triggers them? Pediatrics 111(1):e17–e25, 2003.

18. Haas DC, Foster GL, Nieto FJ, et al: Age-dependent associations between sleep-disordered breathing and hypertension: importance of discriminating between systolic/diastolic hypertension and isolated systolic hypertension in the Sleep Heart Health Study. Circulation 111(5):614–621, 2005.

19. Jacobs GD, Pace-Schott EF, Stickgold R, Otto MW: Cognitive behavior therapy and pharmacotherapy for insomnia: a randomized controlled trial and direct comparison. Arch Intern Med 164(17):1888–1896, 2004.

20. Javaheri S: Acetazolamide improves central sleep apnea in heart failure: a double-blind, prospective study. Am J Respir Crit Care Med 173(2):234–237, 2006.

21. Kushida CA, Littner MR, Morgenthaler T, et al: Practice parameters for the indications for polysomnography and related procedures: an update for 2005. Sleep 28(4):499–521, 2005.

22. Lockley SW, Evans EE, Scheer FA, et al: Short-wavelength sensitivity for the direct effects of light on alertness, vigilance, and the waking electroencephalogram in humans. Sleep 29(2):161–168, 2006.

23. Lu J, Greco MA: Sleep circuitry and the hypnotic mechanism of GABA-A drugs. J Clin Sleep Med 2(2):S19–S26, 2006.

24. Massimini M, Ferrarelli F, Huber R, et al: Breakdown of cortical effective connectivity during sleep. Science 309(5744):2228–2232, 2005.

25. McKeith IG, Dickson DW, Lowe J, et al: Diagnosis and management of dementia with Lewy bodies: third report of the DLB Consortium. Neurology 65(12): 1863–1872, 2005.

26. Mignot E, Chen W, Black J: On the value of measuring CSF hypocretin-1 in diagnosing narcolepsy. Sleep 26(6):646–649, 2003.

27. Mignot E, Nishino S: Emerging therapies in narcolepsy-cataplexy. Sleep 28(6):754–763, 2005.

28. Mochizuki T, Crocker A, McCormack S, et al: Behavioral state instability in orexin knock-out mice. J Neurosci 24(28):6291–6300, 2004.

29. Mundey K, Benloucif S, Harsanyi K, et al: Phase-dependent treatment of delayed sleep phase syndrome with melatonin. Sleep 28(10):1271–1278, 2005.

30. Nofzinger EA, Buysse DJ, Germain A, et al: Functional neuroimaging evidence for hyperarousal in insomnia. Am J Psychiatry 161(11):2126–2168, 2004.

31. Pirelli P, Saponara M, Guilleminault C: Rapid maxillary expansion in children with obstructive sleep apnea syndrome. Sleep 27(4):761–766, 2004.

32. Punjabi NM, Shahar E, Redline S, et al: Sleep-disordered breathing, glucose intolerance, and insulin resistance: the Sleep Heart Health Study. Am J Epidemiol 160(6):521–530, 2004.

33. Reichmuth KJ, Austin D, Skatrud JB, Young T: Association of sleep apnea and type II diabetes: a population-based study. Am J Respir Crit Care Med 172(12):1590–1595, 2005.

34. Saper CB, Cano G, Scammell TE: Homeostatic, circadian, and emotional regulation of sleep. J Comp Neurol 493(1):92–98, 2005.

35. Silber MH: Clinical practice. Chronic insomnia. N Engl J Med 353(8):803–810, 2005.

36. Silber MH, Ehrenberg BL, Allen RP, et al: An algorithm for the management of restless legs syndrome. Mayo Clin Proc 79(7):916–922, 2004.

37. Simantirakis EN, Schiza SE, Chrysostomakis SI, et al: Atrial overdrive pacing for the obstructive sleep apnea-hypopnea syndrome. N Engl J Med 353(24):2568–2577, 2005.

38. Tinuper P, Provini F, Bisulli F, Lugaresi E: Hyperkinetic manifestations in nocturnal frontal lobe epilepsy. Semeiological features and physiopathological hypothesis. Neurol Sci 26(Suppl 3):s210–s214, 2005.

39. Van Dongen HP, Maislin G, Mullington JM, Dinges DF: The cumulative cost of additional wakefulness: dose-response effects on neurobehavioral functions and sleep physiology from chronic sleep restriction and total sleep deprivation. Sleep 26(2):117–126, 2003.

40. Veasey SC, Davis CW, Fenik P, et al: Long-term intermittent hypoxia in mice: protracted hypersomnolence with oxidative injury to sleep-wake brain regions. Sleep 27(2):194–201, 2004.

41. White DP: Pathogenesis of obstructive and central sleep apnea. Am J Respir Crit Care Med 172(11):1363–1370, 2005.

42. Wyatt JK: Delayed sleep phase syndrome: pathophysiology and treatment options. Sleep 27(6):1195–1203, 2004.

43. Yaggi HK, Concato J, Kernan WN, et al: Obstructive sleep apnea as a risk factor for stroke and death. N Engl J Med 353(19):2034–2041, 2005.

44. Yokoe T, Minoguchi K, Matsuo H, et al: Elevated levels of C-reactive protein and interleukin-6 in patients with obstructive sleep apnea syndrome are decreased by nasal continuous positive airway pressure. Circulation 107(8):1129–1134, 2003.

45. Young T, Finn L, Austin D, Peterson A: Menopausal status and sleep-disordered breathing in the Wisconsin Sleep Cohort Study. Am J Respir Crit Care Med 167(9):1181–1185, 2003.

Valuable Resources*

*Compiled by Mikhael Loots, MPAS, PA-C from Internet (public domain) resources.
Note: This section contains resources that may change. The reader is advised to check for updated information as indicated.

PROFESSIONAL SLEEP ASSOCIATIONS/ SOCIETIES

1. American Academy of Sleep Medicine (AASM)
   One Westbrook Corporate Center, Ste. 920
   Westchester, IL 60154
   Phone: 708-492-0930
   Fax: 708-492-0943
   Web address: *http://www.aasmnet.org*

2. American Society of Electroneurodiagnostic Technologists (ASET)
   6501 East Commerce Avenue, Ste. 120
   Kansas City, MO 64120
   Phone: 816-931-1120
   Fax: 816-931-1145
   Email: info@aset.org
   Web address: *http://www.aset.org*

3. Sleep Research Society (SRS)
   One Westbrook Corporate Center, Ste. 920
   Westchester, IL 60154
   Phone: 708-492-1093
   Web address: *www.sleepresearchsociety.org*

4. Association of Polysomnographic Technologists (APT)
   One Westbrook Corporate Center, Ste. 920
   Westchester, IL 60154
   Phone: 708-492-0796
   Fax: 708-273-9344
   Email: apt@aptweb.org
   Web address: *http://www.aptweb.org*

5. The National Center on Sleep Disorders Research (NCSDR)
   NIH/NHLBI/NCSDR
   6705 Rockledge Drive
   One Rockledge Center, Ste. 6022
   Bethesda, MD 20892-7993
   Phone: 301-435-0199
   Fax: 301-480-3451
   Email: ncsdr@nih.gov
   Web address: *http://www.nhlbi.nih.gov/about/ncsdr/index.htm*

6. National Sleep Foundation
   1522 K Street, NW, Ste. 500
   Washington, DC 20005
   Phone: 202-347-3471
   Fax: 202-347-3472
   Email: nsf@sleepfoundation.org
   Web address: *http://www.sleepfoundation.org*

7. Associated Professional Sleep Societies (APSS)
   One Westbrook Corporate Center, Ste. 920
   Westchester, IL 60154
   Phone: 708-492-0930
   Fax: 708-273-9354
   Web address: *http://www.apss.org*

8. Academy of Dental Sleep Medicine
   One Westbrook Corporate Center, Ste. 920
   Westchester, IL 60254
   Phone: 708-273-9366
   Fax: 708-492-0943
   Email: info@dentalsleepmed.org
   Web address: *http://www.dentalsleepmed.org*

9. Kentucky Sleep Society
   667 Elsmere Park
   Lexington, KY
   Phone: 859-252-6447
   Fax: 859-313-3021
   Web address: *http://www.kyss.org*

10. Society for Research on Biological Rhythms (SRBR)
    Karen Nichols
    University of Illinois at Urbana-Champaign
    Phone: 217-333-2880
    Fax: 217-333-9561
    Web address: *http://www.srbr.org*

11. Society of Light Treatment and Biological Rhythms (SLTBR)
    4648 Main Street
    Chincoteague, VA 23336
    Fax: 757-336-5777
    Email: sltbrinfo@aol.com
    Web address: *http://www.sltbr.org*

INTERNATIONAL SLEEP ORGANIZATIONS

1. Austrian Sleep Research Society
   Web address: *http://www.schlafmedizin.at*
2. British Sleep Society
   Web address: *http://www.british-sleep-society.org.uk*

3. Club del Sueño (Sleep Club)
Web address: *http://www.rems.com.ar*
4. Die Deutsche Gesellschaft für Schlafforschung und Schlafmedizin (The German Sleep Society)
Web address: *http://www.uni-marburg.de/sleep/dgsm/welcome.html*
5. The Irish Sleep Apnoea Trust
Web address: *http://www.isat.ie*
6. International Directory of Sleep Researchers and Clinicians
Web address: *http://www.websciences.org/directory*
7. Sleep Chapter of the Spanish Society of Clinical Neurophysiology (Grupo Sobre Transtornos del Sueno de la Sociedad Espanola de Neurofisiologia Clinica)
Web address: *http://www.neurofisiologia.org*
8. World Federation of Sleep Research Societies
Web address: *http://www.wfsrs.org/1generalinfo.html*

The WFSRS is a Federation of the following societies:
a. Asian Sleep Research Society (ASRS)
Web address: *http://www.wfsrs.org/iasrs.html*
b. Australasian Sleep Association (ASA)
Web address: *http://www.wfsrs.org/iasa.html*
c. Canadian Sleep Society (CSS)
Web address: *http://www.css.to*
d. European Sleep Research Society (ESRS)
Web address: *http://www.wfsrs.org/iesrs.html*
e. Latin American Sleep Society (LASS)
Web address: *http://www.wfsrs.org/ilass.html*
f. Sleep Research Society (United States) (SRS)
Web address: *http://www.srssleep.org*

SLEEP MEDICINE BOARDS/EDUCATION

1. American Board of Sleep Medicine (ABSM)
One Westbrook Corporate Center, Ste. 920
Westchester, IL 60154
Phone: 708-492-1290
Fax: 708-492-0943
Web address: *http://www.absm.org*
2. American Academy of Sleep Medicine (AASM)
One Westbrook Corporate Center, Ste. 920
Westchester, IL 60154
Phone: 708-492-0930
Fax: 708-492-0943
Web address: *http://www.aasmnet.org*
3. American Board of Medical Specialties (ABMS)
1007 Church Street, Ste. 404
Evanston, IL 60201-5913
Phone: 847-491-9091
Fax: 847-328-3596
Web address: *http://www.abms.org*

ABMS is the umbrella organization that represents 24 medical specialty boards including the ones responsible for future sleep medicine candidates for sleep board examinations from:
a. American Board of Internal Medicine
510 Walnut Street, Ste. 1700
Philadelphia, PA 19106-3699
Phone: 215-446-3500
Phone: 800-441-2246
Fax: 215-446-3633
Web address: *http://www.abim.org*
b. American Board of Psychiatry and Neurology, Inc.
500 Lake Cook Road, Ste. 335
Deerfield, IL 60015-5249
Phone: 847-945-7900
Fax: 847-945-1146
Web address: *http://www.abpn.com*
c. American Board of Pediatrics
111 Silver Cedar Court
Chapel Hill, NC 27514
Phone: 919-929-0461
Fax: 919-929-9255
Web address: *http://www.abped.org*
d. American Board of Otolaryngology
5615 Kirby Drive, Ste. 600
Houston, TX 77005
Phone: 713-850-0399
Fax: 713-850-1104
Web address: *http://www.aboto.org*

CURRENT PHYSICIAN SLEEP MEDICINE FELLOWSHIPS FALL 2006

Programs previously accredited by the AASM
**Listed as current ACGME-accredited programs as of December 2006
Because this list will be changed with the transition to ACGME-accredited fellowship programs, please look for updated information at: *http://www.aasmnet.org/FellowshipTraining.aspx*

1. Stanford, CA
Stanford University; Stanford Sleep Disorders Clinic
401 Quarry Road, Ste. 3301
Stanford, CA 94305-5547
Phone: 650-723-6601 or 415-725-5911
Fax: 650-725-8910
2. Norwalk, CT
Norwalk Hospital Sleep Disorders Center
34 Maple Street
Norwalk, CT 06856
Phone: 203-855-3632
Fax: 203-852-2945

3. Gainesville, FL
   University of Florida College of Medicine**
   1600 SW Archer Road
   Gainesville, FL 32610
   Phone: 352-392-2666
   Fax: 352-379-4155

4. Jacksonville, FL
   Mayo Clinic/Mayo Graduate School of Medicine, Jacksonville Mayo Clinic
   4500 San Pablo Road, Room 172 W
   Jacksonville, FL 32224
   Phone: 904-953-2000
   Fax: 904-953-2082

5. Miami Beach, FL
   Mount Sinai Sleep Disorders Center
   4300 Alton Road
   Miami Beach, FL 33140
   Phone: 305-674-2613
   Fax: 305-674-2647

6. Iowa City, IA
   University of Iowa Hospital**
   200 Hawkins Drive
   Iowa City, IA 52242
   Phone: 319-356-2538
   Fax: 319-356-4505

7. Chicago, IL
   Children's Memorial Hospital Sleep Medicine Center
   2300 Children's Plaza, Box 43
   Chicago, IL 60614
   Phone: 773-880-8230
   Fax: 773-880-4057

8. Chicago, IL
   Rush-Presbyterian-St. Luke's Medical Center Sleep Disorders Center**
   1653 West Congress Parkway
   Chicago, IL 60612-3833
   Phone: 312-942-5440
   Fax: 312-942-8961

9. Chicago, IL
   McGaw Medical Center of Northwestern University**
   251 East Huron Street
   Chicago, IL 60611
   Phone: 312-908-5633
   Fax: 312-908-5073

10. Indianapolis, IN
    Sleep Medicine and Circadian Biology Program/ Indiana University School of Medicine, Department of Medicine
    550 N. University Boulevard
    University Hospital/UH5450
    Indianapolis, IN 46202
    Phone: 317-274-2136
    Fax: 317-274-4224

11. Lexington, KY
    University of Kentucky
    MN-614, UKMC; 800 Rose Street
    Lexington, KY 40536-0084
    Phone: 859-323-5419
    Fax: 859-323-1020

12. Louisville, KY
    University of Louisville School of Medicine**
    323 East Chestnut
    Louisville, KY 40202
    Phone: 502-852-2323
    Fax: 502-852-2215

13. New Orleans, LA
    Tulane University School of Medicine
    1430 Tulane Avenue; Department of Pediatrics, SL-37
    New Orleans, LA, 70112
    Phone: 504-588-5601
    Fax: 504-588-5490

14. Boston, MA
    Brigham & Women's Hospital**
    Division of Sleep Medicine, Sleep Research at BI
    75 Francis Street
    Boston, MA 02115
    Phone: 617-732-5778
    Fax: 617-732-7337

15. Boston, MA
    Beth Israel Deaconess Medical Center**
    CC-866, Sleep Unit
    330 Brookline Avenue
    Boston, MA 02115
    Phone: 617-667-5864
    Fax: 617-667-4849

16. Brighton, MA 02135
    St. Elizabeth's Medical Center
    736 Cambridge Street
    Brighton, MA 02135
    Phone: 617-789-2545

17. Burlington, MA
    Lahey Clinic; 41 Mall Road
    Burlington, MA 01805
    Phone: 781-744-8480
    Fax: 781-744-3443

18. Worcester, MA
    Worcester Medical Center Campus at St. Vincent Hospital; Department of Neurology
    20 Worcester Center Boulevard
    Worcester, MA 01608
    Phone: 508-363-6066
    Fax: 508-363-6373

19. Baltimore, MD
    Johns Hopkins University/Bayview Medical Center**
    5501 Hopkins Bayview Circle
    Baltimore, MD 21224

Phone: 410-550-0572
Fax: 410-550-3374

20. Ann Arbor, MI
Michael S. Aldrich Sleep Disorders Laboratory
UH 8D8702-0117
University of Michigan Medical Center**
1500 East Medical Center Drive
Ann Arbor, MI 48109-0117
Phone: 734-647-9064
Fax: 734-647-9065

21. Detroit, MI
Detroit VA Medical Center
Neurology Section 11M-NEU; 4646 John R.
Detroit, MI 48201
Phone: 313-576-3311
Fax: 313-576-1377

22. Detroit, MI
Wayne State University; Detroit Medical Center; Harper University Hospital**
3990 John R., 3-Hudson
Detroit, MI 48323
Phone: 313-745-6033
Fax: 313-745-2481

23. Detroit, MI
Henry Ford Hospital HFH Sleep Disorders & Research Center**
2799 W. Grand Boulevard; CFP-3
Detroit, MI 48202-2691
Phone: 313-916-5173
Fax: 313-916-5150

24. Minneapolis, MN
Hennepin County Medical Center**
701 Park Avenue South
Minneapolis, MN 55415
Phone: 612-873-2611
Fax: 612-904-4680

25. Rochester, MN
Mayo School of Graduate Medical Education (Rochester)**
Mayo Clinic College of Medicine
200 First Street SW
Rochester, MN 55905
Phone: 507-284-4500

26. Columbia, MO
University of Missouri—Columbia School of Medicine**
M 178 Medical Sciences Bldg.
One Hospital Drive
Columbia, MO 65212
Phone: 573-882-2260
Fax: 573-884-4249

27. Kansas City, MO
University of Missouri at Kansas City
2411 Holmes
Kansas City, MO 64108

Phone: 816-756-2466
Fax: 816-756-5015

28. St. Louis, MO
Washington University; B-JH/SLCH Consortium Program**
212 N. Kingshighway, Ste. 237
St. Louis, MO 63108
Phone: 314-362-4342
Fax: 314-747-3814

29. Jackson, MS
University of Mississippi Medical Center Sleep Disorders Center**
2500 North State Street
Jackson, MS 39216-4505
Phone: 601-984-6925
Fax: 601-984-4828

30. Chapel Hill, NC
University of North Carolina Hospital**
3114 Bioinformatics Building, Department of Neurology
CB 7025, UNC
Chapel Hill, NC 27599
Phone: 919-966-3707

31. Durham, NC
Duke University Medical Center (DUMC)**
Box 3678; 202 Bell Building
Durham, NC 27710
Phone: 919-684-8485
Fax: 919-684-8955

32. Winston-Salem, NC
Wake Forest University Health Sciences
Medical Center Boulevard
Winston-Salem, NC 27157
Phone: 336-716-7228
Fax: 336-716-9489

33. Omaha, NE
University of Nebraska Medical Center (UNMC)
Box 985300, Nebraska Medical Center
Omaha, NE 68198-5300
Phone: 402-559-4087
Fax: 402-559-8210

34. Lebanon, NH
Dartmouth-Hitchcock Medical Center**
Mary Hitchcock Memorial Hospital Sleep Disorders Center
One Medical Center Drive
Lebanon, NH 03756
Phone: 603-650-7534
Fax: 603-650-7820

35. Newark, NJ
Newark Beth Israel Sleep Disorders Center
201 Lyons Avenue
Newark, NJ 07112
Phone: 973-926-7163
Fax: 973-282-0821

36. Edison, NJ
Seton Hall University School of Graduate Medical Education**
Center for Sleep Disorders Treatment; Research and Education
400 South Orange Avenue
South Orange, NJ 07079
Phone: 732-632-1685

37. Hackensack, NJ
Hackensack University Medical Center—Institute for Sleep/Wake Disorders
30 Prospect Avenue
Hackensack, NJ 07601
Phone: 201-996-3732
Fax: 201-498-1163

38. Albuquerque, NM
New Mexico Center for Sleep Medicine**
4700 Jefferson NE, Ste. 800
Albuquerque, NM 87109
Phone: 505-872-6000
Fax: 505-872-6003

39. Bronx, NY
Albert Einstein College of Medicine**
Yeshiva University
111 East 210th Street
Bronx, NY 10467
Phone: 718-920-4841
Fax: 718-798-4352

40. Buffalo, NY
University of Buffalo**
Buffalo General Hospital Department of Medicine
Buffalo, NY 14203
Phone: 716-859-2271
Fax: 716-859-1491

41. Buffalo, NY
SUNY Buffalo School of Medicine
Geriatric Psychiatry & Sleep Medicine Fellowships
Office of Graduate Medical Education, ECMC Room 144
462 Grider St.
Buffalo, NY 14215
Phone: 716-961-6955
Fax: 716-961-6960

42. Manhasset, NY
NSLIJHS-North Shore University Hospital**
NYU School of Medicine
North Shore University Hospital
410 Lakeville Road, Ste. 105
New Hyde Park, NY 11042
Phone: 516-465-3899
Fax: 516-616-4124

43. Mineola, NY
Winthrop-University Hospital**
259 First Street
Mineola, NY 11501
Phone: 516-663-2004
Fax: 516-663-4888

44. New Hyde Park, NY
Long Island Jewish Medical Center
Division of Pulmonary and Critical Care Medicine
270-05 76th Avenue
New Hyde Park, NY 11040
Phone: 516-470-6400
Fax: 516-488-7162

45. New York, NY
CliniLabs, Inc., Sleep Disorders Institute
1090 Amsterdam Avenue
New York, NY 10025
Phone: 212-523-1700
Fax: 212-523-1704

46. Stony Brook, NY
Center for the Study of Sleep and Waking; SUNY Stony Brook
University Hospital MR 120-A
Stony Brook, NY 11794-7139
Phone: 631-444-2916
Fax: 631-444-7851

47. Cincinnati, OH
Cincinnati Children's Hospital Medical Center**
University of Cincinnati College of Medicine
3333 Burnet Avenue, MLC #2021
Cincinnati, OH 45229
Phone: 513-636-7945
Fax: 513-636-4615

48. Cleveland, OH
Cleveland Clinic Foundation Sleep Disorders Center**
9500 Euclid Avenue; S-51
Cleveland, OH 44195
Phone: 216-445-2990
Fax: 216-445-6205

49. Cleveland, OH
Case Western Reserve University**
University Hospitals of Cleveland
11100 Euclid Avenue
Cleveland, OH 44106
Phone: 216-844-3201
Fax: 216-844-8708

50. Columbus, OH
Ohio State University Hospital**
410 West Tenth Avenue
125 Doan Hall
Columbus, OH 43210
Phone: 614-247-7707
Fax: 614-293-4799

51. Philadelphia, PA
Drexel University College of Medicine/Hahnemann Program**
245 N. 15th Street
Philadelphia, PA 19102
Phone: 215-762-7011
Fax: 215-762-8728

52. Philadelphia, PA
    Thomas Jefferson University Hospital**
    1015 Walnut Street, Ste. 319
    Philadelphia, PA 19107
    Phone: 215-955-6175
    Fax: 215-955-9783
53. Philadelphia, PA
    Temple University Hospital**
    3401 N. Broad Street
    Philadelphia, PA 19140
    Phone: 215-707-4678
    Fax: 215-707-6867
54. Philadelphia, PA
    University of Pennsylvania Sleep Medicine Fel-
       lowship Program**
    3400 Spruce Street
    975 Maloney Building
    Philadelphia, PA 19104
    Phone: 215-615-3699
    Fax: 215-662-7749
55. Pittsburgh, PA
    University of Pittsburgh Medical Center**
    Medical Education Program
    200 Lothrup Street
    NW628, MUH
    Pittsburgh, PA 15213
    Phone: 412-692-2880
56. Johnson City, TN
    Center for Sleep Disorders at Johnson City
       Medical Center
    310 N. State of Franklin Road, Ste. 303
    Johnson City, TN 37604
    Phone: 423-926-8181
    Fax: 423-926-8652
57. Nashville, TN
    Vanderbilt University**
    Department of Neurology
    2100 Pierce Avenue
    Nashville, TN 37212
    Phone: 615-322-0283
    Fax: 615-936-0223
58. Dallas, TX
    University of Texas Southwestern Medical
       School**
    5323 Harry Hines Blvd.
    Dallas, TX 75390
    Phone: 214-648-7364
    Fax: 214-648-7370
59. Houston, TX
    University of Texas Health Science Center
       at Houston
    Division of Pulmonary, Critical Care, and Sleep
       Medicine
    6431 Fannin Street, Ste. 1260
    Houston, TX 77030
    Phone: 713-500-6823

    Fax: 713-500-6829
60. Temple, TX
    Scott & White Memorial Hospital and Clinic
    2401 South 31st Street
    Temple, TX 76508
    Phone: 254-724-2554
    Fax: 254-724-2497
61. Salt Lake City, UT
    Intermountain Sleep Disorders Center at
       LDS Hospital**
    University of Utah
    325-Eighth Avenue & C Street
    Salt Lake City, UT 84143
    Phone: 801-408-3617
    Fax: 801-408-5110
62. Burlington, VT
    University of Vermont
    Fletcher Allen Health Care
    111 Colchester Avenue Patrick 5
    Burlington, VT 05401
    Phone: 802-847-5338
63. Seattle, WA
    University of Washington
    325 9th Avenue; Box 359803
    Seattle, WA 98104-2499
    Phone: 206-731-5703
    Fax: 206-731-5657
64. Madison, WI
    University of Wisconsin**
    University of Wisconsin Hospital and Clinics
    600 Highland Avenue, K4/926
    Madison, WI 53792
    Phone: 608-256-1901
    Fax: 608-280-7291
65. Huntington, WV
    St. Mary's Medical Center/Ultimate Health
       Services
    2900 First Avenue
    Huntington, WV 25702
    Phone: 304-526-1880
    Fax: 304-526-1886

PICKWICK POSTDOCTORAL FELLOWSHIP

From the National Sleep Foundation website: "Since 1995, the Pickwick Postdoctoral Fellowship program has provided funds to enable young researchers to devote full-time professional effort to mentored research in sleep or sleep disorders."

For more information:

National Sleep Foundation
1522 K Street NW, Ste. 500
Washington, DC 20005
Phone: 202-347-3471

Fax: 202-347-3472

Web address: *http://sleepfoundation.org/activities/index. php?id=23*

Sleep Continuing Medical Education (CME) and Sleep Conferences

1. The American Society of Electroneurodiagnostic Technologists
   6501 East Commerce Avenue, Ste. 120
   Kansas City, MO 64120
   Phone: 816-931-1120
   Fax: 816-931-1145
   Email: info@aset.org
   Web address: *http://www.aset.org*
2. The Atlanta School of Sleep Medicine
   5780 Peachtree-Dunwoody Road, Ste. 150
   Atlanta, GA 30342-1513
   Phone: 404-303-3385
   Fax: 404-252-0311
   Web address: *http://www.sleepschool.com*
3. The School of Sleep Medicine, Inc.
   260 Sheridan Avenue, Ste. 100
   Palo Alto, CA 94306
   Phone: 650-326-1296
   Fax: 650-326-1295
   Web address: *http://www.sleepedu.net*
4. American Academy of Sleep Medicine (AASM)
   One Westbrook Corporate Center, Ste. 920
   Westchester, IL 60154
   Phone: 708-492-0930
   Fax: 708-492-0943
   Web address: *http://www.aasmnet.org*
5. Associated Professional Sleep Societies (APSS)
   One Westbrook Corporate Center, Ste. 920
   Westchester, IL 60154
   Phone: 708-492-0930
   Fax: 708-273-9354
   Web address: *http://www.apss.org*
6. California College for Health Sciences Polysomnography Certificate
   2423 Hoover Avenue
   National City, CA 91950
   Phone: 619-477-4800
   Fax: 570-961-4150
   Web address: *cchsinfo@cchs.edu*
7. Synapse Media, Inc.
   School of Clinical Polysomnography
   4702 Cloudcrest Drive
   Medford, OR 97504
   Phone: 541-608-0381
   Fax: 541-608-6139

Web address: *http://www.synapsemedia.com*
8. National School of Sleep Medicine
   Fairlawn, Ohio
   Web address: *http://sleepmedicine.org*

PATIENT EDUCATIONAL MATERIALS

There are multiple organizations that provide sleep medicine education and support for patients. This is a *sample* of the organizations available:

1. American Sleep Apnea Association at *www.sleepapnea.org*
2. Florida Narcolepsy Association at *www.flnarcolepsy.org*
3. Narcolepsy Network at *www.narcolepsynetwork.org*
4. Restless Legs Syndrome Foundation at *www.rls.org*
5. Sleep/Wake Disorders Canada at *www.swdca.org*
6. AAA Foundation for Traffic Safety at *http://www.aaafoundation.org/home*
7. American Fibromyalgia Syndrome Association at *http://www.afsafund.org*
8. Association for the Study of Dreams at *http://www.asdreams.org*
9. Better Sleep Council at *http://www.bettersleep.org/index.html*
10. Drowsy Driving links, from the AAA Foundation for Traffic Safety at *http://www.aaafoundation.org/resources/index.cfm?button=links*
11. Encyclopaedic Directory of Neurosciences and Mental Health at *http://www.nsm.es/directorio*
12. Medline Plus Health Information (a service of the National Library of Medicine) *http://www.nlm.nih.gov/medlineplus/sleepdisorders.html*
13. MedSupport FSF International at *http://www.medsupport.org*
14. National Center on Sleep Disorders Research at *http://www.nhlbi.nih.gov/about/ncsdr*
15. National Enuresis Society at *http://www.peds.umn.edu/Centers/NES*
16. National Heart, Lung and Blood Institute at *http://www.nhlbi.nih.gov*
17. NHLBI Garfield "Star Sleeper" at *http://starsleep.nhlbi.nih.gov*
18. NIH's Clinical Trials at *http://clinicaltrials.gov*
19. National Organization of Rare Disorders, Inc. at *http://www.rarediseases.org/cgi-bin/nord*
20. Sleep for Science Program at *http://www.sleepforscience.org/bradley*
21. Sleep Home Pages at *http://www.sleephomepages.org*

22. Sleeping Like a Baby at *http://www.tau.ac.il/~sadeh/baby*

23. SleepQuest at *http://www.sleepquest.com*

24. SLEEP-The Journal of Sleep and Sleep Disorders Research at *http://www.journalsleep.org*

25. Stanford University Center of Excellence for the Diagnosis and Treatment of Sleep Disorders at *http://www.med.stanford.edu/school/psychiatry/coe*

26. Sudden Infant Death Syndrome Alliance at *http://www.sidsalliance.org*

27. Teaching Sleep Medicine: MedSleep Educational Materials at *http://www.aasmnet.org/MEDSleep/medsleephome.HTM*

Sleep Stage Scoring

ALON Y. AVIDAN

Sleep stage scoring is based on criteria derived from several physiologic signals, usually as outlined by Rechtschaffen and Kales (R-K) (1968). The R-K method divides sleep into five stages: non-rapid eye movement (NREM) stages 1, 2, 3, and 4 and stage REM sleep. Physiologic signals of interest are generated from the cerebral cortex (electroencephalogram [EEG]), eye movements (electro-oculogram [EOG]), and the muscles of the face (chin electromyography [EMG]). Table A1-1 summarizes sleep stages according to the R-K criteria.

This appendix includes a discussion of the specific parameters required for staging sleep. Unless otherwise stated, all polysomnogram (PSG) samples are recorded at a paper speed of 10 mm/sec, where one page equates to 30 seconds and is defined as one epoch.

ABBREVIATIONS USED IN THE PSG SAMPLES PROVIDED HERE INCLUDE:

LOC-A2, ROC-A1 = Left and right EOG referred to right and left mastoid leads.
LOC-AVG = Left and EOG referred to an average reference electrode
Chin1-Chin2 = Chin EMG electrode
EEG Monitoring: The exploring reference electrode (F3, F4, C3, C4, O1, and O2) is chosen on the opposite side of the head from the mastoid electrode (A1, A2) or average (AVG)
LAT1-LAT2, RAT1-RAT2 = Leg (anterior tibialis) EMG electrode (L = Left, R = Right)
N/O = Nasal/oral airflow channel
THOR1-THOR2 = Thoracic effort channel
ABD1-ABD2 = Abdominal effort channel

PARAMETERS FOR STAGING HUMAN SLEEP

The following three physiologic parameters are universal to all PSG monitoring:

- EOG leads—left eye and right eye
- EEG leads—a minimum of one central EEG lead and one occipital EEG lead
- EMG lead—one submental EMG channel

EOG Recording

- The EOG signals measure changes in the electric potential of the (+) anterior aspect of the eye, the cornea, relative to the (–) posterior aspect, the retina.
- EOG voltages are higher than the EEG signal. Because the eye is outside of the skull structure, there is no bone to attenuate signal.
- Cornea (front) has a positive polarity. The retina (back) has a negative polarity.
- EOG placement (LOC and ROC) is on the outer canthus of the eye—offset 1 cm below (= LOC) and 1 cm above (= ROC) the horizon.
- EOG picks up the inherent voltage of the eye. During eyes-open wakefulness, sharp deflections in the EOG tracing may indicate the presence of eye blinks.

EEG Recording Criteria

- Wakefulness and sleep are determined by the characteristic patterns of the scalp EEG signals and are of fundamental importance in interpreting PSG studies.
- EEG is a record of electric potentials generated by the cortex but can reflect the influence of deeper brain structures, such as the thalamus.
- Two centrocephalic and two occipital cortical channels are recorded: The PSG references the left and right centrocephalic electrodes (C3, C4) or the left and right occipital electrodes (O1, O4) to electrodes on the opposite right and left ears (A2, A1).
- Measurement of the EEG signal is possible because of the relative difference in potential between two recording electrodes.
- A (–) discharge, by convention, is represented by an upwardly deflecting wave.
- Minimum paper speed of 10 mm/sec. One page equates to 30 seconds and is defined as one epoch.
- Time constant (TC) of 0.3 seconds and/or low-frequency filter (LFF) of 0.3 Hz.
- Pen deflections of 7.5–10 mm for 50 µV are recommended.
- Electrode impedances should not exceed 10 kw.

TABLE A1-1 ■ Synopsis of Sleep Stages According to the Rechtschaffen and Kales Criteria

Properties	Stage Wake (W)	Stage 1	Stage 2	Stages 3 & 4 Sleep	Stage-REM Sleep
Duration		10 minutes	20 minutes	30–45 minutes	The first REM period is very short, (lasting ~5 minutes), the second is about 10 minutes, and the third is roughly 15 minutes. The final REM period usually last for 30 minutes (but can last up to an hour)
% Total sleep time	2–5%	3–8%	44–55%	10–15%	20–25%
EEG	Eyes open: Low voltage, mixed frequency. *Alpha* attenuates. Eyes closed: Low voltage, high frequency. More than 50% *alpha* activity	Low voltage, mixed frequency. *Theta activity.* *Vertex sharp waves*	Low voltage, mixed frequency. At least one *K-complex/sleep spindle*	Stage 3 = 20–50% high-amplitude delta activity. Stage 4 = >50% high-amplitude delta activity	Low-voltage, mixed frequency. Presence of *sawtooth waves.* *Desynchronized EEG* (In all other stages, the EEG is *synchronized*)
EOG	Eye blinks, voluntary control, *SREM* when drowsy	*SREM*	Occasional *SREM*	Mirrors EEG	Phasic REM
EMG	Tonic activity, High EMG activity. Under voluntary control	Tonic activity, High-medium EMG activity	Tonic activity, Low EMG activity	Tonic activity, Low EMG activity	*T-REM:* Relatively reduced. *P-REM:* Episodic EMG twitching
Arousal threshold	Lowest		Lower	Highest	Low
Physiologic changes		Progressive reduction of physiologic activity, blood pressure, heart rate slows down			*T-REM* = Muscle paralysis, increased cerebral blood flow. *P-REM* = Irregular breathing, variable heart rate, REM, phasic muscle twitching
Dreaming				Diffuse dreams	Vivid, bizarre, and detailed dreams
Parasomnias	Hypnic jerks in transition to stage 1	Hypnic jerks	Confusional arousals, somniliquy	Sleep walking, night terrors	REM-sleep behavior disorder, REM nightmares

Adapted from Rechtschaffen A, Kales A (eds): *A Manual of Standardised Terminology, Techniques and Scoring System for Sleep Stages of Human Subjects.* Los Angeles: Brain Information Service/Brain Research Institute, 1968.
Modified after Avidan AY: Recognition of sleep stages including scoring techniques. In Chokroverty S, Thomas R, Bhatt, M (eds): *Atlas of Sleep Medicine.* Philadelphia, Elsevier, 2005, pp 95–121.
The following are abbreviations used in the sleep montage recordings: LOC, left electro-oculogram; ROC, right electro-oculogram; Chin, chin electromyogram; ECG, electrocardiogram; LAT, left anterior tibialis surface electromyogram; RAT, right anterior tibialis surface electromyogram; SNORE, snore sensor; N/O, nasal/oral airflow; THOR, thoracic respiratory effort; ABD, abdominal respiratory effort; NPRE, nasal pressure recording effort; SpO₂, pulse oximetry.
*For Stage MT (movement time, please see text): EEG, electroencephalography; EOG, electro-oculography; EMG, electromyography; REM, rapid eye movements (T-REM, tonic REM; P-REM, phasic REM); SREM, slow rolling eye movements.

EMG Recording

- The EMG signals are muscle twitch potentials that are used in PSG to distinguish between sleep stages based on the fact that EMG activity diminishes during sleep.
- Mental, submental, and masseter placements are acceptable. This is a mandatory recording parameter for staging sleep.
- They are used to detect muscle tone changes for scoring REM versus NREM sleep.
- Muscle tone is high during wakefulness and NREM sleep. It is lower in NREM sleep, progressively lower in slow wave sleep (SWS) and lowest in REM sleep.
- Submental EMG records muscle tone.

EEG ACTIVITY DURING WAKEFULNESS AND SLEEP

Cortical activity can be characterized by its specific frequencies. Frequency is noted as cycles per second (i.e., Hertz, Hz). EEG activity has been divided into four bands based on the frequency and amplitude of the waveform and are assigned Greek letters (alpha, beta, theta, delta). The EEG frequencies are defined slightly differently according to the reference used.

Beta Activity

- Beta EEG—defined as a waveform of 14–30 Hz.
- Originates in the frontal and central regions.
- Present during wakefulness and drowsiness.
- May become persistent during drowsiness, diminish during SWS, and reemerge during REM sleep.
- Enhanced or persistent activity suggests use of sedative-hypnotic medications.

Alpha Activity

- Alpha EEG defined as a waveform of 8–14 Hz.
- Originates in the parietooccipital regions bilaterally
- A normal alpha rhythm is synchronous and symmetrical over the cerebral hemispheres.
- Seen during quiet alertness with eyes closed.
- Eye opening cause the alpha waves to "react" or decrease in amplitude.
- Has a crescendo-decrescendo appearance.
- Diminished frequency with aging.

Theta Activity

- Theta frequency is defined as a waveform of 4–8 Hz.
- Originates in the central vertex region.
- Lacks an amplitude criteria for theta.
- The most common sleep frequency.

Sleep Spindles

- Defined as a waveform of 12–14 Hz.
- Originates in the central vertex region.
- Has a duration criterion of 0.5 to 2–3 seconds.
- Typically occurs in stage 2 sleep but can be seen in other stages.

K-Complexes

- Defined as sharp, slow waves, with a biphasic morphology (negative then positive deflection).
- Predominantly central-vertex in origin.
- Duration must be at least 0.5 seconds.
- Lacks an amplitude criteria.
- Indicative of stage 2 sleep.

Delta Activity

- Defined as a waveform of 0.5–2 Hz.
- Seen predominantly in the frontal region.
- Delta activity has an amplitude criterion of >75 μV.
- Lacks a duration criterion.
- Stage 3 sleep is defined when 20–50% of the epoch is scored as delta activity.
- Stage 4 sleep is defined when >50% of the epoch is scored as delta activity.

STAGES OF SLEEP

Stage Wake (Figure A1-1)

- Typically, the first several minutes of the record will consist of wake (W) stage.
- Stage W is recorded when more than 50% of the epoch has scorable alpha EEG activity.
- The EEG will show mixed beta and alpha activities as the eyes open and close and predominantly alpha activity when the eyes remain closed.
- Submental EMG is relatively high tone and will reflect the high-amplitude muscle contractions and movement artifacts.
- The EOG channels will show eye blinking and rapid movement. The record will slow in frequency and amplitude as the subject stops moving and becomes drowsy.

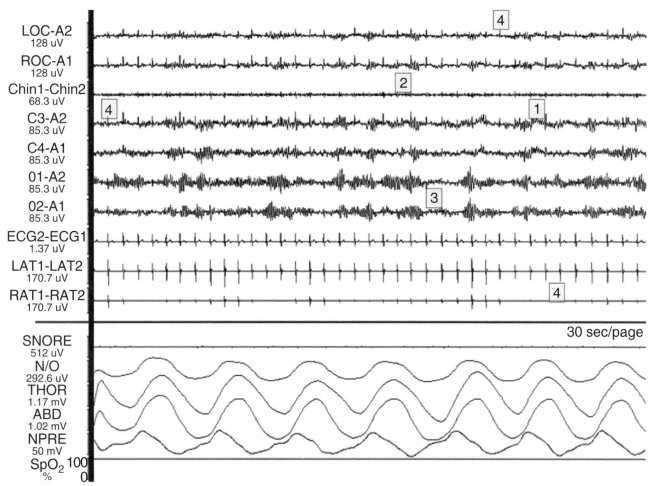

FIGURE A1-1 ■ Stage Wake (30-second epoch). Wakefulness, eyes open. More than 50% of the epoch has scorable alpha EEG activity (1). EMG activity is reduced, consistent with relaxed wakefulness (2). Note the posterior dominant alpha frequency in the O1-A2 and O2-A1 leads (3). An ECG artifact is noted in the EOG, EEG, and EMG leads (4). N/O, Nasal/oral airflow; NPRE, nasal pressure recording effort; SPO_2, pulse oxymetry.

■ As the patient becomes drowsy, with the eyes closed, the EEG will show predominant alpha activity, while the EMG activity will become less prominent.

Stage 1 NREM Sleep (Figures A1-2, A1-3)

■ Stage 1 sleep is scored when more than 15 seconds (>50%) of the epoch is made up of theta activity (3–7 Hz), sometimes intermixed with low-amplitude delta activity replacing the alpha activity of wakefulness.

■ Characterized by low-voltage fast EEG activity with an amplitude of less than 50–75 µV.

■ The alpha activity in the EEG drops to less than 50%.

■ Vertex sharp waves may occur towards the end of stage 1 sleep. They are characterized by high voltage sharp surface negative followed by surface positive component and are maximal over the Cz electrode.

■ Sleep spindles or K-complexes are never a part of stage 1. Vertex waves are.

■ The EMG shows less activity than in wake stage and is relatively high.

■ Arousals defined by paroxysms of EEG activity (typically to a faster alpha or theta activity) lasting 3 seconds but less than 15 seconds. If an arousal occurs in stage 1 sleep, and if the burst results in alpha activity for greater than 50% of the record, then the epoch is scored as stage W.

■ The eyes begin to show slow rolling eye movements (SREM).

■ The time spent in stage 1 may increase with age.

Stage 2 NREM (Figure A1-4)

■ Characterized by predominant theta activity and minimal alpha activity, stage 2 NREM accounts for the bulk of a typical PSG recording (up to 50% in adult patients).

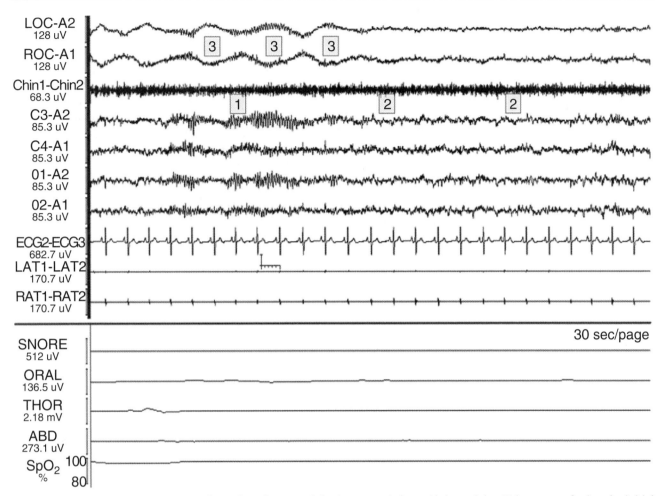

FIGURE A1-2 ■ Stage 1 sleep (30-second epoch). The record depicts stage 1 sleep. Alpha activity (1) is present during the initial 10 seconds of the epoch and is gradually replaced by low-voltage, mixed-frequency theta activity (2). SREMs become more prominent (3).

- K-complexes and sleep spindles occur for the first time and are typically episodic.
- Predominantly central-vertex in origin, K-complexes are sharp, biphasic slow waves, with a sharply negative (upward) deflection followed by a slower positive (downward) deflection. They characteristically stand out from the rest of the background.
- K-complexes have a duration criterion of at least 0.5 seconds but lack an amplitude criterion.
- K-complexes, even without the presence of sleep spindles, are sufficient for scoring stage 2 sleep.
- The EOG leads mirror EEG activity.
- Submental EMG activity is tonically low.
- Delta is only allowed to occur for less than 19% of the epoch. The threshold-triggering SWS scoring is reached if 20% of the epoch is composed of delta activity.
- Excessive spindles activity may indicate the presence of medications (such as benzodiazepines).

- Sleep spindles are 12–14 Hz sinusoidal EEG activity in the central vertex region and must persist for at least 0.5 seconds. They are generated in the midline thalamic nuclei and represent an inhibitory activity.
- Central nervous system (CNS) depressant drugs (i.e., benzodiazepines) often increase the frequency of the spindle activity in the record, whereas advancing age often diminishes their frequency.

Stages 3 and 4 NREM Sleep

- Stages 3 and 4 NREM sleep may also be termed *deep sleep*, *slow wave sleep (SWS)*, or *delta sleep*. Traditional R-K scoring classifies stages 3 and 4 separately, but many sleep laboratories classify stages 3 and 4 together and do not make this distinction.
- SWS is marked by high-amplitude slow waves.
- SWS tends to diminishes with age.

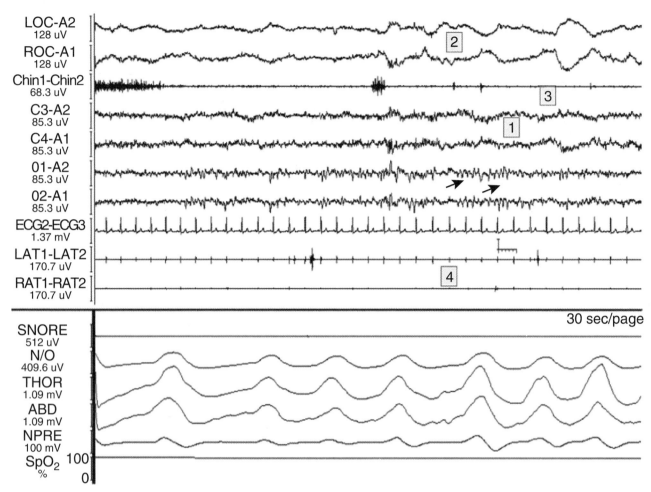

FIGURE A1-3 ■ Stage 1 sleep (30-second epoch). There is presence of low-voltage, mixed-frequency theta activity demarcated by the arrows (1). SREMs are evident (2), and so is a more substantial reduction in chin EMG tone (3), which happens to capture activity from the ECG leads in the form of an ECG artifact (4).

Stage 3 NREM Sleep (Figure A1-5)

- Stage 3 NREM sleep marks the beginning of slow wave (deep) sleep, occurring about 30–45 minutes after sleep onset.
- It is characterized by slow, large-amplitude EEG activity (at the rate of 0.5 to 4 per second-delta wave), with peak-to-peak amplitudes greater than 75 μV for between 20% and 50% of the epoch.

Stage 4 NREM Sleep (Figure A1-6)

- Characterized by delta activity of 4 Hz or slower activity, with peak-to-peak amplitudes greater than 75 μV for at least 50% of the epoch.

Stage REM Sleep (Figures A1-7, A1-8)

- REM sleep typically occurs 90–120 minutes after sleep onset and occupies 20–25% of the night.

- The EEG activity of REM sleep is characterized by relatively low-amplitude, mixed-frequency EEG theta waves, intermixed with some alpha waves, usually 1–2 Hz slower than waking. It resembles waking state more than it does the sleeping state.
- The EMG should show the lowest tone in the record, but no specific amplitude or frequency criteria are in place.
- The EOG of REM shows paroxysms of conjugate high-amplitude activity, which is relatively sharply contoured and occurs in all eye leads simultaneously.
- The EOG activity is not needed to mark the start of an REM period, REM epochs may be recognized by EEG activity before EOG movements start.
- Any two of the previous three criteria (mixed-frequency EEG, minimal EMG tone rapid, and rapid eye movements) must be present to score REM sleep.

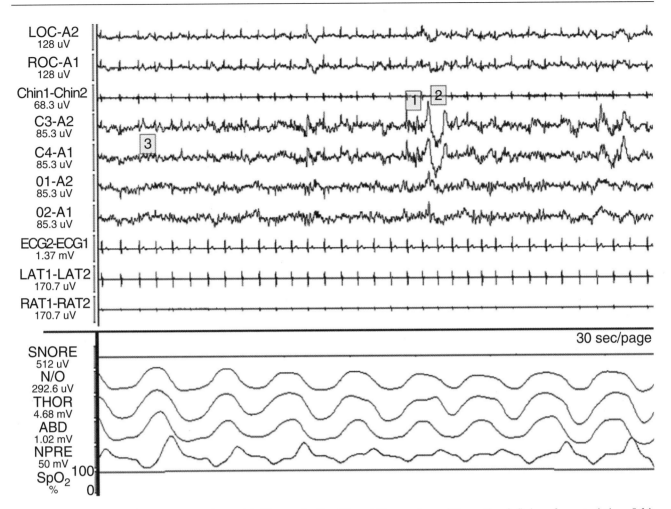

FIGURE A1-4 ■ Stage 2 sleep (30-second epoch). Sleep spindles (1) and K-complexes (2) are the defining characteristics of this sleep stage. No specific criteria exist for EOG and EMG in this stage. There is evidence of theta activity (3).

- The first REM period is typically brief with subsequent REM period, becoming progressively more robust.
- The *sawtooth wave* pattern characterizes stage REM sleep. These are 2–6 Hz, sharply contoured triangular, and jagged-like in morphology and evenly formed EEG pattern.
- They may occur serially for few seconds and are highest in amplitude over the vertex region (Cz and Fz electrodes). REM sleep may be preceded by a series of sawtooth waves.
- REM sleep is sometimes divided into *phasic* (P) and *tonic* (T) components.
  - P-REM sleep is characterized by phasic twitching in the EMG channel occurring concurrently with bursts of rapid eye movements, suggestively correlated with dream content. The phasic EMG twitching in this stage is very short muscle twitches that may occur in the middle ear muscles, genioglossal muscle, and facial muscles.

- T-REM sleep generally consists of low-voltage activated EEG and is characterized by a marked decrease in skeletal muscle EMG activity, without obvious EOG activity. Tonic REM appears to be mediated by areas near the locus coeruleus.

STAGE MOVEMENT TIME (FIGURE A1-9)

- Movement time (MT) is a scorable sleep stage identified by amplifier blocking or excessive EMG activity that obscures the EEG and EOG tracing in more than 50% of the epoch.
- Scorable stage of sleep must occur before and after stage MT.
- The duration of MT is generally greater than 15 seconds but less than 1 minute. When the MT is immediately preceded and followed by stage W, the epoch is scored as stage W, rather than stage MT.

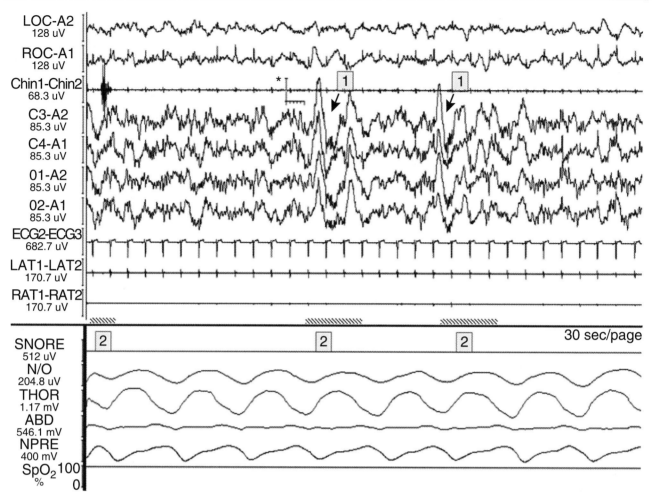

FIGURE A1-5 ■ Stage 3 sleep (30-second epoch). Stage 3 NREM sleep is characterized by slow, large-amplitude delta activity (1) at the rate of 0.5 to 4 per second with peak-to-peak amplitudes greater than 75 μV. The ruler provided (*) is at 1 second and 75 μV units. Delta activity should occur for more than 20% but less than 50% of the epoch, as demarcated by the patterned lines (2).

EEG AROUSALS, RANDOM BODY MOVEMENTS, OR MOVEMENT AROUSAL (FIGURE A1-10)

- Arousals are paroxysms of activity lasting 3 seconds or longer, but less than 15 seconds of the record. Sleep must be maintained before and after the arousal.

- If an arousal obscures the record for more than 15 seconds, then the epoch is scored as MT.
- The minimum arousal is simply a paroxysmal burst in the EEG channel to a faster alpha or theta activity. If the burst results in alpha activity for greater than 50% of the record, then the epoch is scored as wake.

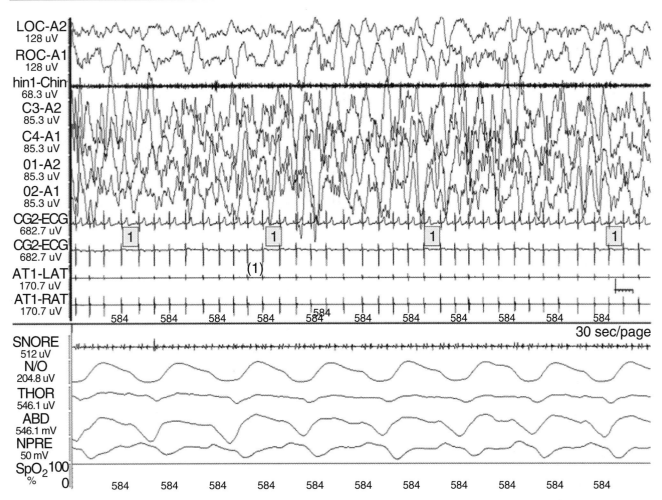

FIGURE A1-6 ■ Stage 4 sleep (30-second epoch). This 30-second epoch depicts stage 4 NREM sleep. The predominant feature in this epoch is that of the high-amplitude delta activity (1).

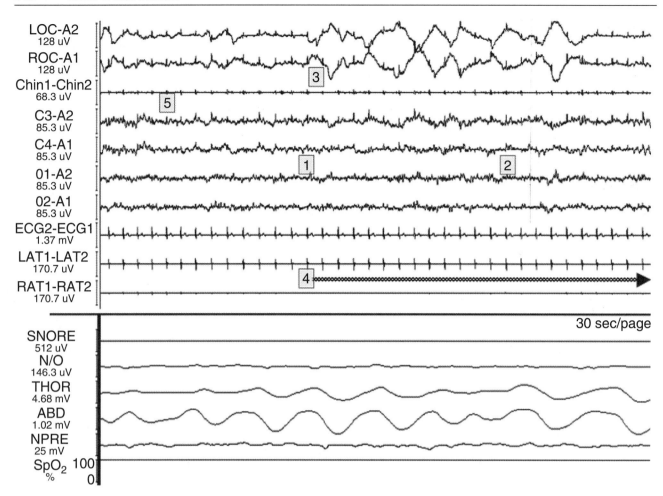

FIGURE A1-7 ■ Stage REM sleep (30-second epoch). Stage REM sleep is characterized by relatively low-amplitude, mixed-frequency EEG theta waves (1), intermixed with alpha waves (2). The EOG leads depict rapid eye movements, which are paroxysmal, relatively sharply contoured, high-amplitude activity occurring in all eye leads simultaneously (3) and are demarcated by the arrow (4). EMG tone (5) should show the lowest tone in the record, but no specific amplitude or frequency criteria are in place.

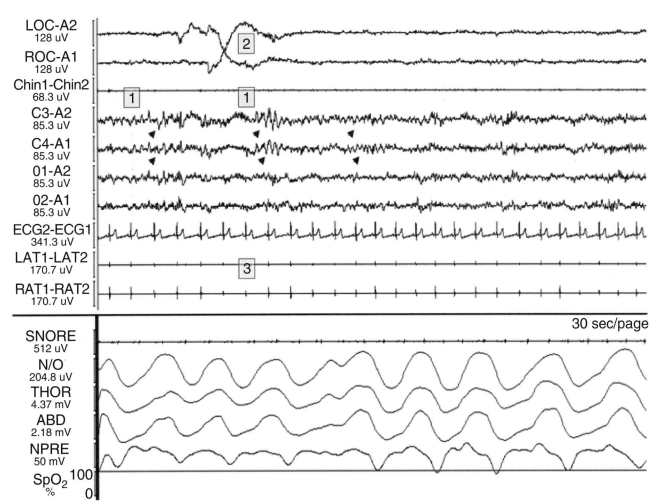

FIGURE A1-8 ▪ Stage REM sleep (30-second epoch). Stage REM sleep is also characterized by the unique *sawtooth wave* pattern (1, arrowheads). These are 2–6 Hz, sharply contoured triangular, jagged-like in morphology and evenly formed EEG pattern. They may occur serially for a few seconds and are best visualized, because of their highest amplitude, over the vertex region (Cz and Fz electrodes). REM sleep may be preceded by a series of sawtooth waves. Other features of REM sleep shown in this epoch are the rapid eye movements (2) and the muscle atonia reflected in the EMG leads (3).

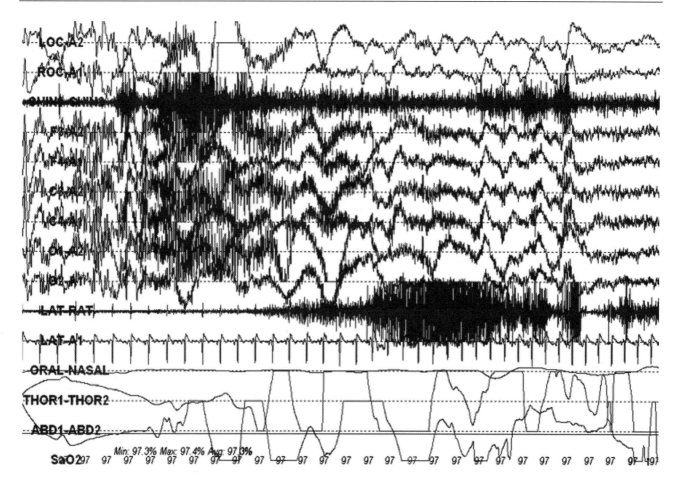

Stage movement time

FIGURE A1-9 ■ Stage-Movement time (30-second epoch). Stage movement time (MT) is characterized by amplifier blocking or excessive EMG activity that obscures the EEG and EOG tracing in more than 50% of the epoch. Scorable stage of sleep must occur before and after stage MT. The duration of MT is generally greater than 15 seconds but less than 1 minute.

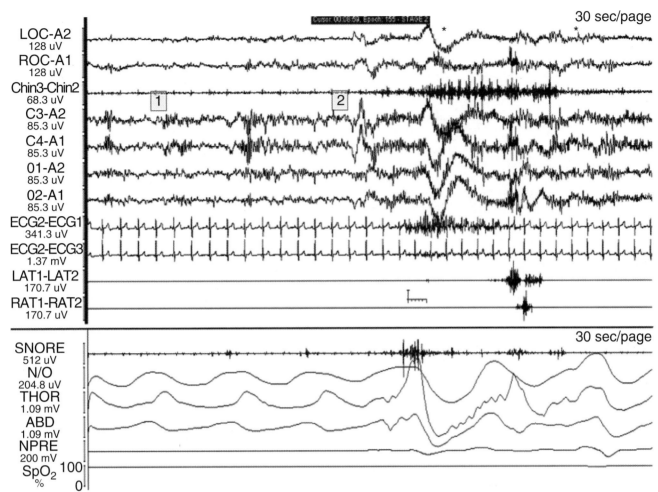

FIGURE A1-10 ■ EEG arousal (30-second epoch). An EEG arousal is not a scorable epoch of sleep but is intended as an aid in the scoring of sleep stages. Its duration activity is short; it must take place for longer than 3 seconds but less than 15 seconds. There should be no EEG obscuring. Sleep must be maintained before and after the arousal. In this 30-second epoch, the patient was in stage 2 sleep just before the arousal (*) as noted by the sleep spindles (1) and K-complex (2). The EEG leads show a shift to a higher frequency. If an arousal obscuring the record occurs for more than 15 seconds, then the epoch is scored as MT (movement time).

BIBLIOGRAPHY

1. Aldrich MS: *Sleep Medicine,* vol 53. New York, Oxford University Press, 1999.
2. Avidan AY: Recognition of sleep stages including scoring techniques. In Chokroverty S, Thomas R, Bhatt M (eds): *Atlas of Sleep Medicine.* Philadelphia, Elsevier Inc., 2005, pp 95–121.
3. Berry RB: *Sleep Medicine Pearls.* Philadelphia, Hanley & Belfus, Inc., 1999.
4. Brown CC: A proposed standard nomenclature for psychophysiologic measures. Psychophysiology 4:260–264, 1967.
5. Butkov N: *Atlas of Clinical Polysomnography,* vol II. Ashland, OR, Synapse Media, Inc. 1996, pp 330–362.
6. Geyer JD, Payne TA, Carney PR, Aldrich MS: *Atlas of Digital Polysomnography.* Philadelphia, Lippincott, Williams & Wilkins, 2000.
7. Jacobson A, Kales A, Lehmann D, Hoedemaker FS: Muscle tonus in human subjects during sleep and dreaming. Exp Neurol 10:418–424, 1964.
8. Jasper HH (Committee Chairman): The 10-20 electrode system of the International Federation. Electroenceph Clin Neurophysiol 10:371–375, 1958.
9. Johnson LC, Nute C, Austin MT, Lubin A: Spectral analysis of the EEG during waking and sleeping. Electroenceph Clin Neurophysiol 23:80, 1967.
10. McCarley RW: Sleep neurophysiology of basic mechanisms underlying control of wakefulness and sleep. In Chokroverty S (ed): *Sleep Disorders Medicine,* 2nd ed. Boston, Butterworth-Heinemann, 1999.
11. Monroe LJ: Inter-rater reliability of scoring EEG sleep records. Paper read at the Association for Psychophysiological Study of Sleep Meeting, Santa Monica, California. April, 1967. Abstract in Psychophysiology 4:370–371, 1968.
12. Pampiglione G, Remond A, Storm van Leeuwen W, Walter WG: Preliminary proposal for an EEG terminology by the Terminology Committee of the International Federation for Electroencephalography and Clinical Neurophysiology. Electroenceph Clin Neurophysiol 1(3):646–650, 1961.
13. Pressman MR: *Primer of Polysomnogram Interpretation.* Boston, Butterworth Heineman, 2002.
14. Rechtschaffen A, Kales A, Rechtschaffen A, Kales A (eds): *A Manual of Standardised Terminology, Techniques and Scoring System for Sleep Stages of Human Subjects.* Los Angeles, Brain Information Service/Brain Research Institute, 1968.
15. Roth B: The clinical and theoretical importance of EEG rhythms corresponding to states of lowered vigilance. Electroenceph Clin Neurophysiol 13:395–399, 1961.
16. Shepard JW: *Atlas of Sleep Medicine.* Armonk, NY, Futura Publishing Co., 1991.
17. Siegel JM: Brainstem mechanisms generating REM sleep. In Kryger MH, Roth T, Dement WC (eds): *Principles and Practice of Sleep Medicine.* Philadelphia, Saunders, 2000, pp 112–133.
18. Walczak T, Chokroverty S: Electroencephalography, electromyography and electrocooculography: general principles and basic technology. In Chokroverty S (ed): *Sleep Disorders Medicine,* 2nd ed. Boston, Butterworth-Heinemann, 1999.

Cardiac Arrhythmias

JON W. ATKINSON

ANATOMY AND PATHWAYS

Arrhythmia recognition and identification is a logical process but is based on a good working knowledge of the anatomy and pathways of the conduction system of the heart. The heart contains areas of specialized tissue that have the primary function of generating electrical impulses or transmitting these impulses to other areas of the conduction system and finally to the cardiac muscle mass. The principal areas of interest are as follows: the sinoatrial (SA) node, the atrioventricular (AV) node, the AV bundle or bundle of His, the left and right bundle branches, and the Purkinje system. The normal sequence of events is as follows:

1. The cycle begins with a discharge of the SA node, which causes the atria to depolarize.
2. The AV node receives input via the internodal pathways and holds the signal for a brief period (a brief pause between atrial and ventricular depolarization that facilitates ventricular filling).
3. The impulse is passed from the AV node to the AV bundle.
4. The signal is sent down the right and left bundles (the left bundle branches to an anterior and a posterior fascicle).
5. The left and right bundles distribute the impulse via the Purkinje system to the ventricular myocardium such that all the cardiac muscles contract simultaneously as a unit.

Figure A2-1 is a graphic illustration of the conducting system.

CARDIAC CYCLE

The cardiac cycle is the repetitive sequence of atrial depolarization, atrial repolarization, ventricular depolarization, and ventricular repolarization and the appearance of the main components of the electrocardiogram (ECG complex), P-QRS-T. There is a relationship between anatomy and physiology of the cardiac cycle and the waveforms and intervals of the ECG. Table A2-1 shows the physiologic event and related ECG component. Figure A2-2 shows a graphic representation.

NORMAL ECG PARAMETERS

The discussion of arrhythmias necessitates an understanding of what is normal. The normal ranges for parameters important in diagnosing arrhythmias are shown in Table A2-2. The basis for observing and identifying arrhythmias is the normal sinus rhythm. Figures A2-3 and A2-4 are samples presented in a 30-second window and a 10-second window for comparison. A beneficial feature of digital recordings is the ability to change display widths without changing how

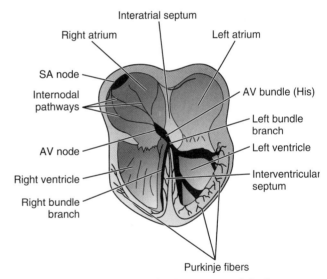

FIGURE A2-1 ■ The conducting system of the heart.

TABLE A2-1 ■ Physiologic Event and Related ECG Waveform	
Physiologic Event	**ECG Waveform**
Atrial depolarization	P wave
Atrial repolarization	None seen (hidden by the timing and magnitude of the QRS complex)
Pause between atrial depolarization and ventricular depolarization	PR interval (the last portion after the P wave, PR segment)
Ventricular depolarization	QRS complex
Ventricular repolarization	T wave

the recording is saved to the hard drive. For the purpose of arrhythmia analysis, it is frequently beneficial to view the detail using a 10-second window rather than the common 30-second window. This demonstrates a basic concept: To view activities that are rapidly occurring (e.g., ECG, electroencephalogram [EEG]), spread the display out; to view repetitive, slowly occurring events (e.g., apnea/hypopneas, periodic leg movements), compress the display. Table A2-3 lists the characteristics of the normal sinus rhythm.

ECG ABNORMALITIES

An ECG abnormality occurs if there is a difference in impulse formation, impulse conduction, or both. Heartbeats that originate outside of the SA node, such as other areas in the atrium, the AV node, or

the ventricle, are examples of impulse formation abnormalities. These abnormal beats do not have a sinus P wave. Abnormal beats with only conduction abnormalities exhibit a sinus P wave, but then show prolonged conduction across the AV node or through the ventricular conduction pathway. The AV blocks and bundle-branch blocks are good examples of impulse conduction abnormalities. When impulse formation and impulse conduction are affected, neither a normal sinus P wave nor a normal QRS complex is present. Any of the ventricular arrhythmias show impulse formation and impulse conduction abnormalities. Essentially an arrhythmia is present if the rate is too fast or too slow, the rhythm is irregular, the site of origin is abnormal, or the movement of the impulse through the conductive system is abnormal.

ARRHYTHMIA ANALYSIS

Often there is the temptation to "'guess'" the type of arrhythmia that is presented on the polysomnogram (PSG). This section presents a systematic method to the more accurate analysis of cardiac rhythm disturbances. If possible, a second, different ECG should be added to the montage. This is generally accomplished easily, unless the manufacturer has a dedicated, two-input amplifier for recording the ECG. Using a second ECG channel may reveal changes in P wave or QRS complex configuration that are difficult to ascertain with a single-channel recording. When examining the ECG for detail, a 10-second or 6-second window should be used to examine the intervals or subtle changes in morphology. Routine use of the following methodical system can improve the accuracy of identifying arrhythmias.

Step 1. Examine the P Wave

Is the P wave absent or present? Absence of a distinct P wave indicates that the arrhythmia is not of atrial origin (except atrial fibrillation or atrial flutter.) Do the P waves all look the same (same morphology)? If an ECG complex starts from the same location and takes the same pathway, it will always look the same. The corollary is if it starts from a different location or takes a

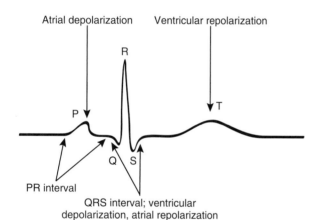

FIGURE A2-2 ■ Graphic representation of the cardiac cycle.

TABLE A2-2 ■ Normal Adult ECG Parameters	
Parameter	**Value**
Heart rate	60–100 beats/min
Rhythm	Regular
PR interval	0.12–0.20 sec
QRS interval	0.04–0.11 sec
SA node discharge rate	60–100/min
AV node discharge rate	40–60/min
Ventricular discharge rate	20–40/min

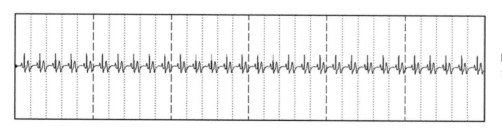

FIGURE A2-3 ■ Normal sinus rhythm, 30-second display.

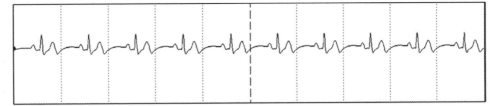

FIGURE A2-4 ■ Normal sinus rhythm, 10-second display.

TABLE A2-3 ■ **Characteristics of the Normal Sinus Rhythm**

Parameter	Value
P wave	Present, each appears the same
QRS complex	Present, each appears the same
PR interval	0.12–0.20 sec
QRS interval	0.04–0.11 sec
P:QRS ratio	1:1
Rhythm	Regular
Rate	60–100

different pathway, the appearance will be different. For lack of a better term, this is called the *rule of differing morphology*.

Step 2. Examine the QRS Complex

Check for absence or presence and similar appearance of the QRS complex. Absence of the QRS complex indicates some type of second-degree or third-degree AV block or severe ventricular disturbance, such as ventricular fibrillation or asystole. Differing morphologies of the QRS complex indicate a shift from a supraventricular origin of the abnormal beat or a different pathway in the ventricle, such as bundle-branch block or multifocal ventricular origin.

Step 3. Examine the P and QRS Relationship

Ask the following questions: Is there a P for every QRS? Is there a QRS for every P? Is there a 1:1 P:QRS ratio? A P:QRS ratio of greater than 1 (more Ps than QRSs) indicates some sort of AV block. A P:QRS ratio of less than 1 (more QRSs than Ps) indicates a junctional or ventricular arrhythmia.

Step 4. Measure the Intervals

Is the PR interval normal, or is it too long or too short? An abbreviated PR interval may indicate a junctional beat (retrograde P wave) or an accessory pathway (e.g., in Wolff-Parkinson-White syndrome). A prolonged PR interval indicates some type of AV block is occurring. Is the QRS interval normal or too long (seldom, if ever,

will it be too short)? A widened QRS complex likely indicates bundle-branch block, a beat of ventricular origin, or, in some cases, an aberrantly conducted beat of supraventricular origin (the beat originates before the ventricular conductive pathway is repolarized during the relative refractory period).

Step 5. Regular or Irregular Rhythm

Examine the PP intervals and the RR intervals. If the intervals are constant, the rhythm is regular. If they vary, the rhythm is irregular. It is not recommended to use calipers on your computer monitor, so either print out the screen and measure with calipers or take a 3- × 5- inch index card and mark a P wave and then the next one on a stationary screen view. Move the card from P to P to P and see if they fall on the marks. Do the same for the R waves.

Step 6. Determine the Rate

The heart rate can be determined in a variety of fashions:

Times 2 method—count the number of beats in a 30-second screen and multiply by 2. This can be cumbersome but is accurate. This should be done in a freezescreen view.

Times 6 method—count the number of beats in 10 seconds and multiply by 6. Use a stationary screen.

Interval method—measure the active screen width in millimeters. If you have a 30-second window, multiply this number by 2 to get the number of millimeters in 60 seconds. If you are using a 10-second window, multiply the active screen width by 6 to obtain the number of millimeters in 60 seconds. Measure the RR interval with a ruler, and divide into the number of millimeters in 60 seconds.

COMMON ATRIAL ARRHYTHMIAS

Representative illustrations (Figures A2-5–20) and a summary of characteristics (Tables A2-4–11) are provided for each arrhythmia in the following list. The reader is advised to consult the tables when examining the illustrations. Common atrial arrhythmias include the following:

Text continued on p. 550

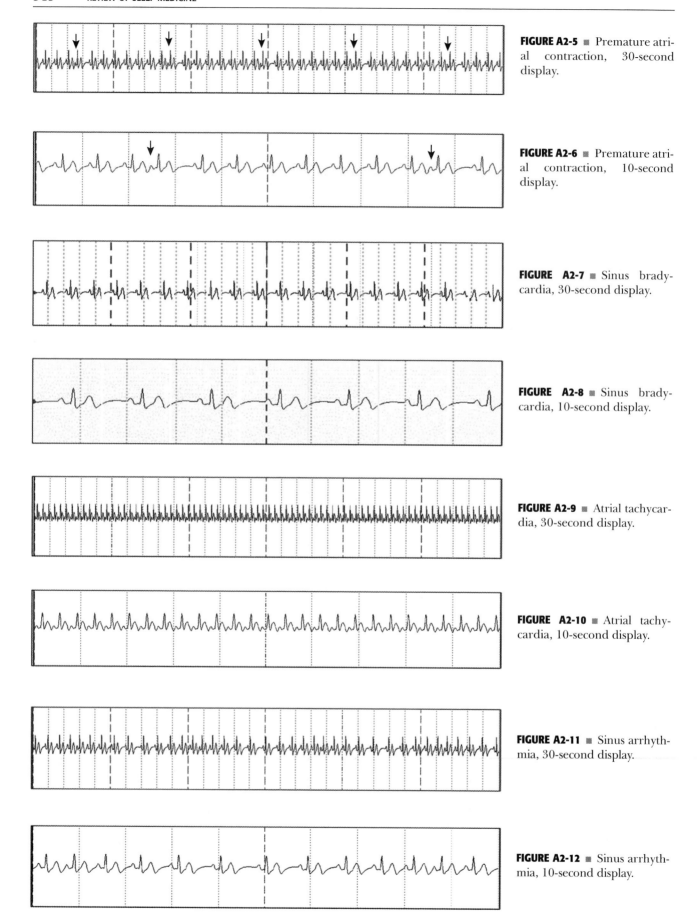

FIGURE A2-5 ■ Premature atrial contraction, 30-second display.

FIGURE A2-6 ■ Premature atrial contraction, 10-second display.

FIGURE A2-7 ■ Sinus bradycardia, 30-second display.

FIGURE A2-8 ■ Sinus bradycardia, 10-second display.

FIGURE A2-9 ■ Atrial tachycardia, 30-second display.

FIGURE A2-10 ■ Atrial tachycardia, 10-second display.

FIGURE A2-11 ■ Sinus arrhythmia, 30-second display.

FIGURE A2-12 ■ Sinus arrhythmia, 10-second display.

FIGURE A2-13 ■ Sinus pause, 30-second display.

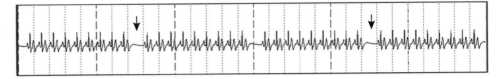

FIGURE A2-14 ■ Sinus pause, 10-second display.

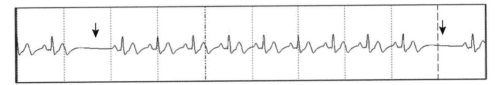

FIGURE A2-15 ■ Paroxysmal atrial tachycardia, paroxysmal supraventricular tachycardia, 30-second display.

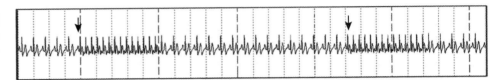

FIGURE A2-16 ■ Paroxysmal atrial tachycardia, paroxysmal supraventricular tachycardia, 10-second display.

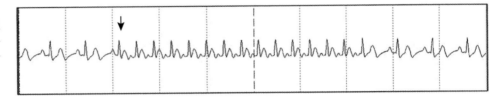

FIGURE A2-17 ■ Atrial fibrillation, 30-second display.

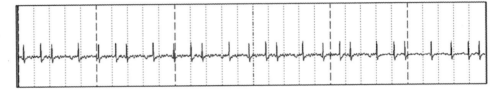

FIGURE A2-18 ■ Atrial fibrillation, 10-second display.

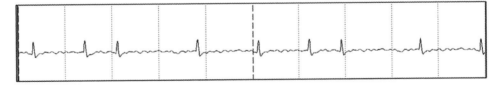

FIGURE A2-19 ■ Atrial flutter, variable block, 30-second display.

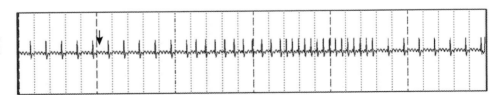

FIGURE A2-20 ■ Atrial flutter, variable block, 10-second display.

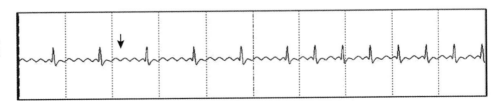

TABLE A2-4 ■ Characteristics of Premature Atrial Contractions*

Parameter	Value
P wave	Present; appearance of the P wave of the abnormal beat is different (it arises from a different location)
QRS complex	Present; each appears the same
PR interval	0.12–0.20 sec, may vary slightly with the abnormal beat
QRS interval	0.04–0.11 sec
P:QRS ratio	1:1
Rhythm	Irregular owing to the premature beat; PP is different, as is RR
Rate	60–100

*Note the different appearance of the P wave (origin is from a different source and travels a different pathway) at the arrows. There also may be subtle PR interval changes. The QRS and the T wave are normal in appearance, unless the ectopic atrial focus fires so early that it captures the ventricle while still relatively refractory to conduction (premature atrial contraction with aberrancy).

TABLE A2-5 ■ Characteristics of Sinus Bradycardia*

Parameter	Value
P wave	Present; each appears the same
QRS complex	Present; each appears the same
PR interval	0.12–0.20 sec
QRS interval	0.04–0.11 sec
P:QRS ratio	1:1
Rhythm	Regular
Rate	<50, some authors say <60

*This looks like normal sinus rhythm except that the rate is slower. It is common in athletes and patients taking beta-blockers.

TABLE A2-6 ■ Characteristics of Tachycardias*

Parameter	Value
P wave	Present; each appears the same; may not be well defined in SVT
QRS complex	Present; each appears the same
PR interval	0.12–0.20 sec
QRS interval	0.04–0.11 sec
P:QRS ratio	1:1
Rhythm	Regular
Rate	>100

*These are rapid, regular rhythms with normal-appearing QRS complexes. Sinus tachycardia has a normal sinus P wave. In atrial tachycardia, the P wave has a different morphology than the sinus P wave. Supraventricular tachycardia does not have a clearly defined P wave. It is difficult to distinguish one from the other on the surface ECG. Electrophysiologic studies may be necessary to determine the precise focus. Sustained tachycardias decrease cardiac output. The patient should be assessed for level of consciousness, chest pain, and blood pressure, and the physician should be notified.

- Premature atrial contractions (Figures A2-5 and -6; Table A2-4)
- Sinus bradycardia (Figures A2-7 and -8; Table A2-5)

TABLE A2-7 ■ Characteristics of Sinus Arrhythmia*

Parameter	Value
P wave	Present; each appears the same
QRS complex	Present; each appears the same
PR interval	0.12–0.20 sec
QRS interval	0.04–0.11 sec
P:QRS ratio	1:1
Rhythm	Irregular
Rate	60–100

*Frequently seen in infants and children. Often seen in obstructive sleep apnea as result of vagal effect of intrathoracic pressure fluctuations.

TABLE A2-8 ■ Characteristics of Sinus Pause*

Parameter	Value
P wave	Absent during pause
QRS complex	Absent during pause
PR interval	Absent during pause
QRS interval	Absent during pause
P:QRS ratio	1:1
Rhythm	Irregular
Rate	60–100, but can occur at any rate

*Cannot distinguish arrest from block on surface ECG. This requires electrophysiologic studies of the heart. If prolonged, notify appropriate medical personnel according to protocol.

TABLE A2-9 ■ Characteristics of Paroxysmal Tachycardias*

Parameter	Value
P wave	Present; aberrant, often hidden
QRS complex	Present; appearance is the same, may be aberrant
PR interval	Not measurable
QRS interval	0.04–0.11 sec
P:QRS ratio	1:1
Rhythm	Regular during paroxysm
Rate	150–250

*Often occurs with reentry phenomena from accessory pathway. The term *paroxysmal* describes a phenomenon that arises abruptly from the background and abruptly returns to that background. Generally the arrhythmia is self-limiting, but if sustained, assess patient and notify appropriate medical personnel according to protocol.

- Atrial tachycardia, sinus tachycardia, supraventricular tachycardia (Figures A2-9 and -10; Table A2-6)
- Sinus arrhythmia (Figures A2-11 and -12; Table A2-7)
- Sinus pause (Figures A2-13 and -14; Table A2-8)
- Paroxysmal atrial tachycardia (Figures A2-15 and -16; Table A2-9)
- Atrial fibrillation (Figures A2-17 and -18; Table A2-10)
- Atrial flutter (Figures A2-19 and -20; Table A2-11)

TABLE A2-10 ■ Characteristics of Atrial Fibrillation*	
Parameter	**Value**
P wave	None per se; chaotic deflections called *fibrillatory waves*
QRS complex	Present; appearance is the same
PR interval	Not measurable
QRS interval	0.04–0.11 sec
P:QRS ratio	Not applicable
Rhythm	Irregularly irregular
Rate	Ventricular rate is highly variable

*Central sleep apnea, Cheyne-Stokes respirations, and mixed apneas (often with a long central component) frequently are seen with atrial fibrillation. This is likely due to decreased cardiac output and a prolonged circulation time, rendering the breathing control centers ineffective. If sustained or previously undocumented, notify appropriate medical personnel according to protocol.

TABLE A2-11 ■ Characteristics of Atrial Flutter*	
Parameter	**Value**
P wave	None per se; saw-tooth deflections called *flutter waves*
QRS complex	Present; appearance is the same
PR interval	Not measurable
QRS interval	0.04–0.11 sec
P:QRS ratio	Variable 2:1, 3:1, 4:1
Rhythm	Regular or irregular depending on variability of block
Rate	Atrial: 250–400; ventricular rate depends on degree of block and atrial rate

*Often occurs with reentry phenomena from accessory pathway. If sustained or previously undocumented, notify appropriate medical personnel according to protocol.

JUNCTIONAL ARRHYTHMIAS

Representative illustrations (Figures A2-21–28) and a summary of characteristics (Tables A2-12–15) are provided for each arrhythmia in the following list. The reader is advised to consult the tables when examining the illustrations. Junctional arrhythmias include the following:

- Premature junctional contraction (Figures A2-21 and -22; Table A2-12)
- Junctional rhythm (Figures A2-23 and -24; Table A2-13)
- Accelerated junctional rhythm (Figures A2-25 and -26; Table A2-14)
- Junctional tachycardia (Figures A2-27 and -28; Table A2-15)

Junctional arrhythmias can occur if the AV nodal tissue fires prematurely or if the atrial mechanism

for initiating the cardiac cycle fails. Key features of junctional arrhythmias are normal-appearing QRS complexes (the pathway distally from the AV bundle is intact). P waves may or may not be seen. If the P waves are seen, they are inverted (a reverse from the normal P wave vector) and can occur before or after the QRS complex. If they occur before the QRS, the PR interval is shorter than normal.

BLOCKS

Representative illustrations (Figures A2-29–40) and a summary of characteristics (Tables A2-16–21) are provided for each arrhythmia in the following list. The reader is advised to consult the tables when examining the illustrations. Blocks include the following:

- First-degree AV block (Figures A2-29 and -30; Table A2-16)
- Second-degree AV block, type 1 (Wenckebach) (Figures A2-31 and -32; Table A2-17)
- Second-degree AV block, type 2 (Figures A2-33 and -34; Table A2-18)
- Third-degree AV block (Figures A2-35 and -36; Table A2-19)
- Left bundle-branch block (Figures A2-37 and -38; Table A2-20)
- Right bundle-branch block (Figures A2-39 and -40; Table A2-21)

VENTRICULAR ARRHYTHMIAS

Representative illustrations (Figures A2-41–60) and a summary of characteristics (Tables A2-22–26) are provided for each arrhythmia in the following list. The reader is advised to consult the tables when examining the illustrations. Ventricular arrhythmias include the following:

- Premature ventricular contractions (Figures A2-41–50; Table A2-22)
- Unifocal premature ventricular contractions
- Multifocal premature ventricular contractions
- Ventricular trigeminy
- Ventricular bigeminy
- Ventricular couplets
- Idioventricular rhythm (Figures A2-51 and -52; Table A2-23)
- Accelerated ventricular rhythm (Figures A2-53 and -54; Table A2-24)
- Ventricular tachycardia (Figures A2-55–58; Table A2-25)
- Runs of ventricular tachycardia

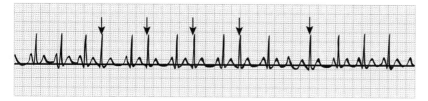

FIGURE A2-21 ■ Premature junctional (nodal) contraction, 30-second display.

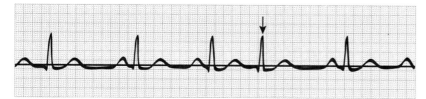

FIGURE A2-22 ■ Premature junctional (nodal) contraction, 10-second display.

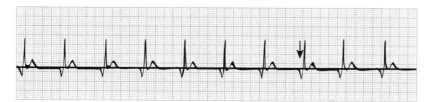

FIGURE A2-23 ■ Junctional (nodal) rhythm, 30-second display.

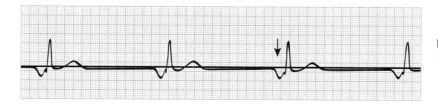

FIGURE A2-24 ■ Junctional (nodal) rhythm, 10-second display.

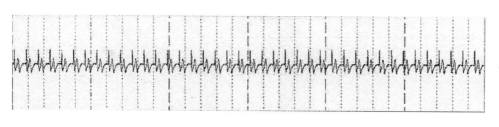

FIGURE A2-25 ■ Accelerated junctional rhythm, 30-second display.

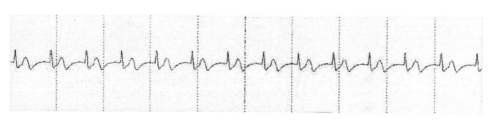

FIGURE A2-26 ■ Accelerated junctional rhythm, 10-second display.

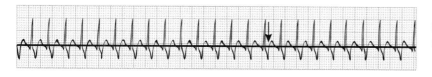

FIGURE A2-27 ■ Junctional tachycardia, 30-second display.

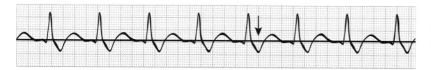

FIGURE A2-28 ■ Junctional tachycardia, 10-second display.

TABLE A2-12 ■ Characteristics of Premature Junctional Contraction*

Parameter	Value
P wave	Premature and abnormal configuration, inverted; can be before (with shortened PR interval), after, or hidden in the QRS
QRS complex	Present; appearance is the same
PR interval	Shorter than normal; <0.12 sec
QRS interval	0.04–0.11 sec
P:QRS ratio	<1:1 if hidden; 1:1 if inverted P is seen
Rhythm	Irregular
Rate	Usually normal but can occur in sinus tachycardia or sinus bradycardia

*The premature beats with normal-appearing QRS complexes and absent or hidden P are shown in Figures A2-21 and A2-22.

TABLE A2-13 ■ Characteristics of Junctional Rhythm*

Parameter	Value
P wave	Premature and abnormal configuration, inverted; can be before (with shortened PR interval), after, or hidden in the QRS
QRS complex	Present; appearance is the same
PR interval	Shorter than normal; <0.12 sec
QRS interval	0.04–0.11 sec
P:QRS ratio	<1:1 if hidden; 1:1 if inverted P is seen
Rhythm	Regular
Rate	40–60

*Often seen as escape rhythm with sinus node dysfunction. Note the inverted P wave and short PR interval in Figures A2-23 and A2-24.

- Sustained ventricular tachycardia
- Ventricular fibrillation (Figures A2-59 and -60; Table A2-26)

INTERVENTIONS

Each facility should have a policy for dealing with severe arrhythmias. Sustained tachyarrhythmias (atrial or junctional tachycardias and ventricular tachycardias), atrial fibrillation and flutter with rapid ventricular response, and sustained ventricular arrhythmias (idioventricular or accelerated ventricular rhythm) require immediate assessment of the patient. This assessment should include level of consciousness; dizziness or lightheadedness; presence of chest, arm, or neck pain; and blood pressure. Emergency protocol for "'code blue'" or activating the emergency medical system should be initiated in the case of unresponsiveness. Other arrhythmias, such as runs of ventricular tachycardia,

TABLE A2-14 ■ Characteristics of Accelerated Junctional Rhythm*

Parameter	Value
P wave	Premature and abnormal configuration, inverted; can be before (with shortened PR interval), after, or hidden in the QRS
QRS complex	Present; appearance is the same
PR interval	Shorter than normal; <0.12 sec
QRS interval	0.04–0.11 sec
P:QRS ratio	<1:1 if hidden; 1:1 if inverted P is seen
Rhythm	Regular
Rate	60–100

*Often seen as escape rhythm with sinus node dysfunction.

TABLE A2-15 ■ Characteristics of Junctional Tachycardia*

Parameter	Value
P wave	Premature and abnormal configuration, inverted; can be before (with shortened PR interval), after, or hidden in the QRS
QRS complex	Present; appearance is the same
PR interval	Shorter than normal; <0.12 sec
QRS interval	0.04–0.11 sec
P:QRS ratio	<1:1 if hidden; 1:1 if inverted P is seen
Rhythm	Regular
Rate	O100

*Note the inverted P wave after the QRS. Assess patient if sustained, and notify appropriate medical personnel according to protocol.

asystoles, second-degree and third-degree blocks, and previously undocumented atrial fibrillation or flutter, warrant a call to the medical director, referring physician, or house officer for direction, according to protocol.

RECORDING AND MONITORING TECHNIQUES

This section contains tips for recording and viewing the ECG in PSG. Discussion is limited to digital PSG. Many sleep centers have a prescribed electrode placement for recording the ECG; this usually involves recording from the right and left subclavicular areas (essentially lead I) or the right subclavicular area and the left abdomen (essentially lead II). One electrode combination may not always show a good P wave and a QRS complex of adequate amplitude, however. The ECG quality should be observed before or during the physiologic calibration procedure. Different lead combinations should be sampled to provide the most adequate sample of the ECG before "'lights out.'"

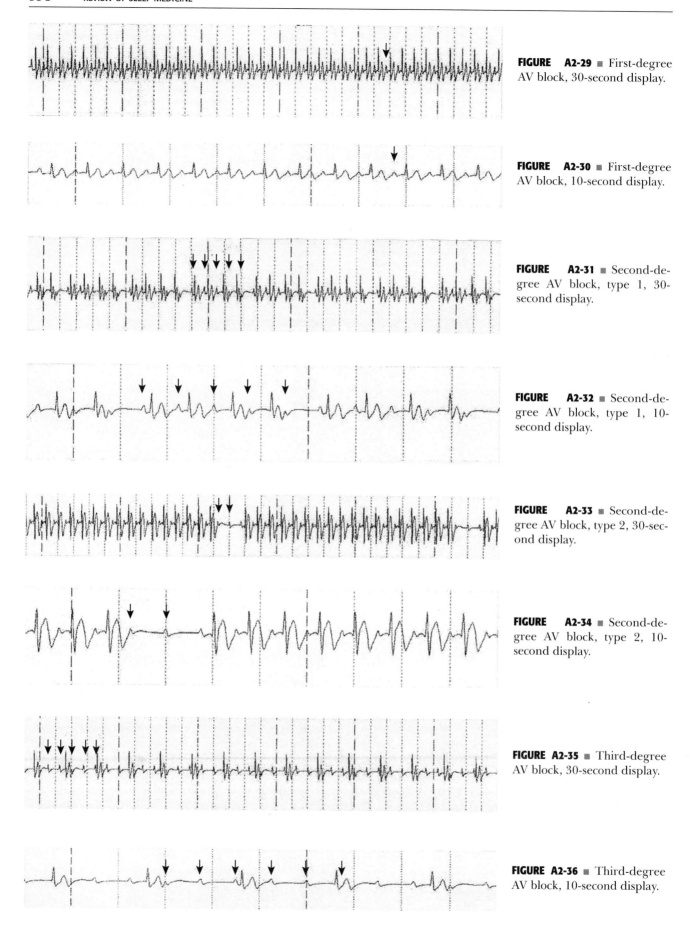

FIGURE   A2-29 ■ First-degree AV block, 30-second display.

FIGURE   A2-30 ■ First-degree AV block, 10-second display.

FIGURE   A2-31 ■ Second-degree AV block, type 1, 30-second display.

FIGURE   A2-32 ■ Second-degree AV block, type 1, 10-second display.

FIGURE   A2-33 ■ Second-degree AV block, type 2, 30-second display.

FIGURE   A2-34 ■ Second-degree AV block, type 2, 10-second display.

FIGURE   A2-35 ■ Third-degree AV block, 30-second display.

FIGURE   A2-36 ■ Third-degree AV block, 10-second display.

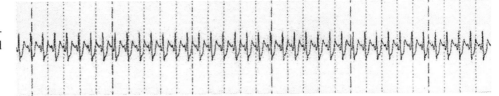

FIGURE A2-37 ■ Left bundle-branch block, 30-second display.

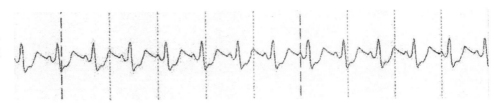

FIGURE A2-38 ■ Left bundle-branch block, 10-second display.

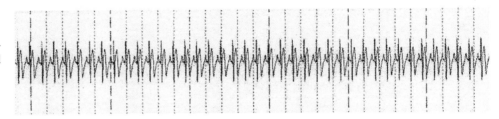

FIGURE A2-39 ■ Right bundle-branch block, 30-second display.

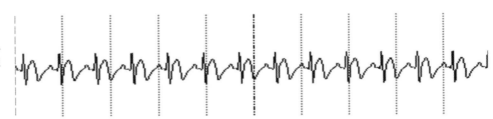

FIGURE A2-40 ■ Right bundle-branch block, 10-second display.

TABLE A2-16 ■ Characteristics of First-Degree AV Block*	
Parameter	**Value**
P wave	Present; appearance is the same
QRS complex	Present; appearance is the same
PR interval	Longer than normal; 0.20 sec
QRS interval	0.04–0.11 sec
P:QRS ratio	1:1
Rhythm	Regular
Rate	Usually normal

*Note the difficulty seeing a prolonged PR interval on a 30-second display and the clarification provided with a 10-second display.

TABLE A2-17 ■ Characteristics of Second-Degree AV Block, Type 1 (Wenckebach)*	
Parameter	**Value**
P wave	Present; normal sinus P, some note followed by QRS
QRS complex	Present; appearance is the same
PR interval	Progressively lengthening
QRS interval	0.04–0.11 sec
P:QRS ratio	>1:1
Rhythm	Irregular
Rate	Usually slow, but can be normal

*The progressively lengthening PR intervals are better appreciated on a 10-second display. This arrhythmia is common. If it occurs repeatedly, notify appropriate medical personnel according to protocol.

Some recording systems have a dedicated paired input for the ECG. In this case, the user must move the electrode physically to another location. Other systems allow the user to reference any recording electrode to another. In this case, it is fairly simple to reference an ECG electrode to another recording electrode (e.g., a left leg electrode) and obtain a different view of the ECG.

A better approach would be to monitor routinely two separate ECG leads (e.g., lead I and lead II) simultaneously. Some recording systems have the capability of averaging recording signals. It is possible in these systems to provide a semblance of the precordial leads by averaging left arm, left leg, and right arm signals as a reference for any of the V leads. Additionally, a

Text continued on p. 559

TABLE A2-18 ■ Characteristics of Second-Degree AV Block, Type 2*

Parameter	Value
P wave	Present; normal sinus P wave, R2 more P waves before QRS
QRS complex	Present; appearance is the same
PR interval	Constant PR interval before dropped QRS; PR interval may be normal or prolonged
QRS interval	0.04–0.11 sec
P:QRS ratio	>1:1
Rhythm	Irregular
Rate	Usually slow, but can be normal

*If prolonged, escape beat may occur. Note the constant PR interval before dropped QRS. May lead to a string of P waves without QRS complexes. Call medical personnel according to protocol.

TABLE A2-20 ■ Characteristics of Left Bundle-Branch Block*

Parameter	Value
P wave	Normal
QRS complex	Present; widened and notched (M-shaped pattern) best seen in V6, lead I, or AVL
PR interval	Normal; can be prolonged with first-degree block
QRS interval	>0.12 sec
P:QRS ratio	1:1
Rhythm	Regular
Rate	Usually 60–100, but can occur with slower or faster rates

*Bundle-branch blocks are difficult to visualize. The key is to use a 10-second display (or less) and look for the increased QRS interval and notching (may be quite subtle).

TABLE A2-19 ■ Characteristics of Third-Degree Block, AV Dissociation*

Parameter	Value
P wave	Present but have no relationship with QRS; often hidden in QRS and T waves
QRS complex	Present; appearance is the same
PR interval	Varies greatly
QRS interval	<0.12 sec if block is in bundle of His; >0.12 sec if block is in bundle branches
P:QRS ratio	>1:1
Rhythm	Regular PP and regular RR, but not the same rate
Rate	40–60 if bundle of His is blocked; 30–40 if bundle branches involved

*Note the constant PP interval and the constant RR interval (i.e., a regular atrial rhythm and a regular ventricular rhythm), just not at the same rate. P waves sometimes are difficult to see when occurring during other waveforms, such as the T wave and QRS complex.

TABLE A2-21 ■ Characteristics of Right Bundle-Branch Block*

Parameter	Value
P wave	Normal
QRS complex	Present; widened and notched (rabbit-eared appearance), best seen in V1 or MCL1, hence not well seen in most sleep studies
PR interval	Normal, can be prolonged with first-degree block
QRS interval	>0.12 sec
P:QRS ratio	1:1
Rhythm	Regular
Rate	Usually 60–100, but can occur with slower or faster rates

*Often difficult to visualize during polysomnography. Use 10-second and look for widened QRS. A W-shaped wave in lead I may be seen.

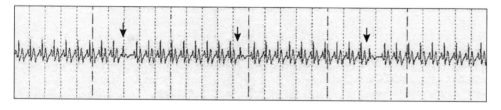

FIGURE A2-41 ■ Unifocal premature ventricular contractions, 30-second display.

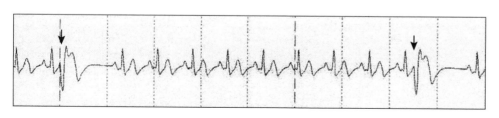

FIGURE A2-42 ■ Unifocal premature ventricular contractions, 10-second display.

FIGURE A2-43 ■ Multifocal premature ventricular contractions, 30-second display.

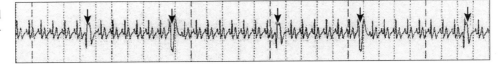

FIGURE A2-44 ■ Multifocal premature ventricular contractions, 10-second display.

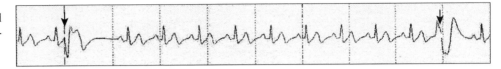

FIGURE A2-45 ■ Trigeminal premature ventricular contractions, ventricular trigeminy, 30-second display.

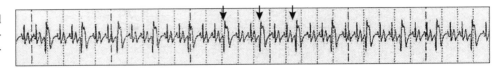

FIGURE A2-46 ■ Trigeminal premature ventricular contractions, ventricular trigeminy, 10-second display.

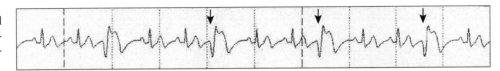

FIGURE A2-47 ■ Bigeminal premature ventricular contractions, ventricular bigeminy, 30-second display.

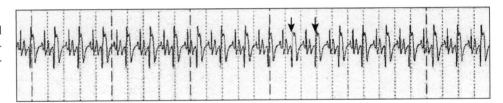

FIGURE A2-48 ■ Bigeminal premature ventricular contractions, ventricular bigeminy, 10-second display.

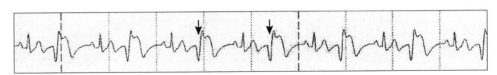

FIGURE A2-49 ■ Ventricular couplets, 30-second display.

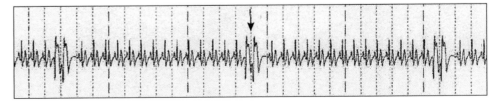

FIGURE A2-50 ■ Ventricular couplets, 10-second display.

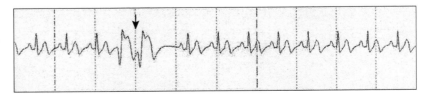

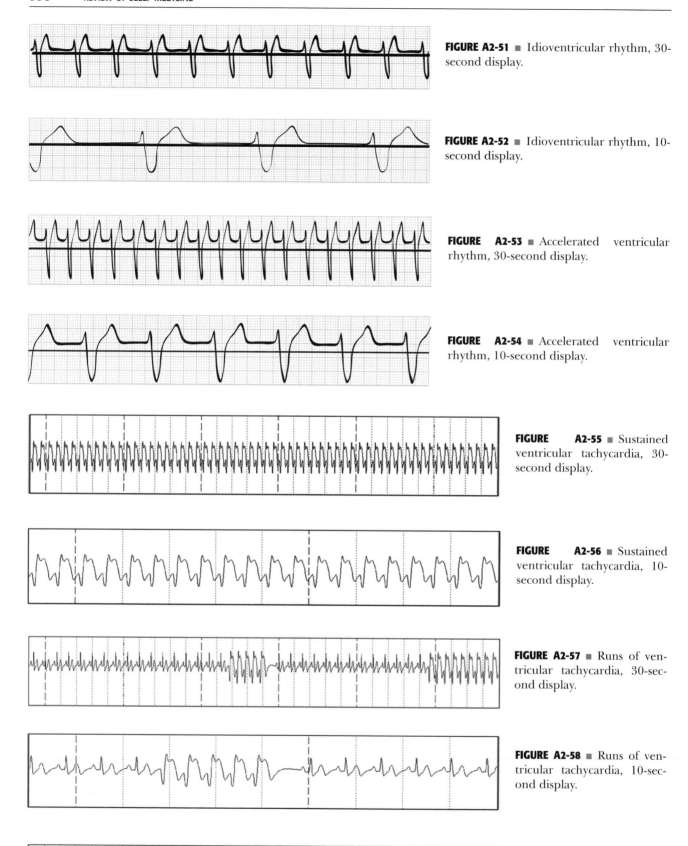

FIGURE A2-51 ■ Idioventricular rhythm, 30-second display.

FIGURE A2-52 ■ Idioventricular rhythm, 10-second display.

FIGURE A2-53 ■ Accelerated ventricular rhythm, 30-second display.

FIGURE A2-54 ■ Accelerated ventricular rhythm, 10-second display.

FIGURE A2-55 ■ Sustained ventricular tachycardia, 30-second display.

FIGURE A2-56 ■ Sustained ventricular tachycardia, 10-second display.

FIGURE A2-57 ■ Runs of ventricular tachycardia, 30-second display.

FIGURE A2-58 ■ Runs of ventricular tachycardia, 10-second display.

FIGURE A2-59 ■ Ventricular fibrillation, 30-second display.

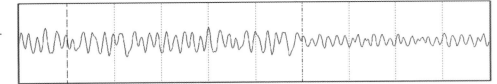

FIGURE A2-60 ■ Ventricular fibrillation, 10-second display.

TABLE A2-22 ■ Characteristics of Premature Ventricular Contractions*

Parameter	Value
P wave	Not present with abnormal beat
QRS complex	Occurs earlier than expected; widened and bizarre appearing in abnormal beat
PR interval	None
QRS interval	>0.12 sec with abnormal beat
P:QRS ratio	<1:1
Rhythm	Irregular
Rate	Usually 60–100, but can occur with slower or faster rates

*Figures A2-41 and A2-42 have different-appearing premature ventricular contractions. This sample was taken from the same recording but using a different lead combination. Figure A2-41 is lead I, and Figure A2-42 is lead II. Changing lead combinations may make the abnormality more apparent. Also note the change in display width. In Figures A2-43 and A2-44, note the different appearance of the premature ventricular contractions. Apply the rule of differing morphology. These beats originate from different areas of the ventricle (separate foci) and are called *multifocal premature ventricular contractions*. Figures A2-45 and A2-46 display premature ventricular contractions every third beat (ventricular trigeminy), and Figures A2-47 and A2-48 present premature ventricular contractions every other beat (ventricular bigeminy). The terms *trigeminy* and *bigeminy* also can refer to atrial and junctional extrasystoles bearing similar patterns. Figures A2-49 and A2-50 show paired premature ventricular contractions (i.e., ventricular couplets). Those shown have the same appearance and the same focus. Multifocal couplets are paired ventricular beats arising from different locations.

TABLE A2-23 ■ Characteristics of Idioventricular Rhythm*

Parameter	Value
P wave	No P waves associated with abnormal
QRS complex	Wide and bizarre
PR interval	None
QRS interval	>0.12 sec
P:QRS ratio	<1:1
Rhythm	Regular
Rate	<40

*Often escape rhythm when sinus node and AV node dysfunction. If sustained, assess the patient and notify appropriate medical personnel according to protocol.

TABLE A2-24 ■ Characteristics of Accelerated Ventricular Rhythm*

Parameter	Value
P wave	No P waves associated with abnormal
QRS complex	Wide and bizarre
PR interval	None
QRS interval	>0.12 sec
P:QRS ratio	<1:1
Rhythm	Regular
Rate	40 ± 100

*Often escape rhythm when sinus node and AV node dysfunction. Cardiac output is generally adequate. If sustained, assess the patient and notify medical personnel according to protocol.

TABLE A2-25 ■ Characteristics of Ventricular Tachycardia*

Parameter	Value
P wave	No P waves associated with abnormal
QRS complex	Wide and bizarre
PR interval	None
QRS interval	>0.12 sec
P:QRS ratio	<1:1
Rhythm	Regular
Rate	100–250

*Nonsustained: notify medical personnel according to protocol. Sustained: assess the patient and activate emergency medical system according to protocol.

TABLE A2-26 ■ Characteristics of Ventricular Fibrillation*

Parameter	Value
P wave	No P waves seen
QRS complex	None; wave deflections are disorganized, chaotic, varying size and shape
PR interval	None
QRS interval	Not measurable
P:QRS ratio	<1:1
Rhythm	Chaotic
Rate	Not measurable

*This is an emergency situation. Assess the patient and activate emergency medical system. When the ECG looks like the EEG, you're in trouble.

reasonable facsimile of the augmented limb leads (aVR, aVL, and aVF) may be obtained by recording the right arm versus the average of the left arm and left leg (aVR).

Viewing of the ECG and arrhythmia recognition are facilitated by "'spreading the recording out'" (i.e., using a 10-second display or less; the author has used

6 seconds to try to find evidence of "'hidden'" P waves). Intervals are all but impossible to assess using a standard 30-second screen width. The PR and QRS intervals can be measured by printing out the 10-

second display and measuring the intervals with a millimeter ruler and dividing this measurement by the number of millimeters per second on the printout. Standard calipers can be used to determine regularity on these printouts. If the system is incapable of printing during recording, it is possible to obtain intervals and test regularity by getting a stationary 10-second window and using an index card. One makes tick marks at the beginning and end of the interval of interest, measures this distance in millimeters, and divides by the number of millimeters per second provided by the display. Regularity can be checked by making tick marks at three successive R waves (or P waves), then moving the card from R wave to R wave (or P wave to P wave.) If the tick marks fall in line, the rhythm is regular.

FURTHER READINGS

1. Dubin D: *Rapid interpretation of EKG*, 6th edition. Tampa, FL, Cover Publishing, 2000. GP notebook. Arrhythmias (cardiac). Available at: http://www.gpnotebook.co.uk/simplepage.cfm?ID=−737804245.
2. GP notebook. ECG changes in bundle-branch block. Available at: http://www.gpnotebook.co.uk/simplepage.cfm?ID=1644560404&linkID=13734&cook=yes.
3. GP notebook. ECG changes in left bundle-branch block. Available at: http://www.gpnotebook.co.uk/simplepage.cfm?ID=288686086&linkID=13685&cook=yes.
4. GP notebook. ECG changes in right bundle-branch block. Available at: http://www.gpnotebook.co.uk/simplepage.cfm?ID=335937542&linkID=13684&cook=yes.
5. Klimes R: EKG review 1. Available at: http://www.ce5.com/ekg100.htm.
6. Klimes R, et al: EKG review. Available at: http://www.learnwell.org/ekg.htm.
7. Bob Nurse: Cardiology in critical care, EKG and arrhythmia recognition. Available at: http://rnbob.tripod.com/ekgandarrhythmiarecognition.htm.
8. Thaller M: *The Only EKG Book You'll Ever Need*, 4th ed. Philadelphia, Lippincott, Williams & Wilkins, 2003.

Index

Page numbers followed by f and t indicate figures and tables, respectively.